Nail Disorders

Nail Disorders
A Comprehensive Approach

Edited by
Archana Singal
Shekhar Neema
Piyush Kumar

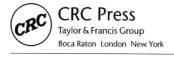

CRC Press
Taylor & Francis Group
Boca Raton London New York

CRC Press is an imprint of the
Taylor & Francis Group, an **informa** business

CRC Press
Taylor & Francis Group
6000 Broken Sound Parkway NW, Suite 300
Boca Raton, FL 33487-2742

First issued in paperback 2020

ISBN 13: 978-0-367-73171-7 (pbk)
ISBN 13: 978-0-815-37834-1 (hbk)

Library of Congress Cataloging-in-Publication Data

Names: Singal, Archana, editor. | Neema, Shekhar, editor. | Kumar, Piyush,
1982- editor.
Title: Nail disorders : a comprehensive approach / [edited by] Archana
Singal, Shekhar Neema, Piyush Kumar.
Description: New York, NY : CRC Press/Taylor & Francis Group, 2019. |
Includes bibliographical references and index.
Identifiers: LCCN 2018055489| ISBN 9780815378341 (hardback : alk. paper) |
ISBN 9781351139724 (ebook)
Subjects: | MESH: Nail Diseases--diagnosis | Nail Diseases--therapy
Classification: LCC RL165 | NLM WR 475 | DDC 616.5/47--dc23
LC record available at https://lccn.loc.gov/2018055489

Visit the Taylor & Francis Web site at
http://www.taylorandfrancis.com

and the CRC Press Web site at
http://www.crcpress.com

Dedication

To my parents, my husband Dinesh and children Suvina, Ramit & Arshia for their unconditional and constant support, love and encouragement.

Archana Singal

My Mother for being a constant source of inspiration and support.

Shekhar Neema

My Family who generously parted with their time to allow me the privilege of working for this book.

Piyush Kumar

Contents

Foreword

Rarely has a book such as *"Nail Disorders: A Comprehensive Approach"* deserved this title. Three eminent editors, Dr. Archana Singal, Dr. Shekhar Neema, and Dr. Piyush Kumar have not only written excellent chapters but have also attracted the most universal recognized onychologists in order to produce this exceptional book—a very original contribution to a rarely discussed topic. I particularly appreciate the diagnostic chapters with lab investigations, imaging in nail diseases, onychoscopy, and the compelling work on histopathology produced by one of the most talented specialists in this field. I feel truly privileged to be able to congratulate the editors and the individual contributors.

Robert Baran
Nail Disease Centre
Cannes, France

Preface

The study of nail disorders (onychology) was in its nascent stage in India, but in less than a decade, we have witnessed a tremendous and rapidly growing interest amongst dermatologists, pathologists, and plastic surgeons alike. Nail disorders are complex and intriguing owing to the anatomically small nail unit that limits the expression of various diseases of diverse etiology. Due to their evident visibility, nails score high on aesthetic and cosmetic value. And on closer examination, the nails may act as a window into the body. Of late, there has been a steady increase in the number of patients seeking dermatological consult for nail disorders. Thus, nail disorders and their management form a significant share of a dermatologists' practice. But nails do not get due importance during a postgraduate curriculum, leaving a lot to be learned later in practice.

The aim of this book is to provide comprehensive information on medical as well the surgical aspect of nail diseases. A wide and exhaustive range of nail disorders including infective, inflammatory, traumatic, drug-induced changes; benign and malignant tumors; nails in different age groups; and nails in dermatological and systemic diseases have been covered. Dedicated chapters on newer diagnostic tools beyond histopathology, onychoscopy, and nail imaging have been included. To keep pace with the present trend and interest of the readers in cosmetology, a special section on nail cosmetics and cosmetic procedures has been included. In addition, a simple stepwise approach to diagnosis, based on the most important clinical features, examination, laboratory investigations, and treatment, is presented.

The chapters have been contributed by authors from all over the globe who are the experts in the field of onychology. Their writing comes from years of practical and academic experience in the field. Since "a picture is worth a thousand words," we have effectively conveyed the essence of this phrase by including a liberal number of quality photographs that will help our valuable readers to identify common and uncommon nail disorders. The information has been presented in a very reader friendly manner with the generous use of tabulations, graphics, and flow charts.

It has been a wholehearted and earnest endeavor on our part to present updated information in a concise manner. We are open to appreciations, suggestions, and criticism from our esteemed readers, so that we can eliminate the errors in the subsequent editions. We hope that this book will generate enough curiosity and interest in not only the dermatological but the medical fraternity and will make it to the list of "must have" manuals for all.

Archana Singal
Shekhar Neema
Piyush Kumar

Acknowledgments

We express our gratitude to the authors for working tirelessly on this project during the last year and completing the assignment on time.

We are grateful to our teachers for showing us the path.

We thank all our patients, who kept faith in us and taught us in the process.

We thank all our students, past and present: we learn more when we teach.

We are thankful to the publishers, and especially Ms. Shivangi, Ms. Mouli, and Ms. Raina, who worked with us during the project.

Editors

Archana Singal is Director professor in the department of dermatology and STI, at University College of Medical Sciences, New Delhi, India. She has 30 years' experience in clinical dermatology. She is a fellow of the National Academy of Medical Sciences (FAMS). She did her clinical and research fellowship at the University of Sydney, Australia (2001–2002). She has a special interest in the diagnosis and management of nail diseases. She is the founder president of the Nail Society of India (NSI). Her other areas of interest include tropical dermatology and genodermatoses. She has to her credit more than 180 scientific publications in indexed journals and has authored nearly 30 chapters pertaining to dermatology in various textbooks. She is editor of *Comprehensive Approach to Infections in Dermatology* and *Atlas of Infections in Dermatology*. She has been awarded the Indian Association of Dermatologist, Venereologist and Leprologist (IADVL) Systopic Oration, Sardarilal Memorial Award for academic excellence and the IADVL teacher par excellence award. She was the organizing president for the second ONYCHOCON conference (Annual National conference of NSI in 2013), third International Summit for Nail Diseases (ISND) and the fourth ONYCHOCON (2015). She was the scientific chairperson for the Dermatology and Allied Specialty Summit (DAAS) during 2014–2018. Dr. Singal also served as president of IADVL, Delhi State Branch, in 2009. She is a regular invited faculty to various national and international dermatology congresses.

Shekhar Neema is an alumnus of the Armed Forces Medical College, Pune, India. He excelled in MBBS with 10 distinctions to his name and was awarded the President Gold Medal for the best academic record in 2006. He was awarded gold medal from Maharashtra University of Health Sciences (MUHS) in MD (Dermatology). He successfully cleared the European Board of Dermatology and Venereology examination. He has done an International Society of Dermatology (ISD) fellowship at Ludwig Maximilian University, Munich. He has more than 30 publications in indexed journals and has authored many chapters in various dermatology textbooks. He is the editor of the books *Dermoscopy in Darker Skin* and *Handbook of Biologics and Biosimilars in Dermatology*. He has been involved as assistant editor of various books, namely the *IADVL Atlas of Dermatology, Clinical Correlations in Dermatology*, and Association of Cutaneous Surgeons of India (ACSI) textbook of procedural dermatology. His areas of special interest are immunodermatology, dermatotherapeutics, dermatosurgery, dermoscopy, and nail diseases. He is presently working as an associate professor at the Armed Forces Medical College, Pune.

Piyush Kumar graduated from the University of Calcutta with a gold medal. He finished his post-graduate studies in Dermatology at the Medical College and Hospital, Kolkata, in 2011, and was judged the best outgoing university medical graduate in Dermatology. He received various scholarships during and after his post-graduation studies to attend and present papers at international conferences. His interest in academics led him to pursue teaching in a medical college as a career and he is currently working as an associate professor. He has published more than 100 papers in indexed national and international journals and works as a reviewer for various national and international specialty journals. He has contributed many chapters to various books and is currently editing three books. His areas of interest are clinical dermatology, dermatopathology, nail disorders, and genital dermatoses.

Contributors

Mohammad Abid Keen MD
Department of Dermatology and STD
Government Medical College
Srinagar, India

Pooja Agarwal MD
Department of Dermatology
Smt. NHL Municipal Medical College
SCL Hospital
Ahmedabad, India

Kartikay Aggarwal MBBS
Dermatology
Maharishi Markandeshwar Institute of Medical Sciences
    and Research
Ambala, India

Aurora Alessandrini
Dermatology
Department of Experimental, Diagnostic and Specialty
    Medicine
University of Bologna
Bologna, Italy

Azzam Alkhalifah MD
Dermatology Department
Unaizah College of Medicine
Qassim University
Buraydah, Saudi Arabia

Balachandra S. Ankad MD
Department of Dermatology
S. Nijalingappa Medical College
Bagalkot, India

Shikha Bansal MD, DNB, MNAMS
Department of Dermatology
Vardhman Mahavir Medical College (VMMC) and
Safdarjung Hospital
New Delhi, India

Sonal Bansal MD
Consultant Dermatologist
DermaSpace Skin Clinic

and

Fortis Memorial Research Institute
Gurgaon, India

Robert Baran MD
Department of Dermatology
Nail Disease Center

and

Consultant Dermatologist
Gustave Roussy Cancer Institute
Cannes, France

Rizwana Barkat MD
Consultant Dermatologist
Gaya, India

Savitha L. Beergouder DDVL
Department of Dermatology
S. Nijalingappa Medical College
Bagalkot, India

Yasmeen Jabeen Bhat MD
Department of Dermatology, STD and Leprosy
Government Medical College
Srinagar, India

Deepak Bhatt DMRD, MD
Consultant Radiologist
UBM Institute and Dr. Bhatt Sonography Center

and

Honorary Consultant Radiologist
JJ Group of Hospitals
Mumbai, India

Kalpana Bhatt DMRE, MD (Radiology)
Consultant Radiologist
UBM Institute and Dr. Bhatt Sonography Centre

and

Honorary Consultant Radiologist
Wadia Hospital
Mumbai, India

Somodyuti Chandra MD, DNB, SCE (UK)
Junior Consultant
The Venkat Centre for Skin and Plastic Surgery
Bangalore, India

Parul Chojer
Department of Dermatology
Government Medical College
Amritsar, India

Vikrant Choubey MD
Department of Dermatology
Maulana Azad Medical College and LNJP Hospital
New Delhi, India

Anupam Das MD
Dermatology
KPC Medical College and Hospital
Kolkata, India

Shukla Das MD, DNB, MNAMS
Department of Microbiology
University College of Medical Sciences and
    GTB Hospital
New Delhi, India

Taru Garg MD
Dermatology and Venereology
Lady Hardinge Medical College and Associated
    Hospitals
New Delhi, India

Chander Grover MD, DNB, MNAMS
Department of Dermatology and STD
University College of Medical Sciences and
    GTB Hospital
New Delhi, India

Sanjeev Gupta MD, DNB
Dermatology
Maharishi Markandeshwar Institute of Medical Sciences
    and Research
Ambala, India

Eckart Haneke MD, PhD
Department of Dermatology
Inselspital University of Bern
Bern, Switzerland

and

Dermatology Practice Dermaticum
Freiburg, Germany

Iffat Hassan MD
Department of Dermatology, STD and Leprosy
Government Medical College
Srinagar, India

Deepak Jakhar MD
Department of Dermatology
Hindu Rao Hospital
New Delhi, India

Hemangi R. Jerajani MD, DVD, FIAD
Department of Dermatology
MGM Medical College and Hospital
Navi Mumbai, India

Shilpa Kapanigowda MD
Department of Dermatology
Bangalore Medical College
Bangalore, India

Vandana Kataria MD
Department of Dermatology
Maulana Azad Medical College and LNJP Hospital
New Delhi, India

Subuhi Kaul MD
Department of Dermatology
All India Institute of Medical Sciences
New Delhi, India

Ishmeet Kaur MD
Department of Dermatology
ESI Medical College and Hospital
New Delhi, India

M. N. Kayarkatte MD
Department of Dermatology
University College of Medical Sciences and
GTB Hospital
New Delhi, India

Sunil K. Kothiwala
Consultant Dermatologist
SkinEva Clinic
Jaipur, India

Neha Kumar MD
Department of Dermatology
VMMC and Safdarjung Hospital
New Delhi, India

Piyush Kumar MD
Department of Dermatology
Katihar Medical College and Hospital
Katihar, India

B. B. Mahajan MD
Department of Dermatology
Government Medical College
Amritsar, India

Neha Meena MD
Dermatologist (DMO)
Central Hospital, North Western Railway
Jaipur, India

Jyotisterna Mittal MBBS, MD
Consultant Dermatologist
Ludhiana, India

Pooja Arora Mrig MD, DNB, MNAMS
Department of Dermatology
Dr. Ram Manohar Lohia Hospital and PGIMER
New Delhi, India

Amiya Kumar Mukhopadhyay MD, PhD, DNB (Derm), DNB (Derm and Vener), MNAMS
Consultant Dermatologist
Kolkata, India

Soni Nanda MD
Consultant Dermatologist
Shine and Smile Skin Clinic
New Delhi, India

Chitra S. Nayak MD, DDV, DHA, AFIH
Department of Dermatology
Topiwala National Medical College and
BYL Nair Hospital
Mumbai, India

Shekhar Neema MD, FEBDV
Department of Dermatology
Armed Forces Medical College
Pune, India

Deepika Pandhi
Department of Dermatology and STD
University College of Medical Sciences and
GTB Hospital
New Delhi, India

Manoj Pawar MD
Department of Dermatology
Dr. V.P. Medical College, Hospital and Research Centre
Nashik, India

Malcolm Pinto MD
Department of Dermatology
Yenepoya Medical College
Mangalore, India

Bianca Maria Piraccini MD, PhD
Dermatology
Department of Experimental, Diagnostic and Specialty
Medicine
University of Bologna
Bologna, Italy

Niharika Ranjan Lal MD
Department of Dermatology
ESI PGIMSR and ESI Medical College
Kolkata, India

Dipali Rathod MBBS, DDV
Consultant Dermatologist
Mumbai, India

Santoshdev P. Rathod MD
Department of Dermatology
Smt. NHL Municipal Medical College and
V. S. Hospital
Ahmedabad, India

Vineet Relhan MD
Department of Dermatology
Maulana Azad Medical College & LNJP Hospital
New Delhi, India

Bertrand Richert MD, PhD
Department of Dermatology
Brugmann, Saint-Pierre and Queen Fabiola Children
University Hospitals
Université Libre de Bruxelles
Brussels, Belgium

Sarita Sanke MD, DNB
Department of Dermatology and Venereology
Lady Hardinge Medical College and Associated
Hospitals
New Delhi, India

A. S. Savitha MD, DNB, FRGUHS
Department of Dermatology
Sapthagiri Medical College and Research Institute
Bangalore, India

Bela J. Shah MD
Department of Dermatology, Venereology and Leprology
B.J. Medical College and Civil Hospital
Ahmedabad, India

Pooja Sharma MD
Department of Pathology
All India Institute of Medical Sciences
New Delhi, India

Sonal Sharma MD
Pathology
University College of Medical Sciences and GTB Hospital
New Delhi, India

B. M. Shashikumar MD, FIADVL
Department of Dermatology
Mandya Institute of Medical Sciences
Mandya, India

Avner Shemer MD
Dermatology Department
Sackler School of Medicine
Tel-Aviv University
Tel-Aviv, Israel

Manjunath M. Shenoy MD, DNB
Department of Dermatology
Yenepoya Medical College
Yenepoya University
Mangalore, India

Archana Singal MD, FAMS
Department of Dermatology and STD
University College of Medical Sciences & GTB Hospital
New Delhi, India

Khayati Singla MD
Department of Dermatology
Government Medical College
Patiala, India

Michela Starace MD
Dermatology
Department of Experimental, Diagnostic and Specialty
  Medicine
University of Bologna
Bologna, Italy

Harsh Tahiliani MD
Visiting Consultant
Dermatology
Bhartiya Arogya Nidhi Hospital
Mumbai, India

Sushil Tahiliani MD, DV&D
Visiting Consultant
Dermatology
Hinduja Hospital
Hinduja Healthcare Surgical and Asian Heart Institute
Mumbai, India

Swagata Arvind Tambe MD, DNB, FCPS, DDV
Consultant Dermatologist
Innovation Skin Clinic & Laser Center
Mumbai, India

Richa Tigga MBBS
Department of Microbiology
University College of Medical Sciences and
GTB Hospital
New Delhi, India

Biju Vasudevan MD, FRGUHS
Department of Dermatology
Base Hospital
Lucknow, India

Vijay Zawar
Department of Dermatology
Dr. V.P. Medical College, Hospital and Research Centre
Nashik, India

PART 1

History and Normal Nail

History of nail diseases

AMIYA KUMAR MUKHOPADHYAY

"Ungues nigri et digiti manuum et pedum frigidi, contracti, vel remissi mortem in, propinquo esse ostendunt".

Hippocrates (Section VIII, Aphorism 12)

[*Trans.* Blackness of the *nail*s, coldness, contraction, or relaxation of the fingers and toes—foreshow the near approach of death.]

INTRODUCTION

Nails, though considered "dead structures," have attracted attention since antiquity. They occupy a very small area of the body, yet play a very significant role. Nails not only act as vital instruments that help picking, scratching, cutting, crushing, gripping, clinging, and many more activities, but they have also remained a target that has attracted people pursuing diverse activities—from artists to archaeologists, sorcerers to crime detectors, doctors to designers, commoners to celebrities, and almost everyone! Any defects in such an important structure have fascinated the common as well as medical men since the early days. This is evident in the diverse archaeological artefacts, votive reliefs, mummies, literatures (both medical and non-medical), paintings, relics, etc.

Nails not only have their own problems in the form of various diseases, but also act as a screen on which the stories of different systemic illnesses are recorded. Even being such a significant part of the body and the fact that the incidence of the diseases of the nail claims a considerable portion of the total dermatological disorders in modern medical science, it has attracted very little interest of the medical world in the remote as well as recent past. However, in modern medicine onychology—the subject dealing with nail diseases and related problems—has secured a noteworthy position. This present scenario is the outcome of accumulation of knowledge since ancient times gathered by the human race from all corners of the globe. The systematic study of the nail and its ailments started only 200 or at the most 300 years back. This present chapter is a brief overview of this evolutionary aspect of the history of nail diseases.

The scientific study of the nail and its diseases has started only some 300 years back as already mentioned, with the study of Robert Boyle, Albrecht Haller, and others, but the evidence of the presence of nail disorders is obtainable in the history of almost all ancient civilizations. For the sake of discussion, the history of nail diseases will be discussed in the following compartments of time periods divided arbitrarily:

1. History of nail diseases in ancient civilizations (pre-historic period–AD 400)
2. The nail and its diseases in the "Dark Period" of the history of medicine (AD 400–AD 1400)
3. Nail diseases in the modern era (AD 1400–present period)

HISTORY OF NAIL DISEASES IN ANCIENT CIVILIZATIONS

The human civilization began its journey from different points on the globe, as did diseases and deformities. For example, the presence of horizontal lines on the nails (Beau's lines) that probably developed after some significant suffering months before death in the oldest preserved European subject (5200 years) is a fascinating instance of nail diseases in ancient days.[1]

From the very early days of life, the need to fight diseases and the necessity to maintain a healthy life were recognized in both animals and plants. As far as human civilization, the observation regarding the causation, course, and remedy of diseases has caught the attention of man since the primeval period. Significantly, diseases of the nail have been mentioned in the early medical literature of various civilizations.

Mesopotamia

In the ancient civilization of the river valleys of Mesopotamia that flourished during the fourth millennium BC, the mention of different diseases and their remedies are evident in clay tablets written in cuneiform scripts.[2] A physiognomic text mentioning the "illness of the nails" shows the knowledge of diseased nails in Mesopotamians.[3] Another clay tablet mentioning ill-nail in the Uruk cuneiform clay tablet needs mention in this regard.[4]

Egypt

Egypt is a treasure trove for medical history lovers. Its tombs and monuments are beautifully drawn with pictures and writings in hieroglyphics on the walls, and the mummies inside with a variety of substances provide pictorial evidence of diseases of that period. Moreover, a number of medical scrolls like the Edwin Smith, the Kahun, the Ebers, the Hearst, the Erman, the London, the Berlin, and the Chester Beatty papyri furnish direct records of diseases of various parts of the body that were prevalent in ancient Egypt. The Hearst papyrus (*c.* BC 1550) makes many mentions of prescriptions for toe- and fingernail diseases. The Ebers papyrus (*c.* BC 1555) similarly described diseases of the nails.

Greece

Modern Western medicine practically started its journey from Greece about 2500 years back. Greek medicine was influenced by the Mesopotamian, Egyptian, and Phoenician medical cultures. The Asclepiad cult dominated the ancient Greek medical world. Hippocrates of Cos (BC 460–BC 370) was the first to visualize diseases in the light of logic instead of the magico-religious point of view, which was customary until then. His description of the nail deformity associated with lung disease (empyema) is remembered in the clinical medicine as "Hippocratic nail" even today. He also described various color changes of the nails as prognostic signs.[5]

Rome

The Romans had their own system of medicine, but it was not well organized. It turned into a highly developed medicine under the Greek influence. Aulus Cornelius Celsus (BC 25–AD 50) was the greatest medical writer of the Roman Empire. In his *De Medicina* he described various diseases. In Chapter 19 of his sixth book of "*De Medicina*," he described chronic paronychia. He also described how the color changes of the nails have prognostic importance.[6,7] Kriton, a modestly known medical writer of the 1st century AD, described the psoriasis of the nails.[8] Galen of Pergamon (AD 129–AD 210) was the next most famous Roman medical authority whose influence prevailed in Western medicine until the 16th century; he noted a variety of changes in the nail in diseases and their prognostication.[5]

India[9]

India, unlike other major ancient civilizations, was the cradle of human progress whose lifeline never died. The shadow of the ancient culture is still palpable in many spheres of common Indian life. As far as the history of diseases of the nails is concerned, nothing is known to us from the Indus valley civilizations that flourished around BC 2500 or even much earlier. The earliest mention of nail involvement in systemic disorder (*Yakshmā* or consumption) can be found in a hymn (163.5) of Book X of the *Rig-Veda*, the oldest religious record of the Indo-Iranian Aryans. Among the four *Veda*s, the *Atharva-Veda* deals more with the diseases and their remedies than the others. Interestingly the mention of ill-nail in verses 65–67 of Book VII of the *Atharva-Veda* remind us of ectodermal dysplasia or porphyria or similar other diseases involving the nails. The *Yajur-Veda* (Book II, Hymn 5.2) mentions that a person making love with a lady suffering from *duscharma* (a scaly skin condition) will develop disorder of the nail and hair along with the other affection of the skin. Was it any communicable disease like ringworm or leprosy or any sexual disorder? That is not certain yet. In the latter part of the Vedic period, the emergence and development of the *Ayurveda* rendered a distinct shape to the ancient rational medicine. The major texts like *Charaka Samhitā* (*c.* BC 400) and *Susruta Samhitā* (6th century BC) described nail disorders and changes of the nails in systemic diseases. In the *Nidānasthānam* of the *Susruta Samhitā* there is clear mention of acute paronychia (*Chipparaoga*) and deformity of the nail following an injury (*Kunakha*). Similar mentions can also be seen in other major compendiums like *Vāgbhat's Astānga Hridaya Samhitā*, and *Mādhava Kara's Nidān*.

THE NAIL AND ITS DISEASES IN THE "DARK PERIOD" OF THE HISTORY OF MEDICINE

With the beginning of the Christian era almost all civilizations either started perishing or declining to a very low ebb. This affected every sphere of science, art, culture, economy, and all other aspects of the civilizations. Nothing much was added in the next 1000 years. Pusey has appropriately designated this period as the "Dark Period" of medicine.[9]

During this period the epicenter of Greco-Roman medicine shifted to the Arabic-speaking countries and as a result medicine flourished there to a great extent. Various authors like Avicenna, Razes, Albucasis, and Al Majusi wrote their famous treatises. They have included their observations on the various changes in the nail in different diseases. Albucasis and Haly Abbas described the treatment of the bruised nails. *Kamil us sana'at* written by Al Majusi (AD 930–AD 994) discussed nails in Book VIII.[10] Ibn-Al Bytar of the 13th century mentioned the nail discoloration in opium poisoning.[11]

During this "dark period" among very few notable works in the Western medicine the compendium of Paulus Aeginita, a Greek physician of the 7th century needs special mention. This work described paronychia, subungual hemorrhage, and their remedies. Aeginita also wrote about the use of sulphur, arsenic, and cantharides in the removal of a diseased nail.[12] Mercurialis in the 15th century wrote a treatise on wound management, pestilent fever, and nails.[13] As for the medical scenario in India, the picture reflects a similar situation. The mentions of nail disorders in medical compendia of this era are only the repetitions of the already gathered knowledge.[14]

NAIL DISEASES IN THE MODERN ERA

The knowledge that was accumulating since antiquity assumed a distinct shape in the last few hundred years, particularly in the last three centuries. Robert Boyle first mentioned the studies regarding nail growth in 1684, but a better scientific study about nail growth came from the studies of Albrecht Heller in 1741, and the first methodical study in detail took another century. It came from the work of Arnold Berthold in his paper entitled *Beobactungen über das Verhälniss der Nägel-und Harbildung beim Menschen* in 1850. Theophil Metecki did the first ever biochemical study of the nail in 1837.[15] Rudolph Albert von Kölliker was the pioneer in the study of the cellular aspect of nails. His famous *Manual of Human Histology*, published in 1852, devoted 15 pages to the detailed description of nail complex.[16] In the similar period, nail anatomy and histology were greatly elaborated by famous authorities like Gustav Simon (1848), Virchow (1854), and others.[15]

Since the early days of Western medicine, the subject of nails was explored mainly by chiropodists and surgeons, who, like Adolphus, Ashton, Reulihet, and Durlache, published a number of detailed treatises on the disorders of the nail with their cause and management.[17–21]

So far as the physicians' and dermatologists' contributions to understanding nail diseases are concerned, Daniel Turner discussed ingrown nails in detail in his famous *De Morbis Cutaneis* in 1726.[22] Joseph Jacob Ritter von Plenck of Vienna was the first ever medical authority to include nail disorders as a distinct class (class XIII – *Morbi Unguium*) in

the classification of dermatologic diseases in his *Doctrina de Morbis Cutaneis* in 1776.[23] In 1796 Johann-Christian Reil, the famous German physician, anatomist, and physiologist, described a cross furrow on the nail following systemic disturbances. This was re-described by Beau and is now known as the Beau–Reil line.[24] The term *onychia mailigna* for the syphilitic nail changes was first used by James Wardrop in 1814.[15] John Hunter in his famous *Treatise on Venereal Diseases* in 1786 gave a detailed account of syphilitic nail changes. He wrote in the section entitled *Of the symptoms of the first stage of Lues venerea* in Chapter 2[25]:

> *This disease, in its first appearance, often attacks the part of the fingers upon which the nail is formed, making that surface red which is shining through the nail, and, if allowed to continue, the separation of nail takes place...*

Robert Willan in 1808 first described the modern finding on psoriasis of the nails as below[26]:

> *The Psoriasis unguium sometimes occurs alone, but it is usually connected with scaly patches on the arms, hands &c. in some cases, nails from the middle appears brown or yellowish; they bend upwards, and are ragged at the ends, and rough on the surface. In other cases, they are thickened, deeply indented and bent downwards over the end of the fingers.*

The early observation on the fungal infection of the nail came from the narrative of Mahon the younger who, though not a trained physician, belonged to a family who took care of the favus and other fungal infections at the L'Hopital St Louis (Paris). They used some undisclosed method to treat their patients.[27] The causative agent of the dermatophytic nail affection was described by George Messiner in 1853 and the term "onychomycosis" was coined by Virchow in the year 1856.[15] Duhring presented a case of *tinea trychophytina unguium* or *onychomycosis trychophytina* to the Philadelphia County Medical Society on 22 April 1878 and described the entity as a "quite rare form of nail disease." Candida infection of the nail was described much later in 1904.

The nail changes in eczematous disorders were first described by Pierre Rayer in 1835 in his *Traité Théorique et Pratique des Maladies de la Peau.*[28] This was the first book to consider nail diseases in an elaborate fashion and also the pioneer to provide the illustration on nail disorders. In the year 1846 Joseph Honoré Simon Beau described the well-known nail sign in internal disorders that disturb the keratin physiology, now known as Beau's line. Blackman's English translation (1855) of Vidal's famous book on *Treatise on Venereal Diseases* described a variety of nail afflictions in syphilis.[29] The nail changes in malignant melanoma were illustrated by Jonathan Hutchinson in 1857 as melanotic whitlow. He also gave the description of nail changes in pityriasis rubra pilaris in the year 1878. Though *leichen planus* was described by

Table 1.1 Various nail abnormalities/signs

Name of the abnormality/sign	Describing authority	Year
Clubbing of nail	Hippocrates of Cos	?
Beau–Reil groove	Johann-Christian Reil	1796
	Honoré Simon Beau	1846
Hutchinson sign	Jonathan Hutchinson	1857
Koilonychia	Radcliffe Crocker	1893
Nail–patella syndrome	EM Little	1897
Pachyonychia congenita	Jadassohn and Lewandowsky	1906
Mees lines	RA Mees	1919
Median canaliform dystrophy	J Heller	1928
Onychotillomania	J Alkiewicz	1934
Lovibond angle	JL Lovibond	1938
Trachyonychia	J Alkiewicz	1950
Curth's modified profile sign	HO Curth	1953
Terry's nail	RB Terry	1955
Muehrcke band	RC Muehrcke	1956
Yellow nail syndrome	PD Samman and WF White	1964
Pincer nail	CE Cornelius and WB Shelly	1968
Bissell's line	GW Bissell	1971
Leukonychia striata longitudinalis	N Higashi, T Sugai, T Yamamoto	1971
Pterigium inversum unguis	ME Caputo, G Prandi	1973
Nutcracker nail	BH Cohen	1975
Twenty-nail dystrophy	DE Hazelrigg, C Duncan, M Jarratt	1977
Congenital malalignment of big toenail	PD Samman	1978
Congenital hypertrophy of the lateral fold of the hallux	Martinet	1984

Source: Samman, P.D. and Fenton, D.A. *The Nail in Disease*, 4th ed., William Heinemann Medical Books, London, UK, 1986; Scher, R.K. and Daniel III, C.R. (Eds). *Nails: Diagnosis, Therapy, Surgery*, 3rd ed., Saunders, Pennsylvania, PA, 2005; Hamm, H., Diseases of nails. In: Burgdorf, W.H.C., Plewig, G., Wolff, H.H., Landthaler, M. (Eds), *Braun-Falco's Dermatology*, 3rd ed., Springer, Heidelberg, Germany, 2010.

Erasmus Wilson in 1869 (perhaps earlier by Hebra as *lichen ruber*), the first description of nail lichen planus came from William Dubreuilh in the year 1901.

Leprosy was a matter of discussion and attention since antiquity. The real advancement of knowledge took place with the discovery of lepra bacilli by Hansen in 1874. Nail changes have been noted by physicians for a long time. As for the nail involvement in leprosy the earlier books like "*A few Observations on the Leprosy of the Middle Ages*" of Shapter (1835) mention observations on nail changes. Regarding the cause, Hansen and Looft (1895) were of the opinion that the reason was "trophic disturbance."

With the beginning of the 20th century the nail got much attention of the dermatologists and physicians. One after another findings of nail disorders that were either primary diseases of the nail structure or their association with the systemic diseases were published in the literature (Table 1.1). The systematic study on the subject of the nail that started in the 17th century gradually enlarged and matured to a separate subject on its own and onychology—the study of nail in health and diseases—was born. If we look back only three centuries, nail involvement in different diseases was touched upon mostly as passing references, but today we have a number of text books and atlases with beautiful illustrations (Figures 1.1 through 1.5) that deal with nails, their disorders, and management—both medical and surgical.

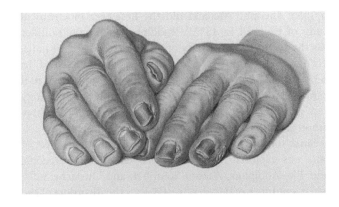

Figure 1.1 Syphilitic paronychia of both hands (1898). (From *Atlas of Syphilis and the Venereal Diseases* including a brief treatise on the pathology and treatment by Franz Marcek. https://wellcomeimages.org/. Copyrighted work available under Creative Commons Attribution only license CC BY 4.0 http://creativecommons.org/licenses/by/4.0/.)

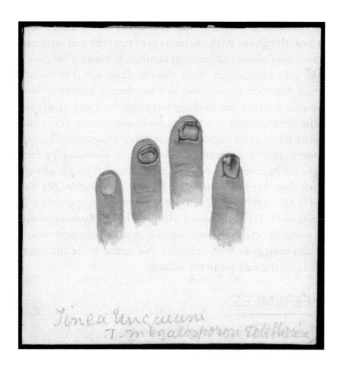

Figure 1.2 Fingers with diseased nails (1899). (From Patients and diseases. Paintings commissioned by Sir Jonathan Hutchinson, ca. 1891–1906. https://wellcomeimages.org/. Copyrighted work available under Creative Commons Attribution only license CC BY 4.0 http://creativecommons.org/licenses/by/4.0/.)

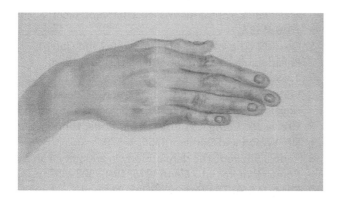

Figure 1.3 Watercolor drawing of the right hand of a boy who had congenital absence of the nails. Patient also suffered from purpura hemorrhagica (1891). (From St Bartholomew's Hospital Archives & Museum. [1891] By: Mark, Leonard Portal. https://wellcomeimages.org/. Copyrighted work available under Creative Commons Attribution only license CC BY 4.0 http://creativecommons.org/licenses/by/4.0/.)

"Nail" in the last 100 years

The last 100 years, or more accurately from the beginning of the last century, a rapid spurt in the research in every field of science, especially in medicine, has resulted in an altogether new thinking regarding the disease, its causation, and its management. For example, the recent concept of "nail unit" as propounded by Zaias in 1990 has changed our

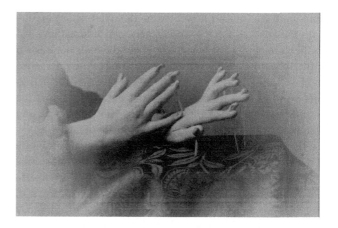

Figure 1.4 Black and white photograph of the hands of a girl affected with congenital deformity of the nails (onychogryphosis) (1887–1888). (From St Bartholomew's Hospital Archives & Museum By: Hadley, George. https://wellcomeimages.org/. Copyrighted work available under Creative Commons Attribution only license CC BY 4.0 http://creativecommons.org/licenses/by/4.0/.)

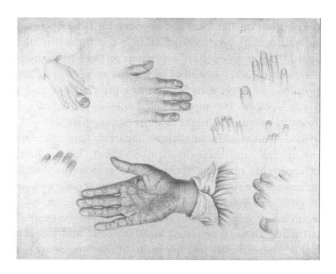

Figure 1.5 Psoriasis diffusa (1878–1888). (From University Hospitals Bristol, NHS Foundation Trust, Wellcome Images.)

vision.[29] The works of Lewis, Zaias, Hashimoto, and others on the embryology of the nail have reinforced our basic knowledge on the early days of formation of the nail unit and the fundamental aspect of congenital nail disorders.[30] The discovery of newer biochemical, biophysical, biomechanical, and histochemical techniques; imaging studies like ultra sound and MRI; and application of knowledge of microbiology and investigation like different kinds of nail biopsy have thrown newer insight onto the disease pattern. For example, better conception about the molecular basis of the keratin biosynthesis (like missense mutation of the initiation peptide of K16) in pachyonychia congenita or the mutation in the R-spondin 4 gene acting as the underlying cause of congenital anonychia has helped us understand the different nail manifestations. Some other factors like abundant use of the newer cosmetics coming every day onto the market along with cosmetic procedures have led to the development of new disorders of the nails not known hitherto. Another important factor leading to the emergence of newer nail disorders is the discovery of newer medicines that are used to treat diverse diseases but at the same time resulting in the development of many side effects causing changes in the structure and morphology of the nails.[31]

The historical aspect of modern-day onychology remains incomplete without acknowledging the enormous contributions of various authorities. As a complete discussion on this topic merits a separate chapter itself, so a brief overview is included here (hence it is obviously not exhaustive). The researches of great personalities like Nardo Zaias, Robert Baran, Peter Samman, Richard Scher, Eckart Haneke, Paul Kechijian, Ralph Daniel, Antonella Tosti, Philip Fleckmen, Phoebe Rich, and many others not only enriched the subject but made it a distinct specialty. Zaias described the embryology of the nail in detail, prescribed a new method of taking longitudinal biopsy, put his observation on the psoriasis of the nails, and did a plethora of researches to develop the subject.[32–34] Samman's contribution on nail changes in psoriasis, lichen planus, and yellow nail syndrome should be mentioned in this regard.[35] Scher noted his observations on the nail changes in various diseases as well as in various ages.[36] Baran did enormous work on nails leading to a great advancement of the subject. He supplemented Zaias's classification of onychomycosis to make it more appropriate. He also divided leukonychia into true, apparent, and pseudo-leukonychia and his description about longitudinal melanonychia resulting from various reasons improved our knowledge significantly. Baran's first ever descriptions on onychmatricoma, color clues for malignancies, nail degloving syndrome, etc. and accounts on congenital nail malalignment, acquired malalignment, and surgery of the proximal nail fold are some of the famous works that deepened the knowledge on onychology. He authored a number of books (37!) that have formed the storehouse of information on the nail and its ailments.[37] The treatises authored by Zaias, Samman, Scher, Haneke, and Piraccini are other treasure troves of nail disorders.[38,39]

The descriptions of newer diseases like shell nail syndrome, pincer nail deformity, yellow nail syndrome, nail–patella syndrome, pachyonychia congenita, etc. have enriched the subject further. The unfolding of the causes of different nail disorders led to newer and better strategies of managing nail diseases and a range of newer modalities of management like surgery, cryotherapy, laser, and prosthetics have opened a number of new avenues in onychology today.

EPILOGUE

Not too long ago, the nail was virtually ignored by the medical community. Nobody ever considered it as a structure that could provide innumerable information on various health concerns. Earlier, the nail was a subject of interest to the chiropodists, a few surgeons, and ladies as an instrument for beautification. With the passage of time the nail attracted attention of almost all medical faculties because it renders a lot of information that offers clues to diagnosis. The history of nail disorders enumerates this fascinating history of how one after another nail findings were observed and finally led to the development of a subject on its own merit. Scher and Daniel III, in their famous treatise *Nails: Diagnosis, Therapy, Surgery*, rightly observed: ....*An area of dermatology long neglected by clinical and basic-science research people as well, onychology has rather suddenly become fashionable. The nail unit is no longer regarded as untouchable or an appendage to be ignored.*[38] Truly, the speed with which the advancement in the research on onychology is going on at the moment means we can anticipate with certainty that many more historical events on the nail are in the offing.

REFERENCES

1. Lidell K. Skin diseases in the antiquity. *Clin Med* 2006; 6(1): 81–86.
2. Biggs RD. Medicine, surgery, and public health in ancient Mesopotamia. *J Assy Acad Studies* 2005; 19(1): 1–19.
3. Böck B. Die Babylonisch-Assyrische morphoskopie. *Archive für Orientforschung* 2000; 158: 142.
4. Geller MJ. *Look to the Stars: Babylonian Medicine, Astrology, Magic and Melothesia*. Berlin, Germany: Max Planck Institut für Wissenschaftsgeschichte; 2010: 1–87.
5. Coxe JR. *The Writings of Hippocrates and Galen*. Philadelphia, PA: Lindsay and Blackstone; 1846: 1–690.
6. Verbov J. Celsus and his contributions to dermatology. *Int J Derm* 1978; 17: 521–523.
7. Greive JA. *Cornelius Celsus of Medicine*. London, UK: Wilson and Durham; 1756: 1–570.
8. Radbill SX. Pediatric dermatology in antiquity. Part II. Roman Empire. *Int J Derm* 1976; 15(4): 303–307.
9. Pusey WMA. *The History of Dermatology*. Springfield, MO: Charles C Thomas; 1933.
10. Browne EG. *Arabian Medicine*. Cambridge, UK: Cambridge University Press; 1962: 109.
11. Hamarneh S. Pharmacy in medieval Islam and the history of drug addiction. *Med Hist* 1972; 16(3): 226–237.
12. Aeginita P. *The Seven Books of Paulus Aeginita*. London, UK: Sydenham Society; 1844.
13. Park R. *An Epitome on the History of Medicine*. Philadelphia, PA: The FA Devis Company; 1899: 80.
14. Mukhoadhyay AK. *Skin Diseases ('Dermatology') in India: History and Evolution*. West Bengal, India: Allied Book Agency; 2011: 1–182.
15. Crissey JT, Parish LC. Historic aspect of nail disease. In: Scher RK, Daniel III CR (Eds.). *Nails: Diagnosis, Therapy, Surgery*. 3rd ed. Pennsylvania, PA: Saunders; 2005: 7–13.

16. Külliker RA. *Manual of Human Histology*. London, UK: Sydenham Society; 1853: 153–168.
17. Adolphus LJ. *A Concise Treatise on the Disorders of Human Foot: Corns, Bunions and Diseased Nails*. London, UK: Mitchell Book Sellers and Publishers; 1865.
18. Ashton TJ. *A Treatise on Corns, Bunions and Ingrowing of the Toenail: Their Cause and Treatment*. London, UK: John Churchill; 1852.
19. Laforest M. *L'art de soigner les peids*. Paris; 1781.
20. Reulihet M. *Maladise cutanées des pieds*. Toulous: Imprierie De Bonnal Et Gibrac; 1845.
21. Durlacher L. *A Treatise on Corns, Bunions and Diseases of the Nails and the General Management of the Feet*. London, UK: Simpkin, Marshall & Co; 1845.
22. Turner D. *De morbis cutaneis*. 3rd ed. London, UK: R & J Bronwicke; 1726: 267–273.
23. Mukhopadhyay AK. On the history of classification in dermatology. *Indian J Dermatol* 2016; 61(6): 588–592.
24. Binder DK, Schaller K, Clusmann H. The seminal contributions of Johann-Christian Reil to anatomy, physiology and psychiatry. *Neurosurgery* 2007; 61: 1091–1096.
25. Hunter J. *A Treatise on the Venereal Diseases*. Philadelphia, PA: Haswell, Barrington & Haswell; 1841: 261.
26. Willan R. *On Cutaneous Diseases*. Philadelphia, PA: Kimber & Conrad; 1809: 129.
27. Mahon Juene M. *Recherchaes sur le siége et la nature des teignes*. Paris: Bailliere Chez JB; 1829.
28. Rayer P. *Traité Théorique et Pratique des Maladies de la Peau*, atlas. Paris: JB Bailliére; 1835.
29. Vidal A. *A Treatise on Venereal Diseases*. 2nd ed. New York: Samuel S & William Wood; 1855.
30. Zaias N. *The Nail in Health and Disease*. 2nd ed. Norwalk, CT: Appleton & Lange; 1990.
31. Holbrook KA. Human epidermal embryogenesis. *Int J Dermatol* 1979; 18: 329–356.
32. Zaias N. Embryology of the human nail. *Arch Dermatol* 1963; 87: 37.
33. Zaias N. The longitudinal nail biopsy. *J Invest Dermatol* 1967; 49: 406.
34. Zaias N. *Psoriasis of the nail. Arch Dermatol* 1969; 99: 567.
35. Samman PD, Fenton DA. *The Nail in Disease*. 4th ed. London, UK: William Heinemann Medical Books; 1986.
36. Scher RK, Daniel III CR (Eds.). *Nails: Diagnosis, Therapy, Surgery*. 3rd ed. Pennsylvania, PA: Saunders; 2005.
37. Baran R. Autobiography of a loner tackling the nail (Zakon Lecture). *Skin Appendage Disord* 2017; 3: 2–6.
38. Zaiac M, Daniel III CR. Pigmentation abnormalities. In: Scher RK, Daniel III CR (Eds.). *Nails: Diagnosis, Therapy, Surgery*. 3rd ed. Pennsylvania, PA: Saunders; 2005: 73–90.
39. Hamm H. Diseases of nails. In: Burgdorf WHC, Plewig G, Wolff HH, Landthaler M (Eds.). *Braun-Falco's Dermatology*. 3rd ed. Heidelberg, Germany: Springer; 2010.

2

Nail anatomy and physiology

POOJA ARORA MRIG AND NEHA MEENA

The nail is an important skin appendage. It is useful, not only for the aesthetic appearance, but also for its role as a diagnostic clue to various cutaneous and systemic disorders. The nail also protects the underlying rich neurovascular supply, which is used for thermoregulation and sensory purposes. Knowledge of nail development, anatomy, and physiology helps us in better understanding of nail disorders and it also guides us in therapeutic interventions and innovations.

ANATOMY OF NAIL UNIT

Embryology and development

The fingernail primordium develops during the 8th embryonic week from the epidermis slightly earlier than the initiation of hair follicle development, as a transverse ridge on the distal dorsal surface of the digit. Development of toenails starts 4 weeks later in similar pattern. The nail fold is delineated by a continuous groove. A group of cells from the proximal part of the nail fold then grows and extends downwards and proximally into the dermis of the digit, stopping approximately 1 mm from the phalanx and giving rise to

the matrix primordium. This site will in turn form the epithelium of the proximal nail fold, the distal and intermediate matrix epithelium. The presumptive nail matrix cells that are present on the ventral side of the proximal invagination differentiate and keratinize to become the nail plate. The distal part of the nail fold forms the distal ridge, which is a visible group of cells, on the dorsum of the distal tip of each digit (Figure 2.1).[1]

At 11 weeks, the dorsal nail bed surface begins to keratinize. At 13 weeks' gestation, the proximal nail fold is formed and the first signs of nail plate growth are observed from the lunula. Moreover, nail fold epithelium starts to keratinize with formation of the stratum granulosum, beginning distally and advancing towards the proximal nail fold. The nail matrix is completely developed by 15 weeks and it starts to produce the nail plate, which will continue to grow until death.[2,3]

The granular layer recedes at 18 weeks' gestation and the nail bed epithelium takes on a postnatal appearance. The process of cellular differentiation and maturation within the matrix is similar to that seen in adult nails at 20 weeks' gestation. By 32 weeks' gestation, the nail plate reaches the tip of the fingers and all the components of the nail are

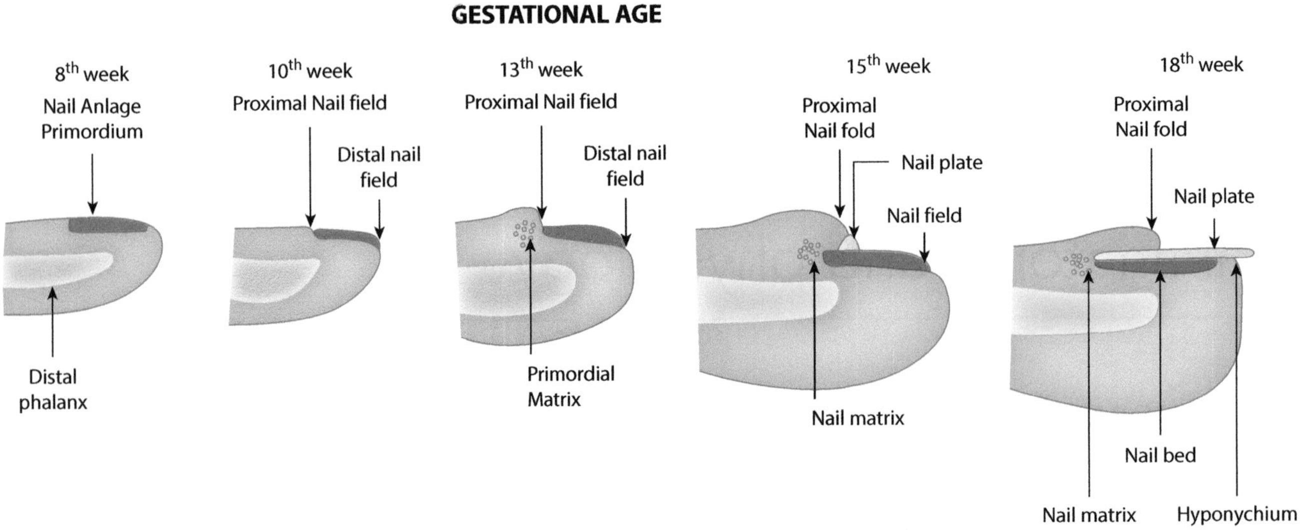

GESTATIONAL AGE

8th week	10th week	13th week	15th week	18th week
Nail Anlage Primordium	Proximal Nail field	Proximal Nail field	Proximal Nail fold	Proximal Nail fold

Distal nail field

Distal nail field

Nail plate

Nail field

Nail plate

Distal phalanx

Primordial Matrix

Nail matrix

Nail bed

Nail matrix   Hyponychium

Figure 2.1 Embryologic development of the nail unit.

recognizable. Nail plate in toenails reaches the tip later at 36 weeks only and absent nail plates at the tips of digits are another indicator of prematurity.[2,3]

Transcription factor R-spondin 4 initiates nail development, and its mutation leads to congenital anonychia. Functional *p63* is required for the formation and maintenance of the apical ectodermal ridge, which is an embryonic signaling center required for limb outgrowth and hand plate formation. So, mutations in *p63* affect nail development in syndromes like ankyloblepharon, ectodermal dysplasia, and cleft lip/palate syndrome as well as ectrodactyly, ectodermal dysplasia, and cleft lip/palate syndrome. Wnt7a is also important for dorsal limb patterning and, hence, nail formation. Primary signaling abnormalities in Wnt7a are also associated with inherited nail dysplasias such as Schöpf–Schulz–Passarge syndrome (*Wnt10a*). *LMX1b* and *MSX1* are important for nail differentiation. *LMX1b* is mutated in nail-patella syndrome and *MSX1* in Witkop syndrome. However, in contrast to follicular development, the Shh gene is not required for nail plate formation. In murine models, *Hoxc13* is also an important homeodomain-containing gene for both follicular and nail development.[2–4]

ANATOMY

The nail unit lies immediately above the distal phalanx and the ligaments, and tendons and ligaments around the distal interphalangeal joints not only help anchoring the nail apparatus to underlying bone, but also are essential for nails' mechanical functions. Moreover, fibers from extensor tendons attach to proximal nail fold, thus further strengthening the attachment of nail unit to bone. Thus, the entire nail apparatus is kept in place over underlying distal phalanx, the size and shape of which greatly determine those of the nail plate.[1,2] Close proximity of nail apparatus to periosteum and relative lack of dermis and subcutaneous fat necessitate strict asepsis and careful handling of tissues during the procedures on nail.

The nail unit consists of a nail plate, four specialized epithelia (the proximal nail fold, the nail matrix, the nail bed, and the hyponychium), and lateral nail folds (Figures 2.2 and 2.3).[1]

Nail plate

The nail plate is a hard, semi-transparent, slightly convex "dead" keratinized structure. It is comprised of tightly packed onychocytes that contain abundant hard hair-type keratins embedded in a matrix of sulfur-rich high-cysteine and high-glycine/tyrosine proteins. The

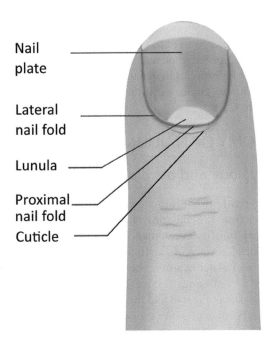

Nail plate

Lateral nail fold

Lunula

Proximal nail fold

Cuticle

Figure 2.2 The nail unit (surface view). (Courtesy of Dr. Sunil Kothiwala.)

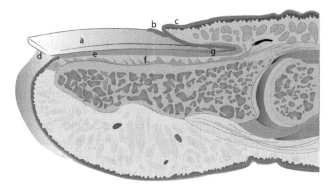

Figure 2.3 The nail unit (longitudinal section) – **(a)** nail plate, **(b)** cuticle, **(c)** proximal nail fold, **(d)** hyponychium, **(e)** nail bed, **(f)** terminal phalanx bone, **(g)** nail matrix. (Courtesy of Dr. Sunil Kothiwala.)

nail plate, analogous to stratum corneum of skin, arises from the lower surface of the proximal nail fold. It is surrounded and partially covered by the proximal and lateral nail folds. Nail plate is a translucent structure but appears pink due to underlying blood vessels except for the free distal margin that appears white. Lunula, a white semi-circular area, may be present in the proximal nail plate. This corresponds to the visible portions of the distal matrix and loose attachment of proximal nail plate to the underlying epithelium. Lunula is most easily visible in thumbnails and great toenails. The natural shape of the free margin of the nail is the same as the contour of the distal border of the lunula. The hyponychium is the gap beneath the free edge of the nail plate distally. Onychocorneal band, a thin distal transverse white band, present in more than 90% of fingernails, represents the last point of firm attachment of the nail plate to the nail bed. Another zone, called onychodermal band, lies just distal to onychocorneal band and is seen as a 1.0–1.5-mm pink (Caucasian) or brown (Afro-Caribbean) colored band.[1,4]

The nail plate is curved in both the longitudinal and transverse axes. This curvature allows nail plates to be embedded in nail folds, providing stronger attachment. The surface of nail plate is not completely smooth, but shows fine longitudinal ridges that correspond to complementary ridges on the underlying nail bed to which it is attached.

The pattern of ridges in childhood is different; short partial oblique ridges are noted in herringbone or chevron pattern. The longitudinal ridges appear as children grow and increase with advancing age. These ridges are considered to be specific to the individual, allowing the distinction between identical twins and, hence, may be used for forensic identification.

Sagittal section of the nail plate shows three portions: (1) dorsal nail plate, derived from keratinization of cells from proximal nail matrix; (2) intermediate nail plate, contributed by distal nail matrix; and (3) ventral nail plate, contributed by nail bed (Figure 2.4). Hence, proximal nail matrix pathology manifests itself in alterations in dorsal nail plate, which are both palpable and visible. On the other hand, distal nail matrix pathology results in alterations in intermediate nail plate, which are visible but not palpable. Understanding this concept is crucial in choosing site of nail biopsy in different conditions.

Nail matrix

Nail matrix is a localized region beneath the proximal nail fold that produces the major part (dorsal and intermediate portions) of the normal nail plate. The width and thickness of the nail plate is determined by the size, length, and thickness of the matrix. The loss of matrix due to surgery or trauma may result in the decreased width of nail plate or split nail plate (depending on the site of tissue loss) and, hence, biopsy with a width more than 3 mm is not desirable. The ventral portion of nail plate is produced by the nail bed. However, above the lunula the nail plate is thinner and consists only of the dorsal and intermediate portions.

When the nail plate is removed and proximal nail is retracted, nail matrix can be visualized as a distally convex crescent-shaped structure with its lateral horns extending proximally and laterally. The proximal margin of the matrix follows the contour of the lunula and reaches up to midpoint of the distance from the proximal nail fold to the central crease of the distal interphalangeal joint. At the lateral horns, a subtle ligamentous attachment can be noticed, arising dorsally from lateral ligaments of the distal interphalangeal joint. Imbalance in symmetrical tension on these attachments results in congenital and acquired malalignment of nail plate.

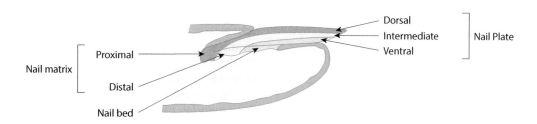

Figure 2.4 Nail matrix and its role in development of nail plate.

Microscopically, nail matrix differs from epidermis by absence of granular layer. Otherwise, nail matrix is similar to epidermis, having columnar, basophilic basal layer and cuboidal, eosinophilic upper layers. The cells of suprabasal layers transits to the uniformly eosinophilic keratogenous zone. The cell nuclei become pyknotic and darker and disappear when the eosinophilic superficial cells turn into onychocytes (analogous to corneocytes of stratum corneum). Melanocytes are present in the lowest three cell layers in the nail matrix, leading to melanization of the keratinocytes. Normal matrix melanocyte distribution is 6.5 melanocytes per millimeter of matrix basement membrane. Nail matrix melanocytes do not express human leukocyte antigen (HLA)-A/B/C antigens, whereas the melanocytes in the proximal nail fold and most other sites do express. Langerhans cells in the matrix are indistinguishable from normal skin.

Nail matrix is the only site of expression of hard keratin proteins especially Ha1 keratin. Cells differentiate with the expression of trichocyte "hard" keratin (K31–40 and K81–86) as they are incorporated into the nail plate along with the normal epithelial keratins. The cells may retain their nuclei called pertinax bodies until more distal in the nail plate. Recent data revealed that fibroblasts derived from the nail matrix may induce hard keratin expression even in non-nail-matrix keratinocytes.[1,4]

Nail bed

The nail bed extends from distal margin of lunula to hyponychium and can be easily differentiated from nail matrix as it is redder and shows surface ridges. Microscopically, nail bed is composed of epidermis, 2–3 cells thick, with underlying connective tissue in close proximity to the periosteum of the distal phalanx. Vertically oriented collagen in the nail bed directly attaches the epidermal basal lamina to the phalanges periosteum. Nail bed is remarkable for capillaries running longitudinally and arranged one above the other in 4–6 rows. This rich vasculature explains pink appearance of the nail plate and unique linear pattern of splinter hemorrhages. There is no subcutaneous fat in the nail bed, but there are many nerves and blood vessels including glomus bodies. Glomus bodies are small, specialized organs, found in great number in the nail bed and matrix dermis, and have an important role in thermoregulation. Skin appendages are usually absent although eccrine sweat glands can be seen in the distal-most part.

Nail bed closely resembles the Henle layer of the internal root sheath of the epidermis as the transitional zone from living keratinocyte to dead ventral nail plate cell is abrupt, occurring in the space of one horizontal cell layer.[1–4]

Hyponychium

The hyponychium is an epithelial area underlying the free edge of the nail plate. Its proximal border is the distal limit of nail bed (the onychodermal band). Distally, it is continuous with normal volar skin and is separated from distal nail groove, with convexity anteriorly. Like any other epidermal areas, hyponychium undergoes normal keratinization and exhibits a granular layer and eccrine glands. The hyponychium is the first site of keratinization in the nail unit and of all epidermis in the embryo. Also, the hyponychium is the initial site of invasion by dermatophytes in the most common type of onychomycosis, distal subungual onychomycosis. In addition, hyponychium and overhanging free nail plate provide a crevice and act as a reservoir for scabies, mites, and microbes.

Nail folds

The proximal nail fold is a continuation of the skin of each digit, forming the dorsal surface that folds underneath itself forming the ventral surface and rests above the nail matrix. The dorsal proximal nail fold is devoid of hair follicles, sebaceous glands, and dermatoglyphic markings; however, there is a normal granular layer. The ventral proximal nail fold also lacks rete ridges. The proximal nail keratinizes by formation of cuticle (Eponychium), which is attached to the upper surface of the nail plate. Cuticle acts as a seal to potential space between proximal nail fold and dorsal nail plate and loss of cuticle compromises the protective role of the proximal nail fold and leaves nail matrix vulnerable to external microbes and allergens. Chronic manipulation, manicure, inflammation, and infection can result in loss of cuticle, which heralds the onset of chronic paronychia.[2]

The lateral nail folds are soft tissues that partially cover the nail plates on radial and ulnar sides and contribute to the firm adherence of the nail plate to the nail bed. They are typically more prominent in the toes than fingers. Loss of volume of lateral nail folds is associated with a tendency for onycholysis. On the other hand, increased bulk of lateral nail folds is incompatible with the curvature and size of the nail plate and is often seen in chronic cases with ingrowing nails.

BLOOD SUPPLY OF NAIL

Nail bed and nail matrix receive their arterial blood supply from paired digital arteries; one of them is a large palmar artery, supplied from the larger superficial and deep palmar arcades, and the other is a small dorsal digital artery on either side. These arteries form three arcades: distal subungual arcade, proximal subungual artery (arcade), and superficial arcade. The main supply passes into the pulp space of the distal phalanx before reaching the dorsum of the digit. The arteries are extremely tortuous and coiled distally, which allows them to be distorted without kinking to occlude supply. The main arterial arches are formed from anastomoses of the branches of the digital arteries supplying the nail bed and matrix (Figure 2.5). Further, they can be categorized into three patterns: (1) vessels that are longitudinal with helical

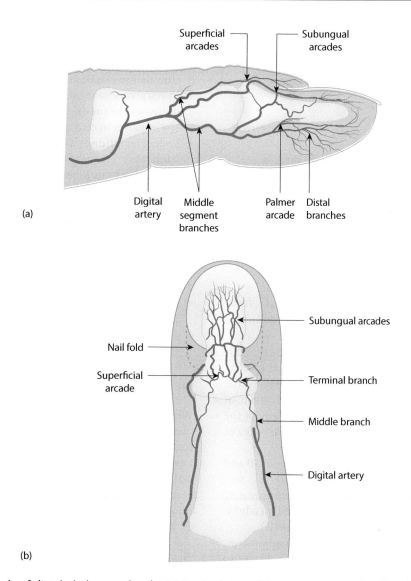

Figure 2.5 Arterial supply of distal phalanx and nail – **(a)** Sagittal view, **(b)** palmar aspect. The digital arteries and nerves arborize or trifurcate near the distal interphalangeal joint.

twisting within the matrix, (2) more longitudinal axis in the nail bed and in the distal proximal nail fold without the tortuosity, and (3) vessels that follow the pattern of the dermatoglyphic in the digit pulp.

Capillaroscopy or dermatoscopic examination of nail fold vessels is used to assess acral microvascular status. Nail vessel video dermoscopy is also used as part of a dynamic and anatomical modeling process establishing the parameters of blood flow and vessel anatomy.[1,4,5]

NERVE SUPPLY OF NAIL

Dorsal branches of the paired digital nerves give rise to the cutaneous sensory nerves that run parallel to the digital vessels. Corresponding palmar and plantar digital nerves innervate the pulp of the distal digit up to the margin with the hyponychium. Fingertips play an important role in the sensory perception with abundant nerve endings that transmit pain (type I fibers), touch (Meissner and Pacinian bodies), and temperature.[4,5]

Clinical implications

Understanding nerve supply of the nail unit is crucial to administering anesthesia in nail surgery, as all relevant nerves need to be blocked. Earlier, use of epinephrine was considered contraindicated for nail surgery; however, recent review of the literature and current experience find the combination of lidocaine and epinephrine safe for both the ring block anesthesia and direct infiltration into digits. Epinephrine also reduces bleeding and prolongs duration of anaesthesia.[6]

PHYSIOLOGY OF NAIL

Function of nail

Nails have various functions[1]:

- Nail plate acts as a protective covering for the fingertips and distal toes.
- Nails also enhance the tactile discrimination of hands and allow precision and delicacy in finger functions.
- Toenails contribute to pedal biomechanics.
- Nails are used for scratching apart from various aesthetic functions.

Nail growth

Nails grow continuously throughout life, unlike hair.

The rate of nail growth depends on various physiological, environmental, and pathological conditions (Table 2.1).[1,4,7]

Rate of nail growth is usually measured as longitudinal elongation of nail plate, using the lunula as a reference structure. However, this does not truly measure the nail-plate production per unit of time. An assessment of nail-plate thickness or mass is required to complement the measures of longitudinal growth, to have a complete idea of rate of nail growth.

The rate of nail growth peaks between the ages of 10 and 14 and then begins a steady decline with age after the second decade. Fingernails have a growth rate of approximately 0.1 mm per day (mean growth rate 3.5 mm/month) in adults. Toenails grow at one-third of this rate (0.03 mm/day).

The nail matrix contributes to most of the nail growth, and the contribution from the nail bed is not significant in healthy state. Diseases of the nail matrix affect nail growth.

The regeneration time for a fingernail is around 100–180 days (6 months) whereas for a toenail it is 12–18 months.

Clinical implications

- Nails free from trauma grow more slowly. Mechanical stimulation can be beneficial in slow-growing nails.
- In refractory cases of onychomycosis, avulsion not only decreases the fungal load but also stimulates growth.
- Use of gloves in cold weather prevents decreased growth.
- Systemic antifungals have a direct effect on nail matrix stimulation and can be used in yellow nail syndrome.
- Biotin, due to its kinetic properties, may be suitable for studies in onychomycosis and yellow nail syndrome.

Methods to assess kinetic activity of nail matrix:

- Immunohistochemistry: using antibodies to detect proliferating cell nuclear antigens and Ki-67. These are antigens associated with proliferating cells.
- Autoradiography: imaging done after injecting labelled thymidine and glycine.
- Direct measurement of matrix product (nail plate) by ultrasound, micrometer, and histology.

Nail morphology

Why do the nails grow flat and not as heaped-up keratinous masses? This question has invited a lot of debate. The exact reason for this is not known but it could be due to various factors like adherence to the nail bed, curtailment by the proximal and lateral nail folds, and the effect of underlying phalanx.

Why are the nails rounded and not pointed? This question remains unanswered. This could be related to the shape of the lunula but the exact cause is not known.[1]

Biochemical composition of nail

Nail plate is composed of both organic and inorganic components. The latter includes trace metals and electrolytes.[1,4]

Table 2.1 Various physiological, environmental, and pathological conditions affecting the rate of nail growth

Faster	Slower
Dominant hand	Non-dominant hand
Fingernails	Toenails
Males	Females
Middle, ring, and index finger	Thumb, little fingernails
Young age (between second and third decade)	At birth, after 60 years of age
Pregnancy	Lactation
Day, warm climate	Night, winter
Localized finger trauma, nail biters, altered nail avulsion	Immobilization of fingers or paralysis
High vascular states (arteriovenous stunts)	Reduced blood supply (peripheral vascular disease)
Hyperthyroidism	Hypothyroidism, fever, poor nutrition, kwashiorkor, acute infections, fever, systemic disorders (renal failure, tuberculosis)
Dermatoses psoriasis, pityriasis rubra pilaris, bullous ichthyosiform erythroderma	Onychomycosis, yellow nail syndrome
Drugs: levodopa, oral retinoids, itraconazole	Chemotherapeutic agents

Table 2.2 Levels of various inorganic elements in nail plate in various conditions

Physiological state/disease	Mineral	Level
Males	Calcium	Higher
	Zinc	Higher
	Magnesium	Lower
Children	Magnesium	Higher
	Sodium	Higher
Children with kwashiorkor	Sodium	Higher
	Calcium	Higher
	Magnesium	Lower
Wilson's disease	Copper	Increased
Iron deficiency anemia	Iron	Decreased/unchanged
Cystic fibrosis	Sodium	Increased
Arsenic intoxication	Arsenic	Increased within hours of exposure
Fluoride	Fluoride content of nail plate reflects dietary fluoride intake	

INORGANIC COMPONENTS

There is a large variation in the values of the inorganic elements of nail reported in various studies. This is due to various factors like accuracy of technique used, environmental contamination, and variation between subjects. Table 2.2 highlights the levels of various inorganic elements in the nail plate in different physiological and pathological conditions.

Nail plate is rich in calcium, which exists as phosphate in hydroxyapatite crystals. Calcium does not contribute to the hardness of the nail significantly. Hardness of the nail plate is imparted by the sulphur protein from the matrix.

ORGANIC COMPONENTS

Carbon, nitrogen, and sulphur are the organic elements found in the nail plate. The nitrogen content of nail is unaffected by nutritional status. Sulphur is a constituent of the amino acid cysteine found in the nail plate. Although the levels of sulphur vary in number of diseases, its estimation is of no value. Nitrogen content is higher in the nails of males whereas the sulphur content is lower. The carbon content is same in both the sexes. With increasing age, the carbon content of nail increases whereas nitrogen content decreases. Sulphur content remains the same.

WATER CONTENT

The water content of the nail plate is around 18% under normal conditions. The water content decreases in winter. The nail plate is highly porous; hence, it can get dehydrated especially in long nails. Decrease in the water content causes brittleness of nails whereas increase (above 30%) leads to softness and opacity of nails.

LIPID CONTENT

The lipid content of nails is less than 5% and mainly found as cholesterol. The levels are regulated by the hormones. Nail plate contains significant amounts of phospholipids that contribute to its flexibility.

NAIL KERATINS

Like all epithelial cells, the nail is also composed of keratins, which are fibrous proteins belonging to the intermediate filament proteins. The nail plate epithelium has 80% "hard" keratin (hair keratin) and 20% epidermal keratins.

The keratins account for 80% of the dry weight of nail plate. The hard hair-type keratins make the nail more ragged and resistant to chemical treatment as they have a large number of sulphur-containing amino acids like cysteine, glutamic acid, and serine. These have the same heterodimer configuration but additional resilience. Hair keratins are also found in hair, tooth, claw, hoof, thymus, and tongue papillae.[3,4]

The pattern of keratin expression in the nail unit is depicted in Figure 2.6.

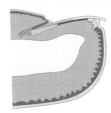

Part of the nail unit	Keratins
Proximal nail fold	BL: K5, K14
	SBL: K5, K6, K10, K14, K16, K17
Proximal nail matrix	BL: K5, K6, K14, K17
	SBL: K5, K6, K10, K14, K16, K17, K85
Distal nail matrix	BL: K5, K14, K17
	SBL: K5, K10, K14, K17, K85
Nail bed	BL: K5, K14, K17
	SBL: K6, K16, K17, K75
Hyponychium	BL: K5, K14, K17
	SBL: K5, K10, K14, K17

BL: Basal layer, SBL: Suprabasal layer, K: Keratin

Figure 2.6 Schematic diagram of keratin expression in the nail unit.

Clinical implications

There are several genodermatoses caused by keratin defects. The type of keratin defect determines the pattern of nail abnormalities. Pachyonychia congenita (PC) is an autosomal dominant disorder caused by mutation in genes encoding keratin 6a or 16 (in PC 1) and 6b or 17 (in PC 2). The condition shows thickening of nail plate and palmoplantar keratoderma.

Biophysical properties of nail

The nail plate is hard and flexible. These physical characteristics and strength of nail are due to its constituents and their orientation in the plane of nail plate. The water content varies between 10% and 30% and decreases with high humidity. The water diffusion constant of nail is 100 times more than the adjacent skin. Thus, the nail is much more permeable than the skin. The loss of water can be stopped by applying nail polish or petrolatum jelly to the nail plate.

The nail also allows permeation of hydrophobic molecules. Hence, anti-fungal nail lacquers can be used as they penetrate the nail to some extent.

The nail plates transmit 30% of grenz rays and 85% of X-rays. Hence superficial X-rays should be used instead of grenz rays to treat diseases of the nail bed.

Innate immunity of nail

The nail has strong innate immunity due to increased local expression of antimicrobial peptide (AMP) human cathelicidin (LL-37). This AMP is not expressed in human skin under normal circumstances but gets induced upon exposure to infection or inflammation.[8] It has potent activity against *Pseudomonas aeruginosa* and *Candida albicans*. However, nail matrix is a site of relative immune privilege, a property contributed by various factors:

- CD4+/CD8+ cells are differentially distributed in and around the nail apparatus. The nail matrix epithelium and its surrounding mesenchyme display lowest CD4+ T cell density. The number of CD8+ T cells are substantially lower than CD4+ T cells.
- Antigen-presenting capacity of Langerhans cells and macrophages in/around the nail matrix may be impaired.
- Capacity of nail matrix dendritic cells (DC) to associate with T cells via DC -specific ICAM-grabbing non-integrin (DC-SIGN) may be impaired.
- NK cells and mast cells are unusually scarce in the vicinity of the nail matrix.
- Major histocompatibility complex (MHC) class I expression is prominently down regulated in the PNM keratinocytes.
- Proximal nail matrix (PNM) melanocytes are MHC class I negative.

- Nail matrix expresses immunosuppressive factors like migration inhibition factor (MIF), IGF-1, alpha MSH, ACTH, and TGF.

Clinical implications

- Acute and chronic inflammatory nail disorders affect primarily the proximal nail fold and not the proximal nail matrix.
- Collapse of the nail immune privilege together with up regulation of MHC Class 1 expression on nail melanocytes can occur in certain conditions such as alopecia areata. This exposes cells to immune recognition and cytotoxic autoimmune attack. This explains the nail changes (trachyonychia, onychodystrophy) seen in patients with alopecia areata.
- The immune privilege may be advantageous in preventing over-reactivity to environmental antigens but it also increases the susceptibility to certain infections, e.g., human papillomavirus.

KEY POINTS

- The fingernail unit starts developing from the 8th week of gestation. At 18 weeks it takes the post-natal appearance. Toenail development occurs 4 weeks later.
- Functional p63, Wnt7a, R-Spondin 4, *LMX1b*, and *MSX1* are important for nail differentiation and development.
- Nail unit comprises nail plate and four specialized epithelia that include the proximal nail fold, the nail matrix, the nail bed, and the hyponychium.
- Major part of the nail plate (dorsal and intermediate) is produced by nail matrix and the rest (ventral part) is by nail bed.
- Nail matrix is the only site of expression of hard keratin proteins.
- Normal matrix melanocyte distribution is 6.5 melanocytes per millimeter of matrix basement membrane.
- Unlike hair, nails grow continuously throughout life.
- The rate of nail growth depends on various factors. Fingernails grow faster than toenails.
- Nail is composed of both organic and inorganic components. Nail plate is rich in calcium.
- The nail plate epithelium has 80% "hard" keratin (hair keratin) and 20% epidermal keratins.
- The nail has strong innate immunity due to increased local expression of AMP human cathelicidin (LL-37). However, nail matrix is a site of relative immune privilege.

REFERENCES

1. de Berker DA, Richert B, Baran R. Acquired disorders of the nail and nail unit. In: Griffith CEM, Barker J, Bleiker T, Chalmers R, Creamer D (Eds.). *Rook's Text Book of Dermatology*, 9th ed. Chichester, UK: John Wiley & Sons; 2016. p. 95.1–95.5.

2. McGrath JA, Uitto J. Structure and function of the skin. In: Griffith CEM, Barker J, Bleiker T, Chalmers R, Creamer D (Eds.). *Rook's Text Book of Dermatology*, 9th ed. Chichester, UK: John Wiley & Sons; 2016. p. 2.9–2.11.

3. Tosti A, Piraccini BM. Biology of nails and nail disorders. In: Goldsmith LA, Katz SI, Gilchrest BA, Paller AS, Leffell DJ, Wolff K (Eds.). *Fitzpatrick's Dermatology in General Medicine*, 8th ed. New Delhi, India: McGraw-Hill; 2012. p. 1009–1012.

4. de Berker DA, Higgins CA, Jahoda C, Christiano AM. Biology of hair and nails. In: Bolognia JL, Jorizzo JL, Schaffer JV (Eds.). *Dermatology*, 3rd ed. Elsevier Saunders; 2012. p. 1085–1089.

5. Haneke E. Surgical anatomy of the nail apparatus. *Dermatol Clin* 2006; 24: 291–296.

6. Hussain SW, Motley RJ, Wang TS. Principles of skin surgery. In: Griffith CEM, Barker J, Bleiker T, Chalmers R, Creamer D (Eds.). *Rook's Text Book of Dermatology*, 9th ed. Chichester, UK: John Wiley & Sons; 2016. p. 20.11–20.12.

7. Geyer AS, Onumah N, Uyttendaele H, Scher RK. Modulation of linear nail growth to treat diseases of the nail. *J Am Acad Dermatol* 2004; 50: 229–234.

8. Ito T, Ito N, Saathoff M, Stampachiacchiere B, Bettermann A, Bulfone-Paus S et al. Immunology of the human nail apparatus: The nail matrix is a site of relative immune privilege. *J Invest Dermatol* 2005; 125: 139–148.

3

Nail unit signs

NIHARIKA RANJAN LAL, PIYUSH KUMAR, AND RIZWANA BARKAT

Before embarking on the journey of nail disorders, it is important to be familiar with various nail signs. Some of these nail signs are specific and help in arriving at a final diagnosis even in the absence of skin lesions. Other nail signs are non-specific but can pinpoint the site of pathological process in the nail unit and thus may direct subsequent investigations and treatment. In this chapter, various nail signs have been summarized along with clinical photographs. The entities have been classified based on their appearance and site of pathology. The entities have been classified based on their appearance and site of pathology.

ALTERATIONS IN THE NAIL PLATE SIZE

Name	Description	Clinical Photographs
Micronychia	• Abnormally small nail (Figure 3.1)	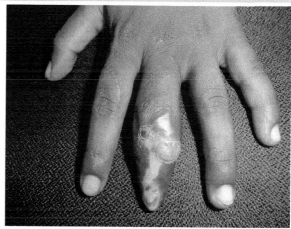

Figure 3.1 Micronychia of middle finger in leprosy.

Brachyonychia/ Racket nail

- Short nail in which the width of the nail plate and nail bed is greater than the length (Figure 3.2)

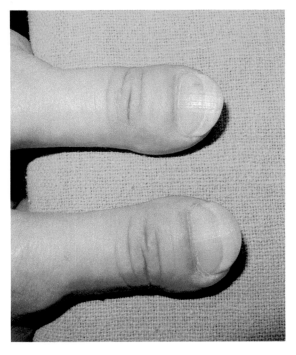

Figure 3.2 Brachyonychia.

Onychoatrophy

- Faulty underdevelopment of the nail in which there is reduction in size and thickness of the nail unit (Figure 3.3)

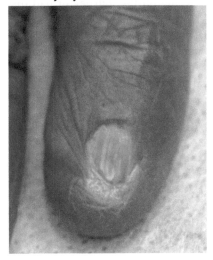
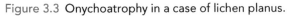

Figure 3.3 Onychoatrophy in a case of lichen planus.

Haplonychia/ Egg shell nail

- Nail plate becomes soft and thin, and breaks. It happens because of malnutrition and debility (Figure 3.4).

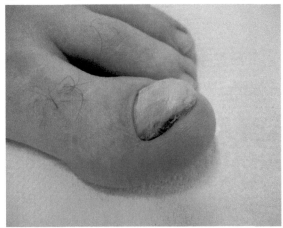

Figure 3.4 Egg shell nail

Onychodystrophy/ Dystrophic nail

- Nails become mis-shapen, thickened, or exhibit a partially destroyed nail plate (Figure 3.5a–c).

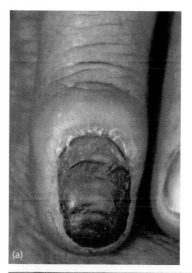

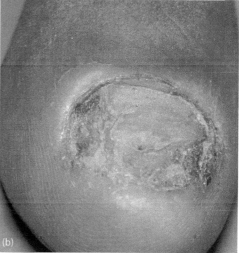

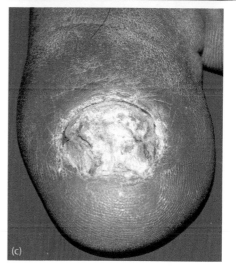

Figure 3.5 **(a)** Onychodystrophy in chronic paronychia; **(b)** Onychodystrophy of toenail; **(c)** Onychodystrophy in tinea unguium.

Macronychia

- Abnormally large nail (Figure 3.6)

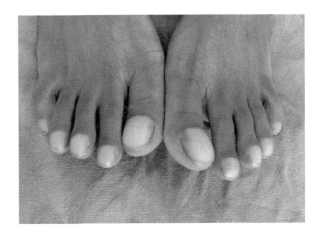

Figure 3.6 Macronychia.

Anonychia

- Complete absence of the nail in one or more fingers or toes (Figure 3.7a–c)

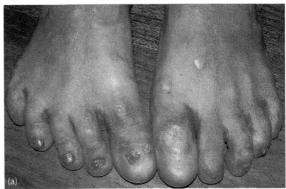

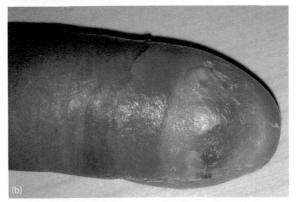

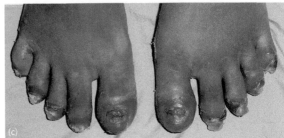

Figure 3.7 **(a)** Anonychia of all toenails in epidermolysis bullosa; **(b)** Anonychia following acrodermatitis continua of hallopeau; **(c)** Anonychia in nail psoriasis with psoriatic arthritis.

ALTERATIONS IN THE NAIL PLATE THICKNESS AND CURVATURE

Pachyonychia
- Thickened nail with an increased transverse curvature (Figure 3.8)

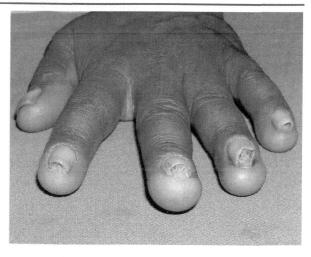

Figure 3.8 Pachyonychia.

Onychochauxis
- Thickened nail with yellowish discoloration without any change in the curvature of the nail plate (Figure 3.9)

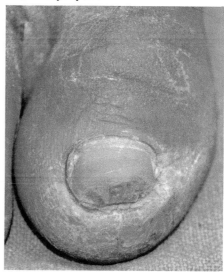

Figure 3.9 Onychochauxis.

Onychogryphosis

- Nail plate thickening with gross hyperkeratosis and increased curvature of the nail plate (Figure 3.10a–c)

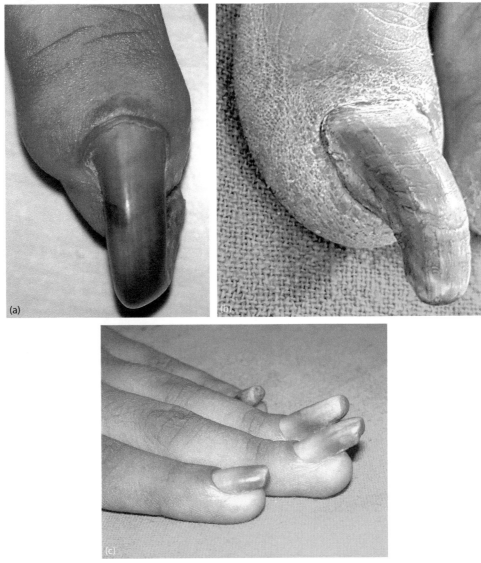

Figure 3.10 **(a, b)** Oyster-like onychogryphosis; **(c)** Ram's horn dystrophy (Onychogryphosis).

Platonychia

- Transverse curvature of nail plate is lost, resulting in an abnormally flat nail (Figure 3.11a and b).

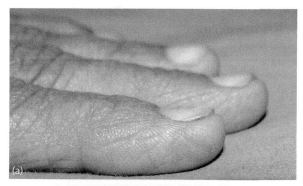

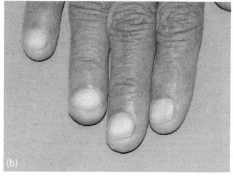

Figure 3.11 **(a, b)** Platonychia.

Koilonychia/Spoon nails

- Abnormally thinned and concave nails with raised edges giving an appearance of spoon (Figure 3.12)

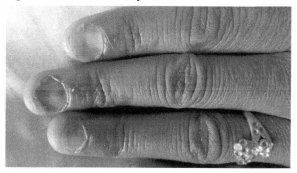

Figure 3.12 Koilonychia in a patient with iron deficiency.

Clubbing

- Swelling of the distal digit with enlarged and excessively curved nail plate resulting in loss of normal angle between proximal nail fold and the nail plate (Figure 3.13)

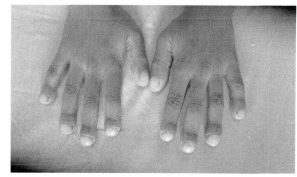

Figure 3.13 Clubbing.

Pincer nail (Omega nails/Trumpet nails)

Excessive transverse curvature of nail plate, resulting in compression of the nail bed and underlying dermis (Figure 3.14a and b)

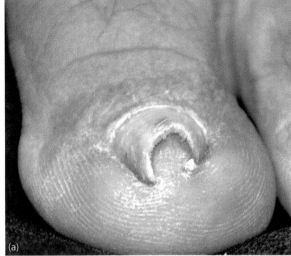

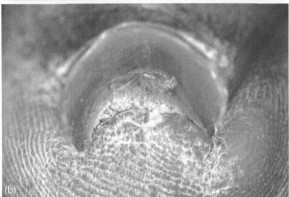

Figure 3.14 **(a)** Pincer nail; **(b)** Pincer nail.

Onychoclavus (Subungual heloma/corn)

Hyperkeratotic tissue in the nail area, mostly under the distal nail margins, due to a bony deformity or repeated minor trauma (Figure 3.14c)

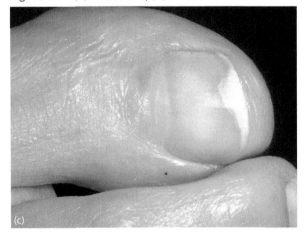

Figure 3.14 **(c)** Subungual corn.

ALTERATIONS IN THE NAIL PLATE COLOR

Chromonychia

- Change in normal "pink translucent appearance" of nail plate (Figure 3.15a–c)

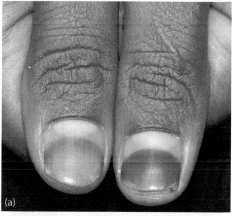

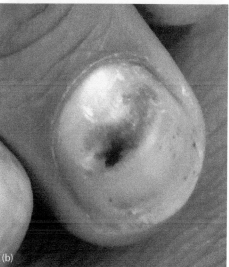

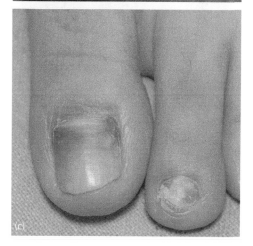

Figure 3.15 **(a)** Exogenous chromonychia following henna application. Note the shape of proximal margin of pigmentation follows the proximal nail fold; **(b)** Endogenous chromonychia due to subungual hematoma. Note the shape of proximal margin of pigmentation follows the lunula; **(c)** Blue green chromonychia due to *Pseudomonas* spp. Colonization.

Leukonychia

- Nail plate appears white. The whole or the part of nail plate may develop leukonychia. It is of three types: true, apparent, and pseudo leukonychia (Figure 3.16a–e).

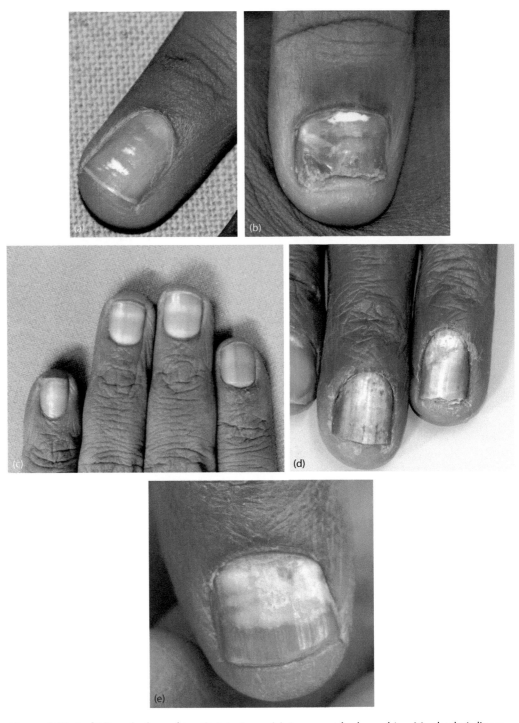

Figure 3.16 (a, b) True leukonychia - Striate type; (c) Apparent leukonychia - Muehrcke's lines; (d, e) Pseudoleukonychia in a case of onychomycosis.

Mees' line

- A single or multiple, transverse, narrow (1–2 mm thick) whitish line running along the width of the nail and parallel to lunula. It is noted to occur at the same level in one or several fingernails (Figure 3.17).

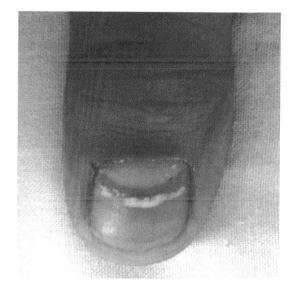

Figure 3.17 Mees' lines.

Melanonychia

- Nail plate develops brown or black discoloration. It may be total or partial, transverse, or linear and may affect one or multiple nails (Figure 3.18a–b).

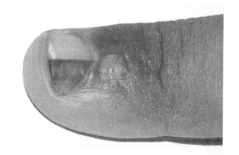

(a)

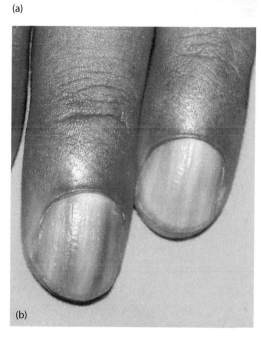

(b)

Figure 3.18 (a) Melanonychia in a child; (b) Multiple bands of melanonychia in an adult.

ALTERATIONS IN THE NAIL PLATE SURFACE

Longitudinal ridge

- Small linear projection extending from proximal nail fold to free distal end of nail plate (Figure 3.19)

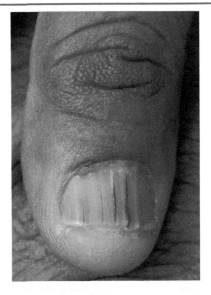

Figure 3.19 Longitudinal ridges.

Nail beads

- Small linear projection may be interrupted at regular intervals, giving rise to beaded appearance (Figure 3.20)

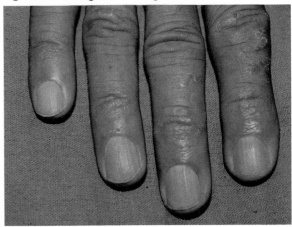

Figure 3.20 Nail beads.

Longitudinal groove

- Shallow furrow on the surface of the nail plate (Figure 3.21a and b)

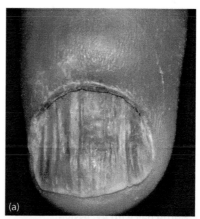

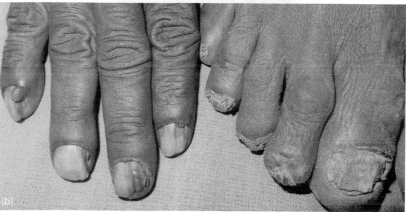

Figure 3.21 **(a)** Longitudinal grooves; **(b)** Longitudinal grooves and koenen tumors in tuberous sclerosis.

Onychorrhexis

- Split or brittle nails with a series of longitudinal ridges (Figure 3.22)

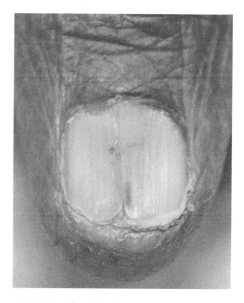

Figure 3.22 Onychorrhexis.

Median nail dystrophy

- Longitudinal defect of the thumb or great toenails in the midline or just off-center, starting at the cuticle and growing out of the free edge. Feathery cracks extend laterally from the split, giving the "inverted fir tree" appearance (Figure 3.23).

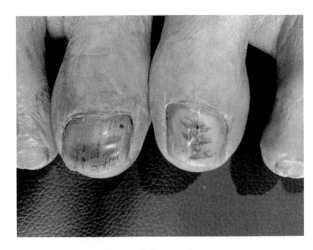

Figure 3.23 Median nail dystrophy.

Trachyonychia

- Brittle nail with excessive longitudinal ridging, imparting a rough surface and "sandpaper-like" appearance in severe cases. Twenty-nail dystrophy is sometimes used synonymously but is not a preferred term as any number of nails may be affected. Two types, shiny and opaque types, have been described (Figure 3.24a–c).

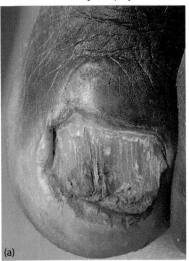

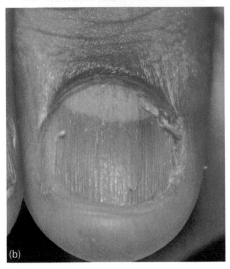

Figure 3.24 **(a)** Opaque trachyonychia with excess longitudinal ridging; **(b)** Shiny trachyonychia.

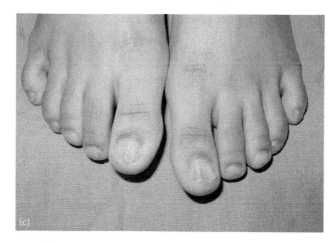

Figure 3.24 (Continued) **(c)** Trachyonychia of multiple digits.

Pitting (Rosenau's depressions)

- Pits are superficial depressions within the nail plate and vary in morphology and distribution (Figure 3.25a and b).

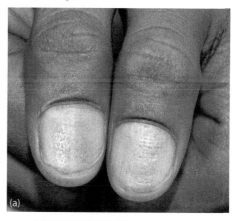

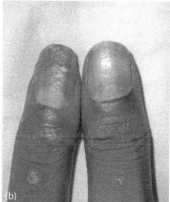

Figure 3.25 **(a)** Fine nail pitting; **(b)** Coarse nail pitting in nail psoriasis.

Elkonyxis

- Very large pits (Figure 3.26).

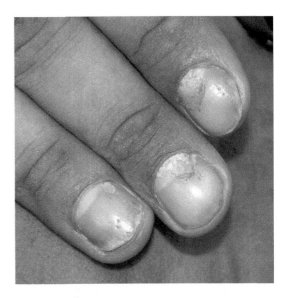

Figure 3.26 Elkonyxis.

Transverse grooves

- Transverse furrow on the surface of nail plate.

Beau's lines

- Transverse groove(s) running from side to side on nail and reflecting temporary reduction in matrix activity (Figure 3.27a–c).

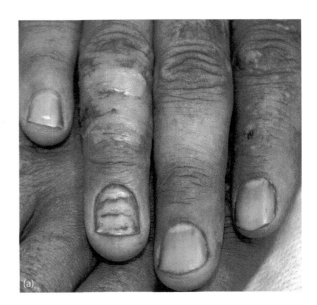

Figure 3.27 **(a)** Beau's lines in allergic contact dermatitis.

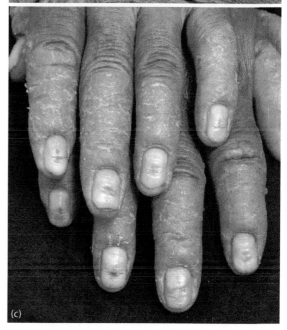

Figure 3.27 (Continued) **(b)** Beau's lines; **(c)** Beau's lines in psoriasis.

Habit tic deformity

- Series of transverse grooves as a result of mechanical injury caused by constant pushing back of cuticle of one or several fingers (Figure 3.28).

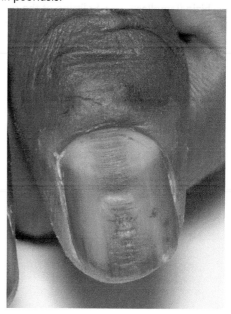

Figure 3.28 Transverse grooves in habit tic deformity.

Onychomadesis

- Spontaneous separation of the nail plate from the matrix area (Figure 3.29a and b).

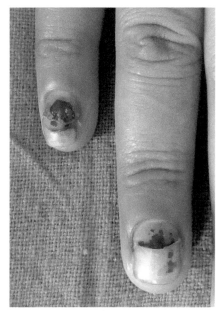

(a)

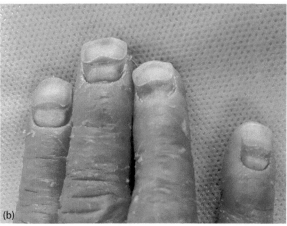

(b)

Figure 3.29 **(a, b)** Onychomadesis.

Onychoschizia (lamellar splitting)

- Splitting of the distal nail plate into layers at the free edge (Figure 3.30).

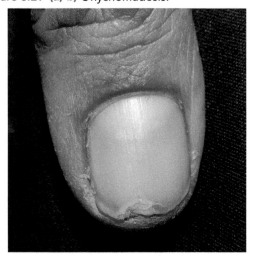

Figure 3.30 Onychoschizia.

**Chevron nail/
Herringbone nail**

- An uncommon transient pattern seen in children that resolves in adulthood. Ridges arise from the proximal nail fold and converge in a V-shaped pattern towards the midpoint distally (Figure 3.31a and b).

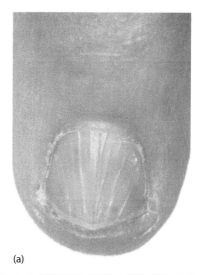

(a)

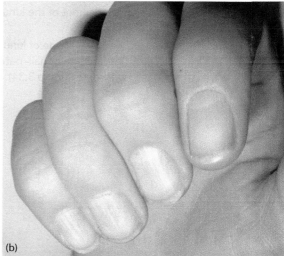

(b)

Figure 3.31 **(a)** Chevron nail; **(b)** Chevron nail in a child.

ALTERATIONS IN LUNULA

Red lunula

- The lunula, which is usually of a ground-glass appearance, may become reddened or suffused. Mostly seen in alopecia and lichen planus (Figure 3.32).

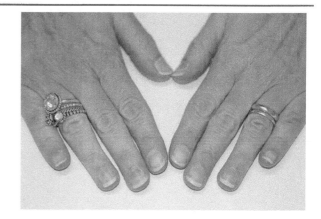

Figure 3.32 Red lunula.

Blue lunula

- Blue color of lunula, seen in Wilson disease, treatment with hydroxyurea (Figure 3.33)

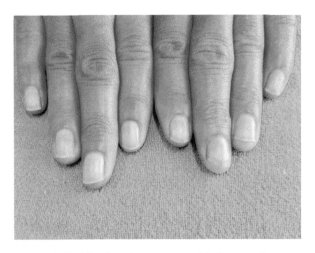

Figure 3.33 Blue lunula in a case with Raynaud's disease.

Macrolunula

- Enlargement of the lunula. Seen in habit tic.

Triangular lunula

- Triangular shape of lunula. Specific sign of nail–patella syndrome (Figure 3.34).

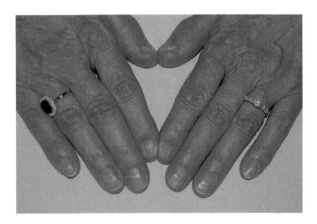

Figure 3.34 Triangular lunula.

NAIL FOLD SIGNS

Paronychia

- Inflammation of the nail folds, with erythema, swelling, pain, and impaired activity. Proximal nail fold involvement is always associated with loss of cuticle in chronic paronychia. (Figure 3.35a–c).

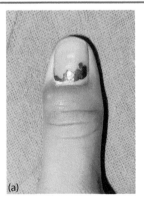

(a)

Figure 3.35 **(a, b)** Acute paronychia.

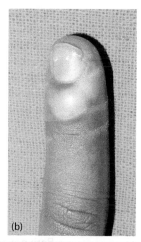

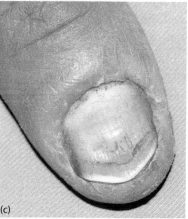

Figure 3.35 (Continued) **(b)** Acute paronychia; **(c)** Chronic paronychia.

Dorsal pterygium

- A linear forward growth of the proximal nail fold, which fuses with the underlying matrix and subsequently with the nail bed, dividing the nail plate in two (Figure 3.36a and b)

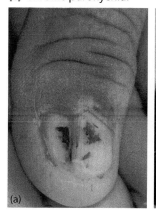
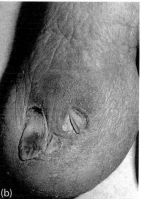

Figure 3.36 **(a)** Dorsal pterygium following trauma; **(b)** Dorsal pterygium in lichen planus.

Ventral pterygium

- Fibrosis extending from the hyponychium, anchoring the undersurface of the distal nail plate to underlying tissue and subsequent obliteration of the distal nail groove (Figure 3.37a and b).

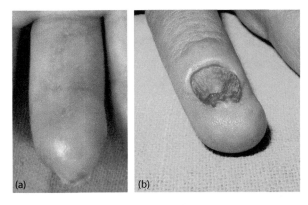

Figure 3.37 **(a)** Ventral pterygium in a case of systemic sclerosis; **(b)** Ventral pterygium.

Hutchinson's sign

- Periungual extension of brown-black pigmentation from longitudinal melanonychia onto the proximal and lateral nail folds. It is an important indicator of subungual melanoma (Figure 3.38).

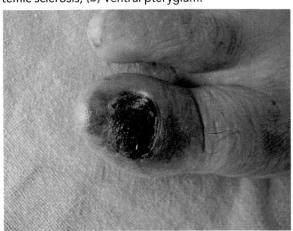

Figure 3.38 Nail bed melanoma with Hutchinson's sign.

Pseudo-Hutchinson's sign

- Pigmentation of nail folds in non-melanoma conditions (e.g., ethnic pigmentation, Laugier–Hunziker syndrome, Bowen's disease, Minocycline induced pigmentation, etc.). In pseudo-Hutchinson's sign, cuticle remains translucent (Figure 3.39).

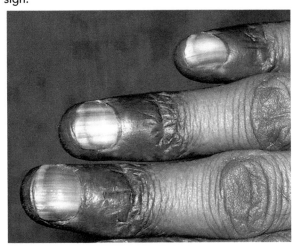

Figure 3.39 Psuedo-Hutchinson sign in a case of Laughier–Hunziker syndrome.

Ingrown nails/ Onychocryptosis	• Periungual inflammation and pain resulting from penetration of part of the nail plate into the soft tissues (Figure 3.40)

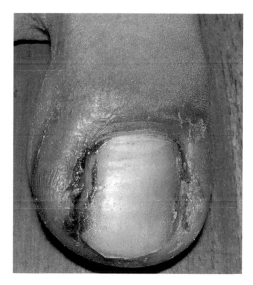

Figure 3.40 Onychocryptosis.

Onychophosis	• Localized or diffuse hyperkeratotic tissue developing within the space between the nail folds and the nail plate

NAIL BED SIGNS

Apparent leukonychia	• Leukonychia due to alterations in nail bed vascularity (e.g., Muehrcke's lines, Terry nails, half-and-half nails)
Muehrcke's lines	• Double white transverse lines in different hypoalbuminemia states (Figure 3.41)

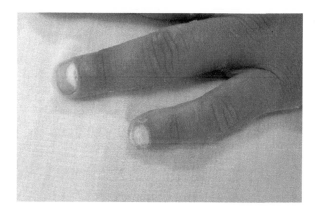

Figure 3.41 Muehrcke's lines.

Terry's nails

- Apparent leukonychia characterized by ground glass opacification of nearly the entire nail, obliteration of the lunula, and a narrow band (0.5–3.0 mm wide) of normal, pink nail bed at the distal border (Figure 3.42).

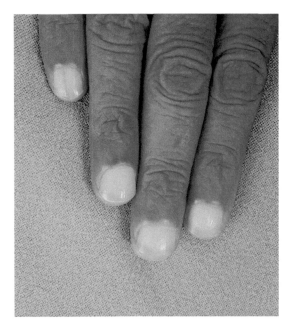

Figure 3.42 Terry's nails.

Half-and-half nail or Lindsay nail

- Nail consists of two segments separated more or less transversely by a well-defined line; the proximal area is dull white, resembling ground glass and obscuring the lunula; the distal area is pink, reddish, or brown (Figure 3.43a and b).

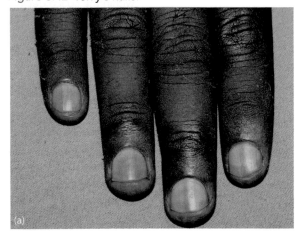

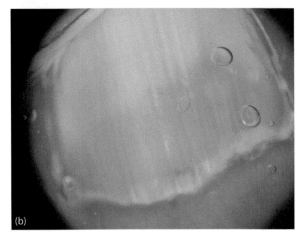

Figure 3.43 (a) Half and half nail; (b) Dermoscopy of half and half nail.

Onycholysis

- Detachment of the nail plate from its bed at its distal end and/or its lateral attachments (Figure 3.44a and b).

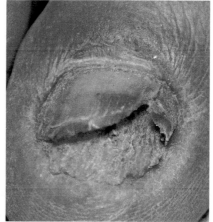

(a)

(b)

Figure 3.44 **(a)** Onycholysis; **(b)** Onycholysis with *Pseudomonas* colonization.

Plummer's nail

- Onycholysis affecting the ring and little fingers, seen in patients with thyrotoxicosis

Photo-onycholysis

- Consists of triad of photosensitization, onycholysis, and dyschromia (Figure 3.45)

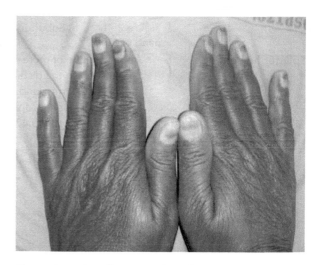

Figure 3.45 Sparfloxacin induced photo-onycholysis.

Nail bed hyperkeratosis/ Subungual hyperkeratosis

- Result of excessive proliferation of nail bed/hyponychium keratinocytes characterized by the accumulation of scales under the nail plate, which is detached and uplifted (Figure 3.46a–c)

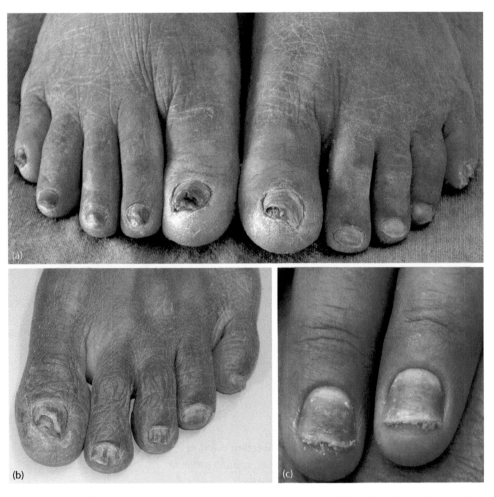

Figure 3.46 **(a, b)** Subungual hyperkeratosis in tinea unguim; **(c)** Nail bed hyperkeratosis in hand eczema.

Splinter hemorrhages

- Appear as one or more red-brown striae in the distal part of the nail and correspond to hemorrhages of the capillaries of the nail bed (Figure 3.47a and b)

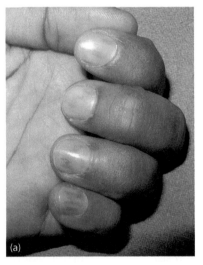

Figure 3.47 **(a)** Splinter haemorrhages in rheumatic heart disease.

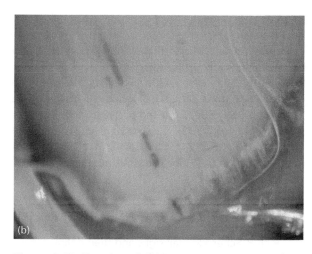

Figure 3.47 (Continued) **(b)** Dermoscopic image of splinter hemorrhage in psoriasis.

Salmon patch

- Yellow-red hue of the nail bed due to glycoprotein of the serum associated with exudative inflammation. It is typical of the psoriatic nail (Figure 3.48).

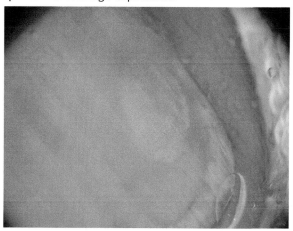
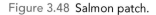

Figure 3.48 Salmon patch.

Subungual hematoma

- Deep-red to black discoloration of the nail due to extravasation of blood between nail plate and nail bed following trauma (Figure 3.49)

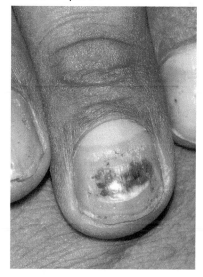

Figure 3.49 Subungual hematoma.

ACKNOWLEDGMENTS

The authors would like to thank Archana Singal (Figures 3.4, 3.8, 3.10, 3.12b, 3.18c, 3.25c, 3.29b, 3.33, 3.35a and b, 3.37a and b, 3.38, 3.41, 3.42, 3.43, 3.48a), Michela Starace (Figures 3.6, 3.31b, 3.32, 3.34), Balachandar Ankad (Figures 3.13a and b, 3.21, 3.30, 3.47a and b, 3.48b, 3.49), Bela J Shah (Figures 3.14 and 3.15), Eckart Haneke (Figure 3.16c), Anil Patki (Figure 3.24), Chander Grover (Figure 3.26b), and Vijay Zawar (3.45) for contributing images from their treasure.

REFERENCES

1. Rich P, Scher RK. Nail signs and their definitions: Non-specific nail dystrophies. In: *An Atlas of Diseases of the Nail.* 1st ed. New York: The Parthenon Publishing Group; 2005. p. 9–45.

2. Rich P, Scher RK. Chromonychias. In: *An Atlas of Diseases of the Nail.* 1st ed. New York: The Parthenon Publishing Group; 2005. p. 47–60.

3. Rubin AI, Baran R. Physical sings. In: Baran R, de Berker DAR, Holzberg M, Thomas L, (eds). *Baran & Dawber's Diseases of the Nails and Their Management.* 4th ed. West Sussex, UK: Wiley-Blackwell; 2012. p. 51–100.

4. Rich P. Nail signs and symptoms. In: Scher RK, Daniel III CR, (eds). *Nails Diagnosis, Therapy, Surgery.* 3rd ed. New York: Elsevier; 2005. p. 1–5.

4

An approach to nail examination

SHIKHA BANSAL AND NEHA KUMAR

INTRODUCTION

A stepwise approach is crucial for diagnosing nail disorders. Most nail diseases can be diagnosed by clinical examination. A careful evaluation of the patient is essential, together with clinical history.

A detailed history and clinical examination of nails, skin, hair, and various systems should be supplemented by simple office procedures, like onychoscopy and light microscopy. All nails should be examined even if the patient presents with a disease involving only one digit.

Normal variations

To arrive at any clinical diagnosis, one should be aware of normal variation in shape and opacity of the nail. The thickness may increase or decrease with age of the patient. Longitudinal ridging and beading are common in elderly persons, though can be a common feature in younger individuals as well.

Nail signs[1]

Nail signs are similar to the skin clinical signs, and their recognition is important for correct diagnosis. Nail signs usually involve the nail plate, which can be altered in shape, size, surface, and color or can be detached and/or uplifted. A nail sign reflects damage to a specific part of the nail unit, according to its role in the normal nail physiology. Nail plate signs can be isolated or associated with abnormalities of the periungual skin, including the nail folds, hyponychium, digital pulp, and skin of the dorsal digit. Changes in periungual tissue can present with clinical symptoms like paronychia, pain, throbbing, etc.

HISTORY TAKING

A detailed history taking is the key to diagnosis of any nail disease.[1] It is important to ask the number of nails affected, as certain conditions like trauma, tumors, etc. usually affect single nails. On the other hand, psoriasis, lichen planus, etc. can affect multiple nails.

A few simple questions can be asked that can provide important clues:

- Time of appearance/duration
- Mode of onset
- Course
- Occupation, hobbies, and habits
- Skin and systemic diseases
- Family history

Time of appearance/duration

Onset at birth or in early childhood would suggest a congenital disorder. As certain nail disorders can be congenital, a few simple questions can be asked, for example, were you born with this problem (e.g., congenital onychodysplasia, anonychia, onychoatrophy, etc.)?

Certain nail disorders can be a manifestation of a more complex entity. For example, Koenen tumors, or periungual and subungual fibromas, are a benign, cutaneous manifestation of tuberous sclerosis (Figure 4.1).

Age of onset is important in evaluation of melanonychia. A band of melanonychia present at birth or during childhood is in fact very likely to be a nevus or a benign melanocytic hyperplasia, while onset in adulthood of a band of melanonychia in a single nail should alert the physician, as it can be a sign of nail melanoma.

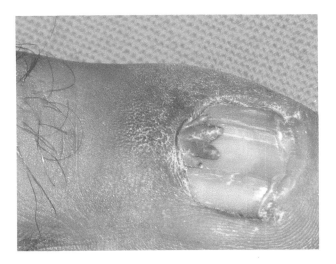

Figure 4.1 Koenen tumors, or periungual in tuberous sclerosis.

Mode of onset

The disorders that cause damage of the nail matrix take 2–3 months of time before becoming evident as nails grow slowly. A patient presenting with Beau's lines on several digits usually gives history of preceding systemic diseases. Acute paronychia, onycholysis, and subungual hematoma may have preceding history of trauma.

Nail psoriasis may be triggered by trauma through the Koebner phenomenon.

Certain nail pigmentations might be associated with long-standing drug intake. For example, a patient of pemphigus vulgaris had long standing history of intake of cyclophosphamide, and he presented in the dermatology department with complaint of grayish discoloration of all fingernails (Figure 4.2a and b).

Course

There are certain nail disorders that undergo spontaneous remission, like psoriasis. On the other hand, Acrodermatitis continua of Hallopeau will have a recurrent course (Figure 4.3).

If acute paronychia is happening in the same digit, it should raise the suspicion of a herpetic infection.

Occupation, hobbies, and habits

Another important history to be taken is the occupation of the patient. The kind of work the patient does—whether he comes in contact with chemicals, irritants, soap/detergent, hair dyes and straighteners, etc.—can be significant. Ask the hobbies of the patient. Do take history of nail trauma. The patient might have hobbies like tennis, jogging, painting, etc., which can induce nail trauma and cause certain characteristic nail changes. Do consider the type of shoes worn by the patient. Poorly fitting shoes have been suggested as one of the most common causes of pincer nails (Figure 4.4).

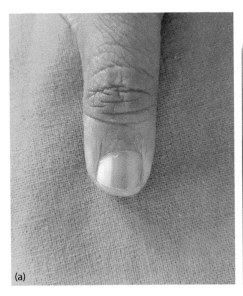

(a)

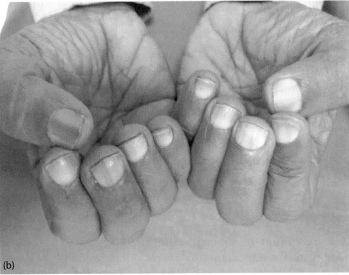

(b)

Figure 4.2 (a, b) Greyish discoloration of fingernails due to cyclophosphamide.

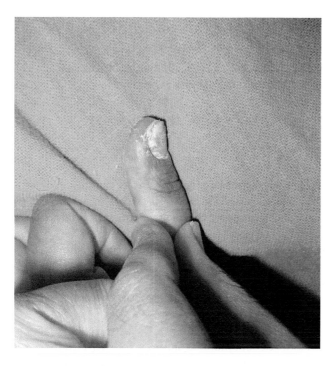

Figure 4.3 Acrodermatitis continua of Hallopeau.

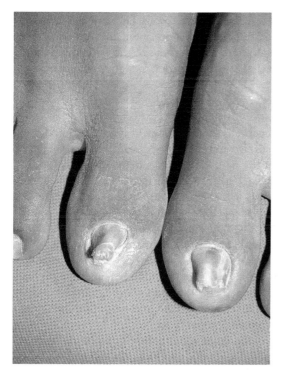

Figure 4.4 Pincer nail deformity of great toenails.

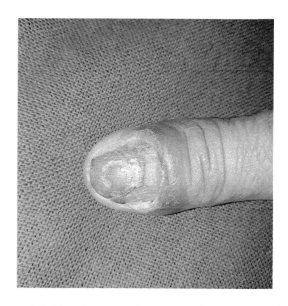

Figure 4.5 Chronic paronychia—compulsive hand washer.

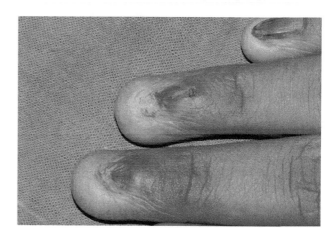

Figure 4.6 Anonychia in a patient with lichen planus.

is in the habit of getting regular manicures and pedicures. In the present day, patients regularly get sculptured nails, artificial/gel nails, nail wraps, and acrylic nails, which have their own set of adverse effects. Hence, a detailed history regarding all the cosmetic procedures is important. Certain common dermatological conditions like lichen planus (Figure 4.6), psoriasis, alopecia areata, etc. have typical nail manifestations as well. Hence, doing a thorough examination of skin and mucosa is a must when dealing with such patients. Do take a history of any hair problems as well.

Skin and systemic disease

History of past medical problems is important—diabetes, heart ailments, thyroid disorders, etc.

Consider any medications patient is taking, e.g., retinoids, taxanes, chloroquine, etc., as they cause characteristic nail

Do consider the personal care habits of the patient, e.g., number of times hands are washed, as compulsive hand washers can present with chronic paronychia (Figure 4.5); use of nail cosmetics; and the instrument used during certain nail cosmetic procedures like scissors, cuticle pushers, etc. It is important to know whether the patient

Table 4.1 Importance of nail signs associated with systemic disorders

S. No.	Nail signs	Systemic disorders
1.	Beau's lines	Certain drugs, high fever, viral illness (hand foot mouth disease, measles), Kawasaki syndrome, peripheral ischemia
2.	Koilonychia	Sideropenic anemia
3.	Periungual erythema	Collagen disorders, infection with HIV or hepatitis-C virus
4.	Lichenoid nail changes with hemorrhage	Systemic amyloidosis
5.	Apparent leukonychia	Renal disorders
	Half-and-half nails	Hepatic disorders
	Terry's nails	Systemic chemotherapy, hypoalbuminemia
	Banded nails (Muehrcke's lines)	
6.	Clubbing	Cardiovascular – aortic aneurysm, congenital/acquired cardiovascular disease
		Bronchopulmonary – intrathoracic neoplasms, chronic intrathoracic-suppurative disorders
		Gastrointestinal – inflammatory bowel disease, gastrointestinal neoplasms, hepatic disorders, multiple polyposis, bacillary dysentery, amoebic dysentery
		Chronic methemoglobinemia
7.	Melanonychia	Acquired immunodeficiency syndrome, inflammatory nail disorders, certain drugs, Addison disease, pregnancy, Laugier–Hunziker syndrome, trauma

changes. Table 4.1 elaborates the importance of examination of nails in systemic disease.

Family history

Do ask regarding family history of nail/skin problems, diabetes, and thyroid disorder.

History of similar nail diseases in family is an important clinical clue in genetic disorders.

CLINICAL EXAMINATION

A thorough clinical examination is a must. Adequate lighting without glare, natural light being the preferred source, is necessary while doing examination of nails. The nail polish needs to be removed (Box 4.1).

Ensure that examination of all nails is done. Pattern of nail involvement needs to be considered, e.g., if only one or

---

very few nails are affected, local factors like trauma, onychomycosis, tumors, circulatory anomalies, etc. are suspected.

In addition, make a note of the part of nail affected—periungual areas, nail bed, nail matrix, and nail plate.

Examination of hands

The fingernails should be looked at with the hand resting on a flat surface and the digits spread. When doing examination of the nail, the patient's digits should be relaxed and not pressed against any surface, as failure to follow these guidelines will alter the hemodynamics of the nail bed and change the appearance of the nails.

An overall appearance of hands may help in making diagnosis: the skin may show dermatitis or callosities, suggesting a particular work or hobby. Check the overall appearance of hands for clues, e.g., dermatitis/corns and calluses in case of laborers or gardeners as a part of work or hobby, respectively. Palmar skin can be afflicted in cases of psoriasis, tinea mannum, contact dermatitis, etc.

Do a thorough examination of inter-phalangeal joints for, e.g., arthritis that can be associated with mucous cysts (Figure 4.7).

Do make an observation regarding how the patient moves the hands while talking. A patient with a habit tic often denies the habit, but unconsciously does it when distracted by talking.

Examination of feet

The toenails should be looked at with the patient seated and the feet parallel and resting flat, in order to

---

BOX 4.1: Certain relevant leading questions can be asked to arrive at a proper diagnosis

Do you:

- Bite or suck on your nails (Onychotillomania)?
- Tear your nails off?
- Have ingrown nails?
- Wear tight, pointed-toe shoes?
- Push the cuticle back? How often?

appreciate the morphology of the feet and the way in which they stay in the shoes.[1]

When the patient presents with an anomaly of toenail, do look at the patient's shoe to see whether they are ill fitting or have pointed toes.

Examine the toenails and feet for traumatic nail dystrophy, calluses, signs of inflammation, traumatic onycholysis, ankle edema, or pedal edema. Onychogryphosis is characterized by thickening and curving of the nails in the finger or toe due to injuries or infection (Figure 4.8). Palmoplantar keratoderma is present in cases of pachyonychia congenita along with typical nail findings.

Skin examination

In many disorders both nail and skin (including mucosae and hair) are affected, e.g., psoriasis, lichen planus, etc. Hence, examination of skin is very important while dealing with a patient of nail diseases. A simple clinical finding of a patch of alopecia areata may be missed by the patient and/or the clinician, in a case of trachyonychia. Certain congenital or hereditary disorders, e.g., Darier's disease (Figure 4.9), pachyonychia congenita, etc. can be associated with classical skin findings as well as with specific nail anomalies.

Correlation of nail findings with anatomical site[2]

Clinical findings suggest the major site of pathology, which further dictates the site of biopsy.

1. Proximal matrix: Beau's lines, pitting, longitudinal ridging, longitudinal fissuring, trachyonychia
2. Distal matrix: True leukonychia
3. Proximal and distal matrix: Onychomadesis, koilonychia, nail thinning
4. Nail bed: Onycholysis, subungual hyperkeratosis, apparent leukonychia, splinter hemorrhages

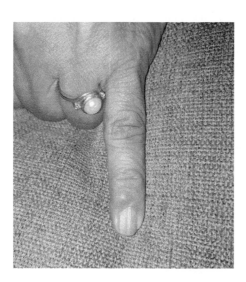

Figure 4.7 Mucous cyst.

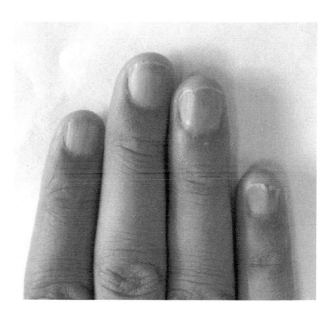

Figure 4.9 Darier's disease.

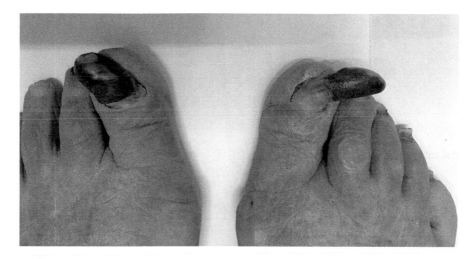

Figure 4.8 Onychogryphosis.

NAIL EXAMINATION

Nail evaluation must include the examination of nail plate, nail bed, and periungual tissue including the distal pulp. Do touch the digit as it will allow perception of temperature. The digit might be painful on palpation, suggesting inflammation or glomus tumor (Figure 4.10).

The clinical examination of nail starts from examination of nail plate.

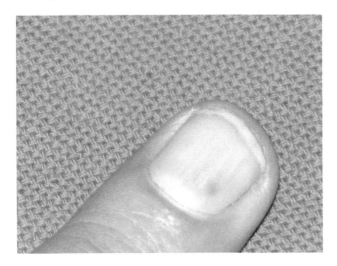

Figure 4.10 Glomus tumor.

Examination of the nail plate[3]

What is the defect?

- Shape
- Size
- Thickness – Is it thick due to nail plate thickening or nail bed hyperkeratosis?
- Transparency – Thickening is always associated with loss of transparency.
- Discoloration of nail plate – The first step is to determine whether the pigment is above, inside, or under the nail plate. In the exogenous pigmentation the proximal margin of the discoloration is proximally convex and follows the margin of the proximal nail fold. Color of the pigment can provide important clues: black discoloration in cases of melanin deposits, green discoloration due to pyocyanin pigment, etc.
- Total leukonychia can be congenital or acquired as well (Figure 4.11).
- Pigmented nail plate – Fungal infection of nail can mimic melanocytic lesions.
- Surface – Think of damage to proximal matrix.
- Adhesion to nail bed – Is the bed healthy or does it present erosions or scales?

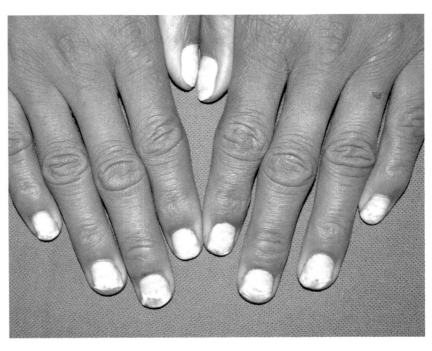

Figure 4.11 Congenital total leukonychia.

- Uplifting – What causes it? Take a detailed look at the nail bed.
- Nail dystrophy may be seen in trauma, psoriasis, lichen planus, alopecia areata, and atopic dermatitis. Complete physical examination of skin and oral mucosa is important in such cases.
- If onychomycotic nail plate covers the bed, examination of the bed is not possible.
- Alignment of nail plate with phalanx should be evaluated: ingrowing or traumatic abnormalities, especially of the big toe, are caused by nail misalignment, characterized by lateral deviation of the nail plate from longitudinal axis of that of the digit.[1]

Examination of nail bed

The nail bed skin can be normal or show accumulation of scales.

- Normal nail bed: In cases of onycholysis where nail bed is normal then trauma is the most common cause.
- Onycholysis is common in onychomycosis (Figure 4.12) too.
- Erosion of epithelium of nail bed present—if several nails are involved consider drugs as the cause. In cases of single digit involved consider squamous cell carcinoma (Figure 4.13), pyogenic

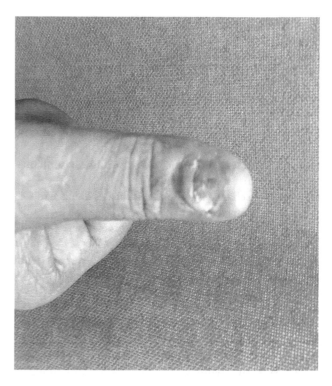

Figure 4.13 Subungual squamous cell carcinoma causing onycholysis.

granuloma, or amelanotic melanoma as differential diagnosis.
- With masses of scale examine the patient for psoriasis or onychomycosis.

Examination of lunula

The lunula can either change shape or color to indicate an underlying disorder.

- Lunula, which is normally white, may become blue in Wilson's disease or argyria.
- It may become red in cardiac failure or carbon monoxide poisoning.
- It normally increases in size in fingers closest to the thumb; however, the lunula becomes smaller or absent in old age.
- It can also be absent in cases of anemia or malnutrition.
- The change in shape can occur in cases of trauma – pyramidal.

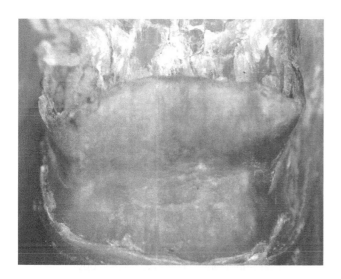

Figure 4.12 Total dystrophic onychomycosis.

Examination of periungual tissue

- Is the skin normal, pink, and healthy?
- Is scaling present (which can indicate chronic inflammation)?
- Is skin red and edematous (which can indicate acute inflammation)?
- Presence of scaling and pustulation over the hyponychium may suggest acodermatitis continua.
- Is cuticle present (as absence of cuticle indicates inflammation or arrest of nail growth)?
- If nail plate change is present, it indicates damage to proximal matrix.
- If a mass is present, it can be a mucous cyst or fibrokeratoma.
- In cases of pyogenic granuloma, do take history of drug intake or ingrown toenail (Figure 4.14).

To conclude, a stepwise approach is very important in the diagnosis of any nail disorder. Certain nail changes are specific for various dermatological disorders. In addition, examination of nails may also provide an insight into more sinister systemic manifestations in the form of subtle as well as specific changes. These findings may present as a defect of various anatomical components of the nail unit: nail matrix, nail plate, and/or nail bed or vasculature. Hence, a detailed history and clinical examination of nails, skin, hair, and various systems is a must. The clinical examination should be supplemented by simple office procedures like onychoscopy and microscopy (Tables 4.2 and 4.3; Box 4.2).

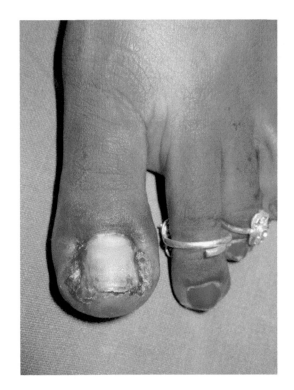

Figure 4.14 Ingrown toenail with granulation tissue.

Table 4.2 Some common nail disorders with investigations[4]

S. No.	Nail disorder	Investigations
1.	Onychomycosis dermatophytic non-dermatophytic yeasts	KOH examination Fungal cultures Onychoscopy, Nail plate biopsy
2.	Psoriasis	Hand-held lens, onychoscopy Nail KOH (to rule out onychomycosis), nail biopsy
3.	Lichen planus	Hand-held lens, onychoscopy nail biopsy
4.	Melanonychia	Dermatoscopy, nail-matrix biopsy
5.	Warts	Onychoscopy, nail biopsy
6.	Twenty-nail dystrophy	Onychoscopy, nail biopsy
7.	Connective tissue disorders Systemic lupus erythematosus, systemic sclerosis, dermatomyositis, rheumatoid arthritis	Hand-held lens, nail-fold capillaroscopy, nail biopsy
8.	Systemic disorders Renal, liver, gastrointestinal, cardiovascular, endocrine, psychological disease	Hand-held lens, nail fold capillaroscopy, dermatoscopy, nail biopsy
9.	Nail tumors	Onychoscopy, X-ray, USG, MRI

Source: Mendiratta, V., Approach to nail disorders, In: S. Sacchidan and A.S. Savitha, Eds., *Nail and Its Disorders*, JP Medical, New Delhi, India, pp. 19–35, 2013.

Table 4.3 Procedures used to aid in diagnosis of nail disorders

S. No.	Procedure	Strength	Limitation
1.	Direct microscopy (KOH mount)	Rapid, simple, inexpensive, easily done in clinical setting, descriptive morphological details of fungus	False negatives, sensitivity of 50%–80% with trained personnel, contaminants
2.	Culture and sensitivity	Gold standard for diagnosing fungus species and deciding treatment. Sensitivity 25%–80%	False negative 30%
3.	Nail biopsy	Nail-bed biopsy is most useful in identifying underlying pathology, ruling out fungal elements	Provides information of limited part of nail-unit histopathology, rare chance of scarring in nail-matrix/proximal nail-plate biopsy
4.	Onychoscopy	Helpful in diagnosing nail pigmentation, melanonychia, onychomycosis, nail psoriasis, lichen planus, traumatic abnormalities, subungual hemorrhage, nail tumor, connective tissue disorders	Knowledge of using dermatoscope, storing images (overcome by USB attachments)
5.	Imaging techniques e.g., X-ray, Ultrasonography, magnetic resonance imaging	Helpful in diagnosis of tumors (e.g., osteoma), connective tissue disorders, calcinosis, erosive arthropathy, osteolysis, involvement of interphalangeal joints	Provides supplemental information
6.	Molecular techniques e.g., Polymerase chain reaction	Fast results, high sensitivity and specificity, no morphological expertise needed	Expensive, not widely available

BOX 4.2: Prerequisites for clinical examination

Adequate lighting
Natural sunlight
All nail polish removed
Surface cleansed with acetone
Examine all 20 nails
Digits should be relaxed and not pressed (alteration of hemodynamics of nail bed)
The feet parallel and laying on plants
Examine the dorsum of feet and hands, as well as palmar and plantar skin.
Use a hand-held lens or a dermatoscope for better visualization.

KEY POINTS

- In a patient presenting with nail disorder, a stepwise approach is essential to arrive at any conclusive diagnosis.
- Detailed history pertaining to signs, drug intake, occupation, and hobbies is often contributory.
- Clinical examination of nails, skin, hair, and various organ systems may be required.
- Clinical examination should be supplemented by simple office procedures like onychoscopy, microscopy, or histopathology.

REFERENCES

1. Piraccini, B.M., (2014). Examination of patients with nail disorders. In: *Nail Disorders: A Practical Guide to Diagnosis and Management*. Milan, Italy: Springer, pp. 23–33.
2. Tosti, A. and Piraccini, B.M. (2012). Nail disorders. In: J. Callen, L. Cerroni, W. Heymann, G. Hruza, A. Mancini, J. Patterson, M. Rocken and T. Schwarz, Eds., *Dermatology*, 3rd ed. London, UK: Elsevier, pp. 1129–1147.
3. Berker, D. and Baran, R. (2010). Disorders of nails. In: D. Burns, S. Breathnach, N. Cox and C. Griffiths, Eds., *Rook's Textbook of Dermatology*, 8th ed. Oxford, UK: Wiley Blackwell, pp. 65.1–65.57.
4. Mendiratta, V. (2013). Approach to nail disorders. In: S. Sacchidanand and A.S. Savitha, Eds., *Nail and Its Disorders*. New Delhi, India: JP Medical, pp. 19–35.

Diagnostics

5

Laboratory investigations of nail diseases

SHUKLA DAS AND RICHA TIGGA

INTRODUCTION

There can be various etiologies for nail disorders, including infections, inflammations, neoplastic, environmental, metabolic, and genetic. History, clinical examination, imaging, microbiological, and histopathological examination of the unit play an important role in the diagnosis of various nail disorders. Diagnosis of infectious diseases requires good laboratory support as different etiological agents can manifest with a similar clinical presentation. Laboratory assistance is of paramount importance for the diagnosis, prognosis, and determination of a cure in nail diseases. Infectious diseases affecting nail unit can be of bacterial, fungal, or viral origin. Various infectious disorders of the nail unit and possible etiology are given in Table 5.1.

One of the major roles of the laboratory diagnosis is the identification of causative fungi in onychomycosis (OM). Major etiological fungi for OM have been summarized in Box 5.1[1]:

Infectious diseases of the nail unit are diagnosed on history, clinical examination, onychoscopy, diagnostic imaging, and laboratory investigations. Onychoscopy and *in vivo* confocal microscopy are non-invasive tests useful especially for onychomycosis.

Table 5.1 Infectious disorders of the nail unit

Acute paronychia	**Bacterial**
	Common – *Staphylococcus aureus, Streptococcus pyogenes, Pseudomonas aeruginosa*
	Rare – *Neisseria gonorrhoeae, Treponema pallidum*
	Viral – *Herpes simplex virus*
Mycobacterial	*Mycobacterium tuberculosis, Mycobacterium marinum*
Chronic paronychia	Candida species, polymicrobial infection
Warty growth	*Human papillomavirus (HPV), Mycobacterium tuberculosis*
Onychomycosis (OM)	Dermatophytes, non-dermatophyte molds, yeast

Source: Tosti, A. and Piraccini, B.M., Biology of nails and nail disorders, In: K. Wolff, L. Goldsmith, S. Katz, B. Gilchrest, A. Paller, D. Leffel, Eds., *Fitzpatrick's Dermatology in General Medicine*, 7th ed, McGraw-Hill Medical, New York; p. 785, 2008.

BOX 5.1: Common causative fungi for onychomycosis

1. Dermatophyte fungi
   a. *Trichophyton rubrum*
   b. *Trichophyton mentagrophytes*
   c. *Epidermophyton floccosum*
   d. *Other Trichophyton species*
2. Non-dermatophyte molds (NDM)
   a. *Acremonium* species
   b. *Alternaria* species
   c. *Aspergillus* species
   d. *Lasiodiplodia theobromae*
   e. *Fusarium* species
   f. *Onycochola canadensis*
   g. *Pyrenochaeta unguis-hominis*
   h. *Scytalidium dimidiatum*
   i. *Scopulariopsis* species
   j. *Scytalidium hyalinum*
3. Yeast
   a. *Candida albicans*
   b. *Non-albicans Candida* spp.

Laboratory investigations include microbiological examination and histopathological examination. Histopathology of nail unit has been dealt with in a separate chapter and we will concentrate mainly on microbiological aspects of laboratory investigations.

ONYCHOSCOPY

Onychoscopy is a dermatoscopic examination of the nail unit and its components, namely, the proximal nail fold, lateral nail fold, hyponychium, nail plate, and bed. It is a potential link between naked-eye examination (clinical onychology) and nail histopathology, opening a valuable second front with a potential to prevent biopsy. Also, onychoscopy aids in the proper selection of the affected area for collection of nail specimen.

IN VIVO CONFOCAL LASER SCANNING MICROSCOPY[2]

In vivo confocal laser scanning microscopy (CLSM) allows us to visualize tissues at different depths and can be done *in vivo* or *ex vivo*. *In vivo* CLSM is very helpful in the diagnosis of OM and can identify the fungal elements (and their density) in the nail plate. It has shown better sensitivity and specificity than that of KOH mount. Also, it offers an advantage of examining the whole nail plate, not just nail plate clipping. The utility of CLSM in the diagnosis of benign versus malignant causes of melanonychia has been well established. Its role in the diagnosis of various inflammatory disorders is being evaluated. Though it seems to be a promising

technology and can reduce the number of nail biopsies, high cost is a limiting factor, especially in developing countries.

MICROBIOLOGICAL INVESTIGATIONS

The microbial investigation includes direct demonstration of the causative agent, culture, and serology and is the major focus of this chapter. Other tests such as antimicrobial susceptibility test (AST) should also be done to guide the treatment. Both direct demonstration and culture are important to establish etiology.

Bacterial infections

Sample collection: In acute paronychia, pus (swab/aspirate) should be collected for gram stain and culture.

GRAM STAIN

Gram stain is simple and one of the most important procedures in microbiology. It is used for detection and classification of bacteria. Gram-positive organisms stain purple while Gram-negative organisms stain pink (Figures 5.1 and 5.2).

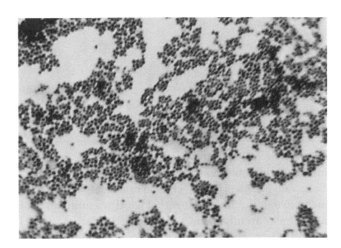

Figure 5.1 Gram-positive cocci. (Courtesy of Dr. Moumita Sarkar, MD.)

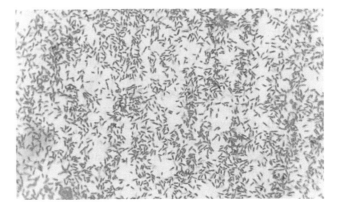

Figure 5.2 Gram-negative bacilli. (Courtesy of Dr. Moumita Sarkar, MD.)

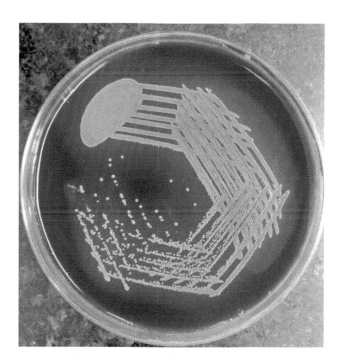

Figure 5.3 Colonies of *Staphylococcus* on chocolate agar.

Gram stain not only classifies the bacteria into Gram-positive and Gram-negative groups but also helps in the identification of the genus based on the morphology. *Staphylococcus* is a Gram-positive coccus that appears as grape-like clusters while *Streptococci* is also Gram-positive cocci but presents in pairs or chains. *Pseudomonas* is a Gram-negative bacillus. Gram-negative kidney-shaped intracellular diplococci are suggestive of *Neisseria gonorrhoeae (Gonococcus)*.

CULTURE

Culture is essential to find out the exact etiological species and to perform antibiotic sensitivity tests. The common basic media that can be used include blood agar, MacConkey agar, chocolate agar, etc. Culture and sensitivity testing become even more important in the era of methicillin-resistant *Staphylococcus aureus* infections (Figure 5.3).

ANTIMICROBIAL SUSCEPTIBILITY TESTING

AST is an important component of laboratory investigation. It not only guides clinicians on how best to treat a case, but also suggests susceptibility of microbes towards antimicrobial agents in a community at a given point of time. Disk diffusion test is the most commonly performed test to detect antimicrobial susceptibility.

Viral infection

Herpes simplex virus (HSV) and human papillomavirus (HPV) can commonly result in the infection of the nail unit. HPV-causing periungual or subungual warts are diagnosed on clinical examination and dermoscopy. Histopathology may sometimes be necessary in doubtful cases. HSV infection can present as acute paronychia and needs to be differentiated from acute bacterial paronychia. Tzanck smear is helpful in the diagnosis.

1. **Tzanck smear**: Tzanck smear is a rapid bedside test for the diagnosis of HSV infection. The vesicle is de-roofed. The blister fluid with floor scraping is smeared on the glass slide, heat fixed or with a fixative like the formol-zenker solution, and stained with Giemsa stain. The presence of ballooning degeneration of the keratinocytes and multinucleated giant cells suggest HSV infection.
2. **Electron microscopy**: Electron microscopy can help in the direct demonstration of DNA viral particles within stratum corneum.
3. **Serology for HSV- ELISA**[3]: IgM- and IgG-based serological assays have been evaluated to detect HSV infection as well as to differentiate between acute and chronic infection. However, there are limitations in the utility of such tests to discriminate between recent and chronic infection. For example, anti-HSV IgM may persist for 48 to 89 days in some instances and can reappear following subsequent HSV episodes in up to one-third of infections. Therefore, recent infection should be considered only if a positive IgM result is accompanied by a negative IgG result. Further, IgM may not be detectable in 50% of culture-confirmed early infections.
4. **Polymerase chain reaction**: Molecular diagnosis of acute HSV can be accomplished via amplification and detection of specific viral genome targets. Early real-time polymerase chain reaction (PCR) assays targets highly conserved regions of the herpes virus DNA polymerase to amplify both HSV-1 and HSV-2.

Histopathological examination: Both HSV and HPV infection show characteristic histopathological findings.

Mycobacterial infection

Nail unit can become infected with *Mycobacterium tuberculosis(Mtb)* or atypical mycobacteria like *Mycobacterium marinum*. Diagnosis of these infections requires direct microscopy, culture, PCR and molecular testing.

DIRECT MICROSCOPY

Mycobacteria may be observed on Ziehl–Neelson staining (ZN stain) of the pus smear or tissue smear, where they appear as acid-fast bacilli (AFB) on the slide.

The diagnostic yield of smears is higher for wet or exudative lesions because they have a higher bacterial load.

CULTURE

There are various culture media available for detection of mycobacteria, which include solid egg-based media like Lowenstein–Jensen (LJ) media, agar-based media such as Middlebrook, and radiometric systems such as BACTEC 460.

A specimen needs to be incubated for a minimum of 8 weeks before it can be declared negative. It generally takes 4 weeks for growth to occur on solid media.

Solid media (LJ) is used to get isolated colonies of *Mycobacterium tuberculosis* to study the morphology of bacilli and perform drug susceptibility testing. It also aids in the differentiation of atypical mycobacteria based on colony growth as well as detection of any contamination grown. Liquid media aids in earlier detection of mycobacterial growth (within 10–12 days) as compared to solid media (4–8 weeks).

Polymerase chain reaction[4]: PCR is mainly used to complement clinicopathological assessment. In this test, *Mycobacterial* DNA present in a sample of fresh tissues, blood, or a paraffin block is amplified many times for easier identification, thus confirming the presence of mycobacteria. However, the results must be understood and interpreted in the context of the clinical presentation.

Genotyping[4]: This is the use of different techniques for molecular typing of *Mtb* strains; it helps in the sequencing of resistance genes to assess mutations and correlate the results of molecular epidemiology with data from classical epidemiology. These data have revolutionized the understanding of tuberculosis's epidemiology. With the amplified DNA, it is also possible to separate atypical mycobacteria from *Mtb*, genotype mycobacteria, and detect mutations that induce resistance to antibiotics. The main molecular typing methods are spacer oligonucleotide typing (Spoligotyping), restriction fragment length polymorphism (RFLP), and mycobacterial interspersed repetitive units-variable number of tandem repeats (MIRU-VNTR). Spoligotyping is considered to be the gold standard for genotyping.

Fungal infection

Fungal infections are the most common infectious diseases affecting the nail unit.

COLLECTING THE NAIL SPECIMEN[5]

For nail lesions where the influence of sampling technique on culture yield is very important,[6] methods differ according to the type of onychomycosis (OM).

1. The first step of the sample collection process is thorough cleansing of the nail area with alcohol to remove contaminants such as bacteria.

   Because the sites of invasion and localization of the infection differ in the different types of OM, different approaches, depending on the presumptive diagnosis, are necessary to obtain optimal specimens (Figure 5.4).

   a. Distal lateral subungual onychomycosis (DLSO)
      i. Dermatophytes in DLSO invade through the hyponychium and then involve the nail plate and nail bed. The specimen must be obtained from the most proximal part of the subungual hyperkeratosis (SUH) area, where the concentration of viable fungi is greatest.

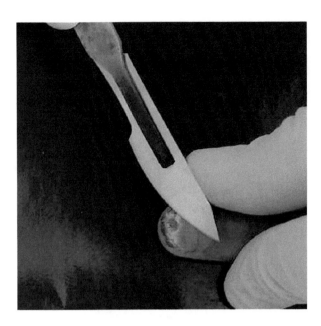

Figure 5.4 Collection of the specimen from the nail plate in OM using a no.23 blade.

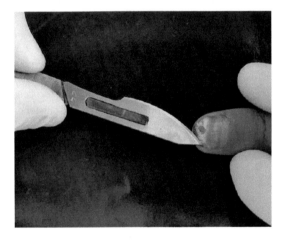

Figure 5.5 Collection of subungal debris in a case of onychomycosis using a no.23 blade.

      ii. The nail clipping for histology should be obtained after discarding the most distal portion of the nail plate. The specimen should be taken from the most proximal region of the SUH with a small curette or a no. 23 scalpel blade (Figure 5.5).
      iii. If debris is insufficient, the material should be obtained by scraping the nail bed.
   b. Proximal subungual onychomycosis.
      i. Because the fungus invades under the cuticle before settling in the proximal nail bed while the overlying nail plate remains intact, the healthy nail plate should be gently pared away with a no. 15 scalpel blade.
      ii. A sharp curette can then be used to remove material from the infected proximal nail bed as close to the lunula as possible.

c. White superficial onychomycosis.
   i. Since the infection affects the nail plate surface, a no. 15 scalpel blade or sharp curette can be used to scrape the white area and remove the infected debris.
d. Candida onychomycosis
   i. The material is needed from the proximal and lateral nail edges.
   ii. If candida onycholysis is suspected, the lifted nail bed should be scraped.
   iii. Scrapings can be taken from the undersurface of the nail if insufficient debris is present in the nail bed.

SPECIMEN ANALYSIS

The specimen should be divided into three portions for performing direct microscopy, histopathological examination, and culture.

The nail sample should be transported in a dry envelope for KOH microscopy and culture. Nail clippings for histopathological examination should be sent in formalin.

MICROSCOPY

In onychomycosis, direct microscopic examination (DME) is the most efficient screening technique with rapid turnaround time.

The specimen can be mounted in a solution of 40% potassium hydroxide (KOH) or sodium hydroxide (NaOH) mixed with 5% glycerol, warmed over Bunsen burner to emulsify lipids, and examined under 40x magnification. Alternately, the nail specimen can be soaked overnight in 20% KOH in a sterile test tube, and a wet mount preparation can be made from the same, the following day. This can be done only for microscopy but not for culture. An alternative formulation consists of 40% KOH and 36% dimethyl sulfoxide. Tetraethylammonium hydroxide (TEAH) can also be used (Figures 5.6 through 5.8).

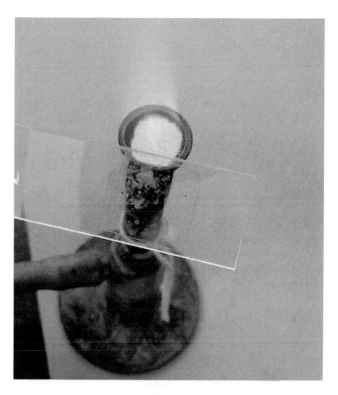

Figure 5.7 Gentle warming of KOH mount over Bunsen burner.

1. **Use of contrast enhancement dyes**:
   a. The specimen may be counterstained with chitin-specific Chlorazol black Eto accentuate hyphae that are present; this is of value if the number of fungal elements is small. This stain is especially useful because it does not stain likely contaminants such as cotton or elastic fibers, which can help prevent false-positive identifications.
   b. **Parker blue-black ink** also can be added to the KOH preparation to improve visualization, but this stain is not chitin-specific.

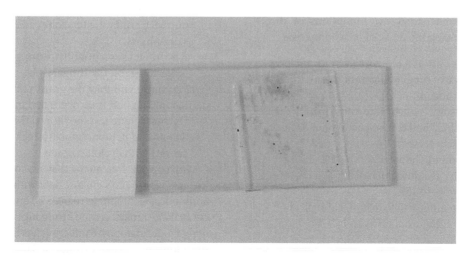

Figure 5.6 KOH mount of the fungal scrapings.

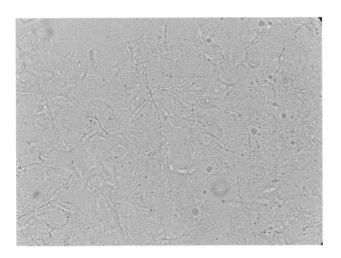

Figure 5.8 Fungal hyphae seen in 400x magnification on KOH mount.

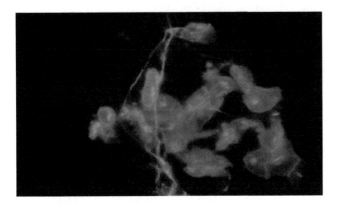

Figure 5.9 KOH mount with calcofluor stain.

c. **Fluorescent staining with optical brighteners (diamino stilbene) like Blankophor® or Calcofluor®** which bind to chitin, the main cell wall component of fungi. This is the most sensitive method for detection via microscopy, i.e., fluorescent microscopy (Figure 5.9).

Limitations

It is important to understand the limitations of direct microscopy in diagnosing the cause of onychomycosis.

a. The test serves only as a screening test for the presence or absence of fungi but cannot differentiate among the pathogens.
b. Direct microscopy is often time-consuming because nail debris is thick and coarse and hyphae are usually only sparsely present.
c. The clinician should be aware of the possibility of false-negative results, which occur at a rate of approximately 5% to 15%.
d. It is difficult to differentiate features of typical of dermatophyte fungi from NDMs.

Although direct microscopy can provide clues about the identity of the microorganism, careful matching of microscopic and culture results is necessary for the clinician to be confident of the diagnosis.[7]

HISTOPATHOLOGICAL EXAMINATION[2]

For diagnosis of onychomycosis, the "gold standard" method is histological examination of a nail plate with direct in situ visualization of fungal elements within the host tissue.

1. Achten's technique with Grocott–Gomori's methenamine silver (GMS) – hyphae appear grey-black.
2. Periodic acid-Schiff (PAS) – hyphae appear red in color.

It may be necessary to perform histopathologic analysis of the nail unit in cases in which the clinical appearance suggests the presence of a fungal nail infection, but the KOH preparation and culture are negative.

While the diagnosis of PSO or PSWO usually requires a punch biopsy from the nail plate, simple nail clippings generally suffice in all other forms of onychomycosis.

Limitations

1. False-negative results may be observed in early nail infections.
2. The histological analysis does not allow species identification.
3. It does not determine the viability of fungi.

Accurate identification of the pathogen cannot be achieved through histology alone, and mycological cultures remain necessary.

CULTURE

This method enables identification of the causative microorganism and confirmation of its identity.[5] Precise identification is useful, as treatment of dermatophyte varies from that of NDM.

1. Specimens should be plated on two different media:
   a. A primary medium that is selective against most non-dermatophytic molds and bacteria, and one with antibiotic (cycloheximide) to avoid saprophytes.
   b. Antifungal susceptibility testing (AFST) may be undertaken on the fungal isolates.
2. Cycloheximide inhibits the growth of non-dermatophytes and is incorporated into media such as:
   a. Dermatophyte test medium (DTM) (Figure 5.10)
   b. Sabouraud peptone-glucose agar (Emmons' modification) with cycloheximide
3. Cycloheximide-free media that are commonly used include Sabouraud's glucose agar with the addition of antibiotics. Gentamicin (0.0025%) and/or chloramphenicol (0.005%) may be added to reduce contamination and, if a dermatophyte infection has been diagnosed, the addition of cycloheximide at 0.04% will inhibit the growth of NDMs.

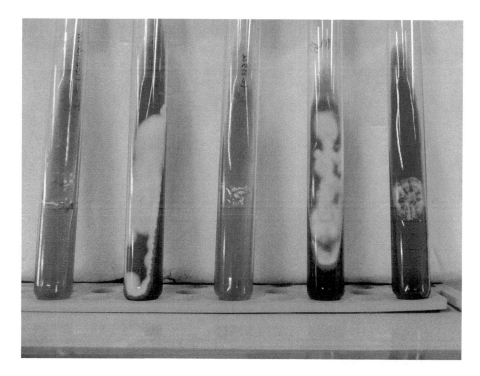

Figure 5.10 Dermatophyte test medium is a specialized agar based on Sabouraud's dextrose agar with added cycloheximide to inhibit saprophytic fungi and phenol red as an indicator. (Courtesy of Dr. Moumita Sarkar, MD.)

The media is inoculated with the material and incubated at room temperature, i.e., 22°C–33°C, for a period of 1–6 weeks. In most dermatophytes, growth and sporulation occur in 7–10 days. When growth becomes evident in the primary culture media, it is examined, and the differentiation of dermatophytes, yeasts, and molds is based on:

1. Macroscopic characteristics (upper and bottom side of colonies as well as pigmentation) (Figures 5.11 and 5.12)
2. Microscopic characteristics (formation of macro and microconidia, respectively, and other growth forms) by Lactophenol cotton blue (LPCB) tease mounts or other methods (Figures 5.13 and 5.14)
3. Physiological tests:
   a. *Biochemical properties (Christensen urea agar for urea hydrolysis)*
      Filter-sterilized urea agar base (Difco) is mixed with sterile molten agar and allowed to set. The medium is then inoculated with the test organism. After incubation at 26°C for 7 days, if urea is degraded the color turns from yellow to magenta red.
   b. *Nutritional tests vitamin and amino acid supplemented Trichophyton agars.*
      Trichophyton agars 1–7 (Difco); Agar 1 is a casein-based, vitamin-free control; agar 2 is supplemented with inositol; agar 3 with thiamine and inositol; and agar 4 with thiamine alone. Agar 5 contains nicotinic acid. Agar 6 is an ammonium nitrate vitamin-free control for agar 7, which is supplemented with histidine.
   c. In vitro *hair perforation tests.*
      Sterile human hair is suspended in sterile distilled water supplemented with yeast extract. The test organism is inoculated onto the hairs. After 2 weeks' incubation at 26°C, hairs are mounted to look for wedge-shaped penetrations perpendicular to the hair axis.

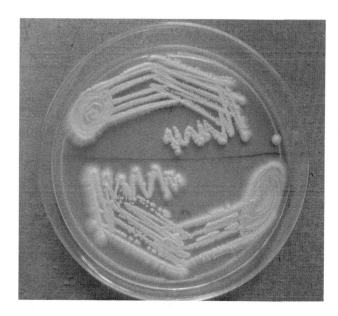

Figure 5.11 Smooth white colonies of *Candida albicans* on Sabouraud's dextrose agar. (Courtesy of Dr. Moumita Sarkar, MD.)

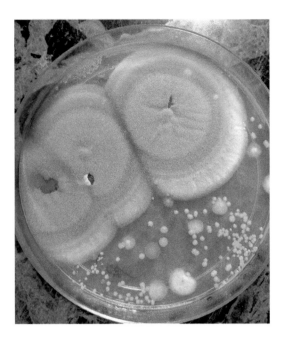

Figure 5.12 Granular to velvety colony of *Aspergillus fumigatus*. (Courtesy of Dr. Moumita Sarkar, MD.)

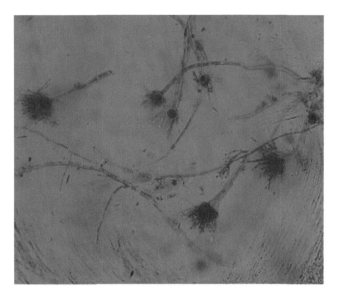

Figure 5.14 Lactophenol cotton blue mount shows biseriate, swept-forward appearance in *Aspergillus terreus*. (Courtesy of Dr Moumita Sarkar, MD.)

FROM CULTURE TO IDENTIFICATION

The growth of a non-dermatophyte alone from a specimen that has tested positive for fungi on direct microscopy does not prove conclusively that the infective agent is a non-dermatophyte. The difficulty in evaluating the role of non-dermatophyte fungi cultured from the nail arises because the same fungi that can be laboratory contaminants are also occasionally found to be pathogens. Reference laboratories should provide data on whether the isolated fungus was a likely pathogen or an unlikely one.

Following principles should be followed during fungal culture:

- All dermatophytes should be considered pathogens.
- All other isolated organisms are probably laboratory contaminants unless KOH or microscopy indicates they have the atypical frondlike hyphae associated with NDMs or if the same organism is repeatedly isolated.

To increase the predictive power of a diagnosis of non-dermatophytic invasion of a nail, Summerbell suggested that non-filamentous non-dermatophytes identified in nail tissue be categorized as a contaminant, commensal organism, or transient colonizer. As for NDM identification,[7] Walshe and English recommended considering any fungus causal if:

- Compatible elements were detected by direct microscopy.
- The fungus grew from 5 or more of 20 inoculum pieces (that is, pieces of nail material planted on fungal growth medium) in the absence of a dermatophyte.
- The fungal agent should grow at least 3 times from 3 different sites sampled from the affected nail.

Figure 5.13 Germ tube formation in *Candida albicans*. (Courtesy of Dr. Moumita Sarkar, MD.)

d. *Growth on rice grains*
   Ordinary white rice is covered with distilled water and autoclaved. The test organisms are then inoculated straight onto the surface, and growth is assessed after 2–3 weeks' incubation at 26°C.

If growth occurs on both types of media, the infective agent is probably a dermatophyte, whereas growth only on the cycloheximide-free medium indicates a contaminant until proved otherwise.

These criteria were based on the premise that an established nail invader would consistently colonize a substantial proportion of the nail material, whereas contaminants would usually consist of one or a few scattered propagules, with any consistency being coincidental and hence unlikely. The criteria were later restricted to filamentous fungi by English since widely dispersed yeast contamination had been found to be common.

- Caution should be exercised in analyzing culture results because nails are nonsterile and fungal and bacterial contaminants may obscure the nail pathogen.
- Culture for identification of yeast requires growth on SDA with antibiotics.
- Any creamy colony suggestive of yeast can be confirmed by gram stain or LPCB mount.
- Identification of yeast by conventional method involves sugar fermentation and assimilation test. Automated VITEK 2 System is rapid tool to identify candida species.
- Cultures often lack sensitivity, they are time-consuming (7–28 days for molds), and identification of filamentous fungi at the species level using morphological characteristics requires an experienced staff.

Subcultures on specific media that stimulate the conidiation and/or production of pigments are often necessary when identification of dermatophyte isolates is not achievable directly from primary cultures like potato dextrose agar (Difco), corn meal agar, etc.

ANTIFUNGAL SUSCEPTIBILITY TESTING

Part of the diagnosis and treatment strategy might include AFST. Susceptibility testing in infections such as onychomycosis becomes more clinically relevant when a choice of effective agents exists.

In addition, susceptibility testing can help distinguish relapse (reinfection by the same agent) from reinfection (by a new agent) and provide evidence about whether the fungus itself is responsible for treatment failure.[8]

Despite the availability of many antifungal agents, antifungal clinical resistance occurs, perhaps because of an infecting organism found to be resistant in vitro to one or more antifungals tested. The role of the AFST is to determine which agents are likely to be effective for a given infection. Thus, if AFST results are timely generated by the clinical microbiology laboratory and communicated to clinicians, they can aid them in the therapeutic decision making, especially for difficult-to-treat chronic dermatophytic infections.

Methods of AFST

Four standard methods for antifungal susceptibility testing (Clinical and Laboratory Standards Institute [CLSI])

- CLSI M27-A3 for macrobroth and microtiter yeast testing
- CLSI M38-A2 for microtiter mold testing

- CLSI M44-A3 for yeast disk diffusion testing
- CLSI M51-P4 for mold disk diffusion testing

Pros

- Disc diffusion for yeast is standardized for Fluconazole and Voriconazole. This can be performed on Mueller–Hinton Agar as per CLSI M44-A and interpreted within 24–48 hours.
- Broth microdilution by E-strip method (commercially available) on Mueller–Hinton Agar can determine the rising MIC in cases with failure to treatment.
- CLSI standardized microbroth dilution guidelines are available for yeast and filamentous fungi and may be performed by trained personnel in a well-equipped laboratory. This may not be used as a routine diagnostic testing for nail infections but can be used to assess treatment failure and correlate with the outcome if desired by the clinicians.
- Surveillance of drug-resistance pattern of predominant pathogens will generate an epidemiological profile and guide treatment modules as per availability of the drug.

Cons

- Broth dilution detection is difficult to standardize by all laboratories. Laboratory personnel having undergone extensive training in performing microdilution AST (by reference lab) can undertake this task. Representative isolates have to be submitted to reference laboratory.
- Variation in performance can result in different readings of the MIC.
- Quality control is to be strictly followed.
- 90/60 rule: all *in-vitro* MIC values may not match clinical outcomes; hence, interpretation of MIC values is to be done carefully.

Procedure

Preparation of antifungal drugs: Fluconazole powder is water soluble, and itraconazole, terbinafine, and all other drugs are soluble in 100% dimethyl sulfoxide (DMSO). Stock solutions of 1,000 µg/mL for each drug can be stored at −20°C until tests are performed. The test is performed on U-bottom microtiter plates. The final concentrations range from 0.0625 to 128 µg/mL for fluconazole, 0.0078 to 16 µg/mL for itraconazole, and 0.0156 to 16 µg/mL for terbinafine. The minimum inhibitory concentration (MIC) corresponds to the lowest drug concentration that resulted in a 100% reduction in growth as compared with their growth control for dermatophytes.

IMMUNODIAGNOSIS[1]

Trichophyton skin antigen (only for dermatophytic skin infection)

Skin test with Trichophyton, a crude extract from dermatophytes, produces a delayed-type hypersensitivity reaction in those afflicted. The reactive component of this dermatophytic antigen is the galactomannan peptide, which is associated with immunity, while the carbohydrate portion is related to immediate response. A skin test reaction with no delayed type and with immediate-type response is indicative of chronicity of the disease.

MOLECULAR METHODS

With recent advances in molecular techniques, direct detection of fungal organisms from the infected sample is quick and reproducible, overcoming the observer's bias.[1] Due to ongoing taxonomic revisions within the fungal kingdom, relying largely on DNA profiles and pathogenicity rather than conventional morphological features, molecular methods of detecting DNA signatures may provide an even higher diagnostic advantage in the future.

Genotypic methods available for fungal identification for yeast and molds targeting ITS 1 & 4 are as follows:

- PCR-polymerase chain reaction[8]
  a. PCR fingerprinting
  b. Random amplification of polymorphic DNA
  c. PCR and restriction fragment length polymorphism analysis
  d. Arbitrarily primed PCR
  e. Real-time PCR for dermatophyte DNA detection

Drawbacks:

  a. Increased contamination
  b. Failure to differentiate between pathogenic and non-pathogenic fungi
  c. Not practical for small-scale or tightly budgeted laboratories
  d. Requires highly skilled personnel
  e. Limited availability
  f. Limited to only discovering targeted species.
- Pan-dermatophyte PCR with Sanger sequencing offers a simple strategy to both detect and identify.
- Apart from direct fungal detection in clinical samples using molecular techniques such as PCR, larger laboratories have established matrix-assisted laser desorption ionization-time of flight (MALDI-TOF) mass spectrometry (MS) as culture confirmation test in the differentiation of dermatophytes, yeast, and other molds. This procedure is immensely timesaving, as it enables simultaneous identification of up to 64 dermatophytes strains, with results coming back within minutes. Although the test's specificity—based on

protein mass fingerprint or mass spectrum—is high, the plausibility of identified species should still always be verified.[9]

Laboratory monitoring is necessary before initiating treatment, as management can be based on the isolated specific pathogen: dermatophytes, yeast, non-dermatophyte mold, or bacterial pathogens.

Simple microscopy and culture are valuable diagnostic tools for infective nail disorders. Appropriate sample collection is extremely important to arrive at the correct diagnosis.

KEY POINTS

- Nail disorders are a growing global problem.
- Appropriate and accurate diagnosis is important to initiate specific management and prevent treatment failures or chronicity.
- The direct microscopy and culture are the gold standard for the diagnosis of nail diseases, especially onychomycosis. However, calcofluor white under fluorescence, nail biopsies and molecular tools are currently being used to optimize early diagnosis and treatment

REFERENCES

1. Chander J. Dermatophytosis. In: *Textbook of Medical Mycology*. 4th ed. New Delhi, India: Jaypee Brothers Medical Publishers; 2018. p. 176.
2. Cinotti E, Fouilloux B, Perrot JL, Labeille B, Douchet C, Cambazard F. Confocal microscopy for healthy and pathological nail. *J Eur Acad Dermatol Venereol* 2014;28(7):853–858.
3. Anderson NW, Buchan BW, Ledeboer NA. Light microscopy, culture, molecular, and serologic methods for detection of herpes simplex virus. *J Clin Microbiol* 2014;52(1):2–8.
4. dos Santos JB, Ferraz CE, da Silva PG, Figueiredo AR, de Oliveira MH, de Medeiros VLS. Cutaneous tuberculosis: Diagnosis, histopathology and treatment—Part II. *An Bras Dermatol* 2014;89(4):545–555.
5. Elewski BE. Onychomycosis: Pathogenesis, diagnosis, and management. *Clin Microbiol Rev* 1998;11(3):415–429.
6. Pihet M, Govic Y Le. Reappraisal of conventional diagnosis for dermatophytes. *Mycopathologia* 2016;182(1):1–12.

7. Gupta AK, Cooper EA, Donald PMAC, Summerbell RC. Utility of inoculum counting (Walshe and English criteria) in clinical diagnosis of onychomycosis caused by nondermatophytic filamentous fungi. *J Clin Microbiol* 2001;39(6):2115–2121.

8. Brillowska-da A, Saunte DM, Arendrup MC. Five-hour diagnosis of dermatophyte nail infections with specific detection of Trichophyton rubrum. *J Clin Microbiol* 2007;45(4):1200–1204.

9. Nenoff P, Krüger C, Schaller J, Ginter-Hanselmayer G, Schulte-Beerbühl R, Tietz H-J. Mycology–An update Part 2: Dermatomycoses: Clinical picture and diagnostics. *J Dtsch Dermatol Ges* 2014;12(9):749–777.

6

Imaging in nail diseases

KALPANA BHATT, SWAGATA ARVIND TAMBE, HEMANGI R. JERAJANI, DEEPAK BHATT, AND CHITRA S. NAYAK

INTRODUCTION

The nail apparatus can be affected as a part of generalized cutaneous disorder, systemic diseases, or diseases which are localized to the nail. Diagnosis of diseases affecting the nail apparatus is often challenging. It can be established by history, clinical examination, imaging and nail biopsy.

Nail biopsy is the gold standard in the diagnosis of nail diseases but it is invasive and often perceived as a painful procedure. Sometimes choosing a wrong site for biopsy and inadequate tissue material may not give the required diagnostic clue. Hence, there is a need of non-invasive imaging techniques to minimize nail biopsies.

Imaging plays an important role in the detection and differentiation of subungual tumors as they are small in size, show nonspecific clinical manifestations, but are of functional significance.[1] History and clinical examination give a clue to the diagnosis. Dermatoscopy is a helpful non-invasive diagnostic tool, but it requires special training and knowledge to identify different diseases and is not always confirmatory.

Radiological imaging methods like X-ray, ultrasonography (USG), computer tomography (CT) scan, magnetic resonance imaging (MRI), and optical coherence tomography (OCT) have been used with variable success. The nail has a special structure, so difficulties and limitations in using these modalities can be attributed to the anatomical and morphological aspects of the nail unit. With newer, better, and higher resolution USG, MRI, and CT scan machines, the role of plain X-ray is limited to diagnosis of bony involvement in nail pathology.

There is a new dimension added to imaging of the nail with the advent of ultrasound biomicroscopy (UBM) using probes of 35 to 50 MHz frequency. The resolution of the image obtained with these probes is 50 microns. The images produced with these probes are comparable to a low-power microscope (but in grayscale). Color and spectral Doppler imaging, multi frequency probes, extended field of vision, use of contrast, and elastography add a new dimension to nail imaging.

With the advent of microcoils in MRI, the nail apparatus can be studied in detail and small lesions can be detected and diagnosed. MRI has an important role in categorizing tumors according to their anatomical location, pathological origin and signal characteristics.

The following imaging techniques have been found to be useful in the diagnosis of infective, inflammatory, and neoplastic nail pathology (Box 6.1).

BOX 6.1: Imaging techniques for nail lesions

- Radiography
- UBM and high frequency ultrasonography (HFUS)
- MRI of nail apparatus

RADIOGRAPHY

Decades ago plain X-ray was the only imaging modality in radiology and played a role in imaging of nail-unit pathologies.

But with the advent of newer modalities like USG, CT scan, and MRI in radiology its role is limited to pathologies involving the distal phalanx and the distal interphalangeal joints (DIPs).

Since a decade, digital X-rays have replaced plain X-rays as the former gives higher resolution of the bony architecture, the cortex, and the medulla as compared to plain X-rays. Digital radiographs in the posterior-anterior (PA), lateral, and oblique views are taken. The conditions where plain X-ray is of diagnostic importance have been summarized in Table 6.1 and have been discussed here.

Table 6.1 X-ray findings in nail diseases

Nail diseases	X-ray findings
Infectious diseases of nail	Periosteal reaction or a lytic lesion involving the cortex
Inflammatory diseases of nails	Increase or decrease in the joint space and peri-articular or bony erosions
Myxoid cysts	DIP osteoarthritis
Keratin cysts	Erosion of the distal phalanx
Glomus tumors	Scalloping of the underlying cortex

(Continued)

Table 6.1 (*Continued*) X-ray findings in nail diseases

Nail diseases	X-ray findings
Vascular malformations	Soft tissue mass with phleboliths/bone erosion
Aneurysmal bone cyst	Lytic lesion with internal linear radio-opaque striations parallel to the shaft of the phalanx
Giant cell tumor of tendon sheath	Soft tissue mass with/without bony erosion of the underlying cortex
Subungual exostoses	Well circumscribed radio-opaque outgrowth without continuity with the medullary cavity and cortex
Subungual osteochondroma	Circumscribed radio-opaque outgrowths showing continuity with cortical and medullary canal
Chondroma	Lobulated radiolucent defects with flecks of calcification
Giant cell tumors of bone	"Soap bubble" appearance
Subungual keratoacanthoma	Lytic, cup-shaped erosion of the distal phalanx
Squamous cell carcinoma	Soft tissue mass with thickening of the periosteum and erosions of the underlying distal phalanx
Malignant melanoma	Soft tissue mass with periosteal reaction

Inflammatory and infectious nail disease

In inflammatory nail diseases like psoriasis, connective tissue disorders, sarcoidosis, dermatomyositis, scleroderma, and infectious disease like abscess, plain X-ray of the digits is done to rule out underlying bone and joint involvement.

In infectious diseases bone involvement is noted in the form of periosteal reaction or as lytic lesions involving the cortex.

In inflammatory diseases, joint involvement on X-rays is seen as an increase in the joint space, which is suggestive of effusion, peri-articular bony erosions, or decrease in the joint space with articular erosions. In severe and long-standing cases acro-osteolysis may also be seen.

Myxoid cysts

Myxoid cysts or mucoid cysts are common benign tumors of the distal digit. They are distinctive, dome shaped and compressible tumors of the periungual skin distal to the DIP and usually occupy some portion of proximal nail fold. Radiographs are mandatory in suspected digital mucoid cysts. Evidence of DIP joint osteoarthritis is a clue to the diagnosis.

The lateral view of the digit shows the dorsal osteophytes on the head of the middle phalanx and the base of the distal phalanx in 70% of cases.[2] In long-standing lesions, joint space reduction with lateral subluxation of the distal phalanx may be seen. In erosive osteoarthritis, joint space narrowing is seen as a seagull pattern often with a large subchondral cystic bone resorption. When there is subungual extension of the tumor, scalloping of the dorsal aspect of the cortex of the distal phalanx is noted.

Keratin cysts

At the onset of the disease, bony changes may not be visible on radiographs but may be seen on USG or MRI. In long standing cases, bony changes like erosion of the distal phalanx may be seen. Bony erosion is seen as a scalloping on the cortex, which appear as round, precisely rimmed lesions without septa or peripheral sclerosis. Pathological fracture, calcification, or ossification of the bone may be associated with this tumor.

Soft tissue tumors

FIBROMAS AND ACQUIRED PERIUNGUAL FIBROKERATOMAS

Plain radiographs of soft tissue tumors like fibroma and fibrokeratoma are seen as a soft tissue mass with/without bony erosion or scalloping. Calcification is absent.

Glomus tumors

Glomus tumors are rare vascular tumors arising subungually in the fingernails. They usually present as small, blue-red papules or nodules in the deep dermis or subcutis in acral location (Figure 6.1a).

Radiographs are not very helpful in the early diagnosis of small glomus tumors.

UBM in the hands of an experienced sonologist and MRI with microcoils for the finger are more sensitive modalities.

In large and long-standing tumors, X-ray shows an abnormal soft tissue mass in the nail bed, erosion or scalloping of the underlying cortex of the distal phalanx (Figure 6.1b).[3]

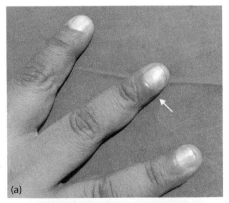

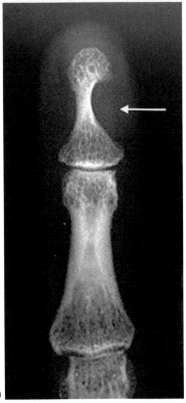

Figure 6.1 Glomus tumor (a) Bluish red tender subungual nodule on the right middle fingernail; (b) X-ray showing scalloping of the distal phalanx due to glomus tumor (left arrow).

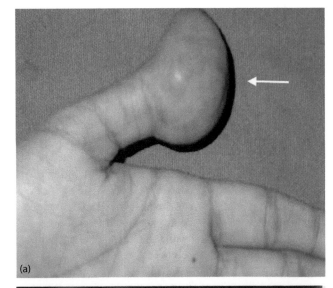

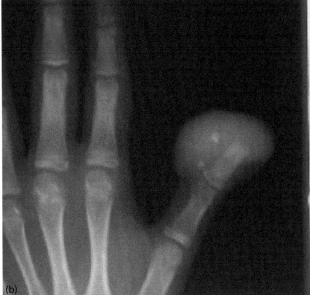

Figure 6.2 Vascular malformation (a) Bulbous compressible swelling of the left thumb with prominent veins on the surface; (b) X-ray shows a soft tissue mass in the distal phalanx of the thumb, with phleboliths. There is erosion of the distal part of the phalanx.

Vascular malformations

Vascular malformations of the fingertip are mainly venous malformations or capillary malformations (Figure 6.2a). UBM and HFUS with color Doppler is the modality of choice.

In large-sized and long-standing lesions, plain X-rays may show a soft tissue mass with phleboliths or bony erosions (Figure 6.2b). Vascular malformation (aneurysmal bone cyst) primarily involving the distal phalanx is seen as expansile osteolytic lesion of the phalanx with internal linear radio-opaque striations parallel to the shaft of the phalanx. Other vascular proliferations like pyogenic granulomas (PGs) do not show X-ray changes.[4]

Neural tumors like neuroma, neurofibroma, and schwannoma rarely show bony involvement.

Giant cell tumor of the tendon sheath

Giant cell tumor (GCT) of tendon sheath is a solitary lesion arising from the tendon sheath of the flexor or the extensor tendons.

Radiographs show a soft tissue mass. Large tumors may be associated with bony erosion of the underlying cortex. These tumors rarely involve the nail apparatus.[5]

Absence of calcification in these tumors differentiates them from synovial sarcomas, which show calcifications on X-ray.

Osteocartilaginous tumors

SUBUNGUAL EXOSTOSES AND OSTEOCHONDROMAS

Subungual exostoses are benign osteocartilaginous tumors that occur beneath the nail bed that commonly affect the great toe and are usually preceded by trauma or infection (Figure 6.3a).

X-ray shows well-defined radio-opaque outgrowth that lacks a clear continuity with the medullary cavity and cortex (Figure 6.3b). HFUS shows a well-defined heterogeneous mass below the skin (Figure 6.3c).

Osteochondroma is the most common benign tumor or tumor-like lesions of the bone that predominantly affect the distal phalanges of the foot. Clinically they present as subungual tumors which usually protrude up through the soft nail bed and appear as firm, slightly lobulated mass lesion (Figure 6.4a). Differentiating osteochondroma from exostosis is difficult but the former usually shows continuity with the cortical and medullary canal (Figure 6.4b).[6,7]

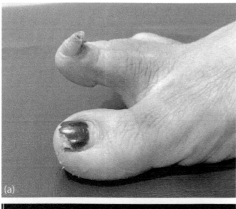

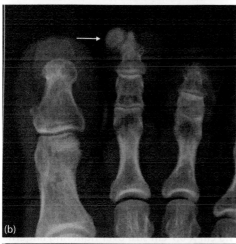

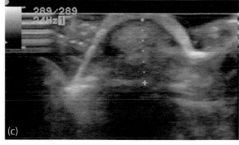

Figure 6.3 Subungual exostosis **(a)** Tender hard subungual nodule on the right second toe; **(b)** There is a round well-defined radio-opaque density seen arising from the cortex of the distal phalanx of the second toe (right arrow); **(c)** HFUS shows a well-defined heterogeneous mass lesion below the skin (marked area).

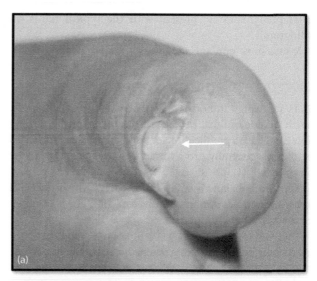

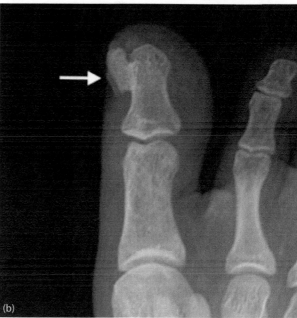

Figure 6.4 Subungual osteochondroma **(a)** Tender, hard subungual nodule causing over-curvature of the great toenail; **(b)** A well-defined sessile radio-opaque mass lesion seen arising from the medial margin of the distal phalanx of the great toe, which is continuous with the underlying cortex and medulla (right arrow).

CHONDROMAS

Enchondromas are the most frequent bone tumors of the hand, accounting for almost 50% of cases. Radiographic findings specific to enchondromas are lobulated expansile lytic lesions with characteristic "rings and arcs" calcifications. Periosteal chondromas (4.6% of all chondromas) appear as well-circumscribed intracortical radiolucencies.[8,9]

OSTEOID OSTEOMAS

Osteoid osteomas are rare in the distal phalanx. Only 8% of osteoid osteomas involve the phalanges. Lesions of the distal phalanx rarely present with the typical nidus on radiographs.

X-rays show non-specific osteosclerosis or periostitis.

GIANT CELL TUMORS OF BONE

GCTs are benign tumors that generally occur in the third or fourth decade of life. They arise from the epiphysis of long bones and have a predilection for the epiphyseal-metaphyseal region and generally grow towards the articular surface of long bones.

The distal phalanx is a rare site for GCTs. The metacarpal bones are more commonly involved. X-ray shows a characteristic "soap bubble" appearance.

The tumor is generally asymptomatic and detected incidentally due to a swelling or a pathological fracture.

Subungual keratoacanthoma

Subungual keratoacanthoma is a low-grade tumor of the pilosebaceous gland that presents as a rapidly growing painful mass.

X-rays show a lytic, cup-shaped erosion of the distal phalanx.[10]

Squamous cell carcinoma

Squamous cell carcinoma (SCC) of the nail bed is a rare malignant subungual tumor. It may arise from the nail bed, matrix, or nail folds. Early clinical manifestations are paronychia, onychomycosis, onycholysis, dyschromia of the nail plate, subungual hyperkeratosis, chronic granulation of the nail bed, ingrown nail and nail deformity. The presence of ulceration, bleeding, and nodule formation indicates its invasive nature (Figure 6.5a).

Bone involvement occurs in 20% of patients. Radiographs show soft tissue mass with thickening of the periosteum and erosion of the underlying distal phalanx in invasive SCC (Figure 6.5b).[11]

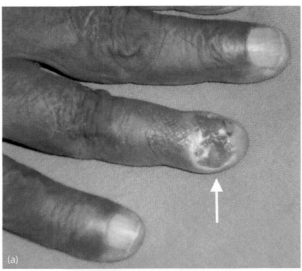

(a)

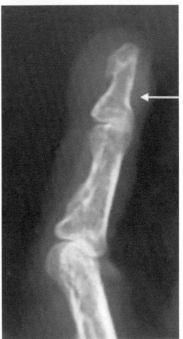

(b)

Figure 6.5 Squamous cell carcinoma (a) Extremely tender ulcer of 1.5 cm × 0.7 cm size over right ring fingernail bed with destruction of nail plate; (b) X-ray shows thickening of the periosteum in the subungual region with a soft tissue mass (left arrow).

Malignant melanoma

Malignant melanoma is a common malignant tumor of the foot and carries a very poor prognosis. Tumor metastasis is common. Therefore, early detection and management is very important.

X-rays are done to rule out bony involvement. On X-rays a soft tissue mass with periosteal reaction is suggestive of bony involvement. Rarely osteolytic lesions can be seen.[12]

X-ray findings of common nail diseases are mentioned in Table 6.1.

ULTRASOUND BIOMICROSCOPY AND HIGH FREQUENCY ULTRASONOGRAPHY

Ultrasound imaging of the nail apparatus is based on the use of high-frequency sound waves in the diagnosis and treatment of patients.

USG machines with high-frequency probes (15 to 50 MHz) are used in the imaging of the nail unit. Ultrasound probes/transducers generate ultrasound beams that originate from the mechanical oscillation of numerous piezoelectric crystals in the transducer, which is excited by electrical pulses. The transducers convert electrical energy to mechanical energy or sound energy and vice versa. The ultrasound waves are transmitted from the transducer, propagate through different tissues and then return to the transducer as reflected echoes. The returned echoes are converted back into electrical impulses by the transducer crystals and are further processed to form the ultrasound image presented on the screen.

The frequency of sound waves produced by a transducer depends on its resonant frequency. As the frequency of the beam increases, the image resolution improves. However, the depth of penetration reduces. Resolution refers to the ability to separate two adjacent tissues or objects. It is in terms of axial and lateral resolution. The frequency and resolution of the transducer are designed for the tissues at a specific depth. For superficial tissues like skin and nail apparatus very high-frequency probes with a frequency range of 35–100 MHz are used.

The term UBM is used for these probes as the image produced can be compared with that of a low-power microscope. Probes with a frequency of 35 and 50 MHz give a lateral resolution of 50 microns and an axial resolution of 40 microns. The depth penetration of these sound waves is only 4 mm (Table 6.2).

Ultrasound waves produced by the transducers are reflected at the surfaces between the tissues of different density, the reflection being proportional to the difference in density or impedance. If the difference in density is increased, the proportion of reflected sound is increased and the proportion of transmitted sound is proportionately decreased. The image formed on the screen depends on the density of the tissue from which the sound is reflected. If the tissue density is high the reflected echoes are bright or hyperechoic, for example, calcifications. If echoes are absent it is anechoic, e.g., fluids like blood, bile, urine, contents of simple cysts, ascites, and pleural effusion are seen as echo-free structures. If there is no difference in a tissue or between tissues it is iso-echoic. If the tissue density is very high then the sound is completely reflected, resulting in total acoustic shadowing, which is characterized by no signals behind the structure that strongly absorb or reflect sound waves. This happens with solid structures; for example, acoustic shadowing is present in thick keratin (thickened nail plate, seborrheic keratosis, verrucous hemangioma), bones, calculi (stones in kidneys, gallbladder, etc.), and air (intestinal gas).

With the availability of multi-frequency probes, high-frequency probes (7 to 20 MHz), color Doppler, elastography, and UBM (35 to 50 MHz), the utility of ultrasound in the imaging of nail unit is possible and gives good results.

UBM uses probe frequency in the range of 35 MHz to 50 MHz. It is called UBM because it gives an image resolution that is comparable to a low-power microscope.[1]

UBM can resolve lesions as small as 50 microns and has a depth penetration of only 4 mm.

It is ideal for superficial lesions.

HFUS can resolve lesions as small as 75 microns and has a depth penetration of 10 to 40 mm. This is ideal for deeper lesions.

Color Doppler studies are done to study the vascularity of a lesion.

Elastography can differentiate between a benign and malignant tumor. Elastography is commonly performed to differentiate benign and malignant tumors in the liver and the breast.

Ultrasound (USG) examination of the nail unit is indicated in infective lesions, inflammatory conditions, and tumors involving the nail unit.

UBM and HFUS can help in the diagnosis, prognosis, and management of lesions. Biopsy sites can be marked accurately. Since it is in real time, dynamic studies and multiple sites can be examined in the same visit. Since it is a non-invasive imaging modality patient compliance is good.

Table 6.2 Ultrasound frequencies/probes used in dermatology

Frequency of probe (MHz)	Depth of penetration (mm)	Resolution (microns)	Structures visualized
7–15	40–60	450	Subcutaneous tissue, muscle, and nail unit
35 (UBM)	6	80	Skin, subcutaneous tissue, and nail unit
50 (UBM)	4	40	Epidermis, dermis, proximal nail fold

Ultrasonography of the normal nail apparatus

The nail unit consists of the proximal and lateral nail folds, the dorsal and ventral nail plates, the nail bed, the nail pulp, the distal phalanx, the DIP, and the tendons attached to the distal phalanx.

The proximal and lateral nail folds overlie the nail plate. The nail folds consist of the skin and sub-cutaneous tissue. The epidermis is visualized as a thin hyperechoic band. The dermis is visualized as the homogenous isoechoic band posterior to the epidermis. The sub-cutaneous tissue is hypoechoic and may show hyperechoic thin lines within it (these are the septae in the subcutaneous tissue). Posterior and proximal to the proximal part of the nail plate, the inter-phalangeal joint and the extensor tendons are visualized. On longitudinal scan, fascicular structure of tendons are seen as multiple closely spaced alternative echogenic and hypoechoic parallel lines. The dorsal and the ventral nail plates are seen as linear hyperechoic bands, one below the other, and are separated by a thin hypoechoic band, which is the interplate space. The nail bed is seen posterior to the nail plates and is hypoechoic. The nail matrix is seen at the proximal end of the nail plate as a thin heterogeneous structure. The cortex of the distal phalanx is posterior to the nail bed and is seen as a hyperechoic band with posterior acoustic shadowing[13-17] (Figure 6.6a and b).

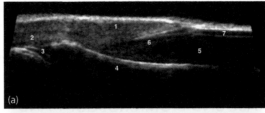

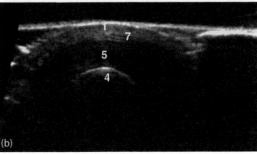

Figure 6.6 Normal longitudinal (a) and transverse; (b) scan of the nail apparatus on UBM. 1. Proximal nail fold; 2. Extensor tendon; 3. Distal interphalangeal joint; 4. Distal phalanx; 5. Nail bed; 6. Nail matrix; 7. Dorsal and ventral nail plate; 8. Root of the nail.

Ultrasonography in nail diseases

UBM and HFUS features of various nail diseases have been summarized in Table 6.3 and have been discussed below.

Table 6.3 Ultrasonography features of benign nail tumors

Nail tumors	UBM and HFUS findings	Color Doppler
Digital myxoid cysts	Well-defined round anechoic structures with internal echoes, which suggests viscous debris, irregularities, or thickening of the nail plates may be seen.	No vascularity
Keratin cysts	Round or oval anechoic or hypoechoic mass with lateral shadowing and internal echoes	Usually no vascularity is seen in the keratin cyst. Increased vascularity is seen in ruptured cysts due to the inflammatory response caused in the surrounding area.
Synovial or ganglion cysts	Anechoic mass lesions in the dermal or sub-dermal region. There is a thin tract seen communicating with the adjacent joint space.	No vascularity
Glomus tumor	Well-defined hypoechoic mass lesions with positive probe tenderness. Larger lesions can cause mass effect and erosion of the underlying cortex of the distal phalanx.	Vascularity noted in the tumor
Lipoma	Well-defined mass lesions in the subcutaneous tissue that are hypoechoic, hyperechoic, or heterogenous in echotexture. Septae in the lipomas when present can be seen as linear hyperechoic bands	No vascularity noted
Neuromas	Well-defined oval or round hypoechoic or heterogenous mass lesions	Absence of vascularity
Soft tissue chondroma	Hypoechoic mass lesion arising from dermis	May or may not show vascularity

(Continued)

Table 6.3 (*Continued*) Ultrasonography features of benign nail tumors

Nail tumors	UBM and HFUS findings	Color Doppler
Onychomatricoma	Well–defined hypoechoic mass lesion arising from the nail matrix with linear hyperechoic lines seen within these mass lesion	No vascularity
Periungual and subungual fibromas	Uniform hypoechoic nodular or oval structure commonly located within the nail bed eccentrically. They may affect the matrix region, including one of its wings. Large tumors may cause remodeling of the bony margin.	Usually hypovascular, with the exception of angiofibromas which may show low-velocity arterial and venous blood flow within the lesion
Giant cell tumor of the tendon sheath	Well-defined heterogenous mass lesions arising from the tendon sheath Real time HFUS: the mass lesion moves with movement of tendon.	Usually avascular
Periungual fibrokeratomas	Hypoechoic structures that may provoke remodeling of the bony margin of the distal phalanx	Hypovascular tumors
Lymphangioma circumscriptum	Multiple well-defined anechoic mass lesions in the epidermal, sub-epidermal, or dermal region. It rules out deeper involvement.	Lymphangiomas are avascular.
AV malformation	Heterogenous mass lesion. Phleboliths are seen as hyperechoic foci with or without posterior acoustic shadowing.	Vascularity present in the mass lesion. Arteries and veins are noted in the mass lesion.
Subungual exostosis and osteochondroma	Nodular hyperechoic calcified mass lesions situated deep in the nail bed and arising from the underlying bone	No vascularity noted

Benign conditions affecting nail apparatus

CONGENITAL HYPERTROPHIC LIP OF HALLUX

This congenital anomaly, characterized by hypertrophy of the lateral nail fold, mostly affects the medial aspect of the hallux, and presents as a red and firm swelling that may resemble recurrent digital fibrous tumors of childhood. On ultrasound, it is seen as an extension of the normal skin of the lateral nail fold without evidence of a mass lesion within it. Additionally, fragments of nail plates may be found embedded in the lateral nail fold.

PACHYONYCHIA CONGENITA

Pachyonychia congenita is a hereditary ectodermal dysplasia with thickening of the nails and subungual hyperkeratosis appearing within the first 6 months of life (Figure 6.7a).

UBM and HFUS show a thickened, hyperechoic, and irregular nail plate. The inter-nail plate space is lost (Figure 6.7b).

ALOPECIA AREATA

Alopecia areata (AA) is an immune-mediated disease presenting with non-cicatricial alopecia occurring in a circumscribed or generalized pattern. The incidence of nail changes in AA is recorded as ranging from 7% to 66%.[17] The nail changes

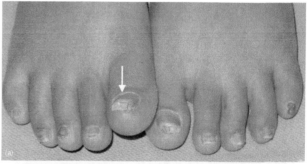
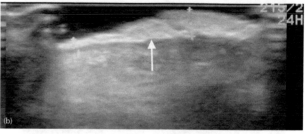

Figure 6.7 Pachyonychia congenita (a) Thickening of the nail plates with yellowish discoloration affecting multiple nails; (b) On HFUS the nail plate is thickened, hyperechoic, and irregular. There is loss of interplate space (up arrow).

observed in AA include diffuse fine pitting (Scotch-plaid appearance), onychorrhexis, Beau's lines, longitudinal ridging, onychodystrophy, and trachyonychia.[18,19]

Ultrasound findings show thickening of the proximal part of the nail bed as compared to the distal nail bed. No vascular changes are noted in the nail bed on color flow study.

INGROWN NAIL OR ONYCHOCRYPTOSIS

An ingrown nail is caused by inflammation of the lateral nail fold due to penetration of the edge of the nail plate resulting in pain, secondary infection, and later the formation of granulation tissue (Figure 6.8a).[20] On UBM and HFUS, the nail plate is noted as an abnormal linear hyperechoic lesion with an irregular surrounding hypoechoic zone. The linear hyperechoic lesion is due to abnormal nail growth, and the hypoechoic zone surrounding it is due to inflammation/granulation tissue or abscess. On color Doppler study abnormal vascular pattern or neovascularity may be noted within the hypoechoic zone (Figure 6.8b–d).

RETRONYCHIA

Retronychia refers to the proximal growth of the nail causing persistent proximal nail fold paronychia. It is characterized by proximal paronychia, elevation of the

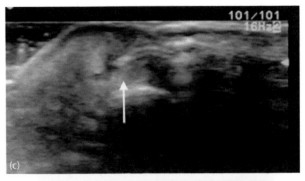

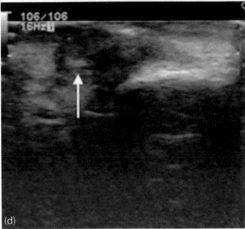

Figure 6.8 (Continued) Ingrown toenail/onychocryptosis: (c) HFUS transverse scan showing ingrown toenail (hyperechoic linear lines, up arrow); (d) Surrounding hypoechoic zone of inflammatory tissue noted (up arrow).

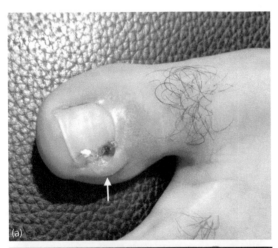

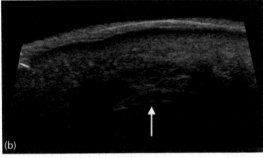

Figure 6.8 Ingrown toenail/onychocryptosis (a) Ingrowth of right great toenail in the lateral nail fold with paronychia and granulation tissue; (b) UBM – transverse scan shows ingrown toenail with surrounding soft tissue inflammation (up arrow)   (Continued)

proximal nail plate, thickening of the proximal portion of the nail plate with multiple layers, yellow nails, granulation tissue arising from the traumatized proximal nail fold, and distal onycholysis.[21]

On UBM and HFUS, the nail plate is closer to the DIP and there may be thickening of the proximal nail fold.[22] Linear calcification is seen in continuity with the nail plate.

ACQUIRED HYPONYCHIA SECONDARY TO TRAUMA

Acquired nail atrophy due to nail matrix injury can result in rudimentary nail. The causes include trauma, systemic diseases, and drugs like etretinate (Figure 6.9a). UBM and HFUS show absence of the nail plate (down arrow) with thickening of the nail bed (Figure 6.9b).

ONYCHOMADESIS

Onychomadesis is an acute non-inflammatory condition affecting the nail matrix that results in spontaneous separation of the nail plate from the matrix starting at the proximal end. A severe systemic illness or trauma may cause

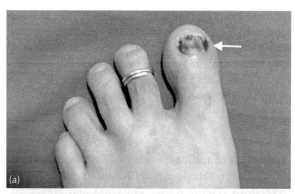

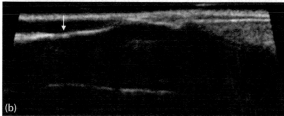

Figure 6.9 Acquired anonychia secondary to trauma
(a) Dystrophic right great toenail with remnant of nail plate at proximal nail fold; (b) UBM transverse scan shows absence of nail plate (down arrow), with thickening of the nail bed.

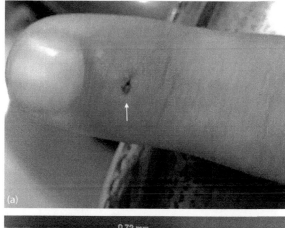

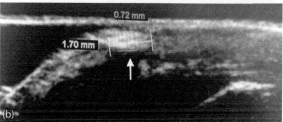

Figure 6.10 Foreign body (lead) in the proximal nail fold
(a) Minimally tender hyperpigmented papule on the dorsum of index finger close to proximal nail fold with surrounding edema; (b) UBM transverse scan shows the hyperechoic foreign body in the epidermis and dermis of proximal nail fold (up arrow).

spontaneous separation of the nail plate from its matrix, which may be due to decrease in the blood supply.

On UBM and HFUS, the nail plate may be fragmented or irregular. Thickening and decreased echogenicity of the proximal nail fold and the proximal nail bed is seen. The role of ultrasound in this condition is to rule out a mass lesion.[22]

MEDIAN CANALIFORM DYSTROPHY

Median canaliform dystrophy of Heller is a rare entity characterized by a midline or a paramedian ridge or split and canal formation in the nail plate of one or both the thumb nails. It is an acquired condition resulting from a temporary defect in the matrix that interferes with the formation of nail. Habitual picking of the nail base may be responsible in some cases.[23]

On UBM and HFUS, median canalicular nail dystrophy is seen as thinning of the central proximal nail bed involving the matrix region, which suggests scarring and chronic inflammatory changes. Distally, the nail plates may show thickening and irregularity. Usually, the nail bed tends to be hypovascular in the affected region on color Doppler ultrasound.

FOREIGN BODY

Foreign bodies may be embedded in the nail bed and periungual area (commonly seen in hands) (Figure 6.10a). There are different types of materials that can be found in the nail bed, both secondary to traumatic events or relating

to the abnormal displacement of surgical materials used for correcting the axis of the toenails. On UBM and HFUS foreign bodies are seen as well-defined hyperechoic lesions with posterior acoustic shadowing. There may be a surrounding hypoechoic zone, in presence of inflammation (Figure 6.10b).

SUBUNGUAL HEMATOMA

Subungual hematoma is characterized by reddish purple discoloration of the nail plate, which can be associated with pain usually following injuries (Figure 6.11a). Hematoma in the nail bed, on UBM and HFUS, is seen as an increase in thickness of the nail bed with a hypoechoic echotexture. Internal echoes may be seen within the hematoma depending on the age of the hematoma (Figure 6.11b).

In the periungual region hematomas are seen as well-defined hypoechoic mass lesions with or without internal echoes. Older hematomas will show an anechoic echotexture.

Infective disorders

ABSCESS

Nail bed abscess is commonly seen under immuno-suppressive conditions, secondary to drugs and/or systemic diseases. It can present as a painful yellowish discoloration of the nail plate with evidence of pus underneath the nail plate (Figure 6.12a).

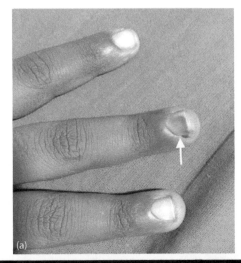

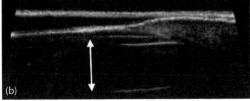

Figure 6.11 Hematoma **(a)** Violaceous discoloration of nail plate of right middle finger; **(b)** UBM longitudinal scan.

On UBM and HFUS, it is seen as an ill-defined heterogenous mass lesion. If the infection is deeper and has reached the underlying bone, periosteal reaction may be noted on the distal phalanx. On color Doppler study, increased vascularity at the periphery of the lesion may be seen (Figure 6.12b and c).

ONYCHOMYCOSIS

Dermatophytic infection of the nail is characterized by nail discoloration, thickening of nail plate, and subungual hyperkeratosis (Figure 6.13a). On UBM and HFUS, there is increase in the nail plate thickness. The nail plate is hyperechoic. There is loss of the inter nail plate space (Figure 6.13b).

FISTULA

Periungual infective fistulous tracts within the soft tissues can directly connect to the bony margin, nail bed or matrix region. Erosions can be seen on the distal phalanx. On UBM and HFUS, a fistula is seen as a thin hypoechoic tract connecting the lesion or abscess to the skin surface.

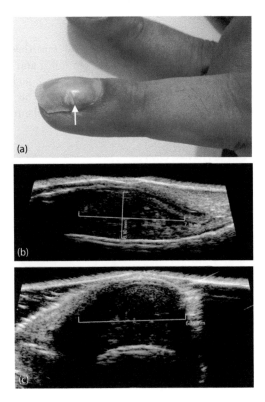

Figure 6.12 Abscess in the nail bed **(a)** Localized yellowish discoloration of right middle fingernail with local tenderness; **(b)** UBM longitudinal scan; **(c)** Transverse scan shows the abscess as a mixed echogenic mass lesion within the marked area. The underlying cortex of the distal phalanx and the overlying nail plate appear normal.

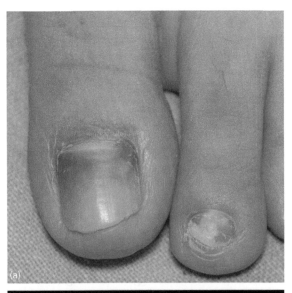

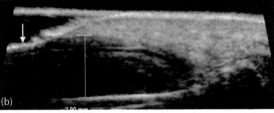

Figure 6.13 Onychomycosis **(a)** Dark greenish discoloration of the nail plate (Courtesy: Piyush Kumar); **(b)** UBM longitudinal scan shows thickened nail plate (down arrow) with increased thickness of the nail bed (marked area).

Inflammatory disorders

PSORIASIS

Psoriatic nail disease usually occurs in patients with clinically evident psoriasis but it can be localized to nails without evidence of cutaneous disease in less than 5% of patients. Varying degrees of alterations are seen in both the nail bed and nail plate (Figure 6.14a). Nail psoriasis as a risk factor for subclinical psoriatic arthritis may have interphalangeal stiffness, pain, and swelling.[24]

When psoriasis affects the proximal nail fold, on UBM the epidermis appears thick and hyperechoic. There is a sub-epidermal hypoechoic band noted. These changes can be seen in sub-clinical state.

If the nail is affected in psoriasis, on UBM and HFUS there is increased thickness of the nail bed and the nail plate (Figure 6.14b). Other findings have been listed in Box 6.2.

UBM improves the diagnostic precision of psoriasis together with clinical examination and thus nail biopsy can be avoided.[25–27]

LUPUS ERYTHEMATOSUS

Focal lesions of DLE occurring over the nail fold can produce nail plate dystrophy with longitudinal ridging and nail bed hyperkeratosis, which may extend on the dorsa of the digits to surround the nails. In chilblains LE, predominantly in women, red-purple patches develop on the fingers and toes that are precipitated by cold and damp climate.

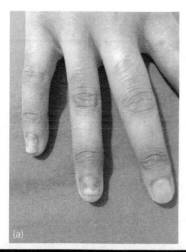
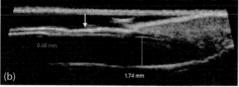

Figure 6.14 Psoriasis **(a)** Yellowish discoloration of nail plate with oil spot and distal onycholysis; **(b)** UBM longitudinal scan shows a thickened (red marker) irregular nail plate (down arrow), with an increase in the thickness of the nail bed (green marker).

> ## BOX 6.2: Nail findings of psoriasis on UBM and HFUS
>
> - Increase in thickness of nail plate and the nail bed
> - Loss of inter nail plate space and the nail plates may be fused.
> - Irregular ventral nail plate
> - Joint involvement – effusion/fluid in interphalangeal joint space
> - Erosion of the bones around the joint space may be seen.
> - Color Doppler study: increase in the blood flow and the resistivity index is high.

Nail changes can be associated with active disease, oral ulceration, and higher incidence of Raynaud's phenomenon. Other findings include nail fold erythema, red lunulae, and nail fold hyperkeratosis with ragged cuticles and splinter hemorrhages.[28]

On UBM and HFUS the nail bed is hypoechoic. The nail bed thickness is variable. The nail plate thickness is irregular and its echotexture is variable. On color Doppler study the nail bed may be hypovascular. The digital vessels may not be visualized due to thrombosis. Areas of variable thickness can be seen in the nail bed including thickening and thinning that is associated with secondary dystrophy.

RHEUMATOID ARTHRITIS

Rheumatoid arthritis (RA) is a chronic inflammatory arthritis with systemic organ involvement.

Clinical nail abnormalities that are commonly described in RA are longitudinal ridging and clubbing.

On UBM and HFUS the nail plates are irregular in thickness. The nail bed is increased in thickness. Soft tissue and bony abnormalities are more commonly observed.

Interphalangeal and peri-articular joint involvement is visualized as anechoic fluid collection in the joint space, presence of bony erosions, and irregularity or atrophy of the tendon and its sheath.

SCLERODERMA

Vascular abnormalities are among the primary pathological components of scleroderma. Proximal nail fold is the most affected site with nail fold erythema and telangiectasia. The frequency of nail fold bleeding and infracts is significantly higher in systemic sclerosis. Nail plates may show increased longitudinal and transverse curvature as well as a white dull discoloration. Complete destruction of the nail apparatus is the final consequence of the dissolution of the terminal phalanges.

On UBM and HFUS, there is thickening and decreased echogenicity of the nail bed with an upward displacement of the nail plate. On color Doppler study, decreased vascularity of the nail bed may be present.

DERMATOMYOSITIS

Periungual capillary changes like dilated and tortuous blood vessels, areas of atrophy, telangiectasias, central areas of hemorrhage, splinter hemorrhages, and bushy capillary loop formation in the proximal nail fold are commonly seen.

On UBM and HFUS calcification may be seen in the dermis of the periungual region. Calcifications are seen as linear or curvilinear hyperechoic bands with distal acoustic shadowing.

On color Doppler study thrombosis of the digital arteries may be seen.

Tumors and pseudotumors

Ultrasound provides additional information about the tumor characteristics that cannot be appreciated on clinical examination alone. Features like origin and exact location, involvement of the nail unit components, surrounding structures, size and composition of the tumor (solid/cystic), and vascularity can be visualized. Effect of mass lesion or erosion on the underlying bone can also be appreciated on USG.

On follow up studies, USG can identify recurrence of the tumor.[1]

LONGITUDINAL MELANONYCHIA

Longitudinal melanonychia can be a presenting feature of various nail diseases including benign and malignant nail tumors like melanoma (Figure 6.15a).

UBM and HFUS is done to rule out tumor in the region of the nail matrix (Figure 6.15b).

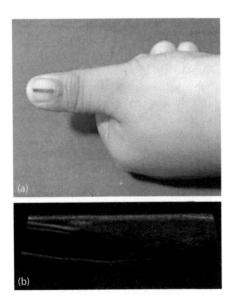

Figure 6.15 Longitudinal melanonychia (a) Single hyperpigmented linear band on the right thumb nail; (b) UBM longitudinal scan shows no mass lesion in the region of the nail matrix or nail bed. The nail plate thickness is normal and the inter-nail plate space is maintained.

DIGITAL MYXOID CYSTS

Clinically they may show as indolent nodules or swelling of the nail and periungual tissues and, when compressing the nail matrix, they can cause dystrophic changes in the nail plates (Figure 6.16a).

On UBM and HFUS they appear as well-defined round anechoic structures sometimes with internal echoes, which suggest viscous debris. On color Doppler study no vascularity is noted. Irregularities or thickening of the nail plates may be detected as signs of a secondary dystrophy (Figure 6.16b and c).[1,29]

KERATIN CYSTS

On UBM and HFUS, the cyst appears as a round or oval, anechoic, or hypoechoic mass with lateral shadowing and internal echoes. No vascularity is noted in the keratin cyst on color Doppler study. Increased vascularity is seen in ruptured cysts due to the inflammatory response caused in the surrounding area.

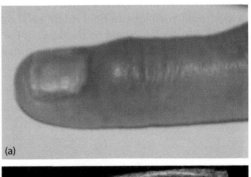

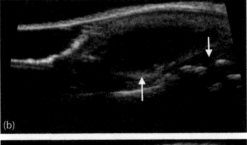

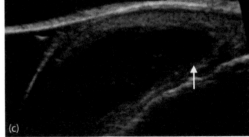

Figure 6.16 Myxoid cyst (a) Solitary skin-colored soft to firm non-tender nodule on the dorsum of right middle finger, extending onto the proximal nail fold; (b) UBM longitudinal scan; (c) UBM transverse scan shows a well-defined oval anechoic mass lesion below the dermis (up arrow). The DIP appears normal (down arrow).

SYNOVIAL OR GANGLION CYSTS

Ganglion cysts are the cysts of excess fluid collection from a tendon or a joint. It is extremely common around the hand and wrist (Figure 6.17a).

On UBM and HFUS a synovial cyst or ganglion cyst is seen as an anechoic mass lesion in the dermal or sub-dermal region. There is a thin tract seen communicating with the adjacent joint space. This helps differentiate a mucoid cyst from a synovial or ganglion cyst. If hemorrhage or rupture occurs, echoes can be seen within the mass lesion (Figure 6.17b and c).

On color Doppler study, there is no vascularity noted in the mass lesion.

Ganglion cyst can be associated with erosion of the bony margins of the underlying joint space.

GLOMUS TUMOR

Glomus tumor presents as a small, reddish blue nodule measuring 3 to 10 millimeters in diameter. Their typical location is the subungual region of the distal phalanges (Figure 6.18 and b).

On UBM and HFUS these tumors are seen as well-defined hypoechoic mass lesions.

On compression with the sonography probe there is tenderness noted (probe tenderness).

If the tumor is more than 4–5 mm in the region of the nail bed, mass effect and erosion of the underlying cortex of the distal phalanx can be seen.

On color Doppler study there is vascularity noted in the mass lesion. Even in the absence of clinically visible tumor or nail changes, the tumor can be diagnosed on UBM (Figure 6.19a and b).[30]

LIPOMAS

Lipoma of distal phalanx can present as a tender and painful swelling with destruction of the distal bony phalanx or as a slowly enlarging swelling on the lateral nail fold or in the subungual location (Figure 6.20a).[31]

On UBM and HFUS lipomas are seen as well-defined mass lesions that are hypoechoic, hyperechoic, or heterogenous

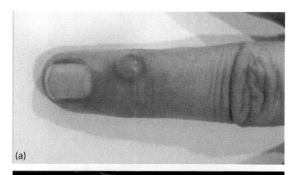

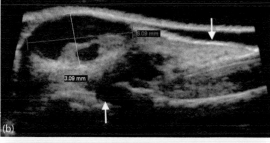

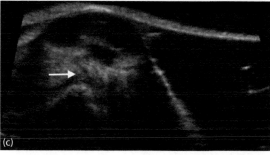

Figure 6.17 Ganglion (a) Firm skin-colored nodule on the dorsum of the finger over the dorsum of the DIP; (b) UBM longitudinal scan shows a well-defined oval anechoic mass lesion with internal echoes (suggestive of hemorrhage or infection) above the DIP (within the markers). There is fluid noted in the DIP space suggestive of effusion (up arrow); (c) UBM transverse scan shows a thin zig-zag communication between the synovial cyst and the underlying joint space (right arrow).

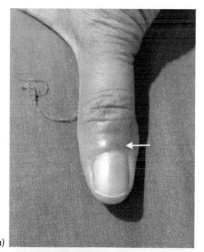

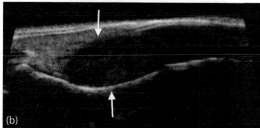

Figure 6.18 Glomus (a) Localized area of tenderness just below the proximal nail fold of right thumb nail; (b) UBM longitudinal scan shows a well-defined oval hypoechoic mass lesion below the proximal nail fold (down arrow). There is scalloping of the underlying distal phalanx (up arrow).

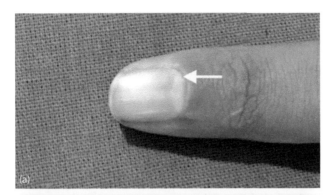

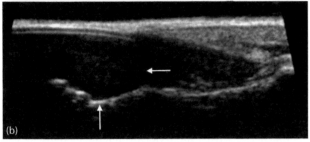

Figure 6.19 Glomus **(a)** Tender bluish subungual nodule just above the lunula; **(b)** UBM longitudinal and transverse scan shows a well-defined round hypoechoic mass lesion in the nail bed (left arrow), with erosion of the underlying distal phalanx (up arrow).

in echotexture. They are generally present in the sub-cutaneous tissue. The septae in the lipomas when present can be seen as linear hyperechoic bands.

On color Doppler study there is no vascularity noted in the lipoma (Figure 6.20b).

NEUROMA

Neuromas develop from the numerous nerve fibers in the nail bed and in the pulp after an injury or repeated microtrauma (Figure 6.21a).

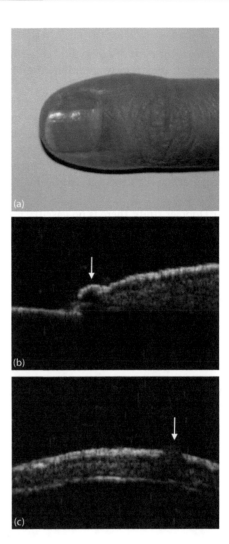

Figure 6.21 Neuroma **(a)** Localized area of tenderness on the proximal nail-fold without any evident mass lesions; **(b** and **c)** UBM longitudinal and transverse scan show a well-defined hypoechoic mass lesion arising from the dermis and causing breach in the continuity of the overlying epidermis (down arrow).

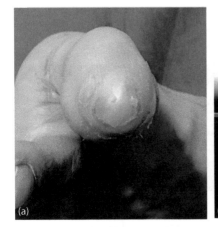

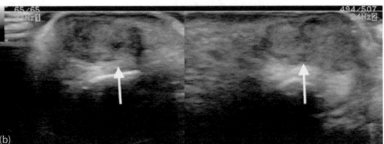

Figure 6.20 Lipoma **(a)** Soft mobile nodule on the hyponychium extending onto the volar aspect of great toe; **(b)** HFUS (longitudinal and transverse scan) shows a well-defined lobulated mixed echogenic mass lesion seen in the pulp of the great toe (up arrow).

On UBM and HFUS these tumors are seen as well-defined oval or round hypoechoic or heterogenous mass lesions with absence of vascularity on color Doppler study (Figure 6.21b and c).[32]

SOFT TISSUE CHONDROMA

Soft tissue chondroma may be purely located in the soft tissues with small nodules of cartilage without any connection to the underlying bone.[33] Fingers are most commonly affected (Figure 6.22a).

On UBM and HFUS soft tissue chondroma is seen as a well-defined hypoechoic mass lesion arising from the dermis. It may or may not show vascularity on color Doppler study (Figure 6.22b and c).

ONYCHOMATRICOMA

Onychomatricoma is a tumor of the nail matrix clinically characterized by the development of longitudinal thick yellow bands in the nail plate accompanied by increased nail curvature (Figure 6.23a and b).

On HFUS it is seen as uniformly thickened nail plate with multiple thin linear hyperechoic bands within it (Figure 6.23c).[34]

KERATOACANTHOMA

Keratoacanthoma is a proliferative benign tumor of the epidermis characterized by a localized proliferation of squamous epithelium with a characteristic central keratin-filled crater.

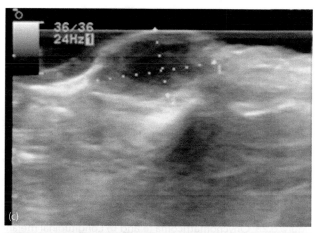

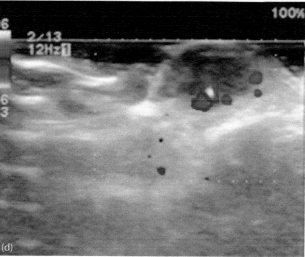

Figure 6.22 (Continued) **(c)** The tumor is causing mass effect on the overlying dermis and the underlying subcutaneous tissue (marked area); **(d)** HFUS with color Doppler showing vascularity in the chondroma.

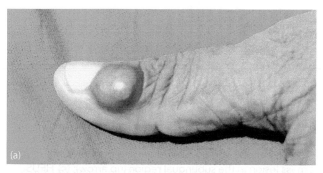

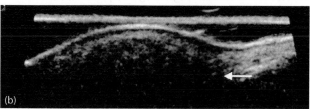

Figure 6.22 **(a)** Soft tissue chondroma: Painless firm to hard nodule on the dorsum of the left thumb impinging on the proximal nail fold; **(b)** UBM longitudinal scan shows a well-defined hypoechoic mass lesion arising from the lower dermis (left arrow). *(Continued)*

On UBM and HFUS keratoacanthoma is seen as a well-defined heterogenous mass lesion in the matrix and the nail bed. These tumors may cause posterior acoustic shadowing due to the presence of keratin in the tumors. Erosion of the underlying distal phalanx is seen.

UBM and HFUS cannot differentiate keratoacanthoma from SCC.

FIBROUS TUMORS

Periungual and subungual fibromas (Koenen tumors) are a benign, cutaneous manifestation of tuberous sclerosis (Figure 6.24a). On UBM and HFUS, fibromas present as uniform hypoechoic nodular or oval structure commonly located within the nail bed eccentrically. They may affect the matrix region, including one of its wings (Figure 6.24b and c). Large tumors may cause remodeling of the bony margin. On color Doppler study, fibrous tumors are usually hypovascular (Figure 6.24d), with the exception of

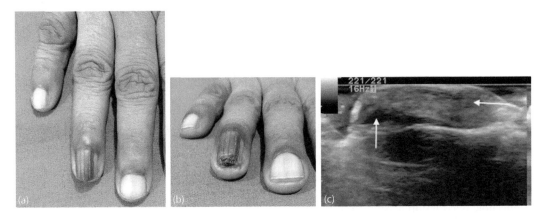

Figure 6.23 Onychomatricoma (a and b) Longitudinal melanonychia with increased transverse over-curvature of the right ring fingernail with thickened subungual mass; (c) HFUS longitudinal scan shows a uniformly thickened nail plate (left arrow) with multiple thin linear hyperechoic bands within it. The underlying hypoechoic nail bed is compressed between the tumor and the distal phalanx (up arrow).

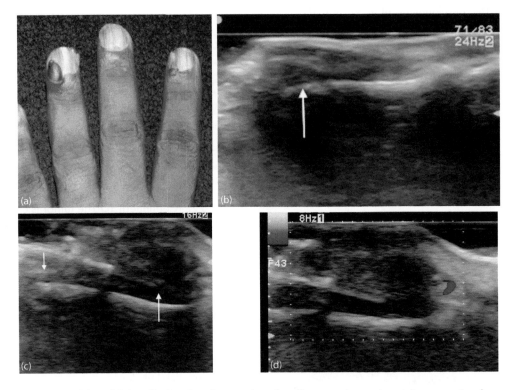

Figure 6.24 Koenen tumors (a) Reddish to flesh-colored, smooth, soft to firm papules and nodules emerging from proximal nail folds; (b) HFUS longitudinal scan shows a well-defined hypoechoic mass lesion in the subungual region (up arrow); (c) HFUS longitudinal scan shows a well-defined mass lesion below the proximal nail fold and superior to the nail plate (up arrow). There is a subungual mass lesion seen anteriorly (down arrow); (d) HFUS with power Doppler study shows no neovascularity.

angiofibromas, which may show low-velocity arterial and venous blood flow within the lesion.[29]

GIANT CELL TUMOR OF THE TENDON SHEATH

It is the second most common subcutaneous tumor of the hand. On the digits, dorsum of the DIP is the most common site and it usually appears as a solitary, often lobulated, slow-growing, skin-colored, and smooth-surfaced nodule that tends to feel firm and rubbery (Figure 6.25a). On HFUS these tumors are well-defined heterogenous mass lesions arising from the tendon sheath. In real time HFUS the tendon is seen to move freely from the mass lesion. The overlying sub-cutaneous tissue and dermis are normal and separate from the mass lesion (Figure 6.25b and c).[35]

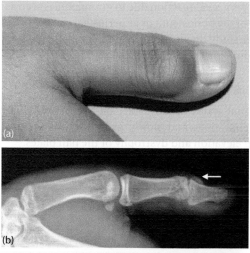

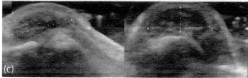

Figure 6.25 Giant cell tumor of the tendon sheath (a) A single hard nodule on the dorsum of right thumbs impinging on to the proximal nail fold; (b) X-ray of the thumb shows a soft tissue mass on the extensor aspect of the distal phalanx (left arrow); (c) HFUS longitudinal and transverse scan shows well-defined heterogenous mass lesion above the extensor tendon and below the sub-cutaneous tissue (marked area).

PERIUNGUAL FIBROKERATOMAS

These are benign fibrous proliferative tumors that lie over the nail plates frequently connect with the proximal or lateral nail folds and may involve the ungual matrix and nail bed.

On sonography, they are seen as hypoechoic structures that are usually hypovascular on color Doppler. Rarely these tumors may provoke remodeling of the bony margin of the distal phalanx.

LYMPHANGIOMA

Lymphangioma circumscriptum is rare on the distal digit and usually presents as a cluster of vesicles resembling frog spawn.

On UBM and HFUS lymphangiomas are seen as multiple well-defined anechoic mass lesions in the epidermal, sub-epidermal, or dermal region.

Lymphangiomas are avascular on color flow studies.

USG is useful to rule out deeper involvement.

AV MALFORMATION

Vascular malformations of the fingertip are mainly venous malformations or capillary malformations (Figure 6.26a).

On UBM and HFUS these tumors are seen as heterogenous mass lesion. Phleboliths are seen as hyperechoic foci with or without posterior acoustic shadowing.

On color and pulsed Doppler study these tumors are very vascular. Arteries and veins are noted in these mass lesions (Figure 6.26b–d).

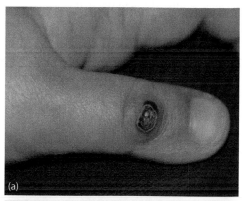

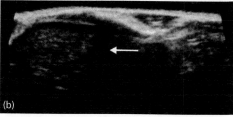

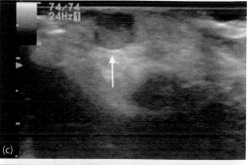

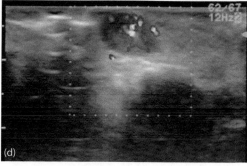

Figure 6.26 Arteriovenous malformation (a) Subcutaneous nodule on dorsum of right thumb with hyperpigmented verrucous surface; (b) UBM longitudinal scan shows a hypoechoic mass lesion in the sub-cutaneous tissue (left arrow); (c) HFUS shows a well-defined hypoechoic mass lesion (up arrow) in the subcutaneous tissue; (d) HFUS with color Doppler shows arterio-venous flow in the mass lesion.

Pseudotumors

GRANULOMAS

Infectious granulomatous diseases caused by mycobacteria and non-infectious granulomatous disease like sarcoidosis[36] can rarely affect the nail apparatus (Figure 6.27a).

On UBM and HFUS granulomas are well-defined mass lesions with irregular margins. When a granuloma is in the nail bed it causes thickening of the nail bed.

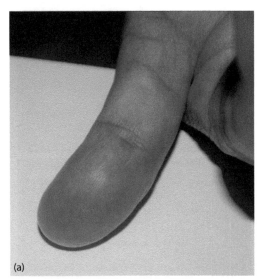

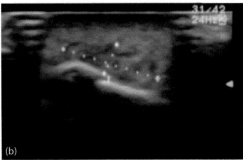

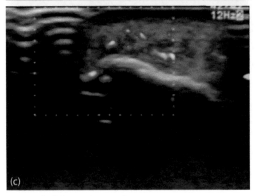

Figure 6.27 Granuloma **(a)** Erythematous tender subcutaneous ill-defined swelling on the volar aspect of the thumb; **(b)** HFUS of the pulp of the thumb shows an ill-defined heterogenous mass lesion anterior to the distal phalanx (marked area); **(c)** HFUS with color Doppler shows telangiectatic vessels.

The periosteal reaction due to granuloma is seen as irregularity of the periosteum or as periosteal elevation. On color Doppler study linear telangiectatic vessels are noted within the granuloma (Figure 6.27b and c).

SUBUNGUAL WARTS

Subungual warts usually start on the hyponychium and periungual areas and slowly grow towards the nail bed, causing elevation and dystrophy of the nail plates.

On UBM and HFUS these lesions are seen as eccentric well-defined hyperechoic masses. The adjacent nail plate may or may not be thickened.

On color Doppler there is no vascularity noted in these lesions.

PYOGENIC GRANULOMAS

Also known as "lobular capillary hemangioma" is a benign vascular proliferation that can arise on the skin or subcutaneous tissue. Periungual PGs can be caused by local trauma, drug intake, or peripheral nerve injury. Clinically it presents as a bright red and rapidly growing mass on the fingertip. Ulceration and bleeding are common complications.

On USG it is seen as a well-defined, mild to moderately echogenic mass lesion with small hypoechoic foci. Increased vascularity is noted in this mass lesion on color Doppler study.[37,38] USG can differentiate the more echogenic lobular capillary granuloma from other subungual vascular malformation (glomus tumor and other vascular malformations).

Osteocartilaginous tumors

SUBUNGUAL EXOSTOSIS AND OSTEOCHONDROMA

On HFUS these are seen as nodular hyperechoic calcified mass lesions situated deep in the nail bed and arising from the underlying bone. There is mass effect noted on the overlying soft tissue. X-ray or CT scan is required to confirm the diagnosis.

Malignant tumors of the nail

BOWEN'S DISEASE, SQUAMOUS CELL CARCINOMA, AND BASAL CELL CARCINOMA

SCC is one of the most common primary malignant tumors of the nail bed. All of them in the subungual location can have atypical presentations resembling inflammatory nail diseases, benign tumors, or pigmentary subtypes.

On UBM and HFUS the lesions are seen as ill-defined hypoechoic mass lesions. Erosions of the bone may be seen with tumor infiltration of the adjacent tissue.

On color Doppler study neovascularity is noted in these mass lesions.

MELANOMA

Subungual melanoma is uncommon, and usually affects the thumb and big toe. Clinical manifestations include ingrown nail, simple split nail, junctional nevus, chronic paronychia with or without pain, and subungual pigmentation (Figure 6.28a).[39] However, subungual melanoma is often amelanotic, which may result in a delayed diagnosis.

On UBM and HFUS melanomas are seen as well-defined hypoechoic lobulated oval or round mass lesions in the sub-epidermal or dermal region. There may be posterior acoustic shadowing due to excessive melanin in the tumor. A peritumoral inflammation may lead to more hypoechoic peripheral areas. The thickness of the cutaneous melanomas can be measured accurately.[40,41] Neovascularity may or may not be seen in the tumor on color Doppler study (Figure 6.28b and c).[1]

UBM and HFUS features of malignant nail tumors are mentioned in Table 6.4.

MAGNETIC RESONANCE IMAGING (MRI) OF NAIL APPARATUS

Recent advances in MRI imaging, with the advent of microcoils for the finger and higher-resolution machines, make imaging of the nail unit pathologies possible. Lesions as small as 2–5 mm can be well imaged and delineated, especially tumors. The size, margins, signal intensity, and enhancement of the tumors on contrast injection and their anatomical relationship to adjoining structures can be well visualized.

Technique

The part to be examined has to be immobilized. The sequences taken are T1 weighted images, T2 weighted images, fat-suppressed images, and post-contrast (gadolinium) preferably dynamic images.

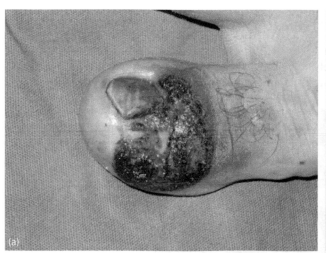
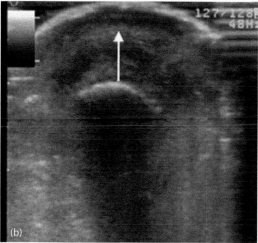
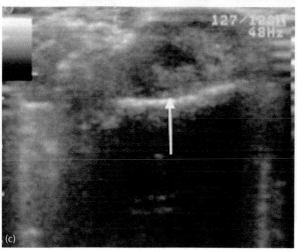

Figure 6.28 Acral lentiginous melanoma: **(a)** Hyperpigmented jet-black-colored plaque on the proximal nail fold of right great toe extending onto the lateral nail fold and surrounding area with yellowish discoloration of nail plate; **(b** and **c)** HFUS shows thickened hyperechoic epidermis and dermis with an ill-defined mixed echogenic mass lesion in the subcutaneous tissue (up arrow).

Table 6.4 Ultrasonography appearance of malignant nail tumors

Nail tumors	UBM and HFUS findings	Color Doppler
Keratoacanthoma	Well-defined heterogenous mass lesions in the matrix and the nail bed. These tumors may cause posterior acoustic shadowing due to the presence of keratin. Erosion of the underlying distal phalanx may be seen due to mass effect.	No vascularity
Bowen's disease, squamous cell carcinoma, and basal cell carcinoma	Ill-defined hypoechoic mass lesions. Erosions of the bone may be seen with tumor infiltration of the adjacent tissue.	Neovascularity is noted in these mass lesions
Subungual melanoma	Well-defined hypoechoic lobulated oval or round mass lesions in the sub-epidermal or dermal lesion. Posterior acoustic shadowing may be seen due to excessive melanin in the tumor. A peri-tumoral inflammation may appear as hypoechoic peripheral areas.	Neovascularity may or may not be seen in the tumor.

MRI in nail diseases

INFANTILE FIBROSARCOMA

Infantile fibrosarcoma is a rare soft tissue tumor in infants and children mostly located in extremities. Clinically presents as a local, progressive mass with no discrete borders.

On MRI, there is osteolysis and resorption of the distal phalanx, which is replaced by a large lobulated intensely enhancing heterogeneous mass showing multiple punctuate intralesional calcifications/ossifications. The mass can also encase the middle phalanx of the ring finger, which appears hypoplastic and shows diffuse sclerosis. The proximal phalanx is relatively spared (Figure 6.29a and b).

GIANT CELL TUMOR

On MRI GCTs are seen as low-signal-intensity tumors on T1 weighed and T2 weighed images. On post-contrast study there is moderate predominantly arterial phase enhancement of the tumor. Bony erosions/scalloping can

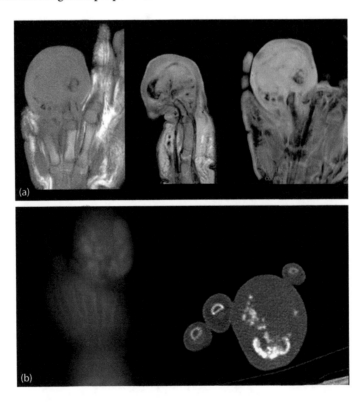

Figure 6.29 (a and b) Infantile fibrosarcoma. There is osteolysis and resorption of the distal phalanx of the left ring finger, which is replaced by a large lobulated intensely enhancing heterogeneous mass showing multiple punctuate intralesional calcifications/ossifications. The mass also encases the middle phalanx of the ring finger, which appears hypoplastic and shows diffuse sclerosis. The proximal phalanx is relatively spared.

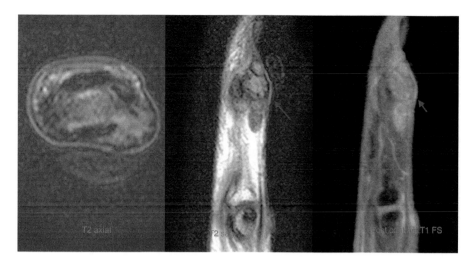

Figure 6.30 Giant cell tumor of tendon sheath. A lobulated heterogeneously enhancing predominantly T2 hypointense mass is seen along the dorso-ulnar aspect of the DIP of the middle finger lying in close approximation to the extensor aponeurosis with focal erosion of the subjacent dorso-ulnar cortex of the middle phalanx as well (red oblique arrow).

be present and are well seen on MRI. MRI is currently the optimal modality for preoperative assessment of tumor size, extent, and invasion of adjacent joint and tenosynovial space (Figure 6.30).[42]

GLOMUS TUMOR

On MRI, glomus tumor is seen as a mass lesion showing low- to medium-intensity signal on T1 weighted images and high signal intensity on T2 weighted images. Uniform intense arterial phase enhancement of the tumor is noted on dynamic contrast images. This arterial enhancement is characteristic of glomus tumor in the nail bed (Figure 6.31).[43]

HEMANGIOMAS AND VENOUS MALFORMATION

On MRI, these tumors show intermediate- to low-intensity signal on T1 weighted images and high-intensity signals on T2 weighted images. High–flow vascular malformations may also show flow voids. On

post-contrast study variable enhancement is noted in the malformations depending on the phase in which the image is captured.

LYMPHATIC MALFORMATION

On MR imaging there is low-intensity signals on T1 weighted images and high-intensity signals on T2 weighted images. On post-contrast study there is minimal/none predominantly rim and septal enhancement noted. The cystic lymphatic filled spaces do not enhance on post-contrast study.

MELANOMA

On MR imaging melanomas are hyperintense on T1 weighted images and hypointense on T2 weighted images. These lesions also show blooming on the gradient sequences.

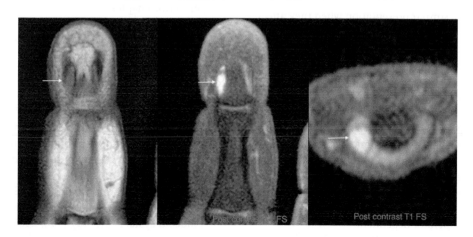

Figure 6.31 Glomus tumor. An intensely enhancing ovoid lesion is seen within the nail bed with otherwise normal subjacent bone (right arrow).

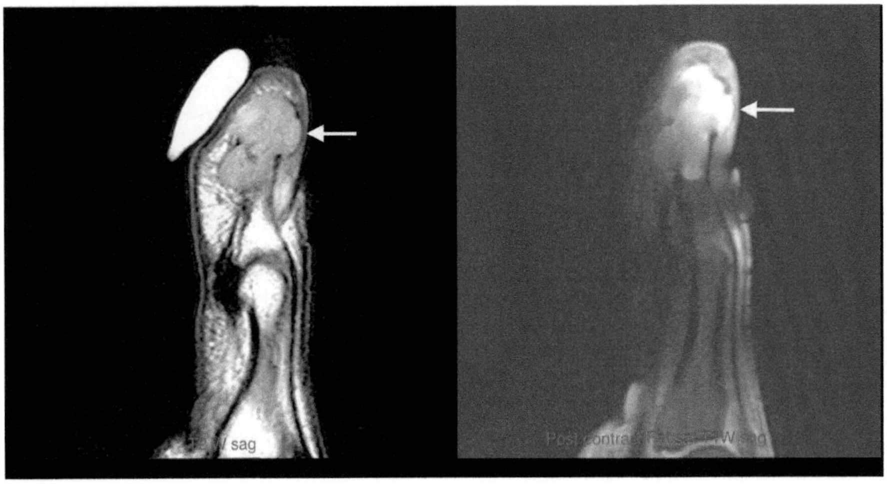

Figure 6.32 Squamous cell carcinoma. Heterogeneously enhancing T1 hypointense and T2 iso to hyperintense osteolytic lesion is seen involving the tip of the distal phalanx of the thumb. The lesion extends into the nail bed as well as the overlying volar subcutaneous fat (left arrow).

The tumor shows uniform enhancement on post-contrast study.[44]

SQUAMOUS CELL CARCINOMA

On MR imaging these tumors show intermediate-to-low-intensity signals on T1 weighted images and high signal intensity on T2 weighted images. On post-contrast study heterogeneous enhancement of the tumor is noted. Bony erosions may be present and are well seen on MRI (Figure 6.32).[44]

CONCLUSION

In conclusion, diagnosis of inflammatory and neoplastic conditions affecting the nail apparatus is often challenging due to the anatomical location of the nail unit. Cutaneous diseases may not have similar presentation when they affect nail unit.

In imaging modalities for nails, X-rays have a limited role in nail pathologies.

The advantage of MRI over UBM and high-frequency USG is in bony tumors.

Bone involvement can be seen well with MRI and cannot be easily picked up on UBM and high-frequency USG. MRI is excellent in visualizing anatomic details and tissue differentiation.

Microcoils for nail unit imaging is mandatory to study nail pathologies without which lesions in the nail unit cannot be resolved on MRI. While MRI is not operator dependent, HFUS and UBM are operator dependent.

There are several advantages of UBM over MRI. Tumors as small as 50 microns can be resolved on UBM. Patient compliance is excellent. Multiple sites can be examined. It is not time consuming.

The dynamic nature of performing UBM and high-frequency USG helps in differentiating tumors on the basis of movements of the structures in the nail apparatus. For example, GCT of the tendon sheath will be static and will not move with the movement of underlying tendon.

But sometimes the thick nail plate may prevent adequate penetration of ultrasound waves in the deeper tissue. Hence a multi-pronged approach is required in imaging of the nail apparatus, where all the modalities have a specific role to play depending on which pathology needs to be imaged and evaluated.

ACKNOWLEDGMENTS

The authors want to thank Dr. Bhavin Jankharia, Consultant Radiologist, for his support and contribution of all the MRI images in this chapter.

The authors want to thank Dr. Vaidehi Bhatt for all the support she gave while writing this chapter.

REFERENCES

1. Bhatt KD, Tambe SA, Jerajani HR, Dhurat RS. Utility of high-frequency ultrasonography in the diagnosis of benign and malignant skin tumors. *Indian J Dermatol Venereol Leprol* 2017; 83: 162–182.

2. Drapé JL, Idy-Peretti I, Goettmann S, Salon A, Abimelec P, Guérin-Surville H, Bittoun J. MR imaging of digital mucoid cysts. *Radiology* 1996; 200(2): 531–536.

3. Vandenberghe L, De Smet L. Subungual glomus tumours: A technical tip towards diagnosis on plain radiographs. *Acta Orthop Belg* 2010; 76(3): 396–397.

4. Wortsman X and Jemec GBE. Ultrasound imaging. In: Baran R, de Berker DAR., Holzberg M, Thomas L editors. *Baran & Dawber's, Diseases of the Nails and their Management*. 4th ed. Chichester, UK; Wiley-Blackwell (John Wiley & Sons), 2012. p. 132–153.

5. Peh WC, Shek TW, Ip WY. Growing wrist mass. *Ann Rheum Dis* 2001; 60(6): 550–553.

6. Sankar B, Ng BY, Hopgood P, Banks AJ. Subungual exostosis following toenail removal: Case report. *Int J Clin Pract Suppl* 2005; (147): 132–133.

7. Gupta S, Mittal A, Gupta S, Mahendra A, Dhull AK. Subungual exostosis of the thumb: First case report in youngest age. *Ind J Dermatol* 2009; 54: 46–48.

8. Feldman F. Primary bone tumors of the hand and carpus. *Hand Clin* 1987; 3: 269–289.

9. Besser E, Roessner A, Brug E, Erlemann R, Timm C, Grundmann E. Bone tumors of the hand. *Arch Orthop Trauma Surg* 1987; 106: 241–247.

10. Levy DW, Bonakdarpour A, Putong PB, Mesgarzadeh M, Betz RR. Subungual Keratoacanthoma. *Skeletal Radiol* 1985; 13: 287–290.

11. Richert B, Lecerf P, Caucanas M, André J. Nail tumors. *Clin Dermatol* 2013; 31: 602–617.

12. Yang Z, Xie L, Huang Y, Sun H, Yuan T, Ma X, Jing C, Liu P. Clinical features of malignant melanoma of the finger and therapeutic efficacies of different treatments. *Oncol Lett* 2011; 2(5): 811–815.

13. Jemec GB, Serup J. Ultrasound structure of the human nail plate. *Arch Dermatol* 1989; 125: 643–646.

14. Wortsman X, Holm EA, Gniadecka M, Wulf HC, Jemec GBE. Real time spatial compound imaging of skin lesions. *Skin Res Technol* 2004; 10: 23–31.

15. Wortsman X, Wortsman J. Clinical usefulness of variable frequency ultrasound in localized lesions of the skin. *J Am Acad Dermatol* 2010; 62: 247–256.

16. Wortsman X, Jemec GBE. Ultrasound imaging of nails. *Dermatol Clin* 2006; 24: 323–328.

17. Cecchini A, Montella A, Ena P, Meloni GB, Mazzarello V. Ultrasound anatomy of normal nails unit with 18 MHz linear transducer. *Ital J Anat Embryol* 2009; 114: 137–144.

18. Modani S, Shapiro J. Alopecia areata update. *J Am Acad Dermatol* 2000; 42: 549–566.

19. Tosti A, Morelli R, Bardazzi F, Peluso AM. Prevalence of nail abnormalities in children with alopecia areata. *Pediatr Dermatol* 1994; 112–115.

20. Baran R, Haneke E, Richert B. Pincer nails: Definition and surgical treatment. *Dermatol Surg* 2001; 27: 261–266.

21. De Berker DA, Richert B, Duhard E, Piraccini BM, André J, Baran R. Retronychia: Proximal ingrowing of the nail plate. *J Am Acad Dermatol* 2008; 58(6): 978–983.

22. Wortsman X, Wortsman J, Guerrero R, Soto R, Baran R. Anatomical changes in retronychia and onychomadesis detected using ultrasound. *Dermatol Surg* 2010; 36: 1615–1620.

23. Beck M, Wilkinson S. Disorders of nails: Median canaliform dystrophy. In: Burns T, Breathnach S, Cox N, Griffiths C, editors. *Rook's Textbook of Dermatology*. 7th ed. Oxford, UK: Blackwell Science; 2004. p. 54–55

24. Balestri R. et al. Natural history of isolated nail psoriasis and its role as a risk factor for the development of psoriatic arthritis: A single-centre cross-sectional study. *Br J Dermatol* 2017; 176(5): 1394–1397.

25. Wortsman X, Holm EA, Jemec GBE, Gniadecka M, Wulf H. [15 MHz high resolution ultrasound examination of psoriatic nails] (Spanish). *Rev Chil Rad* 2004; 10: 6–9.

26. Gutierrez M, Wortsman X, Filippucci E, de Angelis R, Filosa G, Grassi W. High-frequency sonography in the evaluation of psoriasis: Nail and skin involvement. *J Ultrasound Med* 2009; 28: 1569–1574.

27. Marina ME, Jid CB, Roman II, Mihu CM, Tătaru AD. Ultrasonography in psoriatic disease. *Med Ultrason* 2015; 17(3): 377–382.

28. Trueb RM. Hair and nail involvement in lupus erythematosus. *Clin Dermatol* 2004; 22: 139–147.

29. Wortsman X, Wortsman J, Soto R, Saavedra T, Honeyman J, Sazunic I, Corredoira Y. Benign tumors and pseudotumors of the nail: A novel application of sonography. *J Ultrasound Med* 201; 29: 803–816.

30. Dedhia A, Tambe S, Jadhav R, Bhatt K, Jerajani H. Unusual location of glomus tumour on the right ring finger. *J Cutan Aesthet Surg* 2014; 7: 179–181.

31. Baran R. Periungual lipoma, An unusual site. *J Dermatol Surg Oncol* 1984; 10: 32–33.

32. Bhatt KD, Fernandes R, Dhurat R. Ultrasound biomicroscopy of the skin to detect a subclinical neuroma of the proximal nail-fold. *Indian J Dermatol Venereol Leprol* 2006; 72: 60–62.

33. Teh J, Whiteley G. MRI of soft tissue masses of the hand and wrist. *Br J Radiol* 2007; 80: 47–63.

34. Soto R, Wortsman X, Corredoira Y. Onychomatricoma: Clinical and sonographic findings. *Arch Dermatol* 2009; 145: 1461–1462.

35. Middleton WD, Patel V, Teefey SA, Boyer MI. Giant cell tumors of the tendon sheath: Analysis of sonographic findings. *AJR Am J Roentgenol* 2004; 183(2): 337–339.

36. Santoro F, Sloan SB. Nail dystrophy and bony involvement in chronic sarcoidosis. *J Am Acad Dermatol* 2009; 60(6): 1050–1052.

37. Derchi LE, Balconi G, de Flaviis L, Oliva A, Rosso F. Sonographic appearance of hemangiomas of skeletal muscle. *J Ultrasound Med* 1989; 8: 263–267.

38. Maddison A, Tew K, Orell S. Intravenous lobular capillary haemangioma: Ultrasound and histology findings. *Australas Radiol* 2006; 50: 186–188.

39. Leppard B, Sanderson KV, Behan F. Subungual malignant melanoma: Difficulty in diagnosis. *BMJ* 1974; 1(5903): 310–312.

40. Cammarota T, Pinto F, Magliaro A, Sarno A. Current uses of diagnostic high-frequency US in dermatology. *Eur J Radiol* 1998; 27: S215–S223.

41. Lassau N, Spatz A, Avril MF, Tardivon A, Margulis A, Mamelle G, Vanel D, Leclere J. Value of high-frequency US for preoperative assessment of skin tumors. *Radiographics* 1997; 17: 1559–1565.

42. Ramos-Pascua LR, Guerra-Álvarez OA, Casas-Ramos P, Arias-Martín F. Giant cell tumor of the tendon sheaths of the fingers. *Reumatol Clin* 2015; 11(4): 252–254.

43. Theumann NH, Goettmann S, Le Viet D *et al.* Recurrent glomus tumors of fingertips: MR imaging evaluation. *Radiology* 2002; 223(1): 143–151.

44. Baek HJ, Lee SJ, Cho KH, Choo HJ, Lee SM, Lee YH, Suh KJ *et al.* Subungual tumors: Clinicopathologic correlation with US and MR imaging findings. *Radiographics* 2010; 30(6): 1621–1636.

7

Onychoscopy and nail fold capillaroscopy

DEEPAK JAKHAR AND ARCHANA SINGAL

INTRODUCTION

Onychoscopy refers to dermatoscopic assessment of the nail unit. It is a science of studying the nail and its diseases with the help of a handheld magnifying device known as a dermatoscope. Although unaided (naked) visual inspection can help us appreciate the gross morphological features like size, shape, contour, and color of the lesion, onychoscopy allows clinicians to visualize the subsurface characteristics of the nail lesions. In other words, onychoscopy serves as an interface between the visual and microscopic examination of the nail unit. In the past few years, onychoscopy has opened up an exciting front in the morphological evaluation of the nail by revealing structures and colors that are not visible to the naked eye.[1]

Initially utilized for the evaluation of nail pigmentation, onychoscopy is now increasingly being used as a diagnostic aid in the inflammatory and infectious onychopathies,[2] and significant progress has been made in defining the onychoscopic features of various nail tumors as well.

WHY ONYCHOSCOPY?

Evaluation of the nail and its diseases is generally based on a detailed clinical examination. However, the unique anatomy of the nail unit as well as lack of expertise among clinicians makes it challenging to accurately diagnose nail diseases. The investigative armamentarium is restricted to microbiological and histopathological examination. Microbiological examination as well as KOH and fungal culture lack sensitivity and specificity.[3,4] Nail biopsy is perceived as a painful procedure by patients, and there is often reluctance on the part of the treating dermatologist to perform the procedure. The lack of expertise among the pathologists in interpreting the nail histopathology further complicates the problem.[1]

Onychoscopy, being a non-invasive and office-based technique, offers a promising investigative tool. Short learning curve, cost-effectiveness, and reproducibility of the technique are distinct advantages. The onychoscopic pictures can be stored and utilized for future references.

INSTRUMENTS AND INTERFACE MEDIUM

Both contact and non-contact dermatoscopes can be used for examination of nail, but non-contact dermatoscopes provide higher magnification and resolution and minimize the risk of cross infections. Non-polarized light is better suited for the surface abnormalities, and polarized light penetrates deeper and provides a detailed evaluation of subsurface structures. It is important to realize that the two light sources complement each other.[1]

Different interface/immersion fluids can be used for onychoscopy, including mineral oil, distilled water, alcohol, or ultrasound gel, the last of which is better suited for nail examination because the gel's viscosity prevents it from rolling down the nail surface.[1-3] However, choice of interface medium is entirely operator dependent.

TECHNIQUE OF ONYCHOSCOPY

It is important to have a thorough knowledge of nail anatomy before performing onychoscopy (Figure 7.1). The exact area of the nail pathology needs to be identified on clinical examination. It is always good to start with a lower magnification (~10–20x) to get a global view of the nail unit and then move to higher magnification (~50–200x) for more details. Onychoscopy should be done first in non-polarized light to see surface changes followed by examination in polarized light that will allow appreciation of pigmentary and vascular changes in the lesion (dry onychoscopy) (Figure 7.2). An interface medium can be used for finer details (wet onychoscopy) (Figure 7.3).

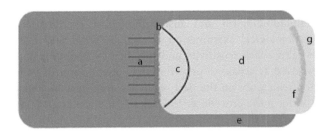

Figure 7.1 Different parts of nail unit. (a) Proximal nail fold with nail fold capillaries; (b) Cuticle; (c) Lunula; (d) Nail plate; (e) Lateral nail folds; (f) Onychodermal band; (g) Free edge of nail plate beneath which lies hyponychium. Two other important components of nail unit are nail matrix and nail bed.

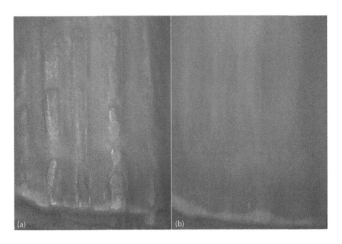

Figure 7.2 (a) Non-polarizing onychoscopy showing the surface changes of the nail plate; (b) Polarizing onychoscopy helps in better visualization of nail bed changes. (DermLite DL3-3Gen;10X.)

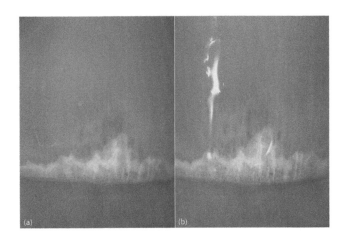

Figure 7.3 (a) Dry onychoscopy with polarizing light helps visualize the nail bed features; (b) Wet onychoscopy with polarizing light improves the delineation of these features. (DermLite DL3-3Gen;10X.)

ONYCHOSCOPY OF HEALTHY NAIL

The proximal nail fold shows regularly and evenly spaced hair-pin loop vessels (Figure 7.4). The cuticle perfectly adheres to the nail plate. Nail plate appears as shiny and translucent. The underlying pink color represents the nail bed and longitudinal capillaries can be visible in the distal nail bed just proximal to the sub-corneal band (Figure 7.5). Nail matrix can only be visible as lunula. The lateral nail fold and the hyponychium shows the normal ridge pattern.

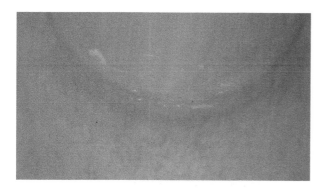

Figure 7.4 NFC of a healthy individual showing regularly and evenly spaced hair-pin loop vessels. (DermLite DL3-3Gen;10X.)

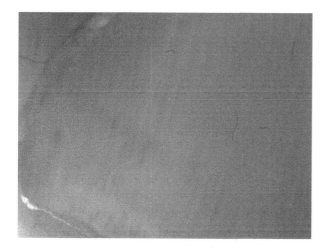

Figure 7.5 Pink color of the healthy nail bed. Note the nail bed capillaries proximal to the sub-corneal band. (DermLite DL3-3Gen;10X.)

INDICATIONS OF ONYCHOSCOPY

The common indications for onychoscopy have been summarized in Table 7.1.

Table 7.1 Indications of onychoscopy

A. Pigmentary conditions
- Melanonychia
  - Subungual hematoma
  - Benign melanonychia: melanocyte activation and proliferation
  - Malignant melanonychia
- Leukonychia
- Erythronychia
B. Inflammatory conditions
- Nail psoriasis
- Nail lichen planus
C. Infectious conditions
- Onychomycosis
- Periungual wart
D. Nail tumors
E. Nail fold capillaroscopy

PIGMENTARY CONDITIONS

Melanonychia

I. Onychoscopy has long been used to study longitudinal pigmentary bands (LPBs). There are well-documented onychoscopic features that differentiate benign LPB from malignant. An international study group on melanonychia published the first ever guidelines (2013) for the use of dermoscopy in the detection and management of nail pigmentation.[5] The group agreed that neither the contact nor the non-contact dermatoscope is superior to the other, and non-polarized and polarized lights are complementary to each other. The use of interface medium is dependent on the expertise of the clinician. The stepwise approach to the nail pigmentation is discussed in Figure 7.6.

II. Subungual hematoma: The most essential step while doing onychoscopy of nail pigmentation is to differentiate blood from melanin. A subungual hematoma is identified as globules of varying sizes, shapes, and colors with or without distal streaks (Figure 7.7). The color of the globules can range from bright red, brown, or black depending on the duration of hemorrhage. Presence of hemorrhage may be the first sign of underlying malignancy and hence does not rule out melanoma.

III. Benign melanonychia: Benign LPB can result from either melanocyte activation or proliferation. Onychoscopy is useful not only in differentiating benign from malignant, but also melanocyte activation from proliferation. A homogenous grey-colored band with thin longitudinal grey lines indicates melanocyte activation (ethnic or drug induced). Melanocyte proliferation as seen in a nevus shows presence of a brown background with regular arrangement of parallel lines. These parallel longitudinal lines are homogenous in color, spacing, thickness, and orientation (known as regular pattern) (Figure 7.8). The color and intensity of bands can vary depending upon the ethnicity, thickness of nail plate, and location of pigment with the nail plate.

IV. Malignant melanonychia: Malignant LPB shows irregular pattern indicated by longitudinal lines that are irregular in color, spacing, thickness, and parallelism. Melanoma may sometimes just show diffuse dark background with barely visible lines. In such a scenario, the variability in hues of pigmentation may indicate the possibility of melanoma. Analogous to the cutaneous melanomas, a diagnostic aid, ABCDEF rule, has been developed for nail melanomas (Table 7.2).

V. Hutchinson's sign: Periungual extension of brown-black pigmentation from longitudinal melanonychia onto the proximal and lateral nail folds is known as Hutchinson's sign and is an important indicator of

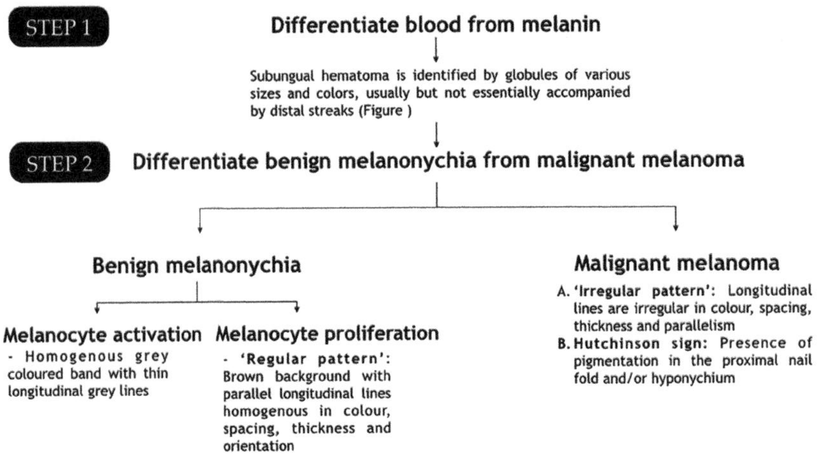

STEP 1 → **Differentiate blood from melanin**

Subungual hematoma is identified by globules of various sizes and colors, usually but not essentially accompanied by distal streaks (Figure)

STEP 2 → **Differentiate benign melanonychia from malignant melanoma**

Benign melanonychia

Melanocyte activation
- Homogenous grey coloured band with thin longitudinal grey lines

Melanocyte proliferation
- 'Regular pattern': Brown background with parallel longitudinal lines homogenous in colour, spacing, thickness and orientation

Malignant melanoma
A. 'Irregular pattern': Longitudinal lines are irregular in colour, spacing, thickness and parallelism
B. Hutchinson sign: Presence of pigmentation in the proximal nail fold and/or hyponychium

Figure 7.6 Stepwise approach to longitudinal melanonychia.

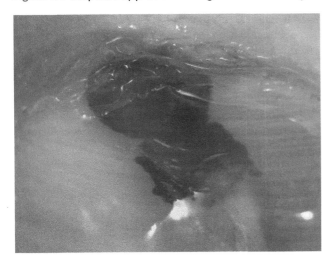

Figure 7.7 Subungual hematomas presenting as homogeneous areas of brown-black discoloration and showing characteristic round red spots/globules at the periphery representing fresh bleed. There is the peripheral fading of the pigmentation. (DermLite DL3-3Gen;10X.)

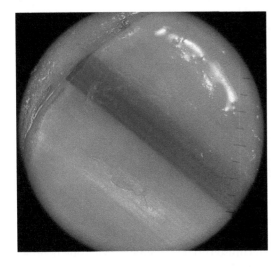

Figure 7.8 Benign melanonychia showing the presence of regular pattern characterized by parallel monochromic lines with uniform thickness. (DermLite DL3-3Gen;10X.)

Table 7.2 ABCDEF rule for nail melanoma

A – Age and race: most melanomas occur between 40–70 years of age. African Americans, native Americans, and Asians have higher percentage of ungual melanomas.

B – Brown to black longitudinal band in the nail; breadth > 3mm; border irregular or blurred

C – Change: rapid increase in width and growth rate. Nail dystrophy does not improve despite adequate treatment.

D – Digit: thumb>big toe>index finger; single digit involvement, two or more nails very rarely affected

E – Extension of pigmentation: Hutchinson's sign

F – Family or personal history of melanoma or so-called dysplastic nevi

subungual melanoma. However, it needs to be differentiated from pseudo-Hutchinson's sign where hyperpigmentation of the nail bed and nail matrix may reflect through the transparent nail folds.[6] An important point to remember is that though Hutchinson's sign is a valuable, though not infallible, predictor of melanoma, it can be seen in non-melanoma skin cancer like Bowen's disease of the nail unit. Ultimately, the diagnosis of subungual melanoma should be made histologically.

VI. Micro-Hutchinson's sign: Visibility on dermoscopy of a pigmentation of the periungual tissues that could not be seen with the naked eye.

VII. Onychoscopy of the distal nail plate also serves as a useful tool to determine the nail pigment origin. Presence of pigment band in the dorsal nail plate indicates its origin in the proximal nail matrix, whereas presence of pigment band in the ventral nail plate indicates its origin in the distal nail matrix. Presence of pigmentary band throughout whole thickness of the nail plate indicates origin of pigment from both proximal and distal matrix.

Leukonychia

White cloud-like structures in the nail plate denote punctate leukonychia (Figure 7.9). A transverse white streak originating from the lunula may be an early sign of Hailey–Hailey disease.[1-3]

Erythronychia

Longitudinal red-colored bands originating from the lunula on onychoscopy can be an indicator of onychopapilloma. Alternating red and white bands are seen in Darier's disease (Figure 7.10).[1-3]

INFLAMMATORY CONDITIONS

Nail psoriasis

Nail changes in psoriasis can be subtle and easily missed out on clinical examination. Various onychoscopic features of nail psoriasis are well documented and have markedly improved the diagnosis (Figures 7.11 through 7.14). The onychoscopic features depend upon the site of psoriatic pathology in the nail unit (Table 7.3).[7-15]

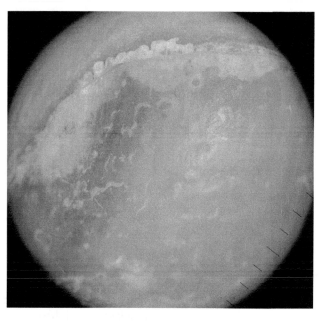

Figure 7.11 Non-polarizing onychoscopy showing the large irregular pits characteristic of psoriasis. (DermLite DL3-3Gen;20X.)

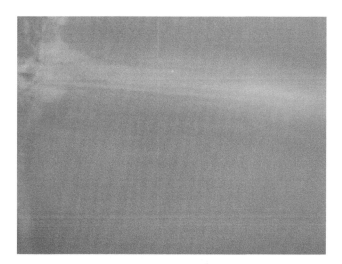

Figure 7.9 Longitudinal leukonychia. (DermLite DL3-3Gen;10X.)

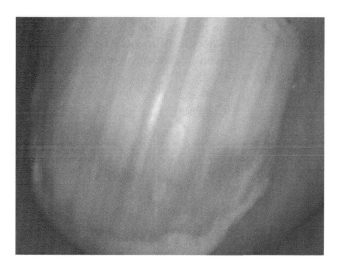

Figure 7.10 Longitudinal erythronychia alternating with longitudinal leukonychia in a case of Darier's disease. (DermLite DL3-3Gen;20X.)

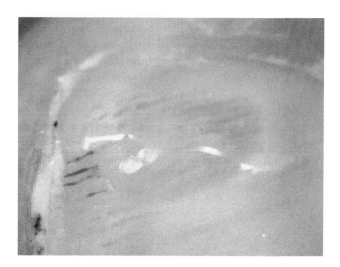

Figure 7.12 Salmon patch visible as orange-colored patch with adjacent longitudinal fusiform streaks characteristic of splinter hemorrhage. (DermLite DL3-3Gen;20X.)

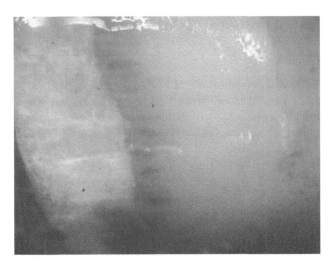

Figure 7.13 Onycholysis with characteristic proximal erythematous band. Also note the fusiform dilated nail bed vessels. (DermLite DL3-3Gen;20X.)

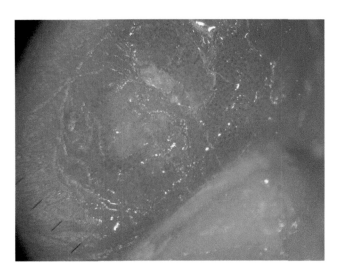

Figure 7.14 Dilated vessels in the hyponychium in a case of nail psoriasis. (DermLite DL3-3Gen;20X.)

Table 7.3 Onychoscopic features of nail psoriasis and nail lichen planus

Part of nail unit affected	Nail psoriasis	Nail lichen planus
Nail matrix	*Pits*: Large, deep, irregular depression *Leukonychia*: White irregular areas within the nail plate	*Pterygium*: Pink band with erythematous and whitish areas *Pits*: Multiple small depressions; sometimes giving rise to trachyonychia *Red lunula*
Nail bed	*Salmon patch*: Red-to-orange-colored patch with irregular size and shape *Splinter hemorrhage*: Longitudinal fusiform streaks of varying colors *Onycholysis*: Erythematous border proximal to the onycholytic band *Nail bed vessels*: Fusiform vessels proximal to the onychodermal band *Nail bed hyperkeratosis*	*Chromonychia*: Multiple-colored appearance of the nail *Splinter hemorrhage* *Nail fragmentation* *Subungual keratosis* *Longitudinal streaks* *Onycholysis*
Nail folds	Regularly distributed glomerular dilated capillaries may be seen in periungual lesion.	Erythema with Wickham's striae may be seen on periungual lesion.
Hyponychium	Dilated tortuous capillaries may correlate with the disease activity.	—
Proximal nail fold capillaries	Mean capillary density is reduced and morphological alterations may be seen.	No changes

NAIL LICHEN PLANUS

Nail involvement is seen in 10% of the cases of lichen planus. Features (Figure 7.15) are based on the involvement of the part of nail unit (Table 7.2).[16–17]

DARIER'S DISEASE

Onychoscopy of nail involvement in Darier's disease shows "V"-shaped nicking and splitting of the nail plate (Figure 7.16). In addition, the alternating red and white bands and splinter hemorrhages can also be seen (Figure 7.17).

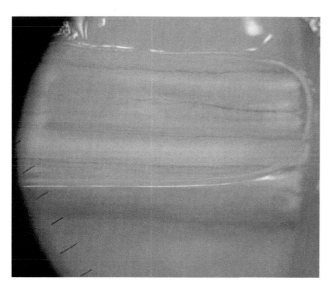

Figure 7.15 Nail lichen planus showing thinning and longitudinal fissures in the nail plate. (DermLite DL3-3Gen;10X.)

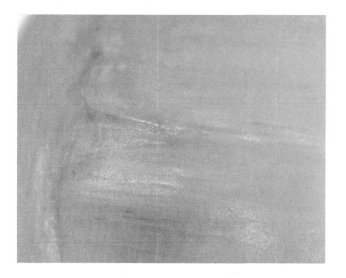

Figure 7.16 Nail involvement in Darier's disease showing the characteristic distal "V"-shaped nicking. (DermLite DL3-3Gen;10X.)

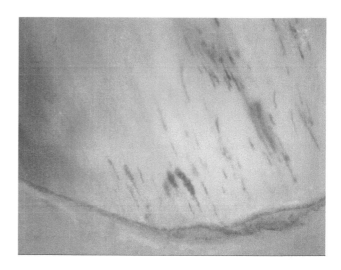

Figure 7.17 Longitudinal splinter hemorrhages in Darier's disease. (DermLite DL3-3Gen;10X.)

INFECTIONS

Onychomycosis

> **BOX 7.1: Onychoscopic features of onychomycosis**
>
> Characteristic onychoscopic features of onychomycosis
>
> - Onycholysis with jagged edges and spikes
> - Aurora Borealis
> - Ruin pattern
> - Distal irregular termination
> - Fungal melanonychia
> - Dermatophytoma

The typical onychoscopic features of onychomycosis include (Box 7.1):[18–22]

- *Onycholysis with jagged edges and spikes*: The proximal end of the onycholytic band shows presence of jagged edges and spikes corresponding to the fungal invasion of the nail plate (Figure 7.18).
- *Aurora Borealis*: Onychoscopic appearance of different colors in the onycholytic nail plate (Figure 7.19a and b)
- *Ruin pattern*: Indented areas on the subungual keratosis and distal pulverization (Figure 7.20)
- *Fungal melanonychia*: It appears as black to brown longitudinal or transverse band with presence of pigment clumps and/or granules within the bands.

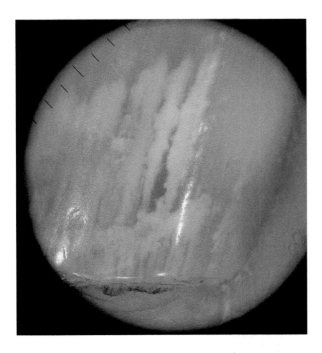

Figure 7.18 Longitudinal streaks with distal onycholysis in OM. (DermLite DL3-3Gen;20X.)

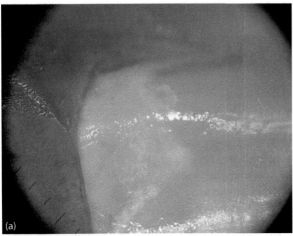

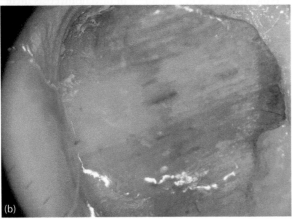

Figure 7.19 (a and b) Onycholysis with jagged spikes at the proximal end of onycholytic bands. Also note the different colors of jagged spikes corresponding to the "Aurora borealis" pattern. (DermLite DL3-3Gen;20X.)

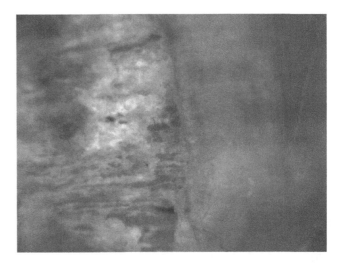

Figure 7.20 Distal onychoscopy showing the ruin pattern. (DermLite DL3-3Gen;20X.)

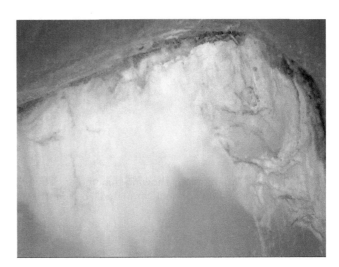

Figure 7.21 Onychoscopy of PSO showing distal jagged edges and spikes corresponding to the fungal invasion. (DermLite DL3-3Gen;10X.)

- Dermatophytoma: Round-shaped yellow-to-orange color patches in the nail plate connected by a narrow channel to the distal nail plate
- Onychoscopy of proximal subungual onychomycosis (PSO) shows distal jagged edges and spikes corresponding to the invasion of the fungal elements from proximal to distal edge of the nail plate (Figure 7.21).
- Onychoscopic differentiation of onycholysis and subungual hyperkeratosis is shown in Figures 7.22 and 7.23. Onychoscopy not only helps in the diagnosis of onychomycosis but also helps in locating the most proximal site for mycological sampling.[23]

PERIUNGUAL WARTS

Onychoscopy shows red to black dots on a hyperkeratotic lesion (Figure 7.24). These dots represent thrombosed vessels. An additional benefit of onychoscopy is that it helps locate the exact proximal extent of wart beneath the nail plate.[1-3]

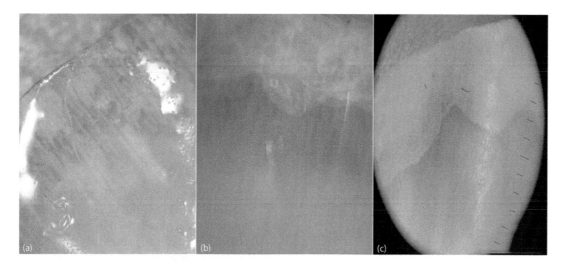

Figure 7.22 Different causes of onycholysis (a) Onychomycosis has jagged edges/spikes proximal to onycholytic band; (b) Psoriasis has an erythematous band proximal to a regular onycholytic band with dilated nail bed vessels; (c) Traumatic onycholysis is characterized by regular onycholytic band with absence of above described features. (DermLite DL3-3Gen;20X.)

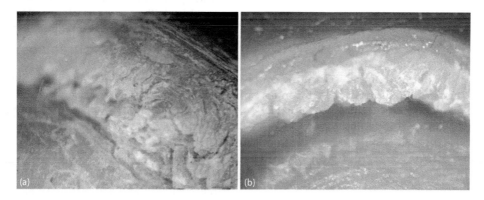

Figure 7.23 Distal end onychoscopy showing differences in subungual hyperkeratosis (a) Onychomycosis has a friable subungual hyperkeratosis, which ultimately leads to the "ruin pattern"; (b) Psoriasis has a compact subungual hyperkeratosis. (DermLite DL3-3Gen;20X.)

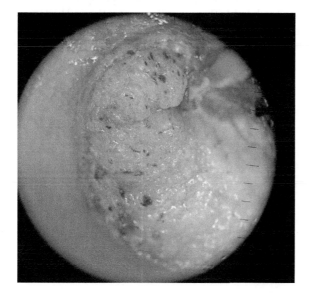

Figure 7.24 Red to brown dots suggestive of thrombosed vessels are characteristic of periungual warts. (DermLite DL3-3Gen;10X.)

TUMORS

Salient onychoscopic features of various nail tumors are discussed below.

Subungual glomus tumor

Glomus tumor is a benign vascular hamartoma arising from the modified smooth muscle cells of the glomus body. Onychoscopic features include:

- Irregular bluish patch with discrete linear vascular structures (Figure 7.25)[24]
- UV light dermoscopy: "Pink glow" indicating vascular nature of the tumor[25]
- Intraoperative onychoscopy: Ramified capillaries over a blue background. This is typically useful for determining the tumor margins as these ramified capillaries disappear abruptly at the margins.[26]

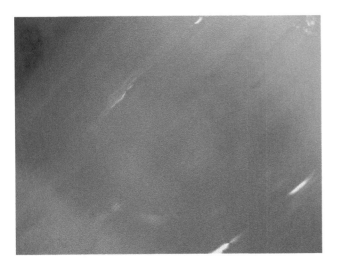

Figure 7.25 Subungual glomus tumor showing irregular bluish patch. (DermLite DL3-3Gen;20X.)

Digital myxoid cyst

When no pressure is applied while doing onychoscopy (non-contact dermoscopy), digital myxoid cyst shows vascular patterns in the form of linear, serpentine, or branched vessels. When pressure is applied (as in contact dermoscopy), the vascular pattern diminishes and only whitish-yellow translucent areas are visible.[3] Wet dermoscopy enhances the visualization of onychoscopic features (Figure 7.26a and b).

Onychopapilloma[27]

- Red bands originating from the lunula with or without splinter hemorrhages.
- Bands typically shows proximal convex border.
- Onychoscopy of the distal edge of nail plate shows a characteristic keratotic subungual mass.

Onychomatricoma[28]

- Parallel lateral edges
- Nail pitting
- Thickening of free edge
- Dark dots
- Splinter hemorrhages
- Longitudinal parallel white bands

Periungual Bowen's disease[1–3]

- White scales and diffusely distributed dotted vessels with whitish halo around these vessels
- The glomerular vessels seen in Bowen's disease at other body sites are typically absent.
- Periungual pigmentation (pseudo-Hutchinson's sign)

Digital fibrokeratoma

- Clumps of homogenous red lacunae divided by white meshwork like septal wall (Figure 7.27)[3]

Periungual pyogenic granuloma

- A reddish homogenous area with white rail lines[3]

"TRANSILLUMINATION DERMOSCOPY" OF THE NAIL[29]

Due to the high reflective nature of the nail plate as compared to the skin, much of the incident light on the nail plate is reflected back and hence the nail bed is not sufficiently illuminated. To overcome this issue, a new technique of performing dermoscopy in the nail, known as "transillumination dermoscopy," has been suggested. In this technique, the palmar/plantar aspect of the fingertip is illuminated with a torch light. This transilluminates the nail bed leading to better visualization of the nail bed pathologies on onychoscopy (Figure 7.28).[29]

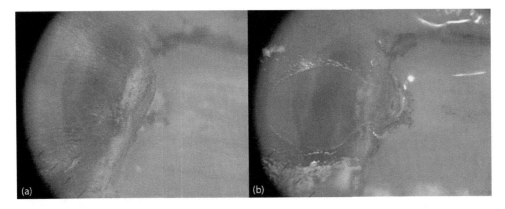

Figure 7.26 (a) Onychoscopy of digital myxoid cyst showing well-defined translucent brownish yellow semilunar area under the proximal nail fold; (b) Note the better delineation of features with wet dermoscopy. (DermLite DL3-3Gen;20X.)

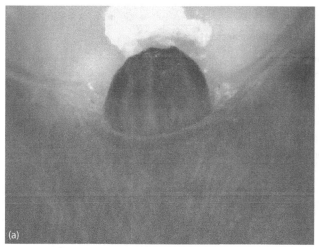
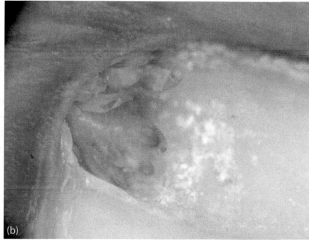

Figure 7.27 (**a** and **b**) Digital fibrokeratoma showing homogenous red lacunae with white meshwork. (DermLite DL3-3Gen;20X.)

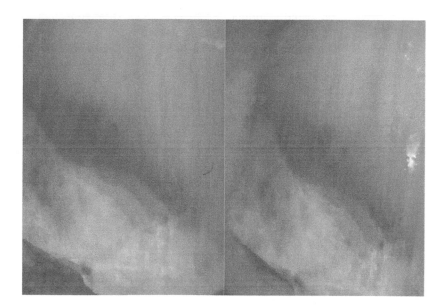

Figure 7.28 Transillumination dermoscopy of the nail. Note the better visualization of nail bed in the second picture. (DermLite DL3-3Gen;20X.)

NAIL FOLD CAPILLAROSCOPY

An *in vivo* assessment of the microcirculation plays an important role in the diagnosis and management of various connective tissue diseases (CTDs).[1–3] Nail fold capillaroscopy (NFC) is a non-invasive technique that helps in the quantitative and qualitative assessment of microcirculation. Quantitative and qualitative parameters recorded in NFC are shown in Table 7.4. Various NFC patterns are summarized in Table 7.5.[30] The role of NFC in systemic sclerosis (SSc) is well established and is now included in the diagnostic criteria of SSc. The level of evidence in other CTDs is still building up. NFC has also been used in systemic diseases like hypertension and diabetes mellitus.[3]

Systemic sclerosis

NFC has been extensively studied in the diagnosis and management of SSc. Three different patterns have been identified, indicating the severity of involvement:[31]

1. "*Early pattern*": Appearance of a few dilated and/or giant capillaries and a few hemorrhages. Capillary distribution is relatively preserved without loss of capillaries (Figure 7.29).
2. "*Active pattern*": Large numbers of giant capillaries, hemorrhages, a moderate loss of capillaries, slight derangement, and diffuse pericapillary edema can be found (Figure 7.30).

Table 7.4 Quantitative and qualitative parameters of NFC

Quantitative parameters	Qualitative parameters
• Capillary density • Capillary width • Capillary length • Capillary diameter • Apex width • Intercapillary distance	• Capillary dilation • Capillary drop out • Avascular area • Microhemorrhages • Capillary shape (bushy, meandering, branched, and tortuous) • Capillary orientation • Subpapillary venous plexus visibility

Table 7.5 Nail fold capillaroscopic patterns

Patterns	Density (capillary/mm)	Length (Microns)	Capillary shape	Capillary arrangement	Pathological hemorrhages
Normal	6–8/ mm	200–500	Hair pin	Parallel rows	−
Minor abnormalities	6–8/ mm	Elongated < 10%	Tortuous < 50%	Parallel rows	−
Major abnormalities	≤ 6–8/ mm	Elongated > 10%	Tortuous > 50%, enlarged meandering, branched	Disarrangement	−/+
Scleroderma pattern	< 6/mm	Elongated > 10%	Tortuous, branched, enlarged, bushy, giant	Disarrangement, with or without avascular area	++

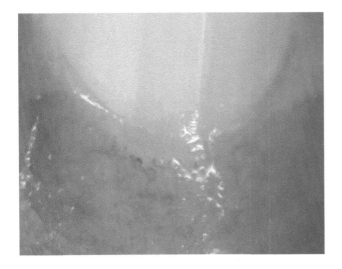

Figure 7.29 Nail fold capillaroscopy showing few dilated and tortuous vessels. (DermLite DL3-3Gen;20X.)

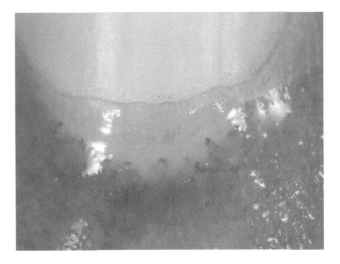

Figure 7.30 Large number of dilated vessels with structural alteration. There is moderate loss of capillaries. (DermLite DL3-3Gen;20X.)

3. *"Late pattern"*: Severe loss of capillaries with extensive avascular areas, bushy and ramified capillaries, or more than one capillary loop in a dermal papilla (Figure 7.31).

Other connective tissue diseases

NFC abnormalities in dermatomyositis have been defined by the presence of two or more capillary architectural changes in at least two nail folds. The changes include capillary loop enlargement, capillary loss, disorganization of the normal distribution of capillaries, "bushy" capillaries, twisted enlarged capillaries, and capillary hemorrhages.[32] NFC has also been studied in systemic lupus erythematosus, mixed CTD, rheumatoid arthritis, and Sjogren's syndrome. Though encouraging, the findings are still to be substantiated.

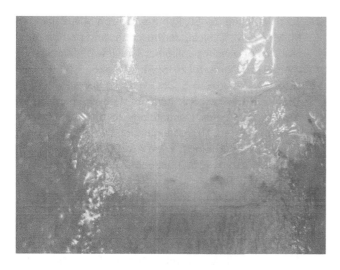

Figure 7.31 Severe loss of capillaries with avascular areas and giant capillaries. (DermLite DL3-3Gen;20X.)

KEY POINTS

- Nail dermoscopy, also known as "onychoscopy," is a very useful technique for the diagnosis and follow-up of numerous nail diseases.
- It is a rapid and noninvasive tool that permits us to recognize morphological structures that are not visible to the naked eye.
- Onychoscopy has a short learning curve.
- The utility of onychoscopy is not limited to pigmentary disorders of the nail unit but has been expanded to inflammatory and infectious disorders and tumors as well.
- NFC has a significant role in the diagnosis and management of CTDs and to assess microcirculation in patients with diabetes mellitus.

REFERENCES

1. Singal A, Jakhar D. Onychoscopy: An overview. *Int J Dermoscop* 2017; 1(2): 41–49.
2. Grover C, Jakhar D. Onychoscopy: A practical guide. *Indian J Dermatol Venereol Leprol* 2017; 83: 536–549.
3. Grover C, Jakhar D. Diagnostic utility of onychoscopy: Review of literature. *Indian J Dermatopathol Diagn Dermatol* 2017; 4: 31–40.
4. Shenoy MM, Teerthanath S, Karnaker VK, Girisha BS, Krishna Prasad MS, Pinto J. Comparison of potassium hydroxide mount and mycological culture with histopathologic examination using periodic acid-Schiff staining of the nail clippings in the diagnosis of onychomycosis. *Indian J Dermatol Venereol Leprol* 2008; 74: 226–229.
5. Di Chiacchio ND, Farias DC, Piraccini BM, Hirata SH, Richert B, Zaiac M et al. Consensus on melanonychia nail plate dermoscopy. *An Bras Dermatol* 2013; 88: 309–313.
6. Baran R, Kechijian P. Hutchinson's sign: A reappraisal. *J Am Acad Dermatol* 1996; 34(1): 87–90.
7. Farias DC, Tosti A, Chiacchio ND, Hirata SH. Dermoscopy in nail psoriasis. *An Bras Dermatol* 2010; 85: 101–103.
8. Yadav TA, Khopkar US. Dermoscopy to detect signs of subclinical nail involvement in chronic plaque psoriasis: A study of 68 patients. *Indian J Dermatol* 2015; 60: 272–275.
9. Yorulmaz A, Artuz F. A study of dermoscopic features of nail psoriasis. *Postepy Dermatol Alergol* 2017; 34: 28–35.
10. Ohtsuka T, Yamakage A, Miyachi Y. Statistical definition of nail fold capillary pattern in patients with psoriasis. *Int J Dermatol* 1994; 33: 779–782.
11. Zaric D, Clemmensen OJ, Worm AM, Stahl D. Capillary microscopy of the nail fold in patients with psoriasis and psoriatic arthritis. *Dermatologica* 1982; 164: 10–14.
12. Bhushan M, Moore T, Herrick AL, Griffiths CE. Nail fold video capillaroscopy in psoriasis. *Br J Dermatol* 2000; 142: 1171–1176.
13. Ribeiro CF, Siqueira EB, Holler AP, Fabr Hol L, Skare TL. Periungual capillaroscopy in psoriasis. *An Bras Dermatol* 2012; 87: 550–553.
14. Iorizzo M, Dahdah M, Vincenzi C, Tosti A. Videodermoscopy of the hyponychium in nail bed psoriasis. *J Am Acad Dermatol* 2008; 58: 714–715.
15. Elfar NN, Abdel-Latif AM, Labeh EA. Role of onychoscopy in differentiation between distal subungual onychomycosis, psoriasis, and traumatic onycholysis. *J Egypt Womens Dermatol Soc* 2015; 12: 145–149.
16. Nakamura R, Broce AA, Palencia DP, Ortiz NI, Leverone A. Dermatoscopy of nail lichen planus. *Int J Dermatol* 2013; 52: 684–687.
17. Friedman P, Sabban EC, Marcucci C, Peralta R, Cabo H. Dermoscopic findings in different clinical variants of lichen planus. Is dermoscopy useful? *Dermatol Pract Concept* 2015; 5: 51–55.
18. Piraccini BM, Balestri R, Starace M, Rech G. Nail digital dermoscopy (onychoscopy) in the diagnosis of onychomycosis. *J Eur Acad Dermatol Venereol* 2013; 27: 509–513.
19. Jesús-Silva MA, Fernández-Martínez R, Roldán-Marín R, Arenas R. Dermoscopic patterns in patients with a clinical diagnosis of onychomycosis-results of a prospective study including data of potassium hydroxide (KOH) and culture examination. *Dermatol Pract Concept* 2015; 5: 39–44.
20. De Crignis G, Valgas N, Rezende P, Leverone A, Nakamura R. Dermatoscopy of onychomycosis. *Int J Dermatol* 2014; 53: e97–e99.

21. Kilinc Karaarslan I, Acar A, Aytimur D, Akalin T, Ozdemir F. Dermoscopic features in fungal melanonychia. *Clin Exp Dermatol* 2015; 40: 271–278.

22. Jesus-Silva MA, Roldan-Marin R, Asz-Sigall D, Arenas R. Dermoscopy. In: Tosti A, Vlahovic T, Arenas R. (Eds) *Onychomycosis*. Springer; 2017 pp. 131–140.

23. Bet DL, Reis AL, Di Chiacchio N, Belda Junior W. Dermoscopy and onychomycosis: Guided nail abrasion for mycological samples. *An Bras Dermatol* 2015; 90: 904–906.

24. Duarte AF, Correia O, Barreiros H, Haneke E. Giant subungual glomus tumor: Clinical, dermoscopy, imagiologic and surgery details. *Dermatol Online J* 2016; 22. pii: 13030/qt66f7b8wt.

25. Thatte SS, Chikhalkar SB, Khopkar US. "Pink glow": A new sign for the diagnosis of glomus tumor on ultraviolet light dermoscopy. *Indian Dermatol Online J* 2015; 6 Suppl 1: S21–S23.

26. Rai AK. Role of intraoperative dermoscopy in excision of nail unit glomus tumor. *Indian Dermatol Online J* 2016; 7: 448–450.

27. Tosti A, Schneider SL, Ramirez-Quizon MN, Zaiac M, Miteva M. Clinical, dermoscopic, and pathologic features of onychopapilloma: A review of 47 cases. *J Am Acad Dermatol* 2016; 74: 521–526.

28. Lesort C, Debarbieux S, Duru G, Dalle S, Poulhalon N, Thomas L. Dermoscopic features of onychomatricoma: A study of 34 cases. *Dermatology* 2015; 231: 177–183.

29. Jakhar D, Kaur I. 'Transillumination Dermoscopy' for nail bed pathology. *J Am Acad Dermatol* 2017. pii: S0190–9622(17)32885–2. doi:10.1016/j.jaad.2017.12.045.

30. Ingegnoli F, Zeni S, Gerloni V, Fantini F. Capillaroscopic observations in childhood rheumatic diseases and healthy controls. *Clin Exp Rheumatol* 2005; 23(6): 905–911.

31. Cutolo M, Sulli A, Pizzorni C, Accardo S. Nail fold videocapillaroscopy assessment of microvascular damage in systemic sclerosis. *J Rheumatol* 2000; 27: 155–160.

32. Klyscz T, Bogenschnsc O, Js M, Rassner G. Microangiopathic changes and functional disorders of nail fold capillaries in dermatomyositis. *Hautarzt* 1996; 47: 289–293.

8

Basics of onychopathology

ECKART HANEKE

INTRODUCTION

The nail apparatus is a unique structure of the skin, but it is also called a musculoskeletal appendage due to its intimate spatial and functional relationship with the distal interphalangeal joint, tendons, and ligaments. Its manifold functions are related, and depend on, its normal anatomy. The nail unit is composed of epithelial and connective tissue components including bones and cartilage as well as the vessels and nerves supplying it.

There are a number of distinct specializations that permit many of these components to be differentiated even when only a part of the nail unit is contained in a slide of nail tissue (Table 8.1). Macroscopically, there are three nail folds, two lateral and one proximal, with special functions. The lateral nail folds give support for the nail and together with the proximal one form a frame, which is open only to the distal direction so as to allow growth of the free edge of the nail plate over the pulp of the finger or toe. The lateral nail folds are like rolls of connective tissue covered with thick acral epidermis without hair follicles and sebaceous glands but with sweat glands. Their connective tissue is constructed in a way that it can abut the lateral nail margin. Long-term irritation, e.g., in an ingrown toenail, may lead to swelling, inflammation, and finally fibrosis with thickening and sclerosis as the end stage. The proximal nail fold is a thin sheet of epidermis-covered connective tissue with a sharp angle at its free margin; it covers most of the matrix. On its dorsal surface, there are no pilo-sebaceous follicles but abundant eccrine sweat glands. Its ventral surface, which is devoid of all skin appendages, is covered with a thin epidermis without rete pegs and with a granular layer and orthokeratin, which is firmly attached to the underlying nail plate. When this grows out the horny layer is pulled out with the nail and forms most of the cuticle. This keratinous structure seals the nail pocket and prevents foreign substances, chemicals, and

Table 8.1 Specific features of the normal nail unit

Proximal nail fold, adjacent to joint	All skin appendages although less numerous hair follicles, except on toes of many men and dark-skinned women.
Proximal nail fold, distal portion	No hair follicles anymore, tendency to deep pigmentation close to the cuticle in dark-skinned persons. Free margin forms the cuticle.
Proximal nail fold, ventral surface	Thin epidermis without rete pegs, but granular layer and orthokeratosis. The keratin forms the bulk of the cuticle. No cutaneous appendages.
Matrix (Figure 8.1a–c)	Epithelium with basophilic basal compartment of several cell layers and eosinophilic superficial keratogenous compartment without a granular layer. Dermis relatively loose, no skin adnexae. Only few adipose cells in the most proximal part.
Nail bed (Figure 8.1d)	Unique epithelium without a granular layer the cells of which enlarge towards the superficial layer. Distal part develops thin granular layer that increases in thickness toward the hyponychium. Dermis very dense and without adipose cells. No adnexae.
Hyponychium (Figure 8.1e)	Circumscribed region with thick horny layer.

microorganisms from entering under the nail fold. In the depth of the nail pocket is the apical matrix that contains the nail stem cells. Here, the so-called true eponychium is formed by an extension of the matrix epithelium that is more similar to nail bed epithelium than to matrix itself, whereas the false eponycium is the product of most of the undersurface of the proximal nail fold epithelium.

The matrix is composed of a highly specialized connective tissue that has a strong morphogenetic potential and the matrix epithelium, which forms the nail plate. The latter is also morphologically unique with two compartments, the basophilic basal and the more eosinophilic superficial ones. The superficial compartment is divided into the prekeratogenous zone, which appears lighter in hematoxylin and eosin (H&E) stains, and the keratogenous zone that is intensely eosinophilic with the nuclei becoming darker and smaller until they disappear completely when the most superficial eosinophilic cells abruptly turn into empty-appearing nail plate cells with faintly stained cell walls that become more obvious in periodic acid-Schiff (PAS) stain demonstrating the glycocalyx of the onychocytes. In the proximal half of the matrix the epithelium is relatively thick but in the distal third it is gradually decreasing in thickness to reach its minimum height where it merges with the nail bed epithelium.

Under normal circumstances, the most superficial layers of the matrix epithelium overlap the thin nail bed epithelium. This is another epithelium without a granular layer. Its basal cells are relatively small and enlarge toward the uppermost layers until they keratinize similar to those of the catagen follicle cyst. They do not form a true nail plate as can be seen by the different staining characteristics, particularly when using Giemsa or Masson's trichrome. The distal portion of the nail bed epithelium develops a regular granular layer; this part is called the nail isthmus. It transits into the hyponychium, which is analogous to the cuticle sealing the virtual subungual space and permitting the nail plate to separate from the nail bed epithelium to which it is normally very firmly attached. The matrix dermis is comparatively loose in contrast to the firm nail bed dermis that does not contain any adipose cells. However, there are abundant blood vessels and glomus bodies as well as nerves in the matrix and nail bed dermis. The nail bed is unique in that it is the sole structure of the body to exhibit parallel rete ridges running from the matrix to the hyponychium. In the connective tissue ridges, three to five longitudinally running capillaries one above the other are found; they are thought to be the cause of the pink color of the nail bed.

The diagnostic gold standard for nail diseases is histopathology. However, there are a number of problems that both the clinician and the histopathologist have to face.[1]

- Good nail biopsies are often difficult to obtain.
- Most dermatologists, general practitioners, and surgeons, including hand and plastic surgeons, are not experienced in taking a nail biopsy.
- Even a technically optimal biopsy is useless if the correct site was missed.
- General pathologists and dermatopathologists rarely get a nail biopsy for evaluation; thus, they lack experience and are unsure about the microscopic nail changes they see under the microscope. Basic clinical knowledge is a must for nail pathologists.
- Most histopathology laboratories fear to get nail specimens as they are difficult to handle and section without tears, folds, and shattering; they require optimal equipment, years-long experience, and patience with each specimen.

Before embarking on nail histopathology, the macro- and microanatomy including some basic physiologic facts must be known. The matrix produces the nail plate (Figure 8.2); the superficial nail plate layer derives from the proximal or apical matrix, and the bulk of the nail plate is produced by the mid and distal matrix whereas the nail bed just adds a very thin layer of keratin that has different chemical and physical properties including its stainability. Thus, changes of the nail surface originate from the apical matrix, changes within the nail plate have their origin in the middle and distal matrix whereas those of the nail bed remain under the nail plate. This has to be known by both the surgeon taking the biopsy as well as the pathologist. The matrix and nail bed

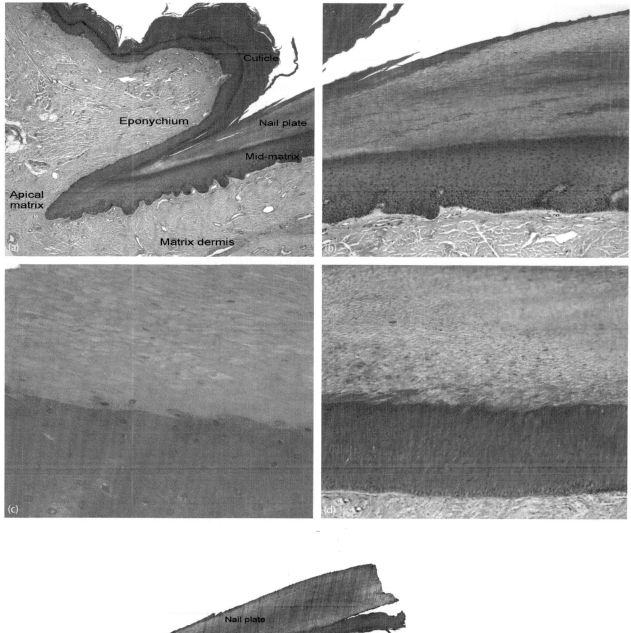

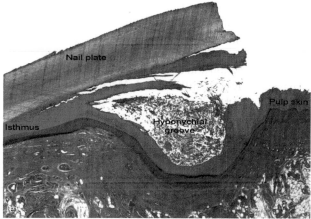

Figure 8.1 (a) Proximal portion of the nail unit with proximal nail fold, cuticle, and matrix; (b) Mid-matrix; (c) Mid-matrix; High power; (d) Nail bed; (e) Hyponychium.

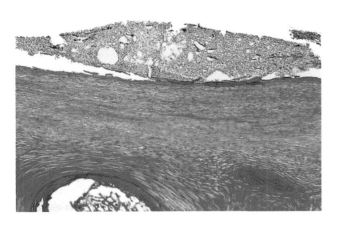

Figure 8.2 Nail plate with nail lacquer on top.

must never be confused or the terms be used interchangeably. The proximal nail fold overlies the matrix except for the halfmoon-shaped whitish area called lunula. The ventral surface of the proximal nail fold is firmly attached to the underlying nail plate. Its epidermis is thin, but keratinizes similar to epidermis with an orthokeratotic horny layer. As this is attached to the underlying nail it is pulled distally with the growing nail and finally appears at the free margin of the nail fold where it forms approximately 80% of the cuticle. It seals the nail pocket and prevents the entrance of foreign substances and microbes. Rounding up of the free margin of the nail fold, stop of nail growth as well as loss of attachment to the nail will cause disappearance of the cuticle as is seen in chronic paronychia or the yellow nail syndrome. The hyponychium is a specialized narrow area at the distal margin of the nail bed where the nail plate physiologically separates from it. The most distal portion of the nail bed just proximal of the hyponychium is called nail isthmus and often shows a granular layer. Both the matrix and the nail bed epithelium although very different biologically and morphologically have no granular layer; whenever this appears this is a sign of irritation and is pathological. The matrix epithelium has a mainly basophilic basal compartment consisting of basal and suprabasal cells that become pale and finally intensely eosinophilic when maturing in the prekeratogenous and keratogenous zones before finally abruptly turning into the nail plate, which is almost completely transparent under routine H&E stains. PAS stain reveals the glycocalyx of the nail plate and thus the cell borders. The matrix epithelium becomes thinner in distal direction until it obliquely overlaps the thinner nail bed epithelium.[1]

A normal fingernail grows approximately 0.1 mm per day with the nail of the longest finger of the dominant hand—in most cases the right middle fingernail—growing fastest. The shorter the fingers and toes the slower the nails grow. Toenails grow only one third the rate of fingernails. Whereas it takes about 6–9 months for a fingernail to grow out the nail of the big toe requires 18 months.[1]

PATIENT SELECTION FOR NAIL BIOPSIES

As in dermatopathology, many, but not all, diseases can be diagnosed histopathologically. Common complaints like brittle and soft nails have no characteristic microscopic changes. Most visible nail changes merit a biopsy; however, the correct site within the nail apparatus must be chosen.

Adequate informed consent is achieved. The patient is advised to bring an extra-large shoe in case of a toenail biopsy and to elevate the extremity for the following 24–48 hours. Except for nail plate biopsies—nail clippings—sterile conditions are a must. The surgeon has to be familiar with digital anesthesias. The patient is asked not to smoke before the biopsy and to wash and brush the digits prior to coming to the operation theater. Post-biopsy pain management and dressing changes are discussed beforehand as well as a potential sick leave.

BIOPSY TECHNIQUES[1]

Principally all different structures of the nail apparatus are amenable for diagnostic biopsies. Nail clippings give invaluable information in case of onychomycosis and can often rule out psoriasis, eczema, and alopecia areata. As much of the nail plate with its underlying keratin is clipped off and sent to the lab. No formalin fixation is necessary.

Punch biopsies are ideal for small lesions of the nail folds. Here, a 4 mm punch is usually sufficient. For nail bed lesions, two possibilities have to be considered: punch without or with prior nail avulsion. As nail bed lesions have no impact on the nail plate this is not needed for the histopathological diagnosis. However, very often parts of the nail bed epithelium remain attached to the avulsed nail. Matrix biopsies should not exceed a diameter of 3 mm.

Fusiform biopsies are performed longitudinally in the nail bed and transversally in the matrix. They are narrow spindles and in order to allow them to be sutured without tension.

Nail changes in lateral position are best biopsied using the lateral longitudinal nail biopsy as they yield the best specimens for the histopathology.

Melanocytic lesions of the nail matrix giving rise to melanonychia can be removed using the superficial tangential biopsy technique. This is also optimal for superficial nail bed lesions as well as combined matrix-nail bed lesions.

Submitting the biopsy specimen[1]

Depending on the size and thickness of the biopsy specimen it is either directly submerged in the container with 10% neutral formalin or gently stretched out on a small piece of filter paper before fixation, particularly if the specimen is a thin sheet of tissue from a tangential biopsy. Lateral longitudinal biopsy specimens are marked so that the median aspect of the specimen will be cut. When submitting the specimen on filter paper it is wise to place it on a drawing showing the exact localization of the lesion within the nail unit.

Softening, embedding, sectioning, and staining[1]

Specimens containing nail plate are notoriously difficult to cut, as the nail is very hard in contrast to the surrounding soft periungual tissue. Immersing the specimen into cedar wood oil for 3 days, in case of very thick nails even longer, renders the nail much softer and easier to cut. It is processed and embedded as usual. 4–6-micron sections are cut and routinely stained with H&E and PAS as well as special stains if necessary. Fontana's silver stained is used for melanin demonstration, but non-specific silver deposits are quite frequent. Immunohistochemistry is performed as needed.

Reading nail slides[1]

In principle there are no differences between reading skin or nail slides. However, the nail reacts in a different way to irritation and a variety of stimuli, which have to be considered. Where parakeratosis is induced in the epidermis a granular layer and some keratinization are induced in the matrix and nail bed. Spongiosis may be seen in the nail where it normally does not occur in the skin, e.g., in nail lichen planus and psoriasis. Severe dense lymphocytic infiltrates may render the differential diagnosis between allergic contact dermatitis and nail lichen planus very difficult. Nail psoriasis and onychomycosis share many features and it is their relation and intensity including the demonstration of fungal elements that finally permits a correct diagnosis. Epithelial alterations of the matrix and nail bed remain visible for a long time whereas they are rapidly shed from the epidermis. Finally, pain although not visible in microscopic slides may be mentioned in the lab form and may be a sign of glomus tumor, keratoacanthoma, or neuroma.

The nail matrix normally contains melanocytes that are far more active in individuals of dark complexion. Matrix melanocytes outnumber nail bed ones. The differential staining with Fontana–Masson and melanocyte marker(s) may be necessary to distinguish between functional melanonychia including racial pigmentation and a lentigo or even melanoma. Obvious melanocytes in the nail bed are suspicious. The diagnosis of very early subungual melanoma can be extremely difficult and may require melanocyte marker studies.

New nail-specific tumors have been observed in recent years and their knowledge is essential for tumor diagnosis. Their terminology is somewhat confusing and requires a consensus discussion among nail pathologists.

CHEMISTRY OF THE NAIL

The nail is a plate of hard keratin overlying the distal dorsal tip of the digits.[2,3] It provides mechanical protection, is a most versatile tool, aids in manual dexterity, is a defense tool, and enhances the digital tips' extremely elaborate sensory functions. It provides counterpressure for the soft tissue of the big toe when, during gait, the whole-body weight that enhances 2.5 times by the forward thrust, is concentrated on the pulp of the toe. When it is lacking or too short it is gradually dislocated dorsally to form a distal bulge. The nail substance consists of α-keratin intermediate filaments imbedded in a sulfur-rich amorphous matrix. The nail keratins belong both to the soft epithelial and the hard hair-nail keratins, which are classified into two groups according to their sequence homology: 11 type I or acidic and 9 type II or basic keratins.[4–6] Disulfide bonds link them to the 7–10 nm thick intermediate keratin filaments.[7] Keratin contains approximately 3% sulfur, 7% hydrogen, 14% oxygen, 15% nitrogen, 45% carbon,[8] and 8%–10% inorganic components. Sulfur and nitrogen occur predominantly in amino acids of the nail plate.[9,10] The water content is between 10% and 30% depending on ambient humidity.[11]

MACROSCOPIC ANATOMY RELEVANT FOR HISTOPATHOLOGY

Four epithelial components intimately linked to connective tissue structures make up the nail apparatus (Figure 8.1)[12,13]:

- The matrix, which forms the nail plate
- The nail bed, which firmly attaches the nail plate to the underlying dermis and terminal phalanx bone
- The hyponychium, which is the transition between the nail bed and the skin of the digital pulp
- The ventral surface of the proximal nail fold, which overlies most of the matrix and forms the true and the false eponychium with the cuticle at its distal margin

The connective tissue of the matrix and nail bed dermis are important for the differentiation of their epithelium. The dermis of the proximal and the paired lateral nail walls as well as the adjacent digital pulp dermis and hypodermis are specialized in the arrangement of their connective fibers. The ligaments and tendons of the distal interphalangeal joints are integral parts of the nail apparatus and indispensable for the nails' mechanical functions as a musculoskeletal appendage.[14,15] The flexor and extensor tendons not only insert at the volar and dorsal base of the terminal phalanx, respectively, but give lateral branches that form together with the lateral ligaments an aponeurosis and ensheath the entire distal interphalangeal joint. Fibers from the extensor tendon radiate into the proximal nail fold forming a holster for the matrix in between.[16,17] The nail apparatus is attached to the underlying terminal phalanx, which greatly determines the shape and size of the nail organ.[18] The distance between the apex of the matrix and the extensor tendon insertion is between 1 and 1.4 mm.[19–21] The extensor hallucis longus tendon inserts all along the dorsal surface of the bone from the base to the tip of the distal phalanx and is thus in between the matrix and the bone.[22]

The proximal nail fold has a concave free margin and the cuticle at its end. The whitish lunula is the most distal portion of the matrix, which is normally only seen in the thumb, index, and middle fingers as well as the big toe, but may be made visible by manicuring such as pushing the cuticle and the proximal nail fold back. A long proximal nail fold protects the underlying matrix from trauma and irritation.[23] The lunula appears when the nail fold is pushed back, which is apparently more attractive for many people, but it often leads to transverse ridges and furrows. Loss of nail shine and median canaliform dystrophy of Heller may develop. The visible pink nail portion is the nail bed. Its color is thought to be the result of the unique arrangement of its rete ridges and its capillaries. The most distal portion of the nail bed is the onychodermal band, which is about 1–1.5 mm wide.[24] Magnification reveals further details: a proximal pink portion, a central white band, and a distal pink zone.[25] Distal of the onychodermal band is the hyponychium, which lies under the free nail margin and is bordered by the distal groove demarcating the transition to the digital pulp skin.

The nail plate has parallel proximal and distal margins, being convex in distal direction and straight laterally. It is gently curved in longitudinal and more markedly curved in transverse direction. The transverse curvature is defined by the shape of the distal phalanx; the longitudinal one is due to the faster proliferation rate of the proximal as compared to the distal matrix. The nail plate develops characteristic longitudinal ridges, increasing and intensifying with age. They even allow monozygotic twins to be distinguished.[26]

NORMAL MICROSCOPIC ANATOMY OF THE NAIL

The macroscopically different parts of the nail unit have their characteristic microscopic appearance, and this may vary in disease. The normal microscopic anatomy of the nail is the basis to evaluate pathological alterations.

Nail matrix

The matrix produces the nail plate. Its visible part is the lunula, which is microscopically identical with the major portion covered by the proximal nail fold. More than 80% of the nail cells are produced by the proximal 50% of the matrix.[27] The matrix has a specialized epithelium with a basal compartment, which is basophilic, and a superficial eosinophilic compartment. The latter remains adherent to the nail plate when this is avulsed. The basal cells are slightly elongated changing to a cuboid shape and later enlarging and flattening in the higher epithelial layers while becoming more eosinophilic. The mid-layer is usually lighter with more pronounced cell walls, which then transits to the uniformly eosinophilic keratogenous or "onychotization" zone. The cell nuclei become smaller and darker and disappear when the eosinophilic superficial cells abruptly turn into nail cells (onychocytes), which appear light in normal H&E-stained sections. There is no granular layer. Often some nuclear remnants remain visible; they are called pertinax bodies.[14] The central matrix has the thickest epithelium.

A PAS stain shows the glycocalyx of the onychocytes, which is barely visible in H&E sections. The so-called dorsal matrix is still a matter of debate. There is a tiny portion of the most proximal part of the proximal nail fold's ventral surface that is similar to the adjacent matrix epithelium in its staining and keratinization pattern. However, on high magnification it can be seen that these cells are different at their border to the underlying nail as compared with the true onychotizing matrix cells and rather resemble nail bed cells. They give rise to the so-called true eponychium. The distal border of the matrix epithelium is thin and appears to overlie the basal layer of the most proximal nail bed in an oblique manner. The matrix expresses cytokeratins 1, 5, 10, and 14 as well as the hard keratin hHa1.[28,29] The upper two-thirds of the matrix epithelium are strongly positive for involucrin,[30,31] but matrix cells also express actin strongly in their cell membranes and weakly in the cytoplasms. Filaggrin is not present in normal nail matrix, neither immunohistochemically nor by electron microscopy.[32] The hair-nail keratin hHb5, but not its type II partner hHa5, is expressed in the keratogenous zone of matrix, where it is co-expressed with K5 and K17. The expression of hHa8 is seen in some cells of the keratogenous zone. When the matrix develops a granular layer under pathological conditions, keratins 1 and 10 are expressed.[32] Stem cells were either detected in the basal cell layer of the matrix adjacent to the nail bed or in the apical-dorsal matrix depending on the methods used.[33,34] Ultrastructurally, the basal compartment of the matrix epithelium is similar to normal epidermis[25,35-37] with many ribosomes and microfibrils that are arranged haphazardly in the basal compartment and become aligned along the nail growth axis in the transitional zone.

Nail bed

The nail bed has an epithelium of regular thickness when sectioned longitudinally, but has very pronounced slender rete ridges of equal length and in close vicinity on transverse cuts. The ridge pattern is unique as this is the only structure where longitudinal ridges run parallel to each other from the matrix to the hyponychium. In the papillary dermis ridges, longitudinally oriented capillaries run parallel to the nail plate and are arranged one above the other in 4–6 rows.[38,39] This particular pattern of capillary arrangement is responsible for the pink color of the nail bed and the reason of the splinter hemorrhages. The longitudinal nail bed ridges end at the hyponychium. The nail bed dermis contains no fat cells and is firmly anchored to the bone. There are many nerves and blood vessels including glomus bodies.

Glomus bodies are small, specialized organs occurring in great numbers in the nail bed and matrix dermis. In the nail bed, between 90–500 glomus bodies are found per mm³. They are encapsulated and have a diameter of about 0.3 mm. They consist of glomus cells and a tortuous vessel linking the arterial with the venous side of the circulation.

For thermoregulation they are arranged parallel to the capillaries.[40]

The nail bed epithelium is similar to the epithelium of the catagen follicle with small basal cells that gradually enlarge while migrating upwards and keratinize abruptly without forming a granular layer. Single cells may protrude into the orthokeratin layer formed by the nail bed epithelium. High magnification reveals that these uppermost cells have very fine indentations that anchor the nail bed cells to the subungual keratin. Immunohistochemistry of the nail bed epithelium shows K6, K16, and K17 and no hard nail keratins.[37] Under normal circumstances, only about 1% of the nail bed cells are labeled with antibodies to proliferation markers such as Ki-67, but this may rise to nearly 30% in nail bed psoriasis and onychomycosis.[32] Electron microscopy shows interdigitations of the uppermost nail bed cells with the overlying nail plate.[80]

Hyponychium

The hyponychium area comprises the onychodermal band until the distal ridge. It allows the nail to physiologically dissolve from the nail bed without leaving a space or onycholysis. The overhanging free nail margin forms a crevice that may harbor both dirt as well as microorganisms.[41] Recently, the proximal portion of the hyponychium was termed nail isthmus.[42–44] Keratins K5, K17 (basal), and K10 (suprabasal) are expressed in the orthokeratinizing eponychium and hyponychium,[37] but the presence of K17 is disputed.

Nail plate

The matrix produces the nail plate that consists of flattened onychocytes, which mostly contain keratin fibers. Under polarized light, they form continuous birefringent fibers. Their arrangement slightly pointing downwards distally allows the growth direction of a nail plate to be determined and also explains the split direction seen in a nail regrowing after a considerable trauma. In histological sections, the most superficial nail plate cells produced by the proximal matrix are the flattest and very densely packed. The height of the corneocytes increases with the depth of the nail plate from 2 μ to up to 15 μ.[80] The longitudinal ridges at the nail's undersurface are not seen on longitudinal sections but form prominent saw-tooth-like structures on transverse sections; this feature is even more pronounced in subungual hyperkeratosis. The dorsal surface of the nail plate is smooth in youngsters but tends to develop longitudinal ridging with age. The fingernail ridges can be best examined using polarized light.[45] Ultrasound suggests a lamellar structure of the nail plate with the superficial layer being dry and the deep compartment being humid.[46] The longer the matrix the thicker the nail plate will be. When the nail cannot grow forward, e.g., due to a distal nail bulge, it becomes thicker, more yellow, and loses its transparency. Histochemically,

the superficial layer of the nail is rich in phospholipids, sulfhydryl groups, and calcium, but the latter is mainly due to adsorption from the environment.[47] High acid phosphatase activity and many disulfide bonds characterize the intermediate layer.[48] Synchroton X-ray microdiffraction also shows a layered nail plate structure that gives the nail its high mechanical rigidity and hardness both in the growth direction as well as the curvature.[49] Scanning electron microscopy of cut surfaces in normal human nails have confirmed that the plastic intermediate nail plate supports the hard dorsal nail plate.[50–52] Transmission electron microscopy shows well-developed cell membranes and intercellular junctions, ampullar dilatations, and anchoring knots. Complete desmosomes are no longer seen[79] but so-called spot desmosomes may be present.[53] The dorsal nail cells are flatter and become gradually thicker toward the deeper layers. At the junction of the nail plate with the subungual keratinocytes of the nail plate, there are many interdigitations firmly anchoring them to each other.[54] The nail plate contains both nuclear and mitochondrial DNA fragments. They are considerably shorter than those of living cells as it is the nail matrix's function to produce large amounts of protein, the keratins. Nuclear fragmentation is complete in the fully matured onychocytes.[55] The nail plate completely blocks ultraviolet B light and only allows a minimum of UV A light, around 0.6%–2.4% (mean 1.65%), to penetrate.[56]

Nail folds

The nail folds are like a frame on three sides of the nail, giving it strong support. The distal nail margin remains free and is used as a versatile tool. The lateral nail folds are connective tissue rolls covered with skin. Hair follicles and sebaceous glands are absent. There may be more hyperkeratosis in the depth of the nail groove; however, this depends on the digit, the shape of the nail, and where the histological section was taken from. The proximal nail fold covers the matrix and only in some digits is the lunula as the most distal part of the matrix visible.[57] It is made up of three compartments. The dorsal aspect is transitory skin with unremarkable epidermis except that there are no pilosebaceous follicles. Its free margin forms the cuticle, which is an extension of the horny layer of the dorsal and the ventral skin of the proximal nail fold. It firmly adheres to the underlying nail plate sealing the nail pocket or cul-de-sac. For a proper cuticle formation, the nail must grow thus pulling the stratum corneum of the ventral surface of the proximal nail fold out, and the free margin of the proximal nail fold must have an acute angle. When it rounds up as in (chronic) paronychia or when the nail stops growing as seen in the yellow nail syndrome, the cuticle disappears spontaneously. The undersurface of the proximal nail fold is covered by a flat epidermis with a well-developed stratum granulosum. The distal two thirds produce the so-called false eponychium, which continues into the cuticle whereas the proximal third gives rise to the true eponychium, which remains adherent to the underlying nail plate also after routine histological processing. The integrity of the proximal nail fold is important for a healthy nail. The proximal nail fold is assumed to have five different functions:

- The dorsal matrix was recently found to harbor the nail stem cells.
- The dorsal matrix may contribute to the nail plate, particularly to the shiny dorsal surface.
- As it is overlying the matrix it may be responsible for the nail growing out and not up.
- Nail fold capillaries exert patterns more or less specific for certain diseases, which can be reproduced by nail fold capillary microscopy.
- A diseased or traumatized nail fold may profoundly alter the clinical appearance of the nail plate.

Immunology of the nail

The nail, and in particular the matrix, is a site of relative immune privilege.[58] Human leukocyte antigen A, B, and C expression is significantly downregulated in the keratinocytes and melanocytes of the proximal matrix whereas it is strongly positive in the periungual epidermis as is β_2-microglobulin. Few CD8+ lymphocytes are present in the nail fold and hyponychium and they are even less frequent in the matrix. Langerhans cells in the nail bed and hyponychium are similar to epidermis,[59] but are very rare in the proximal matrix. Mast cells and NK cells as markers of innate immunity are scarce in the matrix. The nail apparatus is assumed to share part of its embryonal and evolutionary origin as well as many structural and functional features with the hair follicle.[60,61] Examination of defined compartments of the nail apparatus demonstrated a down-regulation of MHC class I as a key feature of immuno-privileged tissue sites[98,99,102] also in the nail matrix epithelium, and most prominently the proximal nail matrix compared to the proximal nail fold, nail bed, and hyponychium. HLA-G a non-classical HLA molecule that is able to downregulate natural killer and CD8+ cytotoxic cells, suppresses NK cell activity against HLA negative cells and is important to establish fetal immune tolerance,[62] is upregulated in the nail matrix.[94] The matrix also produces immunosuppressive factors. The relative immune privilege may explain the therapeutic problems of a variety of nail infections, such as ungual warts and onychomycoses.

Melanocytes of the nail unit

The normal nail matrix contains up to 300 melanocytes per mm².[63,64] They are mostly dormant in fair-skinned persons whereas in deeply pigmented individuals they usually produce enough melanin to cause physiological nail pigmentation. They are much more numerous in the matrix than in the nail bed[65–67] and more active in the distal than in the proximal matrix. In the proximal matrix,

the quiescent melanocytes are DOPA negative and cannot synthesize melanin under normal conditions, but they can be demonstrated by monoclonal antibodies to tyrosine-related protein 1. Immunohistochemical studies showed a melanocyte density of 237/mm² in the matrix, which is far lower than in the epidermis. Most matrix melanocytes are found in suprabasal position, which is an important normal finding in respect to exclude or confirm melanocytic dysplasia.[68] Matrix melanocytes, like fetal melanocytes and melanoma cells, are normally positive for HMB45, another potentially confusing fact. The matrix melanocytes are HLA negative, those in the nail bed and proximal nail fold are strongly HLA positive. Collapse of this immune privilege may expose matrix melanocytes to autoimmune attacks and provoke nail matrix involvement in alopecia areata. Matrix melanocytes are strongly decorated with antibodies like MelanA and HMB45, they often do not or only weakly stain with protein S100, Sox10, and MITF antibodies.[69] Melanocytes are much less numerous in the nail bed or not even demonstrable with immunohistochemical techniques. They retain their distribution in the basal layer. In light-skinned individuals, no melanin is normally seen in the plate. However, when present it derives from matrix melanocytes and is seen as melanin granules. This is a normal phenomenon in darkly pigmented individuals, in whom the presence of melanin pigmentation increases with age.[70,71] Ten to twenty percent of Japanese individuals develop longitudinal melanonychia.[72] Melanin is seen as light brown round granules and stains dark with Fontana–Masson's argentaffin reaction. In contrast, most fungal melanins are soluble and stain the nail diffuse light yellow; in our experience they are not argentaffin positive.

Merkel cells in the nail

Merkel cells are positive for keratins 8 and 20. They were found in the adult nail matrix[73] and in infantile accessory digits.[29]

Blood supply of the nail apparatus[1]

The microscopy of nail blood supply shows many arteries in the nail bed and matrix dermis. Some blood vessels with thin to medium-thick walls have a cushion-like thickening of smooth muscle cells in one circumscribed area, usually in direct relation to the normal muscular layer or directly next to it. The function of these muscle pads is not known, but may have to do something with thermoregulation in analogy to the glomus bodies.[1]

Innervation of the nail

The innervation of the nail unit is very rich. The nail considerably contributes to tactile sensation[74] and sensibility.[75] About 3000 endoneurial tubes enter the pulp of the index finger.[76] Vater–Pacini bodies and Meissner bodies are usually seen directly around the nail unit.

HISTOPATHOLOGY OF CHARACTERISTIC INFLAMMATORY NAIL DISEASES[1]

Many inflammatory skin diseases also involve the nail. If skin lesions are present they may allow the clinical diagnosis to be made and a nail biopsy is not performed. This is the reason that the knowledge of specific nail changes in some inflammatory conditions is limited. It is risky to generalize nail histopathology from a few anecdotal descriptions.

Nail psoriasis

Nail involvement is most frequent in psoriasis. Isolated nail psoriasis is seen in 1%–5%.[77] Although the main histopathological criteria of cutaneous psoriasis also apply to the nail, some differences and features not seen in skin elsewhere are remarkable.[78] Psoriasis may affect any part of the nail.

Pits and whitish-to-ivory-colored spots are very characteristic for nail psoriasis. They are due to tiny psoriatic foci in the most proximal matrix. The apical matrix epithelium develops a slight spongiosis and parakeratosis, but neutrophil exocytosis is rare and may cause a slightly different aspect.[79] Pits are small, superficial depressions developing from parakeratotic mounds in the nail plate surface. They break out when the plate emerges from under the proximal nail fold. Parakeratosis remaining part of the nail plate is clinically seen as a small whitish-to-yellowish dot. The parakeratosis fills a shallow saucer-like depression. The more proximal the pit the more parakeratosis is usually still present.[80] A lesion in the middle of the matrix often causes a leukonychia.[81,82] This is either due to interspersed parakeratotic cells with leukocytes in the nail plate, or to orthokeratosis without leukocytes. Red spots in the lunula show spongiosis, parakeratosis, and leukocyte exocytosis. Salmon spots represent psoriatic plaques of the nail bed. The epithelium develops moderate acanthosis, spongiosis with mononuclear exocytosis and often a spotty granular layer. Parakeratosis forms obliquely-distally ascending columns. Leukocytes usually form Munro's micro abscesses, often in the summits of the parakeratotic mounds.[83] Subungual hyperkeratosis may be very marked and exhibits several layers of hyperkeratosis consisting mostly of parakeratosis with interspersed orthokeratosis. Pyknotic neutrophils are arranged in layers. PAS stain very clearly shows the neutrophils and is important for the differential diagnosis of subungual onychomycosis. Salmon or oil spots, subungual hyperkeratosis, and onycholysis are due to the same fundamental process, a subungual psoriasis lesion, which in case of onycholysis has reached the hyponychium. Subungual splinter hemorrhages are recognized as small intracorneal blood inclusions at the tip of a subungual keratosis directly under the nail plate.

Psoriasis of the proximal nail fold is identical to chronic cutaneous psoriasis. There is acanthosis with club-shaped or rectangular rete ridges, lack of the granular layer, and parakeratosis, but little leukocyte exocytosis. The capillaries are dilated and go high up to the thinned suprapapillary epidermal plate. When the free margin is involved it is rounded up and the cuticle is lost. Involvement of the undersurface of the proximal nail fold is commonly associated with slight to moderate spongiosis. When both the dorsal and the ventral surface are affected the clinical picture of chronic paronychia is seen, which is common in psoriatic arthritis of the distal interphalangeal joint.

Pustular psoriasis frequently involves the nail, both in the localized form of Barber–Königsbeck, in the generalized form of von Zumbusch, and above all in acrodermatitis continua suppurativa of Hallopeau. The latter was once thought to be a different entity but is now accepted as being a variant of pustular psoriasis with insidious onset and recalcitrant course finally leading to complete nail destruction. Histopathologically, Reiter's disease remains almost indistinguishable. Pustular psoriasis is characterized by the development of large spongiform pustules in the matrix and nail bed, often also in the periungual skin. These lakes of pus are seen as yellow spots under the nail plate. There is often considerable spongiosis. Particularly in acrodermatitis continua suppurativa, the nail becomes destroyed and a clinical diagnosis is difficult to be made. When a biopsy is taken at this time psoriatic alterations are still seen.

Acrodermatitis continua suppurativa has three histological appearances: the classical spongiform pustule, a spongiotic variant, and a mixed form with spongiform pustules and spongiosis. Spongiform pustule formation is very pronounced and leads to necrosis of the superficial layers of the nail bed and matrix epithelium, which may be the reason for the progressive and permanent nail atrophy.

In our opinion, palmar plantar pustulosis, also called pustular bacterid of Andrews,[84] is different from palmar plantar psoriasis, both clinically and histologically as well as immunogenetically.[85] Histopathologically, it is not characterized by spongiform pustules but has round-to-oval, well-circumscribed unilocular pustules with sometimes a spongiform shoulder.[86] Nail involvement is very rare.

Nail lesions of Reiter's disease are virtually identical to pustular psoriasis but there are more extravasated erythrocytes giving the lesions clinically a more brownish aspect, and the pits may be deep.[87] The nail fold may be swollen and red.[88]

The histological differential diagnosis comprises parakeratosis pustulosa of Hjorth, pityriasis rubra pilaris, acrokeratosis paraneoplastica of Bazex, crusted (Norwegian) scabies, some drug reactions, and above all onychomycosis, the exact histopathological diagnosis of which requires the demonstration of invasive fungi.

Eczema

The histological hallmarks are spongiosis, lymphocytic exocytosis, and spongiotic vesicles, but to a widely varying degree. Depending on the nail structure involved, the matrix, nail bed, proximal nail fold epidermis or hyponychium, and/or digital pulp become slightly acanthotic, the intercellular spaces of the epithelia widen, and the serum collections increase to form small spongiotic vesicles often with lymphocytes. When this happens in the nail matrix the plasma and lymphocytes are transported up through the keratogenous zone, which often disappears, and are included into the nail plate. A granular layer may develop in the matrix.[32] The nail becomes thicker, brittle, loses its transparency, and its surface loses its shine. Involvement of the most proximal matrix causes a superficial localization of these serum inclusions that break out of the nail and leave small depressions, the characteristic pits of nail eczema. This is also the mechanism how eczematous trachyonychia develops. Nail bed eczema leads to subungual hyperkeratosis that contains serum inclusions and lymphocytes. The hyperkeratosis is mostly orthokeratotic in contrast to skin.

Chronic allergic contact dermatitis of the matrix and nail demonstrates a very dense lichenoid lymphocytic epidermotropic infiltrate, particularly in patients with persistent allergen exposure as in sculptured nails. The matrix and nail bed may develop papillomatosis and a granular layer with irregular hyperorthokeratosis.

Chronic contact dermatitis of the hyponychium and the immediately adjacent pulp skin may lead to thick hyperkeratosis that is cracked and contains dried globules of plasma. When it is more rhagadiform, split-like fissures extend from the surface to the basal layer with eosinophilic homogenous necrosis of the keratinocytes neighboring it.

Nummular eczema is characterized by small red plaques on the proximal nail fold with tiny small papules topped with a minute serous crust. This may sometimes contain a few neutrophils.

Nails in atopic eczema are often shiny, but histologically no apparent changes are seen, although pits are occasionally present. Chronic rubbing may cause thickening of the epidermis with slight papillomatosis and hyperkeratosis as well as dense collagen in the upper dermis, features also seen in knuckle pads. Spongiotic trachyonychia in children is often an atopic manifestation.

Chronic paronychia causes thickening of the proximal nail fold with rounding up of its free margin and spontaneous loss of the cuticle. The eponychium is split off the nail. Spongiosis and spongiotic vesicles may be seen in the epidermis of both the dorsal and the ventral surface of the proximal nail fold. The fibrous tissue contains mainly perivascular lymphocytic infiltrates and a variable degree of fibrosis.

Alopecia areata

Alopecia areata is a relatively common autoimmune disorder thought to be due to the collapse of immune privilege of the hair and nail.[89] Association with other dermatological autoimmune disorders is common.[90,91] Nail involvement is frequent, correlates with the severity of alopecia areata,[92] and is said to be a sign of poor prognosis.[93] The nails in children are affected more frequently.[94,95] Alopecia areata of the nails can occur isolated without hair loss. Histopathologically, the nail demonstrates a spongiotic dermatitis with a

lymphocytic epitheliotropic infiltrate in the dermis of the matrix, spongiosis of the matrix epithelium, lymphocytic exocytosis, and often small spongiotic vesicles.[96] These are taken into the higher epithelial layers and finally included into the newly formed nails. This proteinaceous exudate is seen as homogenously stained, slightly eosinophilic, but PAS-positive inclusions in the nail plate and sometimes in the subungual keratin. They make the nail lose their shine and transparency and may also be responsible for the thickening and friability of the nail. The nail keratin arrangement is irregularly wavy with shallow surface depressions, which do not contain parakeratosis in contrast to psoriatic pits.[97–99] As the proximal matrix is more severely affected, the nail plate changes are more pronounced in the superficial layers. The clinical differential diagnosis comprises all conditions that may cause an irregular or rough nail surface, i.e., psoriasis, lichen planus, eczema, etc. Histologically, the spongiotic dermatitis may be indistinguishable from a mild to moderate eczematous dermatitis. This often shows involvement of the eponychium and nail folds, which is not seen in alopecia areata.[32,92]

Lichen planus of the nail

Approximately 10% of lichen planus patients have nail lesions.[100] Isolated nail lichen planus is observed in 1%–4%.[101–103] Nail involvement is also seen in lichen plano-pilaris.[104] It may cause twenty-nail dystrophy[105] and "idiopathic atrophy of the nails."[99,106,107] Thinning, longitudinal ridges, loss of nail shine, distal splitting, and trachyonychia are common in matrix lichen planus, whereas onycholysis and subungual hyperkeratosis are a sign of nail bed involvement. Pterygium formation highlights irreversible scarring of the matrix. Histopathology of nail lichen planus is usually typical and diagnostic.[106,108,109] The most common histological appearance of nail lichen planus is apical matrix involvement. There is a dense band-like epidermotropic lymphocytic infiltrate from the middle of the ventral surface of the proximal nail fold to the matrix and toward the nail bed. It causes marked hydropic degeneration of the basal cell layer, particularly of the proximal matrix, and a granular layer as well as orthohyperkeratosis instead of a normal nail plate. This is the reason for the longitudinal ridging and loss of nail shine as the proximal matrix is responsible for the latter. In dark-skinned persons, pigmentary incontinence as well as longitudinal melanonychia may develop.[110] This is often overlooked as it is not obvious in histological sections. When the more distal matrix and nail bed are involved subungual hyperkeratosis is a leading feature. The epidermotropic infiltrate that virtually eats up the epithelium causes progressive obliteration of the nail pocket until it is completely obstructed, resulting in a cicatricial pterygium. An even more severe matrix involvement may lead to ulcerative nail lichen planus.[111,112] Severe hydropic degeneration of the basal layer of the matrix and nail bed with a band-like lymphocytic infiltrate is seen in bullous lichen planus of the nail.[113] The irreversible scarring may be a result of the involvement of the most proximal to dorsal matrix where the nail stem cells were located.[34] Involvement of the skin of the proximal nail fold shows a thickened orthokeratotic horny layer with focal hypergranulosis. The rete ridges are saw-tooth like due to a dense lymphocytic epidermotropic infiltrate leading to vacuolar degeneration of the basal layer with a variable number of apoptotic cells. In contrast to skin, spongiosis is very often present and sometimes so pronounced that an eczema may be suspected. Differential diagnosis comprises lichen striatus, drug-induced lichenoid eruption with nail involvement, graft-versus-host disease, amyloidosis, disseminated lichenoid papular dermatosis with nail changes in AIDS,[114] a subungual tumor when only one nail is affected,[115] yellow nail syndrome,[115] and lichen sclerosus et atrophicans.[116] Post-lichen nail dystrophy is difficult to differentiate from nail dystrophy after Stevens–Johnson syndrome (SJS), Lyell syndrome, impaired peripheral circulation, radiodermatitis, after bacterial infections, bleomycin injection, and mechanical trauma to the matrix[117] as there are usually no diagnostic features anymore. Betablockers may induce lichenoid-psoriasiform changes.

Nail lichen striatus

Lichen striatus mainly affects children and adolescents, with about 3% of the cases showing nail involvement.[118] There may also be isolated nail involvement.[119,120] Usually, the disease clears spontaneously[121] with the nail lesions lagging behind, but nail plate alterations may persist for a period of several years.[122] It may be a manifestation of mosaicism characterized by the presence of genetically abnormal keratinocyte clones. Histopathology of lichen striatus exhibits a superficial perivascular lymphocytic infiltrate with some histiocytes. There is a focal band-like lymphocytic infiltrate with epidermotropism and some spongiosis of the proximal nail fold, the matrix, and the nail bed. The basal cell layer shows variable degrees of vacuolar degeneration and necrotic epidermal cells in the spinous layer. The matrix epithelium may show some apoptotic cells,[123] and there may also be focal parakeratosis. Immunohistochemically, the epidermotropic infiltrate was shown to be made up of CD8+ and CD7+ T lymphocytes.[124,125] The differentiation from ungual lichen planus is only possible in the context with the clinical picture.[126] The clinical differential diagnoses are linear lichen planus, lichenoid linear drug eruption,[127] linear epidermal nevus, inflammatory linear verrucous epidermal nevus (ILVEN),[128–130] and linear porokeratosis.[131] Histologically, mainly nail lichen planus has to be excluded, although rarely other interface dermatitides are considered.

Lichen nitidus

Lichen nitidus predominantly affects children and young adults with multiple, very small, flat-topped, mostly skin colored papules, sometimes occurring in groups but not coalescing. Nail involvement is mainly seen as longitudinal ridging, pitting, or fine rippling.[132,133] The nails tend to become fragile. Also, the proximal nail fold may develop small papules. Histopathology of lichen striatus of the nail fold shows small granulomas that are located in a dermal papilla, which becomes widened and finally gives the impression of the epidermal rete ridges embracing the granuloma. The granulomas consist of lymphocytes, histiocytes, and some giant cells. The overlying epidermis is thinned and parakeratotic. Often vacuolar changes of the basal layer and small areas of clefting are seen on top of the granuloma. Lesions in the matrix and nail bed mimic lichen planus with giant cells.[134] The histological differential diagnosis is lichen planus.

Erythema multiforme, Stevens–Johnson syndrome, and toxic epidermal necrolysis of Lyell

For practical reasons, erythema multiforme (EM), bullous erythema multiforme, SJS, and toxic epidermal necrolysis, also called Lyell's syndrome, are often regarded as pathogenetically similar diseases with increasing severity. EM is relatively common and self-limited with symmetrical round red lesions often evolving into typical target lesions with a central bulla. Bullous EM is a more severe yet localized form. SJS is a severe disease with more extensive skin and mucous membrane involvement, fever, and malaise. Toxic epidermal necrolysis involves more than 30% of the body surface. It is characterized by full-thickness epidermal necrosis. SJS/toxic epidermolysis overlap is when between 10% and 30% of the body surface are affected. The most common causes are drugs (allergic EM, SJS, or TEN),[135,136] recurrent herpes simplex (postherpetic EM, SJS, or TEN), and infections (postinfectious EM, SJS, or TEN). Nail involvement in EM and SJS is usually seen as blisters whereas in TEN the surrounding skin is denuded. The nail may fall out[137] and dystrophic nails may regrow[138] or the entire nail organ may be degloved.[139] Particularly after TEN, the nail loss may lead to permanent scarring, pterygium formation, and cicatricial anonychia.[140,141,159] The histopathology of EM depends on the structure involved. The most common localization is periungual skin. The hallmark is a vacuolar interface dermatitis. In the early phase, the basal cells appear vacuolar through lymphocytes that are aligned at the dermo-epidermal junction. There are mild spongiosis in the lower epidermis and a sparse superficial perivascular infiltrate. Some papillary edema and often extravasated erythrocytes are found. Necrotic keratinocytes are present. The stratum corneum is usually orthokeratotic as the process is acute. With time, the infiltrate becomes more lichenoid band-like with more apoptotic cells both in the infiltrate as well as the epidermis. In pronounced cases, the epidermis splits from the dermis and a bulla is formed. The blister roof may become completely necrotic. The SJS/TEN overlap syndrome shows more necrotic keratinocytes, increasing in number until focal full-thickness epidermal necrosis. TEN exhibits extensive full-thickness epidermal necrosis almost without an inflammatory infiltrate. A quick diagnosis from the blister roof: full-thickness necrotic epidermis is in favor of TEN whereas when only horny layer is seen with a few neutrophils this hints at staphylococcal scalded skin syndrome or bulla repens around the nails (run-around).

Granuloma annulare

Granuloma anulare is a fairly common granulomatous disorder mainly of young persons. Rings of small, flat, flesh-colored nodules mainly occur on the extremities, but variant forms exist. Nail fold involvement may occur. Histopathologically, it is characterized by an infiltrate of histiocytes and few lymphocytes. In the center, there may be necrobiotic material, which sometimes stains moderately eosinophilic and often mucin is found here.

Erythema elevatum diutinum

Erythema elevatum diutinum (EED) is clinically characterized by red-to-violaceous, later brown, persistent plaques, and nodules in symmetrical arrangement on the extensor surfaces of the extremities. Periungual lesions exhibit small plaques and nodules.[142] Nail involvement with subungual hemorrhage, onycholysis, and paronychia has been described.[143] Histopathologically, EED is now regarded as a rare type of chronic fibrosing leucocytoclastic vasculitis.[144] It starts with a so-called lymphocytic perivasculitis, which soon develops into a dense diffuse mixed infiltrate, sometimes granulomatous, with abundant neutrophils and often signs of karyorrhexis.[145] The capillaries may be thickened with fibrinoid material and there is often a concentric lamellar perivascular fibrosis. The grenz zone may be spared or not. Old lesions become fibrotic with an orderly array of spindle cells and collagen fibers that may run parallel to the skin surface.

Dermatomyositis

Dermatomyositis is a rare autoimmune disease of muscle and skin. It is a serious condition with up to one quarter to a half being paraneoplastic.[146] Edematous livid-red discoloration of the face, called heliotropic edema, and severe muscle weakness are typical. Gottron's papules are whitish flat lesions on the dorsa of the fingers, particularly on the distal phalanges. The capillaries of the proximal nail fold may be altered.[147] The cuticles are often hyperkeratotic and ragged.[148,149] The lunulae may be red[150] and the nail beds show splinter hemorrhages.[151] Pterygium inversum occurs at the hyponychium.[152] Nail histopathology in dermatomyositis was rarely reported. Periungual erythema usually shows mild inflammatory changes not distinguishable from those of systemic lupus erythematosus. Epidermal atrophy, vacuolar degeneration of basal cells, basal membrane degeneration, and a sparse to moderate perivascular lymphocytic infiltrate are seen. No immune complexes are

observed along the basement membrane, but fibrin deposition may be present in severe inflammation. Vasculitic changes were repeatedly described. The proximal nail fold shows capillary dilatation, numerous epidermal and dermal colloid bodies, basal lamina thickening, and immunoglobulin deposits, which are also seen in lupus erythematosus, scleroderma, and Raynaud's phenomenon.[153] Gottron papules demonstrate acanthosis or epidermal atrophy with orthokeratosis, vacuolar changes in the basal cell layer, cytoid bodies, melanophages in dark-skinned individuals, a mild perivascular mononuclear infiltrate, and mucin deposition in the upper dermis.

Lupus erythematosus

Lupus erythematosus is an autoimmune disease that rarely affects the nail, both in the chronic cutaneous (discoid) (CDLE) as well as the systemic forms (SLE).[154,155] There may be longitudinal ridging[156] and splitting, subungual hyperkeratosis, and finally even total nail loss.[157,158] Longitudinal leukonychia was seen in an African patient who had scarring discoid lupus erythematosus with complete loss of pigment in many of his LE scars on the face and the scalp. Often the nail lesions are not specific.[159] SLE shows periungual erythema due to dilated and tortuous loops of capillaries and prominent dermal venous plexus, nail fold telangiectasiae, splinter hemorrhages, red lunulae,[160] sometimes bluish nail pigmentation,[161] onycholysis, focal nail fold necroses, vasculitis, thrombosis of dermal vessels, digital ulcers, and gangrene.[162] Further non-specific skin lesions associated with active SLE are cuticle abnormalities such as ragged cuticles.[163,164] Splinter hemorrhages may be a hint at antiphospholipid syndrome. Cuticular abnormalities and nail fold telangiectasiae are often encountered in other autoimmune disorders, in particular dermatomyositis, the differential diagnosis of which with SLE can be very difficult, in particular in early disease manifestations.[165] In chilblain lupus[166] being the form to involve the nails most frequently, the tip of the digit—mostly toes—turns livid red, easily ulcerates, is tender, and the nail becomes more and more destroyed.[167,168] Familial chilblain lupus is due to a mutation in the TREX1 gene that encodes a 3′-5′ DNA exonuclease, which inhibits initiation of autoimmunity.[169] Histology greatly depends on the clinical type of lesion. Many are nonspecific and would not allow the diagnosis of lupus erythematosus to be made without the clinical context as well as laboratory and immunological investigations. Mild to moderate epidermal atrophy, hyperkeratosis, hydropic degeneration of the basal cells, thickening of the PAS positive basal membrane, an epidermotropic and perivascular lymphocytic infiltrate, edema, and dilatation of the papillary capillaries are seen in the periungual skin.[170] Nail bed involvement causes hyperkeratosis, development of a granular layer, atrophy of the prickle cell layer, and an interface dermatitis with liquefaction degeneration of basal cells due to the epidermotropic lymphocytic infiltrate. Some hyaline bodies may be seen in the upper dermis as remnants of necrotic keratinocytes.[171,197] The histopathological alterations in early chilblain lupus are very subtle. There may be some ectatic capillaries in the upper dermis and perivascular lymphocytic infiltrates in the middle to deep dermis faintly reminding of perniosis. In full-blown chilblain lupus, the histological features of chronic cutaneous lupus erythematosus are usually very well developed. There is severe nail dystrophy due to matrix and nail bed involvement. A band-like lymphocytic infiltrate leading to atrophy of the matrix and nail bed epithelium, sometimes even to shallow ulceration, is seen with liquefaction degeneration of the basal cells, necrotic keratinocytes, Civatte bodies in the upper dermis, and marked irregular thickening of the PAS-positive basal membrane. Mucin stain may reveal increased amounts of mucin.

Pemphigus vulgaris

Pemphigus represents a group of autoimmune blistering diseases characterized by autoantibodies to desmogleins 3 and 1, which leads to acantholysis, the histopathological hallmark of the pemphigus diseases. Autoantibodies are demonstrable in more than 80% of the cases and their titers correlate with disease activity. Five pemphigus types are generally accepted: pemphigus vulgaris including pemphigus vegetans, pemphigus foliaceus including pemphigus erythematosus and fogo selvagem (endemic Brazilian pemphigus), drug-induced pemphigus, IgA pemphigus, and paraneoplastic pemphigus. Except for IgA pemphigus, IgG is the main immunoreactant. Nails are mainly involved by pemphigus vulgaris,[172] rarely in Brazilian type of pemphigus foliaceus.[173] Nail involvement is rare, but correlates with the severity of (muco)cutaneous lesions and the duration of the disease.[174,175] One fifth exhibit nail lesions as the only sign of their pemphigus.[176] High anti-desmoglein 3 titers may be responsible for paronychia and onychomadesis in pemphigus vulgaris.[177] Secondary infection with *Staphylococcus aureus* and *Candida albicans* exacerbate the paronychia.[178] Beau's lines and onychomadesis are the consequence of matrix involvement.[179] Subungual hemorrhage, nail discoloration, subungual hyperkeratosis, trachyonychia, nail pitting, onycholysis, onychodystrophies, and nail loss are less common.[180–184] Hemorrhagic nail lesions were associated with poor prognosis.[185–188] Paraneoplastic pemphigus, or paraneoplastic autoimmune multiorgan syndrome, is characterized by intractable erosive lesions and blisters, sometimes with severe erosive nail lesions.[189] It is mostly associated with malignant lymphomas, chronic lymphocytic leukemia, Castleman's syndrome, thymoma, and a number of other less common malignancies.[190] Histopathology is diagnostic in most cases although the diagnosis is made with a nail biopsy only when nail involvement is the sole localization. A Tzanck test is easily performed from a fresh bulla, an erosive lesion or in paronychia by gently squeezing the nail fold and collecting the exudate on a slide. A Tzanck cell is a rounded keratinocyte with a round nucleus, light perinuclear cytoplasm, and a condensation of the peripheral

cytoplasm in Giemsa stain. An early lesion, whether a full-blown lesion or just a red spot, should be selected for biopsy. Punch biopsies are not recommended as the blister roof is most often torn off. The earliest change is spongiosis, sometimes eosinophilic. Acantholysis is seen as suprabasal clefting with the basal cells standing in line on the basement membrane like a "row of tombstones," but often also some acantholytic cells are seen above them and look like Tzanck cells. In non-infected blisters the inflammatory infiltrate is mild, but in case of eosinophilic spongiosis it contains many eosinophils, a finding also seen in early bullous pemphigoid. Pemphigus vegetans when occurring on the nails may clinically mimic acrodermatitis continua suppurativa of Hallopeau.[191] Histologically, spongiform pustules with neutrophilic cell infiltration occur in a hyperkeratotic epithelium. The dermal inflammatory cell infiltration is dense and mainly consists of neutrophil granulocytes and many eosinophils. Acantholysis may not be obvious and further sections or biopsies may be necessary.[192] Immunofluorescence shows intercellular antibodies. In the Brazilian type of pemphigus foliaceus, which is believed to be, at least in part, due to stings of the black fly *Simulium pruinosum*, plus sunlight,[193] there is subtle acantholysis in or just beneath the granular layer. This may easily escape notice if there is no clinical information. Whenever possible the diagnosis of pemphigus vulgaris should be confirmed by immunofluorescence, which shows a lacelike intercellular fluorescence of the epidermis with immunoglobulin G and complement 3 in the matrix[183] and nail bed[180,194] and also allows the distinction between pemphigus vegetans and acrodermatitis continua suppurativa.[116] Histology of paraneoplastic pemphigus varies according to the polymorphous clinical lesions. Three main patterns are observed: suprabasal intraepithelial acantholysis similar to pemphigus vulgaris, necrosis of single keratinocytes as in a variety of drug reactions, and vacuolar changes of the basal cell layer similar to lichen planus. There is an intercellular fluorescence of the epidermis plus immunoglobulin and/or complement along the basal membrane.[195]

Bullous pemphigoid and cicatricial pemphigoid

Bullous pemphigoid is mainly seen in elderly patients and characterized by tense bullae on an urticarial erythematous base. Nail involvement was infrequently described. Clear blisters are seen around the nail with consecutive paronychia, onycholysis, Beau's lines, onychomadesis, onychodystrophy, and nail loss.[196–202] Pterygium formation was recently observed.[203] Histologically, a subepidermal blister formation usually with abundant eosinophils is seen. Immunofluorescence demonstrates a linear immunoglobulin G and complement deposition. The targets are mainly bullous pemphigoid antigen (BPAg) 1 (BP230) and BPAg2 (BP180). Cicatricial pemphigoid involving the nail is very rare.[204] Immunofluorescence of the nail bed in bullous pemphigoid shows the typical linear fluorescence along the basement membrane.[205]

Scleroderma

Scleroderma is characterized by progressive hardening of the skin. Of the several variants, acrosclerosis and CREST syndrome are important for nail pathology. The histologic alterations of diffuse scleroderma and morphea are virtually identical. Differences depend on the severity and depth of the changes. Early lesions exhibit a dense perivascular lymphocytic infiltrate. With time, the collagen bundles change to large, eosinophilic, hyaline, swollen ones. In nail pathology, proximal nail fold biopsies have been used for diagnostic purposes.[206] They show perivascular lymphocytic infiltrates, splitting of the basal lamina, broadening of the perivascular connective tissue and immunoglobulin deposits,[207] that are easily identified by PAS.[208] Pterygium inversum unguis shows a hyperkeratosis of the hyponychium reaching farther distal and adhering to the nail plate. The isthmus appears to extend to the medial third of the nail bed.[209-211]

Lichen sclerosus et atrophicans of the nail area is a very rare condition. It may affect the nail fold[212] but nail involvement is exceptional.[116,213,214] One case showed compact hyperkeratosis, vacuolar degeneration of the basal cell layer and a homogenized edematous, light appearing papillary dermis of the nail bed.

Cutaneous vasculitis

Leukocytoclastic vasculitis is sometimes seen on the nail folds and rarely as dark red to black spots under the nail.[215] It is a reaction pattern involving mainly the superficial dermal postcapillary venules. An infiltrate around these vessels predominantly consisting of neutrophils penetrates the vessel walls with fibrinoid change, endothelial cell swelling, and fragmentation of the neutrophil nuclei. Depending on the severity of vessel damage, extravasated erythrocytes may obscure the neutrophils. Severe vessel injury causes circumscribed necroses, occasionally with small ulcerations. Sometimes, there are so many neutrophils that the aspect of a pustular vasculitis develops. Severe edema may cause a blister-like appearance. In fresh lesions, complement factor 3 can be demonstrated in the vessel walls by immunofluorescence.[216] Immunoglobulin A is found in Henoch-Schönlein purpura.[217]

Pyoderma gangrenosum

Pyoderma gangrenosum is a rare neutrophilic dermatosis of unknown etiology. Gastrointestinal, rheumatic, and other diseases are often associated linking it to the group of auto-inflammatory disorders.[218] It is characterized by progressive cutaneous ulceration that may start with a tiny tender papule or pustule, which rapidly enlarges. Differentiation from an infection is crucial and may sometimes be difficult.[219,220] The pathogenesis includes immune complexes mediating neutrophilic vascular lesions. Trauma and Koebner phenomenon may elicit new lesions. Nail involvement was observed in association with cyclosporin A treatment.[221,222] The histopathology of pyodermia gangrenosum is nonspecific and requires clinical data. In the beginning, there is an infiltrate mainly composed of neutrophils. This develops into a necrotizing and suppurative lesion with a lymphocytic margin with perivascular and intramural lymphocytes. Around these, cuffs of neutrophils may be seen. Sometimes, a sweet-like aspect is present.

Inflammatory linear verrucous epidermal nevus

ILVEN is a rare condition presenting with linear, pruritic, persistent lesions most commonly on the limbs, mainly the legs. It often starts in childhood,[128] but adult-onset cases were also reported.[223] Psoriasiform lesions with cuticle loss and onycholysis around the nail without nail pitting were observed. Nail involvement is rare.[130,224] The histopathology shows hyperkeratosis with focal parakeratosis, moderate acanthosis, elongated and thickened rete pegs, and occasional spongiosis with lymphocytic exocytosis. Sometimes, alternating ortho- and parakeratosis with sharp delimitation are present. Then, the parakeratosis is slightly elevated and the orthokeratosis slightly depressed. Involucrin is reduced in the parakeratotic epidermis whereas it is present in psoriasis.[225] Despite its name, the inflammatory infiltrate is usually mild to moderate.

REFERENCES

1. Haneke E. *Histopathology of the Nail— Onychopathology*. CRC Press, Boca Raton, FL, 2016.
2. Achten G. L'ongle normal et pathologique. *Dermatologica* 1963;126:229–245.
3. Achten G. Normale Histologie und Histochemie des Nagels. In: Jadassohn J, editor. *Handbuch der Haut- und Geschlechtskrankheiten, Erg-Werk*, vol. 1. Springer, Berlin, Germany, 1968: pp. 339–376.
4. Langbein L, Rogers MA, Winter H, Praetzel S, Beckhaus U, Rackwitz HR, Schweizer J. The catalog of human hair keratins. I. Expression of the nine type I members in the hair follicle. *J Biol Chem* 1999;274:19874–19884.
5. Langbein L, Rogers MA, Winter H, Praetzel S, Schweizer J. The catalog of human hair keratins. II. Expression of the six type II members in the hair follicle and the combined catalog of human type I and II keratins. *J Biol Chem* 2001;276:35123–35132.
6. Langbein L, Schweizer J. Keratins of the human hair follicle. *Int Rev Cytol* 2005;243:1–78.
7. Alibardi L, Dalla Valle L, Nardi A, Toni M. Evolution of hard proteins in the sauropsid integument in relation to the cornification of skin derivatives in amniotes. *J Anat* 2009;114:560–586.
8. Dittmar M, Dindorf W, Banerjee A. Organic elemental composition in fingernail plates varies between sexes and changes with increasing age in healthy

humans. *Gerontol/Int J Exp Clin Behav Gerontol* 2008;54:100–105.

9. Fleckman P. Basic science of the nail unit. In: Scher R, Daniel III C, editors. *Nails: Therapy Diagnosis Surgery*, 2nd ed. WB Saunders Company, Philadelphia, PA, 1997: pp. 37–54.

10. Schumacher E, Dindorf W, Dittmar M. Exposure to toxic agents alters organic elemental composition in human fingernails. *Sci Total Environ* 2009;407:2151–2157.

11. Baden HP, Goldsmith LA, Fleming B. A comparative study of the physicochemical properties of human keratinized tissues. *Biochim Biophys Acta* 1973;322:269–278.

12. Morgan AM, Baran R, Haneke E. Anatomy of the nail unit in relation to the distal digit. In: Krull E, Zook E, Baran R, Haneke E, editors. *Nail Surgery: A Text and Atlas*. Lippincott Williams & Wilkins, Philadelphia, PA, 2001: pp. 1–28.

13. Haneke E. Surgical anatomy of the nail apparatus. *Dermatol Clin* 2006;24:291–296.

14. McGonagle D, Tan AL, Benjamin M. The nail as a musculoskeletal appendage—implications for a better understanding of the link between psoriasis and arthritis. *Dermatology* 2009;218:97–102.

15. McGonagle D, Fontana NP, Tan AL, Benjamin M. Nailing down the genetic and immunological basis for psoriatic disease. *Dermatology* 2010;221(Suppl):15–22.

16. Hoch J, Fritsch H, Frenz C. Gibt es einen knöchernen Strecksehnenab- oder -ausriß? Plastinations histologische Untersuchungen zur Insertion der Streckaponeurose und deren Bedeutung für die operative Therapie. *Chirurg* 1999;70:705–712.

17. Frenz C, Fritsch H, Hoch J. Plastination histologic investigations on the inserting pars terminalis aponeurosis dorsalis of three-sectioned fingers. *Anat Anz* 2000;182:69–73.

18. Baran R, Juhlin L. Bone dependent nail formation. *Br J Dermatol* 1986;114:371–375.

19. Shum C, Bruno RJ, Ristic S, Rosenwasser MP, Strauch RJ. Examination of the anatomic relationship of the proximal germinal nail matrix to the extensor tendon insertion. *J Hand Surg [Am]* 2000;25:1114–1117.

20. Schweitzer TP, Rayan GM. The terminal tendon of the digital extensor mechanism: Part I, anatomic study. *J Hand Surg [Am]* 2004;29:898–902.

21. Kim JY, Jung HJ, Lee WJ, Kim do W, Yoon GS, Kim DS, Park MJ, Lee SJ. Is the distance enough to eradicate in situ or early invasive subungual melanoma by wide local excision? From the point of view of matrix-to-bone distance for safe inferior surgical margin in Koreans. *Dermatology* 2011;223:122–123.

22. López PP, Becerro de Bengoa Vallejo R, López López D, Prados Frutos JC, Murillo González JA, Losa Iglesias ME. Anatomic relationship of the proximal nail matrix to the extensor hallucis longus tendon insertion. *J Eur Acad Dermatol Venereol* 2015;29:1967–1971.

23. Muto H, Yoshioka I. Relationship between the degree of coverage of the nail root by the posterior nail wall and the length of the visible part of the nail in human toes. *Kaibogaku Zasshi* 1977;52:269–276.

24. Terry RB. The onychodermal band in health and disease. *Lancet* 1955;1:179–181.

25. Sonnex TS, Griffiths WA, Nicol WJ. The nature and significance of the transverse white band of human nails. *Sem Dermatol* 1991;10:12–16.

26. Diaz AA, Boehm AF, Rowe WF. Comparison of fingernail ridge patterns of monozygotic twins. *J Forens Sci CA* 1990;35:97–102.

27. de Berker DAR, McWhinney B, Sviland L. Quantification of regional matrix nail production. *Br J Dermatol* 1996;134:1083–1086.

28. Haneke E. The human nail matrix—flow cytometric and immunohistochemical studies. *Clin Dermatol Year* 2000, Abstr.

29. De Berker D, Wojnarowska F, Sviland L, Westgate GE, Dawber RP, Leigh IM. Keratin expression in the normal nail unit: Markers of regional differentiation. *Br J Dermatol* 2000;142:89–96.

30. Haneke E. Histology, immunohistochemistry and histopathology of the nail. Abstract, VIII. *International Congress of Dermatologic Surgery*, Barcelona, Spain, October 10–13, 1987.

31. Baden H. Common transglutaminase substrates shared by hair, epidermis and nail and their function. *J Dermatol Sci* 1994;7 Supp:S20–S26.

32. Fanti PA, Tosti A, Cameli N, Varotti C. Nail matrix hypergranulosis. *Am J Dermatopathol* 1994;16:607–610.

33. Nakamura M, Ishikawa O. The localization of label-retaining cells in mouse nails. *J Invest Dermatol* 2008;128:728–730.

34. Sellheyer K, Nelson P. The ventral proximal nail fold: Stem cell niche of the nail and equivalent to the follicular bulge—A study on developing human skin. *J Cutan Pathol* 2012;39:835–843.

35. Hashimoto K. Ultrastructure of the human toenail: Cell migration, keratinization and formation of the intercellular cement. *Arch Dermatol Forsch* 1970;240:1–22; Hashimoto K. The marginal band: A demonstration of the thickened cellular envelope of the human nail cell with the aid of lanthanum staining. *Arch Dermatol* 1971;103:387–393.

36. Hashimoto, K. Ultrastructure of the human toenail. II. *J Ultrastruct Res* 1971;36:391–410.

37. Hashimoto K. Ultrastructure of the human toenail. I. Proximal nail matrix. *J Invest Dermatol* 1971;56:235–246.

38. Inoue H. Three-dimensional observations of microvasculature of human finger skin. *Hand* 1978;10:144–149.

39. Sangiorgi S, Manelli A, Congiu T, Bini A, Pilato G, Reguzzoni M, Raspanti M. Microvascularization of the human digit as studied by corrosion casting. *J Anat* 2004;204:123–131.

40. Masson P. *Les Glomus Neurovasculaires*. Hermann et Cie, Paris, France, 1937.

41. Dowsett SA, Archila L, Segreto VA, Gonzalez CR, Silva A, Vastola KA, Bartizek RD, Kowolik MJ. Helicobacter pylori infection in indigenous families of Central America: Serostatus and oral fingernail carriage. *J Clin Microbiol* 1999;37:2456–2460.

42. Perrin C. Peculiar zone of the distal nail unit: The nail isthmus. *Am J Dermatopathol* 2007;29:108–109.

43. Perrin C. Expression of follicular sheath keratins in the normal nail with special reference to the morphological analysis of the distal nail unit. *Am J Dermatopathol* 2007;29:543–550.

44. Perrin C. The 2 clinical subbands of the distal nail unit and the nail isthmus. Anatomical explanation and new physiological observations in relation to the nail growth. *Am J Dermatopathol* 2008;30:216–221.

45. Apolinar E, Rowe WF. Examination of human fingernail ridges by means of polarized light. *J Forens Sci CA* 1980;25:154–161.

46. Jemec GBE, Serup J. Ultrasound structure of the human nail plate. *Arch Dermatol* 1989;125:643–646.

47. Forslind B, Wroblewski R, Afzelius BA. Calcium and sulfur location in human nail. *J Invest Dermatol* 1976;67:273–275.

48. Jarrett A, Spearman JIC. The histochemistry of the human nail. *Arch Dermatol* 1966;94:652–657.

49. Garson C, Baltenneck F, Leroy F, Riekel C, Muller M. Histological structure of human nail as studied by synchrotron X-ray microdiffraction. *Cell Mol Biol (Noisy-le-grand)* 2000;46:1025–1034.

50. Forslind B, Thyresson N. On the structure of the normal nail. A scanning electron microscope study. *Arch Dermatol Forsch* 1975;251:199–204.

51. Dawber RPR. The ultrastructure and growth of human nails. *Arch Dermatol Res* 1980;269:197–204.

52. Meyer JC, Grundmann HP. Scanning electron microscopic investigation of the healthy nail and its surrounding tissue. *J Cutan Pathol* 1984;11:74–79.

53. Arnn Y, Stoehelin IA. The structure and function of spot desmosomes. *Int J Dermatol* 1981;20:331–339.

54. De Berker DAR, André J, Baran R. Nail biology and nail science. *Int J Cosm Sci* 2007;29:241–275 s.46.

55. Bengtsson CF, Olsen ME. Brandt LØ, Bertelsen MF, Willerslev E, Tobin DJ, Wilson AS, Gilber, MTP. DNA from keratinous tissue, Part I: Hair and nail. *Ann Anat* 2010. doi:10.1016/j.aanat.2011.03.013.

56. Stern DK, Creasey AA, Quijije J, Lebwohl MG. UV-A and UV-B penetration of normal human cadaveric fingernail plate. *Arch Dermatol* 2011;147:439–441.

57. Reardon CM, McArthur PA, Survana SK, Brotherston TM. The surface anatomy of the germinal matrix of the nail bed in the finger. *J Hand Surg [Br]* 1999;24:531–533.

58. Ito T, Ito N, Saathoff M, Stapachiacchiere B, Bettermann A, Bulfone-Paus S, Takigawa M, Nickoloff B, Paus R. Immunology of the human nail apparatus: The nail matrix is a site of relative immune privilege. *J Invest Dermatol* 2005;125:1139–1148.

59. Tosti A, Piraccini BM. Biology of nails. In: Freedberg IM, Eisen AZ, Wolff K, Frank Austen K, Goldsmith LA, Stephen K, editors. *Fitzpatrick's Dermatology in General Medicine*. McGraw-Hill, New York, 2003: pp. 159–163.

60. Chuong CM, Noveen A. Phenotypic determination of epithelial appendages: Genes, developmental pathways, and evolution. *J Invest Dermatol Symp Proc* 1999;4:307–311.

61. Wu P, Hou L, Plikus M, Hughes M, Scehnet J, Suksaweang S, Widelitz R, Jiang TX, Chuong CM. Evo-Devo of amniote integuments and appendages. *Int J Dev Biol* 2004;48:249–270.

62. Fuzzi B, Rizzo R, Criscuoli L, Noci I, Melchiorri L, Scarselli B, Bencini E, Menicucci A, Baricordi OR. HLA-G expression in early embryos is a fundamental prerequisite for the obtainment of pregnancy. *Eur J Immunol* 2002;32:311–315.

63. Higashi N. Melanocytes of nail matrix and nail pigmentation. *Arch Dermatol* 1968;97:570–574.

64. Tosti A, Cameli N, Piraccini BM, Fanti PA, Ortonne JP. Characterization of nail melanocytes with anti-PEP1, anti-PEP8, TMH-1, and HMB-45 antibodies. *J Am Acad Dermatol* 1994;31:193–196.

65. De Berker D, Dawber RPR, Thody A, Graham A. Melanocytes are absent from normal nail bed; the basis of a clinical dictum. *Br J Dermatol* 1996;134:564.

66. Perrin C, Michiels JF, Pisani A, Ortonne JP. Anatomic distribution of melanocytes in normal nail unit: An immunohistochemical investigation. *Am J Dermatopathol* 1997;19:462–467.

67. Amin B, Nehal KS, Jungbluth AA, Zaidi B, Brady MS, Coit DC, Zhou Q, Busam KJ. Histologic distinction between subungual lentigo and melanoma. *Am J Surg Pathol* 2008;32:835–843.

68. Rodríguez G, Vargas EJ, Abaúnza MC, Díaz Quijano DM, Melo-Uribe. Immunohistochemical identification of nail matrix melanocytes. *J Eur Acad Dermatol Venereol* 2018, Epub ahead of print.

69. Theunis A, Richert B, Sass U, Lateur N, Sales F, André J. Immunohistochemical study of 40 cases of longitudinal melanonychia. *Am J Dermatopathol* 2011;33:27–34.

70. Monash, S. Normal pigmentation in the nails of negroes. *Arch Dermatol* 1932;25:876–881.

71. Leyden JJ, Spot DA, Goldsmith H. Diffuse banded melanin pigmentation in nails. *Arch Dermatol* 1972;105:548–550.

72. Kopf AW, Waldo F. Melanonychia striata. *Australas J Dermatol* 1980;21:70.

73. Lacour JP, Dubois D, Pisani A, Ortonne JP. Anatomical mapping of Merkel cells in normal human adult epidermis. *Br J Dermatol* 1991;125:535–542.

74. Wu JZ, Dong RG, Rakheja S, Schopper AW, Smutz WP. A structural fingertip model for simulating of the biomechanics of tactile sensation. *Med Eng Phys* 2004;26:165–175.

75. Dumontier C. Distal replantation, nail bed, and nail problems in musicians. *Hand Clin* 2003;19:259–272, vi.

76. Wallace WA, Coupland RE. Variations in the nerves of the thumb and index finger. *J Bone Joint Surg Br* 1975;57:491–494.

77. Lavaroni G, Kokelj F, Pauluzzi P, Trevisan G. The nails in psoriatic arthritis. *Acta Derm Venereol (Suppl) (Stockh)* 1994;186:113.

78. Lewin K, Dewit S, Ferrington RA. Pathology of the fingernail in psoriasis. A clinicopathological study. *Br J Dermatol* 1972;86:555–563.

79. DiChiacchio N, André J, Haneke E, DiChiacchio NG, Noriega LF, Ocampo-Garza J. Pseudo-pitting of the nail in psoriasis. *J Eur Acad Dermatol Venereol* 2017;31:e347–e348.

80. Haneke E. Pathology. In: Rigopoulos D, Tosti A, editors. *Nail Psoriasis.* Springer, Berlin, Germany, 2014: pp. 15–21.

81. Alkiewicz J. Psoriasis of the nails. *Br J Dermatol* 1948;60:195–200.

82. Alkiewicz J, Pfister R. *Atlas der Nagelkrankheiten: Pathohistologie, Klinik und Differential Diagnose.* FK Schattauer, Stuttgart, Germany, 1976.

83. Ackerman AB. Subtle clues to diagnosis by conventional microscopy. Neutrophils within the cornified layer as clues to infection by superficial fungi. *Am J Dermatopathol* 1979;1:69–75.

84. Andrews G, Machacek G. Pustular bacterid of the hands and feet. *Arch Dermatol* 1935;32:835–837.

85. Ammoury A, El Sayed F, Dhaybi R, Bazex J. Palmoplantar pustulosis should not be considered as a variant of psoriasis. *J Eur Acad Dermatol Venereol* 2008;22:392–393.

86. Hornstein OP, Haneke E. Pustular psoriasis (palms and soles) vs. recalcitrant pustular eruption (palms and soles). Histological Differential Diagnosis of Skin Diseases. *International Dermatopathology Symposium*, Munich, Germany, June 16–18, 1978; ref *Skin & Allergy News* 10, 1978.

87. Samman P. *The Nails in Disease*, 3rd ed. Heinemann, London, UK, 1978.

88. Zandieh F, Loghmani M. Reiter's syndrome in a patient with polyarthritis and nail involvement. *Iran J Allergy Asthma Immunol* 2008;7:185–186.

89. Ito T, Meyer KC, Ito N, Paus R. Immune privilege and the skin. *Curr Dir Autoimmun* 2008;10:27–52.

90. Alkhalifah A, Alsantali A, Wang E, McElwee KJ, Shapiro J. Alopecia areata update: Part I. Clinical picture, histopathology, and pathogenesis. *J Am Acad Dermatol* 2010;62:177–188, quiz 189–190.

91. Brenner W, Diem E, Gschnait F. Coincidence of vitiligo, alopecia areata, onychodystrophie, localized scleroderma and lichen planus. *Dermatologica* 1979;159:356–360.

92. Haneke E. Non-infectious inflammatory disorders of the nail apparatus. *J Dtsch Dermatol Ges* 2009;7:787–797.

93. Cho HH, Jo SJ, Paik SH, Jeon HC, Kim KH, Eun HC, Kwon OS. Clinical characteristics and prognostic factors in early-onset alopecia totalis and alopecia universalis. *J Korean Med Sci* 2012;27:799–802.

94. Tosti A, Morelli R, Bardazzi F, Peluso AM. Prevalence of nail abnormalities in children with alopecia areata. *Ped Dermatol* 1994;11:112–115.

95. Sharma VK, Kumar B, Dawn G. A clinical study of childhood alopecia areata in Chandigarh, India. *Ped Dermatol* 1996;13:372–377.

96. Haneke E. Pathology of inflammatory nail diseases. *7th Colloquium of the International Society for Dermatopathology*, Graz, Austria, May 23–25, 1984.

97. Alkiewicz J. Pathologische Reaktionen an den epithelialen Anhangsgebilden. Nagel. In: *Jadassohns Handbuch der Haut- und Geschlechtskrankheiten, ErgWerk*, Vol I/2. Springer, Berlin, Germany, 1964: pp. 299–343.

98. Laporte M, André J, Stouffs-Vanhoof F, Achten G. Nail changes in alopecia areata, light and electron microscopy. *Arch Dermatol Res* 1988;280(Suppl):585–589.

99. Achten G, André J, Laporte M. Nails in light and electron microscopy. *Sem Dermatol* 1991;10:54–64.

100. Samman P. The nails in lichen planus. *Br J Dermatol* 1961;73:288–292.

101. Marks R, Samman PD. Isolated nail dystrophy due to lichen planus. *Trans St John Hosp Dermatol Soc* 1972;58:93–97.

102. Scott MJ Jr, Scott MJ Sr. Ungual lichen planus. *Arch Dermatol* 1979;115:1197–1199.

103. Tosti A, de Padova MP, Tuffarelli M, Passarini B, Varotti C. Lichen planus limited to the nails. *Cutis* 1987;40:25–26.

104. Mehregan DA, Van Hale HM, Muller SA. Lichen planopilaris: Clinical and pathologic study of forty-five patients. *J Am Acad Dermatol* 1992;27:935–942.

105. Scher RK, Fischbein R, Ackerman AB. Twenty-nail dystrophy. A variant of lichen planus. *Arch Dermatol* 1978;114:612–613.

106. Samman PD. Idiopathic atrophy of the nails. *Br J Dermatol* 1969;81:746–749.

107. Colver GB, Dawber RPR. Is childhood idiopathic atrophy of the nails due to lichen planus? *Br J Dermatol* 1987;116:709–712.

108. Zaias N. The nail in lichen planus. *Arch Dermatol* 1970;101:264–271.

109. Tosti A, Peluso AM, Fanti PA, Piraccini BM. Nail lichen planus. Clinical and pathological study of 24 patients. *J Am Acad Dermatol* 1993;28:724–730.

110. Juhlin L, Baran R. Longitudinal melanonychia after healing of lichen planus. *Acta Derm-Venereol* 1989;69:338–339.

111. Oberste-Lehn H, Kühl M. Lichen planus pemphigoides mit Ulzerationen und Anonychie. *Z Haut GeschlKr* 1954;17:195–199.

112. Weidner F, Ummenhofer B. Lichen ruber ulcerosus (dystrophicans). *Z Hautkr* 1979;54:1008–1017.

113. Haneke E. Isolated bullous lichen planus of the nails mimicking yellow nail syndrome. *Clin Exp Dermatol* 1983;8:425–428.

114. Büchner SA, Itin P, Rufli T, Hungerbühler U. Disseminated lichenoid papular dermatosis with nail changes in acquired immunodeficiency syndrome: Clinical, histological and immunohistochemical considerations. *Dermatologica* 1989;179:99–101.

115. Lambert DR, Siegle RJ, Camisa C. Lichen planus of the nail presenting as a tumor. *J Dermatol Surg Oncol* 1988;14:1245–1247.

116. Kossard S, Cornish N. Localized lichen sclerosus with nail loss. *Australas J Dermatol* 1998;39:119–120.

117. Norton LA. Diseases of the nails. In: Conn HF, editor. *Current Therapy.* WB Saunders, Philadelphia, PA, 1982: p. 664.

118. Patrizi A, Neri I, Fiorentini C, Bonci A, Ricci G. Lichen striatus: Clinical and laboratory features of 115 children. *Pediat Dermatol* 2004;21:197–204.

119. Karp DL, Cohen BA. Onychodystrophy in lichen striatus. *Ped Dermatol* 1993;10:359–362.

120. Al-Niaimi FA, Cox NH. Unilateral lichen striatus with bilateral onychodystrophy. *Eur J Dermatol* 2009;19:511.

121. Sandreva T, Bygum A. Lichen striatus with nail abnormality is a self-limiting condition. *(Dan) Ugeskr Læger* 2012;174:652–653.

122. Niren NM, Waldman GD, Barski S. Lichen striatus with onychodystrophy. *Cutis* 1981;27:610–613.

123. Tosti A, Peluso AM, Misciali C, Cameli N. Nail lichen striatus: Clinical features and long term follow up. *J Am Acad Dermatol* 1997;36:906–913.

124. Gianotti R, Restano L, Grimalt R, Berti E, Alessi E, Caputo R. Lichen striatus–chameleon: A histopathological and immunohistological study of forty-one cases. *J Cutan Pathol* 1995;22:18–22.

125. Zhang Y, McNutt NS. Lichen striatus. Histological, immunohistochemical and ultrastructural study of 37 cases. *J Cutan Pathol* 2001;28:65–71.

126. Herd RM, McLaren KM, Aldridge RD. Linear lichen planus and lichen striatus–opposite ends of a spectrum. *Clin Exp Dermatol* 1993;18:335–337.

127. Muñoz MA, Pérez-Bernal AM, Camacho FM. Lichenoid drug eruption following the Blaschko lines. *Dermatology* 1996;193:66–67.

128. Altman J, Mehregan AH. Inflammatory linear verrucous epidermal nevus. *Arch Dermal* 1971;104:385–389.

129. Laugier P, Olmos L. Naevus linéaire inflammatoire et lichen striatus. Deux aspects d'une même affection. *Bull Soc Franc Dermatol Syph* 1976;83:48–53.

130. Landwehr AJ, Starink TM. Inflammatory linear verrucous epidermal naevus, report of a case with bilateral distribution and nail involvement. *Dermatologica* 1983;166:107–109.

131. Rahbari H, Cordero AA, Mehregan AH. Linear porokeratosis. *Arch Dermatol* 1974;109;526–528.

132. Munro CS, Cox NH, Marks JM, Natarajan S. Lichen nitidus presenting as palmoplantar hyperkeratosis and nail dystrophy. *Clin Exp Dermatol* 1993;18:381–383.

133. Bettoli V, De Padova MP, Corazza M, Virgili A. Generalized lichen nitidus with oral and nail involvement in a child. *Dermatology* 1997;194:367–369.

134. Fanti PA, Tosti A, Morelli R, Bardazzi F. Lichen planus of the nails with giant cells: Lichen nitidus? *Br J Dermatol* 1991;125:194–195.

135. Wanscher B, Thormann J. Permanent anonychia after Stevens–Johnson syndrome. *Arch Dermatol* 1977;113:970.

136. Moisidis C, Möbius V. Erythema multiforme major following docetaxel. *Arch Gynec Obstet* 2005;271:267–269.

137. Fellahi A, Zouhair K, Amraoui A, Benchikhi H. Sequelles cutanéo-muqueuses et oculaires des SJS et de Lyell. *Ann Dermatol Venereol* 2011;138:88–92.

138. Magina S, Lisboa C, Leal V, Palmares J, Mesquita-Guimarães J. Dermatological and ophthalmological sequels in toxic epidermal necrolysis. *Dermatology* 2003;207:33–36.

139. Baran R, Perrin C. Nail degloving, a polyetiologic condition with 3 main patterns: A new syndrome. *J Am Acad Dermatol* 2008;58:232–237.

140. Lyell A. A review of toxic epidermal necrolysis in Britain. *Br J Dermatol* 1967;79:662–672.

141. Hansen RC. Blindness, anonychia and mucosal scarring as sequelae of the Stevens–Johnson syndrome. *Ped Dermatol* 1984;1:298–300.

142. Soubeiran E, Wacker J, Haußer I, Hartschuh W. Erythema elevatum diutinum with unusual clinical appearance. *J German Soc Dermatol* 2008;6:303–305.

143. Futei Y, Knohara I. A case of erythema elevatum diutinum associated with B-cell lymphoma: A rare distribution involving palms, soles and nails. *Br J Dermatol* 2000;142:116–119.

144. El Fekih N, Belgith I, Fazaa B, Remmah S, Zéglaoui F, Zermani R, Kamoun MR. Erythema elevatum diutinum: An "idiopathic" case. *Dermatol Online J* 2011;17(7):7.

145. Navarro R, de Argila D, Fraga J, García-Diez A. Erythema elevatum diutinum or extrafacial granuloma faciale? *Actas Dermosifiliogr* 2010;101:814–815.

146. Fardet L, Dupuy A, Gain M, Kettaneh A, Chérin P, Bachelez H, Dubertret L, Lebbe C, Morel P, Rybojad M. Factors associated with underlying malignancy in a retrospective cohort of 121 patients with dermatomyositis. *Medicine (Baltimore)* 2009;88:91–97.

147. De Angelis R, Cutolo M, Gutierrez M, Bertolazzi C, Salaffi F, Grassi W. Different microvascular involvement in dermatomyositis and systemic sclerosis. A preliminary study by a tight video capillaroscopic assessment. *Clin Exp Rheumatol* 2012;30(Suppl 71):S67–S70.

148. Samitz MH. Cuticular changes in dermatomyositis. *Arch Dermatol* 1974;110:866–867.

149. Ekmekci TR, Ucak S, Aslan K, Koslu A, Altuntas Y. Exaggerated changes in a patient with dermatomyositis. *J Eur Acad Dermatol* 2005;19:135–136.

150. Jorizzo JL, Gonzalez EB, Daniels JC. Red lunulae in a patient with rheumatoid arthritis. *J Am Acad Dermatol* 1983;711–714.

151. Tunc SE, Ertam I, Pirildar T, Turk T, Ozturk M, Doganavsargil E. Nail changes in connective tissue diseases: Do nail changes provide clues for the diagnosis? *J Eur Acad Dermatol Venereol* 2007;21:497–503.

152. Caputo R, Cappio F, Rigoni C, Scarabelli G, Toffolo P, Spinelli G, Crosti C. Pterygium inversum unguis. Report of 19 cases and review of the literature. *Arch Dermatol* 1993;129:1307–1309.

153. Schnitzler L, Baran R, Verret JL. La biopsy du repli sus-unguéal dans les maladies dites du collagène. Etude histologique, ultrastructurale et en immunofluorecence. *Ann Dermatol Vénéréol* 1980;107:777–785.

154. Urowitz MB, Gladman DD, Chalmers A, Ogryzlo MA. Nail lesions in systemic lupus erythematosus. *J Rheumatol* 1978;5:441–447.

155. Obermoser G, Sontheimer RD, Zelger B. Overview of common, rare and atypical manifestations of cutaneous lupus erythematosus and histopathological correlates. *Lupus* 2010;19:1050–1070.

156. Matsumura M, Suzuki Y, Yamagishi M, Kawano M. Prominent ridged nail deformity in systemic lupus erythematosus. *Intern Med* 2012;51:1283–1284.

157. Kint A, Van Herpe L. Ungual anomalies in lupus erythematosus discoides. *Dermatologica* 1976;153:298–302.

158. Heller J. Lupus erythematodes der Nägel. *Dermatol Z* 1906;13:613–615.

159. Trüeb RM. Involvement of scalp and nails in lupus erythmatosus. *Lupus* 2010;19:1078–1086.

160. Wollina U, Barta U, Uhlemann C, Oelzner P. Lupus erythematosus-associated red lunula. *J Am Acad Dermatol* 1999;41:419–421.

161. Kapadia N, Haroon TA. Cutaneous manifestations of SLE. *Int J Dermatol* 1996;35:408–409.

162. Hashimoto H, Tsuda H, Takasaki Y. Digital ulcers/gangrene and immunoglobulin classes complement fixation of anti-dsDNA in systemic lupus erythematosus. *J Rheumatol* 1983;10:727–732.

163. Cardinali C, Caproni M, Bernacchi E, Amato L, Fabbri P. The spectrum of cutaneous manifestations in lupus erythematosus—the Italian experience. *Lupus* 2000;9:417–423.

164. Kuhn A, Sticherling M, Bonsmann G. Clinical manifestations of cutaneous lupus erythematosus. *J Dtsch Dermatol Ges* 2007;5:1124–1137.

165. Bouaziz JD, Barete S, Le Pelletier F, Amoura Z, Piette JC, Francès C. Cutaneous lesions of the digits in systemic lupus erythematosus: 50 cases. *Lupus* 2007;16:163–167.

166. Hutchinson J. Harveian lectures on lupus: The varieties of common lupus. *BMJ* 1888;1:58–63.

167. Millard LG, Rowell NR. Chilblain lupus erythematosus (Hutchinson). *Br J Dermatol* 1978;98:497–506.

168. Sifuentes Giraldo WA, Ahijón Lana M, García Villanueva MJ, González García C, Vázquez Diaz M. Chilblain lupus induced by TNF-α antagonists: A case report and literature review. *Clin Rheumatol* 2012;31(3):563–568.

169. Günther C, Meurer M, Stein A, Viehweg A, Lee-Kirsch MA. Familial chilblain lupus: A monogenic form of cutaneous lupus erythematosus due to a heterozygous mutation in TREX1. *Dermatology* 2009;219:162–166.

170. Mackie RM. Lupus erythematosus associated with finger clubbing. *Br J Dermatol* 1973;89:533–535.

171. Sannicandro F. Contributo alla conoscenza clinica ed istologica del lupus eritematoso cronico del complesso ungueale. *Min Dermatol* 1960;35:32–34.

172. Serratos BD, Rashid RM. Nail disease in pemphigus vulgaris. *Dermatol Online J* 2009;15:2.

173. Azulay RD. Brazilian pemphigus foliaceus. *Int J Dermatol* 1982;21:122–124.

174. Habibi M, Mortazavi H, Shadianloo S, Balighi K, Ghodsi SZ, Daneshpazhooh M, Valikhani M, Ghassabian A, Pooli AH, Chams-Davatchi C. Nail changes in pemphigus vulgaris. *Int J Dermatol* 2008;47:1141–1144.

175. Schlesinger N, Katz M, Ingber A. Nail involvement in pemphigus vulgaris. *Br J Dermatol* 2002;146:836–839.

176. Cahali JB, Kakuda EY, Santi CG, Maruta CW. Nail manifestations in pemphigus vulgaris. *Rev Hosp Clin Fac Med São Paulo* 2002;57:229–234.

177. Laffitte E, Panizzon RG, Borradori L. Orodigital pemphigus vulgaris: A pathogenic role of anti-desmoglein-3 autoantibodies in pemphigus paronychia? *Dermatology* 2008;217:337–339.

178. Lee HE, Wong WR, Lee MC, Hong HS. Acute paronychia heralding the exacerbation of pemphigus vulgaris. *Int J Clin Pract* 2004;58:1174–1176.

179. Patsatsi A, Sotiriou E, Devliotou-Panagiotidou D, Sotiriadis D. Pemphigus vulgaris affecting 19 nails. *Clin Exp Dermatol* 2009;34:202–205.

180. Baumal A, Robinson MJ. Nail bed involvement in pemphigus vulgaris. *Arch Dermatol* 1973;107:751.

181. De Berker D, Dolziel K, Dawber RPR, Wojnarowski F. Pemphigus associated with nail dystrophy. *Br J Dermatol* 1993;129:461–464.

182. Rivera Diaz R, Alonso Llamazares J, Rodriguez Peralto JL, Sebastian Vanaclocha F, Iglesias Diez L. Nail involvement in pemphigus vulgaris. *Int J Dermatol* 1996;35:581–582.

183. Kolivras A, Gheeraert P, André J. Nail destruction in pemphigus vulgaris. *Dermatology* 2003;206:351–352.

184. Mascarenhas R, Fernandes B, Reis JP, Tellechea O, Figueiredo A. Pemphigus vulgaris with nail involvement presenting with vegetating and verrucous lesions. *Dermatol Online J* 2003;9(5):14.

185. Böckers M, Bork K. Multiple gleichzeitige Hämatome der Finger und Zehennägel mit nachfolgender Onychomadesis bei Pemphigus vulgaris. *Hautarzt* 1987;38:477–478.

186. Szepietowski JC, Różycka B, Baran E. Subungual haemorrhages in fatal pemphigus vulgaris. *J Eur Acad Dermatol Venereol* 2001;15:87–88.

187. Reich A, Wisnicka B, Szepietowski JC. Haemorrhagic nails in pemphigus vulgaris. *Acta Derm Venereol* 2008;88:542.

188. Tosti A, André M, Murrell DF. Nail involvement in autoimmune bullous disorders. *Dermatol Clin* 2011;29:511–512.

189. Jansen T, Plewig G, Anhalt GJ. Paraneoplastic pemphigus with clinical features of erosive lichen planus associated with Castleman's tumor. *Dermatology* 1995;190:245–250.

190. Czernik A, Camilleri M, Pittelkow MR, Grando SA. Paraneoplastic autoimmune multiorgan syndrome: 20 years after. *Int J Dermatol* 2011;50:905–914.

191. Leroy D, Lebrun J, Maillard V, Mandard JC, Deschamps P. Pemphigus végétant à type clinique de dermatite pustuleuse chronique de Hallopeau. *Ann Dermatol Venereol* 1982;109:549–555.

192. Török L, Husz S, Ócsai H, Krischner Á, Kiss M. Pemphigus vegetans presenting as acrodermatitis continua suppurativa. *Eur J Dermytol* 2003;13:579–581.

193. Lombardi C, Borges PC, Chaul A, Sampaio SA, Rivitti EA, Friedman H, Martins CR et al. Environmental risk factors in endemic pemphigus foliaceus (fogo selvagem). *J Invest Dermatol* 1992;98:847–850.

194. Fulton RA, Campbell L, Carlyle D, Simpson NB. Nail bed immunofluorescence in pemphigus vulgaris. *Acta Derm-Venereol* 1983;63:170–172.

195. Anhalt GJ, Kim SC, Stanley JR, Korman NJ, Jabs DA, Kory M, Izumi H et al. Paraneoplastic pemphigus: An autoimmune mucocutaneous disease associated with neoplasia. *N Engl J Med* 1990;320:1729–1735.

196. De Berker D, Nayar M, Dawber R, Wojnarowska F. Beau's lines in immunobullous disorders. *Clin Exp Dermatol* 1995;20:358–361.

197. Esterly NB, Gotoff SP, Lolekha S, Moore ES, Smith RD, Medenica M, Furey NL. Bullous pemphigoid and membranous glomerulonephropathy in a child. *J Ped* 1973;83:466.

198. Barth JH, Wojnarowska F, Millard PR, Dawber RP. Immunofluorescence of the nail bed in pemphigoid. *Am J Dermatopathol* 1987;9:349–350.

199. Delaporte E, Piette F, Janin A, Cozzani E, Joly P, Thomine E, Nicolas JF, Bergoend H. Pemphigoïde simulant une épidermolyse bulleuse acquise. *Ann Dermatol Venereol* 1995;122:19–22.

200. Namba Y, Koizumi H, Kumakiri M, Hashimoto T, Muramatsu T, Ohkawara A. Bullous pemphigoid with permanent loss of the nails. *Acta Derm Venereol* 1999;79:480–481.

201. Tomita M, Tanei R, Hamada Y, Fujimura T, Katsuoka K. A case of localized pemphigoid with loss of toenails. *Dermatology* 2002;204:155.

202. Gualco F, Cozzani E, Parodi A. Bullous pemphigoid with nail loss. *Int J Dermatol* 2005;44:967–968.

203. Haneke E, Borradori L. Pterygium in bullous pemphigoid. Submitted.

204. Burge SM, Powell SM, Ryan TJ. Cicatricial pemphigoid with nail dystrophy. *Clin Exp Dermatol* 1985;10:472–475.

205. Sinclair RD, Wojnarowska F, Leigh IM, Dawber RP. The basement membrane zone of the nail. *Br J Dermatol* 1994;131:499–505.

206. Von Bierbrauer AF, Mennel HD, Schmidt JA, von Wichert P. Intravital microscopy and capillaroscopically guided nail fold biopsy in scleroderma. *Ann Rheuma Dis* 1996;55:305–310.

207. Maeda M, Matubara K, Kachi H, Mori S, Kitajima Y. Histopathological and capillaroscopical features of the cuticles and bleeding clots in ring or middle fingers of systemic scleroderma patients. *J Dermatol Sci* 1995;10:35–41.

208. Scher RK, Tom DW, Lally EV, Bogaars HA. The clinical significance of periodic acid-Schiff-positive deposits in cuticle-proximal nail fold biopsy specimens. *Arch Dermatol* 1985;121:1406–1409.

209. Oiso N, Kurokawa I, Tsuruta D, Narita T, Chikugo T, Tsubura A, Kimura M, Baran R, Kawada A. The histopathological feature of the nail isthmus in an ectopic nail. *Am J Dermatopathol* 2011;33:841–844.

210. Oiso N, Narita T, Tsuruta D, Kawara S, Kawada A. Pterygium inversum unguis: Aberrantly regulated keratinization in the nail isthmus. *Clin Exp Dermatol* 2009;34:e514–e515.

211. Oiso N, Kurokawa I, Kawada A. Nail isthmus: A distinct region of the nail apparatus. *Dermatol Res Pract* 2012;2012:925023.

212. Steff M, Toulemonde A, Croue A, Lemerle E, Le Corre Y, Verret JL. Lichen scléreux acral. *Ann Dermatol Venereol* 2008;135:201–204.

213. Ramrakha-Jones VS, Paul M, McHenry P, Burden AD. Nail dystrophy due to lichen sclerosus? *Clin Exp Dermatol* 2001;26:507–509.

214. Noda Cabrera A, Sáez Rodríguez M, García-Bustínduy M, Guimerá Martín-Neda F, Dorta Alom S, Escoda García M, Fagundo González E et al. Localized lichen sclerosus et atrophicus of the finger without nail dystrophy. *Dermatology* 2002;205:303–304.

215. Carlson JA, Ng BT, Chen KR. Cutaneous vasculitis update: Diagnostic criteria, classification, epidemiology, etiology, pathogenesis, evaluation and prognosis. *Am J Dermatopathol* 2005;27:504–528.

216. Grunwald MH, Avinoach I, Amichai B, Halevy S. Leukocytoclastic vasculitis- correlation between different histologic stages and direct immunofluorescence results. *Int J Dermatol* 1997;36:349–352.

217. Magro CM, Crowson AN. A clinical and histologic study of 37 cases of immunoglobulin A-associated vasculitis. *Am J Dermatopathol* 1999;21:234–240.

218. Crowson AN, Mihm MC Jr, Magro C. Pyoderma gangrenosum: A review. *J Cutan Pathol* 2003;30:97–107.

219. Weenig RH, Davis MDP, Dahl PR. Skin ulcers misdiagnosed as pyoderma gangrenosum. *N Engl J Med* 2002;347:1412–1418.

220. EL-Kehdy J, Haneke E, Karam P. Pyoderma gangrenosum: A misdiagnosis. *J Drugs Dermatol* 2013;12:228–230.

221. Reich A, Maj J, Cisło M, Szepietowski JC. Periungual lesions in pyoderma gangrenosum. *Clin Exp Dermatol* 2009;34:e81–e84.

222. Bashir SJ, McGibbon D. Subungual pyoderma gangrenosum complicated by myopathy induced by ciclosporin and tacrolimus. *Clin Exp Dermatol* 2009;34:530–532.

223. Goldman K, Don PC. Adult onset of inflammatory linear verrucous nevus in a mother and her daughter. *Dermatology* 1994;189:170.

224. Saraswat A, Sandhu K, Shukla R, Handa S. Unilateral linear psoriasis with palmoplantar, nail, and scalp involvement. *Pediatr Dermatol* 2004;21:70–73.

225. Ferreira FR, DiChiacchio NG, de Alvarenga ML, Mandelbaum SH. Involucrin in the differential diagnosis between linear psoriasis and inflammatory linear verrucous epidermal nevus: Report of one case. *An Bras Dermatol* 2013;88:604–607.

9

Onychopathology of common nail diseases

SONAL SHARMA AND POOJA SHARMA

INTRODUCTION

Nails are composed of both epithelial and connective tissue components. Like any other tissue of the body, several pathologies can affect nails. Nail abnormality can arise due to local inflammatory, infectious, or neoplastic diseases. In addition, certain systemic conditions may initially manifest as subtle nail signs that can provide important clues for timely diagnosis. Many conditions elude diagnosis by simple history, clinical inspection, and routine mycology.[1] In these situations, nail microscopy can be an important aid to diagnosis.[2]

RATIONALE OF NAIL BIOPSY

The nail has a limited repertoire of clinical expressions. Hence, nail biopsies (NB) are often necessary to reach an accurate diagnosis, especially when there is no associated skin, mucosa, or hair involvement. However, the interpretation of NB is often difficult because some parakeratosis, some spongiosis, and rare neutrophils are present in almost all NB. In inflammatory nail conditions, longitudinal NB, which allow examination of the entire nail apparatus, are much more useful than punch biopsies.[3]

Nail is biopsied in numerous clinical situations: histological examination of the nail is required to demonstrate pathological fungal infection, even though the study of KOH preparation is usually sufficient to reach a diagnosis

of onychomycosis.[4] The reported sensitivity of fungal culture for identifying dermatophytes in onychomycotic nail varies from 25% to 80%.[2,5] There is an approximately 30% false negative rate with culture and KOH studies. NB with Periodic acid–Schiff (PAS) staining has been reported to be the most sensitive method for diagnosis.[6]

NB is required for the diagnosis of inflammatory diseases affecting only the nail. For example, NB has a definite diagnostic utility in cases with twenty-nail dystrophy, where absence of cutaneous associations makes a definite clinical diagnosis difficult. Similarly, 1%–5% of the cases with psoriasis may present with purely nail manifestations only.[7-9] 1%–10% of LP cases present as isolated nail lichen planus. Histopathological confirmation of diagnosis is essential to ensure an effective management of the condition. Of note, NB has been helpful in establishing diagnosis in isolated nail lichen striatus[10] and sarcoidosis.[11]

Pigmented nail lesions result from four histopathologically different matrix lesions: epithelial hyperpigmentation, simple lentigines, junctional nevus, and malignant melanoma, besides the obvious hemorrhage, which can also mimic these lesions clinically. NB is a very important tool for evaluation of pigmented nails.

Also, NB is particularly useful in case of nail tumors and is considered the gold standard. Nail matrix is the most common site for glomus tumor. An excision biopsy not only provides histological diagnosis but is also therapeutic and provides relief from pain.[12] Squamous cell carcinoma is the other malignancy common in the nail bed that can be diagnosed easily with a NB, though clinically it mimics many non-tumoral pathologies, namely, onychomycosis, warts, dystrophic nail, onycholysis, paronychia, and melanonychia.[13-16]

Nail also provides a "window" into systemic hematologic or metabolic abnormalities. Gout may be monitored by means of the simple and non-invasive histological processing of nail clippings.[17]

NAIL DISORDERS

Inflammatory diseases of the nail

Inflammatory diseases of the nail are quite common. Different diseases can have very similar clinical appearances.

PSORIASIS

Psoriasis is an inflammatory dermatosis that most frequently affects nail apparatus.

Nail involvement is seen in almost 40% of psoriasis patients and in up to 80% of patients of psoriatic arthropathy.[18] Histological examination of NB is essential to confirm diagnosis of psoriasis and to rule out the differential diagnoses. The best results are obtained with longitudinal biopsies.[2] Histologically the changes are like those observed in psoriatic plaques on the skin: hyperkeratosis, parakeratosis, psoriasiform hyperplasia, dilated and tortuous vessels in papillary dermis, and presence of neutrophils. However, in contrast to the skin, the nail commonly shows evidence of spongiosis and serous exudates and hypergranulosis may be observed (Figures 9.1 and 9.2).[4]

Matrix involvement manifests as spongiosis and lymphocytic exocytosis. Neutrophils are found in upper layers of matrix epithelium. Parakeratotic columns run diagonally supero-distally and often contain neutrophils that become

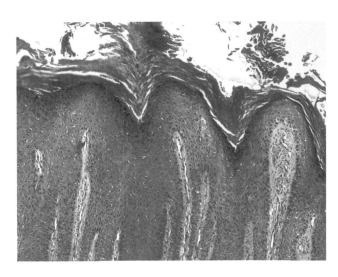

Figure 9.2 Nail psoriasis: section shows dilated capillaries in papillary dermis, H&E x100.

pyknotic and form Munro's micro abscesses. Involvement of the distal nail bed and the hyponychium is usually accompanied by formation of a granular layer with intermittent areas of parakeratosis. Occasionally the dilated capillaries bleed and the blood is carried distally by the nail growing over it producing parallel deep brown striations measuring 0.2–0.5 mm wide in the middle to distal nail bed.[19] Psoriatic leukonychia arises when parakeratosis affects only distal matrix. The affected area appears whitish because of internal desquamation of parakeratosis cells.[20-22] Space between nail and nail bed is often colonized by micro-organisms. Onychomycosis is quite common in psoriasis and both provoke quite similar histological changes (Table 9.1). A PAS stain should always be done to exclude the presence of fungi. However, fungal detection on histology does not rule out psoriasis. The presence of serous exudates, which are common in psoriasis and rare in onychomycosis, is a

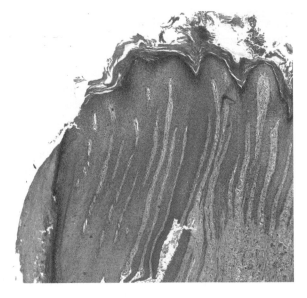

Figure 9.1 Nail psoriasis: section from nail shows part of nail plate with underlying hyperkeratosis, hypergranulosis, marked epithelial psoriasis from hyperplasia, H&E x100.

Table 9.1 Clinical signs of nail psoriasis and corresponding histological changes

Part of nail unit affected	Clinical signs	Histological findings
Nail matrix	Nail pitting, Beau's lines, onychomadesis, trachyonychia, nail dystrophy, and leukonychia	Spongiosis, lymphocytic exocytosis, neutrophils in upper layers of epidermis, Munro's micro abscesses in parakeratotic columns
Nail bed	Onycholysis, oil drop patches, subungual hyperkeratosis, and splinter hemorrhages	Formation of granular layer with intermittent areas of parakeratosis, dilated capillaries

Table 9.2 Differential diagnosis of histology of psoriasis and onychomycosis

Histology	Psoriasis	Onychomycosis
	Marked hyperkeratosis with accumulation of neutrophils and pockets of serum, often columns of layers of parakeratosis containing pyknotic neutrophils	Marked hyperkeratosis with collections of neutrophils and pockets of serum
	Patchy hypergranulosis	May be seen
	Hyperplasia of the nail bed	Papillomatous hyperplasia of the nail bed
	Spongiosis and mononuclear exocytosis	Spongiosis and mononuclear exocytosis
	PAS staining – usually negative for fungus, maybe seen in superadded fungal infection	PAS – Hyphae and spores in subungual hyperkeratotic tissue and the underside of the nail plate

Source: Haneke, E., J. Dtsch. Dermatol. Ges., 7, 787–797, 2009.

histological feature that can help to differentiate the two conditions (Table 9.2).[4]

Hanno et al. proposed diagnostic criteria of nail psoriasis that includes presence of neutrophils in the nail bed epithelium (major criterion), hyperkeratosis with parakeratosis, serum exudates, focal hypergranulosis, and nail bed epithelium hyperplasia (minor criteria).[23] Diagnosis of psoriasis requires the presence of one major criterion with or without minor criteria. Grover et al. have suggested that PAS negativity for fungal hyphae should be included as a major criterion for the diagnosis of nail psoriasis as both show similar features.[9]

LICHEN PLANUS

Lichen planus is a subacute or chronic dermatosis that involves skin, mucous membranes, hair follicles, and nails.[24] Incidence of nail involvement ranges from 1% to 10%.[25] Fingernails are more commonly affected than toenails.[26] Like psoriasis, lichen planus can affect various parts of the nail unit and clinical manifestations are determined by the part of nail unit affected. Matrix involvement leads to nail dystrophy and trachyonychia. Nail bed involvement produces subungual hyperkeratosis and onycholysis. Characteristic features are rough nail surface with longitudinal ridging. It is caused by an inflammatory infiltrate, usually at the proximal tip of the matrix spreading to the underside of the proximal nail fold. If the central portions of the proximal nail fold are completely obliterated, or the adjacent areas, pterygium develops, which divides the nail into two portions. Over the course of the disease, all nails may be lost.[27] LP-associated nail atrophy involves scarring and is thus irreversible.[22]

Pathological examination is required in clinically suspected cases of nail lichen planus to confirm the diagnosis before administering systemic corticosteroids.[28] The histological changes observed are similar to those of affected skin.[29] There is a dense, band-like, epidermotropic infiltrate that spreads into the deep portion of the proximal nail fold from the underside of the proximal nail wall around the matrix toward the nail bed. This leads to hydropic basal cell degeneration of the matrix epithelium with subsequent thinning, formation of a granular layer without real nail formation, and frequently to spongiosis and flattening of the proximal nail fold, which can ultimately lead to pterygium formation. However, the nail can present certain additional features,

such as parakeratosis and serous exudates.[22] In the matrix and nail bed, a compact horny layer replaces the normal nail plate above the zones of hypergranulosis (Figures 9.3 and 9.4).[2] The changes described are not pathognomonic of lichen

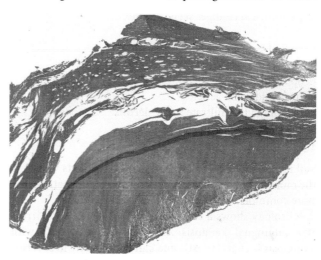

Figure 9.3 Nail lichen planus: section showing hyperkeratosis, serum exudates in nail plate, irregular acanthosis with focal hypergranulosis, and dense inflammation at epidermal-dermal junction, H&E x40.

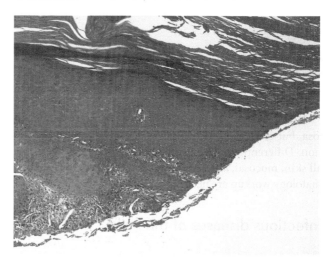

Figure 9.4 Nail lichen planus: higher power view showing interface inflammatory infiltrate, H&E x100.

planus, as they can also be observed in other conditions, such as lichenoid drug reaction, graft versus host disease, amyloidosis, lichen sclerosus et atrophicans, alopecia areata (AA), psoriasis, atopic eczema, sarcoidosis, Darier disease, Hailey–Hailey disease, ichthyosis vulgaris, incontinentia pigmenti, immunoglobulin A deficiency, and in response to trauma.[22] Goettmann et al. analyzed the positivity rate of NB in patients of nail lichen planus. It varied according to the site of biopsy: 85.5% of specimens of matrix biopsy were positive, whereas 95.5% of bed biopsy showed histological features of nail lichen planus. One hundred percent of biopsy from nail fold was contributive.[28]

ECZEMA

All types of eczema can affect the nails. The nail changes should be considered in relation to the skin changes, which usually affect the fingers, hands, or other regions of the body.

Histological changes seen include[4]:

- Foci of parakeratosis
- Formation of a granular layer
- Spongiosis
- Intraepidermal vesicles
- Lymphocytic infiltrate in the dermis

ALOPECIA AREATA

Nail involvement occurs in about 20% of patients with AA. The more severe the disease and the younger the patient, the more common and severe are the nail changes.[22]

Histology shows a compact, wavy nail plate with irregular subungual keratosis. Lymphocytic exocytosis with spongiosis is characteristic and can vary greatly in severity, making differentiation from eczema difficult.[22] The typical changes are limited to the proximal matrix and give rise to pitting of the nail plate. Histologically, these pits resemble those that develop in psoriasis, but are shallower and present a geometric distribution.[7]

REITER DISEASE

Reiter disease is a triad of ocular, oral, and genital mucosal changes, sometimes with mutilating arthritis and psoriasiform skin changes. Involvement of the nail is quite common.[30]

Histological features resemble those of psoriasis pustulosa, but often there is also marked erythrocyte extravasation. Differentiation, however, is very difficult. Analysis of all skin, mucosal, and constitutional symptoms and a rheumatology workup are necessary.

Infectious diseases of the nail

FUNGAL INFECTIONS

Onychomycosis is a chronic infection that is difficult to treat and leads to gradual destruction of the nail plate. It is the most common nail disease.[31] Dermatophytes are the most frequently implicated causative agents (approximately 90% in toenail and 50% in fingernail). Trichophyton rubrum (T. rubrum) is the most common causative agent followed by T. mentagrophytes.[32] Non-dermatophytic molds have also been implicated and molds are considered pathogens when the following criteria are fulfilled:

1. Nail abnormalities consistent with diagnosis
2. Hyphae visualized in the nail keratin on direct microscopy
3. Failure to isolate a dermatophyte in the culture
4. Growth of more than five colonies of the same mold in at least two consecutive nail samplings[23]

Early diagnosis is essential to prevent total nail dystrophy. Histopathological evaluation of PAS-stained nail clippings has a higher sensitivity (91.6%) compared to direct microscopy (77.1%) or mycological culture (70%) and is thus considered the gold standard in the diagnosis of onychomycosis. However, histology and microscopy together provide the most precise diagnostics of onychomycosis.[33] Histopathology can demonstrate whether a fungus is invasive or merely colonizing subungual debris. Also, nail histopathology with PAS staining takes less time than culture and histological slides can be preserved for future reference.[34]

Distal and lateral subungual onychomycosis (DLSO): Histologically, the hyphae are usually found in the keratinized part of the nail bed or in the deepest part of the nail plate. A superficial biopsy of the nail plate may therefore give a false negative result. Thus, a full-thickness biopsy of the nail plate is more reliable than a superficial biopsy for the diagnosis of onychomycosis and is indicated in the case of a negative culture from a superficial sample.[35,36] The epithelium of the nail bed shows the formation of a granular layer and compact hyperkeratosis. Long-standing lesions will also show inflammatory changes such as spongiosis and lymphocyte and neutrophil exocytosis.[37,38] Demonstration of fungi in the biopsy material is essential for confirmation of diagnosis (Figures 9.5 and 9.6).

Proximal subungual onychomycosis: Biopsy must be taken from the whitish areas and must be deep and shows histological changes similar to those described for distal onychomycosis, though serous crusts, extravasation of blood, and more marked hyperkeratosis are also usually observed.[4]

Superficial white onychomycosis: Histologically, yeast-like fungal forms (rather than hyphae) can be seen in the superficial part of the nail. The biopsy must be taken from the most superficial part of the whitish areas of the nail plate.[4]

Endonyx: Endonyx onychomycosis is invasion of the nail plate where the infection starts from the pulp as in DLSO but instead of infecting the nail bed, the fungus penetrates the distal nail keratin of nail plate where it forms milky white patches without subungual hyperkeratosis or

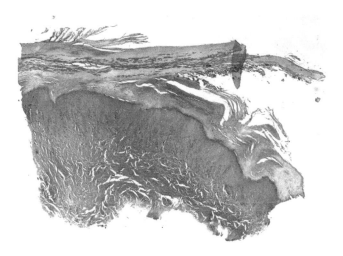

Figure 9.5 Onychomycosis: nail biopsy with hyperkeratosis and fragmented nail plate, H&E x40.

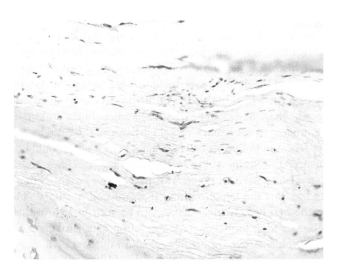

Figure 9.6 Onychomycosis: high power view of nail plate with numerous fungal hyphae, PAS x400.

onycholysis. It has been described with *T. soudanense* and *T. violaceum* infections.[39]

Total dystrophic onychomycosis (TDO): There is destruction of the nail plate where the nail crumbles and disappears leaving a thickened abnormal nail bed retaining keratotic nail debris. It may occur secondarily as the end result of any of the four main patterns. Primary TDO is observed only in patients suffering from chronic mucocutaneous candidiasis (CMC) or the immunodeficient states.[39]

Candida onychomycosis: Histologically, in candida onychomycosis the entire nail is invaded by pseudohyphae and inflammatory changes are present in the epithelium.[7,40]

Zaikovska et al. found VEGF in the connective tissue in the nails affected by onychomycosis, implying vasculogenesis and angiogenesis. Also, significant amounts of the metalloproteinases were detected in nails affected by onychomycosis implying extracellular remodeling of matrix and apoptosis of cells.[33]

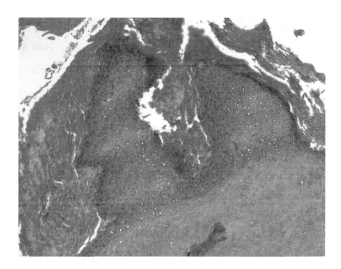

Figure 9.7 Viral wart: nail bed epithelium showing hyperkeratosis, hypergranulosis, and papillomatosis. Epidermal cells with koilocytic change can be seen, H&E x100.

VIRAL WARTS

Viral warts develop in the areas of the nail apparatus that possess a granular layer (nail folds and hyponychium).[4] They are caused by one of the many human papillomaviruses, mainly serotypes 1, 2, and 47.[41,42] Common warts are fibroepithelial papillomatous lesions and commonly show prominent granular layer and occasional koilocytic changes. Papillae usually show tortuous and dilated blood vessels and parakeratosis in vertical tiers at the tip of the papillae is another morphologic sign (Figure 9.7).[42]

Melanonychia

Melanonychia or nail pigmentation can be longitudinal, transverse, or total. Total melanonychia and transverse melanonychia are rare lesions. Longitudinal melanonychia is the result of melanin in the nail plate.[43]

Of note, nail unit melanocytes differ from epidermal melanocytes in the number, density, distributions, functions, and S100 protein expressions as summarized in Table 9.3. Understanding these differentials is critical in evaluation of nail unit melanocytic lesions.

The melanin produced by the matrical melanocytes is degenerated by the matrical keratinocytes, so nail plate is not pigmented under normal conditions. Pigmentation occurs when production of melanin increases to overwhelm the keratinocytes' capacity for degradation.[42]

LONGITUDINAL MELANONYCHIA

Linear pigmentation of the nail apparatus can result from either simple activation of matrical melanocytes or from benign (lentigo or nevus) or malignant (melanoma) melanocyte hyperplasia, and distinction requires a pathological examination.[2,44] It may be the first sign of a nail apparatus melanoma (NAM), especially when it involves a single digit and therefore, is biopsied. Matrix biopsy should be

Table 9.3 Difference in the nail and epidermal melanocytes

	Nail melanocytes			Epidermal melanocytes
	Nail matrix		Nail bed	
Number	Much lower			More in number
Density	200/mm^2		Absent-50/mm^2	1150/mm^2
Distribution	Lower two to four germinative cell layers in proximal matrix First and second layers in distal matrix			Basal layer
Function	Most are dormant in proximal matrix 50% are dormant and 50% are active in distal matrix		They are dormant	Most are active
S100 protein expression	Many intraepithelial nail melanocytes do not express this antigen			Epidermal melanocytes express this antigen

Source: André, J. et al., *Clin. Dermatol.*, 31, 526–539, 2013.

performed, after proximal nail avulsion and direct visualization of the matrix pigmented area.[2]

In melanocytic hyperactivity, melanocytes are seen in the suprabasal location and show an increase in the cytoplasmic pigment. Pigmented granules are seen in the nail plate. Fontana–Masson staining should be performed to enhance visualization of scant pigment.[2]

NAIL LENTIGO

There is a slight to moderate increase in the number of matrix melanocytes (10–31 per mm).[45] They are non-atypical, arranged in single units and located mainly in the basal layer, and also in the immediate suprabasal layer.[46] There is usually no pagetoid extension. If present, it is mild, focal, and always caused by non-atypical cells.[42] The epidermal rete ridges are less prominent than in skin lentigo. Mild cytologic atypia can be seen. Pigmentation is usually limited to the lower third of the nail epithelium but can be seen throughout the thickness. Melanophages may be seen in the superficial dermis.[45–47]

It is important to distinguish melanocytic activation from lentigo because of different clinical management (Table 9.4).

MELANOCYTIC NEVUS

Any type of nevus can present in the nail apparatus-congenital, acquired, blue, or spitz nevus. Melanocytic nevi, histologically, show lentiginous proliferation of melanocytes at the dermo epidermal junction. Nests of melanocytes form with progression of disease to more advanced stages. These nests can be irregular and confluent and may be situated in epithelial layers slightly above the basal layer. If present in the upper layers, a malignant lesion should be suspected.[4] The nests are in the matrix. Sometimes, they may also be seen in the ventral part of the proximal nail fold and/or the hyponychium. It is unusual to find them in the nail bed. Nuclear atypia can be seen in 15% of the lesions and mild melanocytic migration in 20% of cases.[47] The problematic issues with evaluation of menocytic nevi are summarized in Table 9.5 and should be kept in mind while reporting such lesions.

IN SITU MELANOMA

It is characterized by an increased number of melanocytes in the basal cell layer. Amin et al. found the mean number of melanocytes was 58.9 per 1 mm stretch of epithelial-stromal junction (range from 39 to 136) while it was 15.3

Table 9.4 Melanocyte activation versus lentigo

S. no.	Feature	Melanocytic activation	Lentigo
1	Melanocyte count[a]	No increase	Slight to moderate increase
2	Location of melanocytes	Suprabasal	Arranged as single cells along the basal layer and focally in the first suprabasal layer
3	Morphology of melanocyte	Have pigmented dendrites[b]	Round appearance with a clear halo of cytoplasmic retraction
4	Pigment	Often sparse	Usually abundant and regularly dispersed

In normal nails, MC ranges from 4 to 9 melanocytes (mean = 7.7) per 1 mm stretch of normal nail matrix epithelium.[45,48,49]
Source: Perrin, C., *Am. J. Dermatopathol.*, 35, 621–636, 2013.
[a] The melanocyte count (MC) = number of intraepithelial melanocytes per 1 mm segment of nail matrix or tumors of nail app (measured with an ocular micrometer).
[b] A sign of the normal dormant status of the nail melanocyte with a failure of the normal process of pigment transfer to the keratinocyte.[46]

Table 9.5 Problems in evaluation of benign melanocytic proliferations in the nail

1	Symmetry is not a helpful feature to differentiate benign from malignant proliferations because biopsies are often partial and small.
2	Nevi are asymmetrical in longitudinal biopsies due to nail architecture.
3	Margins are often unevaluable.
4	Mild atypia can sometimes be seen in benign lentigo.

Source: André, J. et al., Clin. Dermatol., 31, 526–539, 2013; Tosti, A. et al., J. Am. Acad. Dermatol., 34, 765–771, 1996.

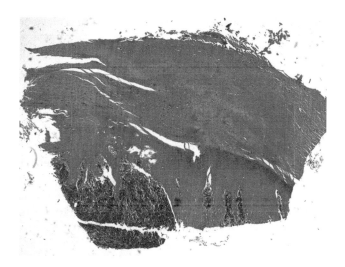

Figure 9.8 Nail malignant melanoma: section from nail showing a tumor in subepithelial tissue with sheets of pigmented cells, H&E x40.

(ranged 5 to 31) for benign melanocytic hyperplasia.[45] Single melanocytes are seen predominantly;[51,52] however, rare small nests may also be seen.[45] Nuclear atypia (nuclear enlargement, pleomorphism, and prominent nucleoli) and pagetoid spread are seen, which in early lesions are focal and moderate. In more advanced lesions, a confluence of single cells is seen with marked nuclear atypia and florid pagetoid migration.[2,42] Individual melanocytes can be spindle-shaped or rounded. Some of them have long pigmented dendrites.[53] Presence of "tumor-infiltrating lymphocytes" is a clue to the diagnosis.[54] The differentiation of in situ melanoma from solar lentigo is difficult at times and the criteria to differentiate these two conditions are given in Table 9.6.

Table 9.6 Criteria proposed to differentiate in situ melanoma from lentigo

1	High melanocyte density
2	Melanocyte multinucleation
3	Multifocal pagetoid spread[a]
4	Cytologic atypia
5	Presence of a moderately dense lichenoid inflammatory infiltrate

Source: André, J. et al., Clin. Dermatol., 31, 526–539, 2013.
[a] Focal pagetoid spread is commonly seen in benign nail lesions.[45]

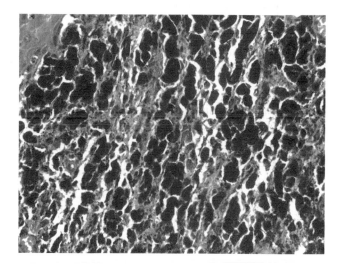

Figure 9.9 Nail malignant melanoma: high power view showing heavily pigmented tumor cells with some having visible vesicular nuclei and prominent nucleoli, H&E x 400.

INVASIVE MELANOMA

Grossly, nodular melanomas vary from a large fungating mass to rather small inconspicuous lesions.[55] Invasive melanoma is characterized by atypical melanocytes invading the dermis (Figures 9.8 and 9.9). There is no adjacent intraepithelial growth of tumoral cells beyond the width of three rete ridges. The key issues in evaluation of malignant melanocytic lesions of the nail unit have been summarized in Table 9.7.

In addition to diagnosis, nail unit biopsy may also help in determining the prognosis of a particular case. The number of dermal mitosis as seen on histology is one of the prognostic factors. The poor prognostic factors have been summarized in Box 9.1.[54]

Among different histologic types of invasive melanoma, the most common subtype was acral lentiginous (60%), followed by nodular (23%) and desmoplastic (7%) as documented in an Australian study. Also, a majority of tumors were locally advanced at presentation, with 79% being Clark Level IV or V. Sentinel lymph node biopsy has been reported to be positive in 17%–24% of patients.[54,69] Observation of osteoid material associated with the tumor is more common in melanomas of the nail compared with those of the skin.[4] Prognosis of nail melanomas is worse than melanoma in other locations, mainly due to delayed diagnosis.[60-66]

Table 9.7 Problems in evaluation of nail apparatus melanomas

1	The histogenic type, the Clark's level, and the Breslow thickness are more difficult to assess because of their peculiar nail anatomy and partial biopsies.[2]
2	It is extremely tough to determine the separation of the papillary from the reticular dermis.[2] Because of the thinness of the papillary dermis, levels III and IV are increased.[56,57]
3	Usually, there is no adipose tissue between the nail bed and periosteum. Therefore, melanoma reaching the periosteum or invading the underlying bone should be classified as Clark level V.[54,55]
4	There is usually no granular layer in the nail matrix and bed and the epithelium can be markedly acanthotic, giving an impression of increased Breslow thickness even if the invasion is limited.[55]
5	An epidermal metaplasia is frequently present that may be partial and of variable thickness.[48,58]
6	The Breslow index is not entirely applicable to the nail apparatus owing to the micro-anatomic particularities of the nail and sectioning artefacts. Further studies are required to quantify the prognostic and therapeutic values of the Breslow index on the nail unit.[46]

BOX 9.1: The poor prognostic factors for nail unit melanoma

Advanced age at diagnosis
High number of dermal mitosis
Tumor-associated ulceration
Amelanosis
Higher stage of disease

Immunohistochemistry

Immunochemistry is particularly useful for the diagnosis of early melanomas and for the determination of margins in acral lentiginous melanomas. For intraepithelial melanocytes, the sensitivity was better with HMB-45 than with Mart-1. S-100 protein was the least sensitive. In invasive NAM, however, S-100 protein was the most sensitive and was the only positive marker in cases of desmoplastic melanoma and in the areas with chondroid differentiation.[49]

Differential diagnosis

It is often difficult to differentiate very early melanoma from other benign conditions such as lentigo. Hematoma is a major differential diagnosis of black nail.[67,68] A prior history of trauma may not always be available. Also, trauma has been implicated in the pathogenesis of melanoma.[43] Hence, an extended non-migratory hematoma is considered suspicious and an iron stain (Perl's stain) is done to confirm old hemorrhage. Benzidine stain can confirm a fresh hemorrhage.

In scenarios where nail histology is not conclusive, certain points as discussed in Box 9.2 guide us in planning further management.

CONCLUSION

Nail histology is an important diagnostic tool in the diagnosis of not only nail tumors but various infective and

---

BOX 9.2: The points to consider when histology is inconclusive

1. If the melanocytic hyperplasia is atypical and the biopsy was partial, an early in situ melanoma cannot be ruled out, and a complete excision of the nail apparatus should be advised.
2. If the intraepithelial component of the melanoma is lacking, immunohistochemistry may be necessary to differentiate an amelanotic melanoma and a desmoplastic melanoma from epithelial or mesenchymal tumors.[69]
3. The possibility of non-representative sampling should always be considered in the assessment of small biopsies and should be clearly stated in the report. A further biopsy should always be considered if clinically appropriate.[54]
4. Biopsy should not be taken from the periungual skin in cases with positive Hutchison's sign because the histological features can be falsely reassuring. Frequently, there is only mild atypical melanocytic hyperplasia with rare melanocytic migration. It may just show epidermal pigmentation.

---

inflammatory nail disorders, especially when there is isolated nail involvement.

REFERENCES

1. Haneke E. Anatomy, biology, physiology and basic pathology of the nail organ. *Hautarzt* 2014;65(4):282–290.
2. André J, Sass U, Richert B, Theunis A. Nail pathology. *Clin Dermatol* 2013;31(5):526–539.
3. Rich P. Nail biopsy: Indications and methods. *Dermatol Surg* 2001;27:229–234.

4. Martin B. Nail histopathology. *Actas Dermo-Sifiliogr* 2013;104:564–578.

5. Fleckman P, Omura EF. Histopathology of the nail. *Adv Dermatol* 2001;17:385–406.

6. Zaias N, Oertel I, Elliot DF. Fungi in toenails. *J Invest Dermatol* 1969;53:140–142.

7. Zaias N. *The Nail in Health and Disease*, 2nd ed. East Norwalk, CT: Appleton and Lange; 1990. pp. 87–105.

8. Suarez SM, Silvers DN, Scher RK, Pearlstein HH, Auerbach R. Histologic evaluation of nail clippings for diagnosing onychomycosis. *Arch Dermatol* 1991;127:1517–1519.

9. Grover C, Reddy BS, Uma Chaturvedi K. Diagnosis of nail psoriasis: Importance of biopsy and histopathology. *Br J Dermatol* 2005;153:1153–1158.

10. Tosti A, Peluso AM, Misciali C, Cameli N. Nail lichen striatus: Clinical features and long-term follow-up of five patients. *J Am Acad Dermatol* 1997;36:908–913.

11. Mann RJ, Allen BR. Nail dystrophy due to sarcoidosis. *Br J Dermatol* 1981;105:599–601.

12. Cigna E, Palumbo F, De Santo L, Edoardo-Zampieri A, Soda G. Short-scar surgical approach for the treatment of glomus tumor of the digit. *J Cut Med Surg* 2011;15:21–28.

13. Saijo S, Kato T, Tagami H. Pigmented nail streak associated with Bowen's disease of the nail matrix. *Dermatologica* 1990;181(2):156–158.

14. Lemont H, Haas R. Subungual pigmented Bowen's disease in a nineteen-year-old black female. *J Am Podiatr Med Assoc* 1994;84(1):39–40.

15. Dalle S, Depape L, Phan A, Balme B, Ronger-Savle S, Thomas L. Squamous cell carcinoma of the nail apparatus: Clinicopathological study of 35 cases. *Br J Dermatol* 2007;156:871–874.

16. Gallouj S, Harmouch T, Soughi M et al. [Subungual verrucous carcinoma of the toe]. *Ann Dermatol Venereol* 2010;137:842–843.

17. Tirado-Gonzalez M, Gonzalez-Serva A. The nail plate biopsy may pick up gout crystals and other crystals. *Am J Dermatopathol* 2011;33:351–353.

18. Raposo I, Torres T. Nail psoriasis as a predictor of the development of psoriatic arthritis. *Actas Dermosifiliogr* 2015;106:452–457.

19. Calvert HT, Smith MA, Wells RS. Psoriasis and the nails. *Br J Dermatol* 1963;75:415–418.

20. Jiaravuthisan MM, Sasseville D, Vender RB, Murphy F, Muhn CY. Psoriasis of the nail: Anatomy, pathology, clinical presentation, and a review of the literature on therapy. *J Am Acad Dermatol* 2007;57:1–27.

21. de Berker DA, Baran R, Dawber RPR. The nail in dermatological diseases. In: Baran R, Dawber RP, editors. *Diseases of the Nail and Their Management*, 3rd ed. Oxford, UK: Blackwell Science; 1991. pp. 172–222.

22. Haneke E. Non-infectious inflammatory disorders of the nail apparatus. *J Dtsch Dermatol Ges* 2009;7(9):787–797.

23. Hanno R, Mathes B, Krull E. Longitudinal nail biopsy in evaluation of acquired nail dystrophies. *J Am Acad Dermatol* 1986;14:803–809.

24. Boyd AS, Neldner KH. Lichen planus. *J Am Acad Dermatol* 1991;25:593–619.

25. Scher RK, Ackerman AB. Lichen planus. *Am J Dermatopathol* 1983;5:375.

26. Tosti A, Peluso AM, Fanti PA et al. Nail lichen planus: Clinical and pathologic study of 24 patients. *J Am Acad Dermatol* 1993;28:724.

27. Pall A, Gupta RR, Gulati B, Goyal P. Twenty nail anonychia due to lichen planus. *J Dermatol* 2004;31:146–147.

28. Goettmann SI, Zaraa I, Moulonguet I. Nail lichen planus: Epidemiological, clinical, pathological, therapeutic and prognosis study of 67 cases. *J Eur Acad Dermatol Venereol* 2012;26:1304–1309.

29. Zaias N. The nail in lichen planus. *Arch Dermatol* 1970;101:264–271.

30. Wu IB, Schwartz RA. Reiter's syndrome: The classic triad and more. *J Am Acad Dermatol* 2008;59:113–121.

31. Andre J, Achten G. Onychomycosis. *Int J Dermatol* 1987;26:481–490.

32. Kaur R, Kashyap B, Bhalla P. Onychomycosis-epidemiology, diagnosis and management. *Indian J Med Microbiol* 2008;26:108–116.

33. Nagar R, Nayak CS, Deshpande S, Gadkari RP, Shastri J. Subungual hyperkeratosis nail biopsy: A better diagnostic tool for onychomycosis. *Indian J Dermatol Venereol Leprol* 2012;78:620–624.

34. Jeelani S, Ahmed Q, Lanker A, Hassan I, Jeelani N, Fazili T. Histopathological examination of nail clippings using PAS staining (HPE-PAS): Gold standard in diagnosis of onychomycosis. *Mycoses* 2015;58:27–32.

35. Haneke E. Fungal infections of the nail. *Semin Dermatol* 1991;10:41–53.

36. Lawry MA, Haneke E, Strobeck K, Martin S, Zimmer B, Romano PS. Methods for diagnosing onychomycosis: A comparative study and review of the literature. *Arch Dermatol* 2000;136:1112–1116.

37. Weinberg JM, Koestenblatt EK, Jennings MB. Utility of histopathologic analysis in the evaluation of onychomycosis. *J Am Podiatr Med Assoc* 2005;95:258–263.

38. Grover C, Reddy BS, Chaturvedi KU. Onychomycosis and the diagnostic significance of nail biopsy. *J Dermatol* 2003;30(2):116–122.

39. Singal A, Khanna D. Onychomycosis: Diagnosis and management. *Indian J Dermatol Venereol Leprol* 2011;77:659–672.

40. Jayayatilake JA, Tilakaratne WM, Panagoda GJ. Candida onychomycosis: A mini-review. *Mycopathologia* 2009;168:165–173.

41. Tosti A, Piraccini BM. Warts of the nail unit: Surgical and nonsurgical approaches. *Dermatol Surg* 2001;27(3):235–239.

42. Fernandez-Flores A, Saeb-Lima M, Martinez-Nova A. Histopathology of the nail unit. *Rom J Morphol Embryol* 2014;55(2):235–256.

43. André J, Lateur N. Pigmented nail disorders. *Dermatol Clin* 2006;24:329–339.

44. Goettman S. Pigmented lesions of the nail apparatus. *Rev Prat* 2000;50:2246–2250.

45. Amin B, Nehal KS, Jungbluth AA et al. Histologic distinction between subungual lentigo and melanoma. *Am J Surg Pathol* 2008;32:835–843.

46. Perrin C. Tumors of the nail unit. A review. Part I: Acquired localized longitudinal melanonychia and erythronychia. *Am J Dermatopathol* 2013;35(6):621–636.

47. Goettmann-Bonvallot S, André J, Belaich S. Longitudinal melanonychia in children: A clinical and histopathologic study of 40 cases. *J Am Acad Dermatol* 1999;41:17–22.

48. Ruben BS. Pigmented lesions of the nail unit: Clinical and histopathologic features. *Semin Cutan Med Surg* 2010;29:148–158.

49. Theunis A, Richer B, Sass U et al. Immunohistochemical study of 40 cases of longitudinal melanonychia. *Am J Dermatopathol* 2011;33:27–34.

50. Tosti A, Baran R, Piraccini BM et al. Nail matrix nevi: A clinical and histopathologic study of twenty-two patients. *J Am Acad Dermatol* 1996;34:765–771.

51. Saida T, Ohshima Y. Clinical and histopathologic characteristics of early lesions of subungual malignant melanoma. *Cancer* 1989;63:556–560.

52. High WA, Quirey RA, Guillén DR et al. Presentation, histopathologic findings, and clinical outcomes in 7 cases of melanoma in situ of the nail unit. *Arch Dermatol* 2004;140:1102–1106.

53. Kwon IH, Lee JH, Cho KH. Acral lentiginous melanoma in situ: A study of nine cases. *Am J Dermatopathol* 2004;26:285–289.

54. Tan KB, Moncrieff M, Thompson JF et al. Subungual melanoma: A study of 124 cases highlighting features of early lesions, potential pitfalls in diagnosis, and guidelines for histologic reporting. *Am J Surg Pathol* 2007;31:1902–1912.

55. Patterson RH, Helwig EB. Subungual malignant melanoma: A clinical pathologic study. *Cancer* 1980;46:2074–2087.

56. Shin HT, Jang KT, Mun GH, Lee DY, Lee JB. Histopathological analysis of the progression pattern of subungual melanoma: Late tendency of dermal invasion in the nail matrix area. *Mod Pathol* 2014;27(11):1461–1467.

57. Thai KE, Young R, Sinclair RD. Nail apparatus melanoma. *Australas J Dermatol* 2001;42:71–81.

58. Dunphy L, Morhij R, Verma Y, Pay A. Missed opportunity to diagnose subungual melanoma: Potential pitfalls! *BMJ Case Rep* 2017;2017. pii:bcr-2016-218785.

59. Cohen T, Busam KJ, Patel A et al. Subungual melanoma: Management considerations. *Am J Surg* 2008;195:244–248.

60. Quinn MJ, Thompson JE, Crotty K, McCarthy WH, Coates AS. Subungual melanoma of the hand. *J Hand Surg Am* 1996;21(3):506–511.

61. Glat PM, Spector JA, Roses DF, Shapiro RA, Harris MN, Beasley RW, Grossman JA. The management of pigmented lesions of the nail bed. *Ann Plast Surg* 1996;37(2):125–134.

62. Haneke E, Baran R. Longitudinal melanonychia. *Dermatol Surg* 2001;27(6):580–584.

63. Metzger S, Ellwanger U, Stroebel W, Schiebel U, Rassner G, Fierlbeck G. Extent and consequences of physician delay in the diagnosis of acral melanoma. *Melanoma Res* 1998;8(2):181–186.

64. Banfield CC, Dawber RP. Nail melanoma: A review of the literature with recommendations to improve patient management. *Br J Dermatol* 1999;141(4):628–632.

65. Grunwald MH, Yerushalmi J, Glesinger R, Lapid O, Zirkin HJ. Subungual amelanotic melanoma. *Cutis* 2000;65(5):303–304.

66. Levit EK, Kagen MH, Scher RK, Grossman M, Altman E. The ABC rule for clinical detection of subungual melanoma. *J Am Acad Dermatol* 2000;42(2 Pt 1):269–274.

67. Baran R, Haneke E, Drapé JL et al. Tumours of the nail apparatus and adjacent tissues. In: Baran R, Dawber RPR, de Berker DAR et al., editors. *Diseases of the Nails and Their Management*, 3rd ed. Oxford, UK: Blackwell Science Ltd; 2001. pp. 607–630.

68. Dawber RPR, Colver GB. The spectrum of malignant melanoma of the nail apparatus. *Sem Dermatol* 1991;10(1):82–87.

69. Parodi PC, Scott CA, De Biasio F et al. Desmoplastic melanoma of the nail. *Ann Plast Surg* 2003;50:658–662.

PART 3

Nail Unit Abnormalities

10

Nail plate abnormalities

BALACHANDRA S. ANKAD AND SAVITHA L. BEERGOUDER

INTRODUCTION

- The nail apparatus consists of nail matrix, nail plate, and the soft tissue around and beneath it. Nail plate is made up of hard keratin and is horny rectangular translucent plate.
- It varies in thickness from 0.5 to 0.7 mm. The surface of nail plate is generally convex although interindividual and interdigital variations are present.
- Histologically, nail plate has three horizontal layers: thin dorsal lamina, thick intermediate layer, and ventral thin lamina.[1]
- The upper surface of nail plate is smooth and longitudinal ridges are present in variable numbers. These are of forensic importance, used to distinguish identical twins.
- Nail plate abnormalities can be classified as abnormalities of nail plate configurations, surface alterations, modifications in the consistency, and soft tissue abnormalities.
- In this chapter, a brief overview of abnormalities of nail plate is discussed.[1]

NAIL PLATE ABNORMALITIES DUE TO SURFACE ALTERATIONS

Longitudinal grooves

- **Introduction:** Longitudinal grooves (LG) are the deep longitudinal defects on the nail surface that run all along the full length of part of nail plate.[2]
- The depth of groove may be full or partial. It should be differentiated from ridges, which are linear elevations on the surface.
- These occur due to long-standing nail abnormalities. LG can be seen in the following clinical scenario (Table 10.1):[1]
  a. Physiological phenomena wherein shallow and delicate furrows are seen running parallel to each other.
  b. Certain pathology such as lichen planus, rheumatoid arthritis, periungual warts, fibromas, myxoma, myxoid cyst, and Darier's disease produce LG.
  c. In some cases, trauma and oral retinoids can be attributed to causation of LG.

Table 10.1 Causes of longitudinal grooves[1]

Physiological	More prominent in old age
Inflammatory conditions	Lichen planus, rheumatoid arthritis
Tumors	Viral warts, myxoid cysts, periungual fibromas
Miscellaneous	Trauma, median canaliform dystrophy of Heller, onychorrhexis

2. Median canaliform dystrophy of Heller (MCDH) is the most distinctive form of LG. This is an uncommon condition consisting of longitudinal defects that start at cuticle or mid-way of nail plate and extend up to free edge of nail plate (Figure 10.1).[3]

Base of the defect may be 2–4 mm wide. Cuticle is normal.[4]

It is usually symmetrical. The thumb is most commonly affected, though other fingers may be involved.

Exact etiology of this condition is not known, but self-inflicted trauma to the nail matrix has been elucidated as one of the causes. Other causes are idiopathic, familial, and subungual tumors.

It may be present in the center or paracentric position. Small fissures or cracks extending from the groove towards periphery that do not reach the edge of nail plate give rise to a "fir-tree" appearance (Figure 10.2). Idiopathic cases revert to normal after months to years. MCDH resulting from self-inflicted trauma is an impulse control disorder and requires psychotropic drugs like selective serotonin reuptake inhibitors (e.g., fluoxetine) for its management.

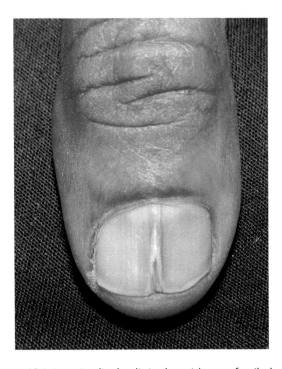

Figure 10.1 Longitudinal split in the mid-way of nail plate in early Heller's dystrophy.

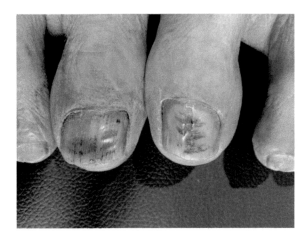

Figure 10.2 Fir-tree appearance in well-established Heller's dystrophy. (Courtesy of Dr Anil Patki, Consultant Dermatologist, Pune, India.)

3. Onychorrhexis is another type of LG wherein series of shallow and narrow furrows are present running parallel on the nail surface (Figure 10.3) (See brittle nail section for details.) (Table 10.2).[2]

4. Tumors at the proximal portion of nail result in longitudinal furrow or canal.

This is due to pressure effect of wart, myxoid cyst, or periungual fibromas. Grooves in it are deep and wide (Figure 10.4).

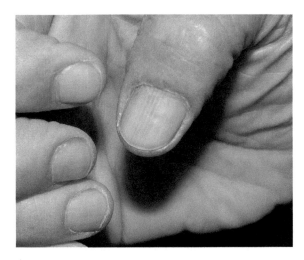

Figure 10.3 Shallow and narrow longitudinal grooves in onychorrhexis.

Table 10.2 Causes for onychorrhexis[2]

Medical causes	Hypothyroidism, bulimia, anemia, anorexia nervosa
Dermatosis	Psoriasis
Trauma	Repeated injuries like keyboard players
Chemical injury	Excessive exposure to soaps and detergents Nail polish removers
Miscellaneous	Exposure to cold, genetics, old age

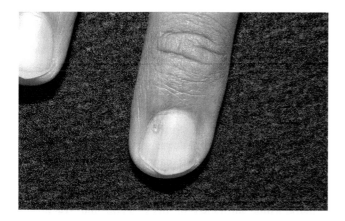

Figure 10.4 Wide and deep canal on the nail plate due to angiofibroma.

- **Pathogenesis:** LG are the result of injury to the cuticle and nail matrix either by repeated pressure resulting from habit tic or tumorous growths pressing upon the nail matrix.[2]
- **Clinical features:** LG are canal like depressions on the nail plate. MCDH appears symmetrical and commonly on the thumbs although other fingernails are affected. After a long period, nail becomes normal but recurrences are not exceptional. Differential diagnosis includes "washboard nail plate" seen in chronic mechanical injury wherein cuticle is pushed back and sometimes there is inflammation of proximal nail folds.
- Nail splits are obvious with sharp free edges in the center and usually seen in pterygium, nail-patella syndrome, trauma, Reynaud's phenomena, and lichen striatus.
- **Diagnosis:** No investigations are necessary as clinical features and history are sufficient for the diagnosis.
- **Treatment:** Some advocate nail splitting, but many authors disagree.[2] Removal of the etiological factors such as tumors and treating the underlying inflammatory conditions like lichen planus and peripheral vascular disease will improve the condition.[1] It should be noted that MCDH may recur even after treatment. Treatment is directed to etiological factors such as any growths in the periungual areas.

Longitudinal ridges and beads

- Beading and ridging on the nail are minor changes on the nail plate. They become prominent with age. They do not indicate any diseases (Figure 10.5).[4]

Transverse grooves

- **Introduction:** Transverse grooves (TG) are horizontal depressions on the nail surface. TG represents injury to the nail matrix. During injury, cessation or interference of nail growth is reflected as groove (Table 10.3).[2]
- **Pathogenesis:** TG results after temporary cessation of nail matrix activity due to various diseases and insults to the matrix. This chronic mechanical injury results in TGs and a large central depression running down the nail.[2]
- **Clinical features:** TG matches arcuate shape of lunula in endogenous injuries. In exogenous origin due to manicure, they assume the shape of the proximal nail fold.[4]

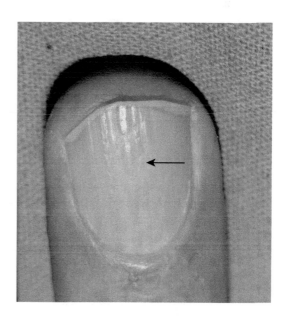

Figure 10.5 Longitudinal ridges in normal individuals. Note the beading (arrow) also.

Table 10.3 Causes for transverse grooves[2]

Causes	Isolated	Multiple
Trauma	Onychotillomania, manicure	Rarely onychotillomania
Inflammatory	Dermatitis, periungual erythema, and paronychia	Eczema, erythroderma
Systemic conditions		Drugs, viral illness (measles), diarrhea, Kawasaki syndrome, peripheral ischemia

Source: de Berker, D.A.R. et al., Acquired disorders of nail and nail unit, in: Griffiths, C. et al., eds., *Rook's Textbook of Dermatology*, 9th ed., Wiley Blackwell, Oxford, UK, pp. 95.1–95.65, 2016.

- **Types**[2]:
  1. Nervous habit of pushing back the cuticle repeatedly results in multiple transverse ridges on a single or multiple nails. When multiple TG is present it is difficult to differentiate habit tic deformity from psoriasis (Figure 10.6).
  2. TGs due to systemic conditions are referred to as Beau's lines. They were first described by Beau in 1846.

     TG may involve single or multiple digits and are usually at the same distance from proximal nail folds when the cause is systemic one.

     Depressions may provide useful information about the duration of illness prior to the appearance of groove. Depressions can involve whole or partial depth of nail plate.[1]

They start at cuticle and progress forward as nail grows and ultimately disappear.

Thumb nail supplies information for the previous 5–6 months whereas great toe gives evidence of disease up to 2 years. Hence, they are called "retrospective indicators" of many pathological states (Figures 10.7 and 10.8).

Depth and width of groove give clues to the severity and duration of illness, respectively. Sometimes very deep Beau's lines will cause total division of nail plate resulting in latent onychomadesis. Beau's lines are analogous to Pohl-Pinkus line found in hairs, which shows loss of medulla and shaft fracture (Table 10.4).[1,2]

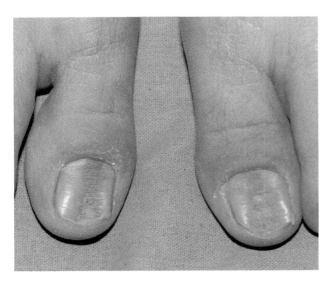

Figure 10.6 Multiple transverse grooves covering entire nail plate. In this case, they are due to repeated trauma.

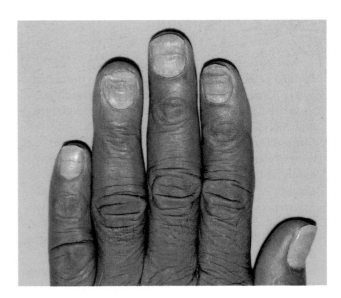

Figure 10.7 Beau's lines on all the nails due to preceding systemic illness.

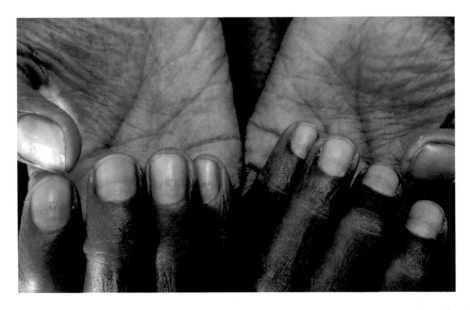

Figure 10.8 Beau's lines, rather shallow as compared to Figure 10.7, represent temporary cessation of nail growth.

Table 10.4 Causes for Beau's lines[1,2]

Physiological	4–5 week babies
	Cyclically with menstruation
Systemic diseases	Coronary thrombosis, pulmonary embolism, renal failure, Kawasaki disease, zinc deficiency
Infections	Measles, mumps, pneumonia
Drugs	Retinoids, Metoprolol, anti-mitotic agents, Dapsone hypersensitivity syndrome
Physical	Severe exposure to cold, carpal tunnel syndrome

Source: Puri, K.J.P.S., Nail and its disorders, in: Sacchidanand, S. et al., Eds., *IADVL Textbook of Dermatology*, 4th ed., Bhalani Publishing House, Mumbai, India, pp. 1588–1647, 2015; Baran, R., and Dawber, R.P.R., Physical signs, in: Baran, R., and Dawber, R.P.R., Eds., *Diseases of Nails and Their Management*, 2nd ed., Blackwell Scientific Publications, Oxford, UK, pp. 35–80, 1994.

TRANSVERSE OVER-CURVATURE OF THE NAIL

Introduction: Nail curvature may exceed the normal limit resulting in nail plate abnormalities.

1. **Pincer nails:** It is also called as trumpet, arched, or omega nail.
   - It is a nail dystrophy characterized by transverse over-curvature, which increases in the longitudinal axis resulting in increased midline growth of nail.
   - Due to over-curvature in the distal edge of nail plate and midline growth, lateral portions overgrow into the nail bed soft tissue (Figure 10.9).
   - In extreme cases, free-growing edges embed and pinch the soft tissues, forming a tunnel (Figure 10.10).[2,5]
   - It is probably due to selective widening of the horns of the lateral matrix by juxta-articular osteophytes.
   - This condition is inherited. Ill-fitting shoes may be contributory. Usually great toes are involved.

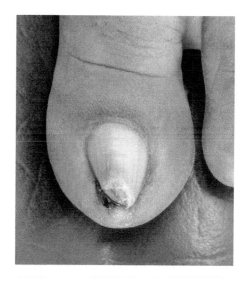

Figure 10.10 Pincer nail deformity: soft tissue is embraced by the overgrown lateral margins of nail plate.

   - However, if fingernails are affected, inflammatory osteoarthritis or subungual exostosis should be looked for. X-ray shows lateral deviation and widened base of base of distal phalanx and also exhibits bony outgrowths pointing distally.
2. **Tile-shaped nails:** There is increase in the transverse curvature but lateral margins remain parallel (Figure 10.11).
   - This is acquired form and associated with degenerative osteoarthritis affecting nails of fingers and toes. Radiography reveals similar changes as that of pincer nails.
3. **Plicated nail:** Surface is flat but the lateral margins are sharply angled forming vertical sides, which are parallel (Figure 10.12).
   - This is due to injury to the distal phalanx and nail organ by psoriasis and total destructive onychomycosis, which causes shrinkage of nail tissue, leading to over-curvature of the involved nail.
   - These deformities may be associated with ingrowing nails but inflammatory edema is absent.

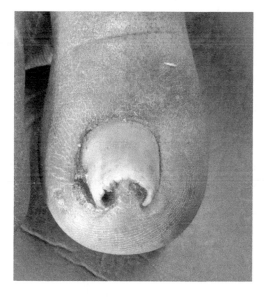

Figure 10.9 Lateral margins overgrowing to embed in the nail soft tissue in pincer nail deformity appearing as trumpet.

Treatment: It depends on the type and duration.[2]

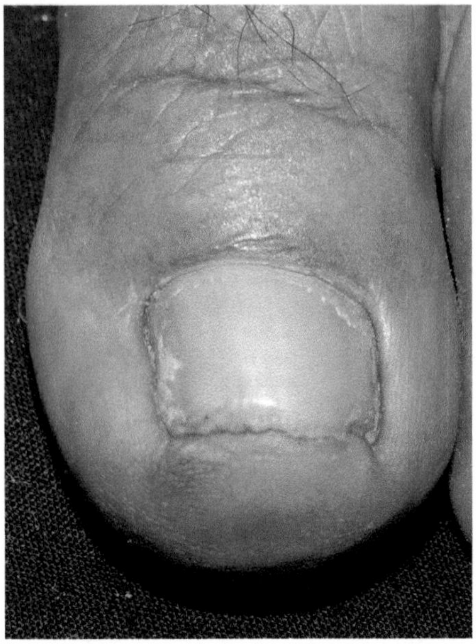

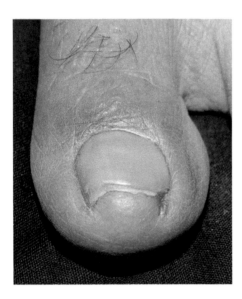

Figure 10.11 Tile-shaped nails showing increased transverse curvature. Note the parallel lateral margins.

Figure 10.12 Plicated nail surface due to over-curvature of nail plate. Vertical growth of lateral margins is evident.

Conservative

- **Clipping:** Clipping off of lateral margin of nail plate as proximally as possible.
- This may be facilitated by application of salicylic acid (3%) application 3–5 days prior to the procedure.
- **Grooving:** For early cases, grooving of involved portion of nail plate with a burr will help. It is usually done from lunula to free edge of nail.
- **Nail brace technique:** This is termed as orthonyx by Fraser, which describes the field of mechanical correction. In this procedure, lateral groves are cleaned and a brace is constructed to fit the curved plate exactly.

Nail plate, being weaker than the steel brace wire, will conform to the shape of brace. Nail plate becomes painlessly flattened within 6 months.

These conservative methods are simple and easy to perform. However, recurrences are common.

Surgical correction

After partial nail avulsion, lateral matrix horns are treated by chemical cautery with 88% phenol. Dorsal osteophytes are removed and nail bed is widened. The various techniques for nail bed widening include Zigzag nail bed flap method and Haneke's method.

PITTING

- **Synonym:** Pits; Rosenau's depressions; erosions; onychia punctata.
- **Introduction:** Pitting of nail plate is defined as punctate indentations due to the parakeratosis of proximal nail matrix. As the nail plate grows beyond the margin of proximal nail fold, abnormal parakeratotic keratinocytes are lost to leave behind tiny depression or pits on the surface.[2]
- Pits more commonly affect fingernails than toenails.
- **Causes:** Pits are seen in many inflammatory conditions that include psoriasis, eczema, pityriasis rubra pilaris, parakeratosis pustulosa, alopecia areata, chronic paronychia, Reiter's disease, lichen planus, and lichen striatus (Table 10.5).[1]
- Pits vary in depth, size, shape, and number depending on the etiology.
- **Clinical features:** In psoriasis, they are small, less than 1mm, but either shallow or deep seated. They are irregular, coarse, and randomly placed on the surface. The presence of more than 20 pits is suggestive of psoriasis (Figure 10.13).[6]
- Sometimes, pits are arranged in regular and uniform pattern or in a grid-like pattern. Samman described pits are arranged in rippling or ridging pattern and these are variants of regular and uniform patterns.
- Rarely a single, larger, and deeper pit is noted in psoriasis and is called elkonyxis. Occasionally, it is also

Table 10.5 Causes of nail pitting[1,6]

• Psoriasis	• Pemphigus vulgaris
• Alopecia areata	• Congenital
• Eczema	• Diabetes mellitus
• Parakeratosis pustulosa	• SLE
• Reiter's disease	• Sarcoidosis
• Chronic paronychia	• Rheumatoid arthritis
• Lichen planus	• Dermatomyositis
• Lichen nitidus	• Drug-induced
• Lichen striatus	erythroderma
• Pityriasis rosea	• Incontinentia pigmenti
• Vitiligo	• Chemical dermatitis

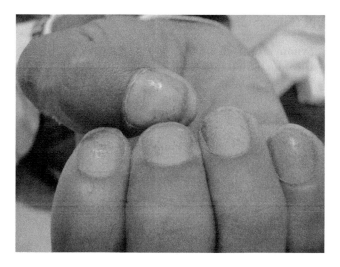

Figure 10.13 Numerous pits in psoriasis. Pits are irregular in size and shape.

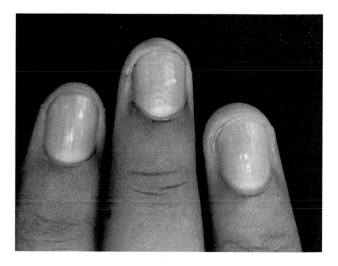

Figure 10.15 Idiopathic pitting in normal individual.

seen in secondary syphilis, Reiter's syndrome, and after etretinate and isotretinoin therapy.[7]

- In alopecia areata, they are small, fine, and regular and arranged in particular pattern making vertical or transverse rows and columns. They are referred to as Glen-plaid or Scotch-plaid pattern.[1]
- However, it is important to note that nail plate pitting in alopecia areata might be an expression of other isolated nail diseases such as nail psoriasis.[8]
- In eczema, coarse and irregular pits are seen in affected fingernails.
- In Reiter's syndrome and secondary syphilis, pits are seen in lunula giving mottled appearance to the lunula.
- In diabetes mellitus, pits are seen as small craters on the middle and ring finger and are referred to as Rosenau's depressions (Figure 10.14).[9]
- It should be noted that pitted nails grow faster than normal nails.

- Occasional pits appear in normal individuals (Figure 10.15) and pits can also appear as a developmental anomaly.

TRACHYONYCHIA

- **Synonym:** Rough nails, twenty-nail dystrophy.
- **Introduction:** Trachyonychia refers to nail plate dystrophy wherein plate loses luster and becomes rough. It was first described by Alkiewicz in 1950.[10]
- It is described aptly as "sand-blasted nails," a French term, which evokes clinical feature of grey roughened surface (Figure 10.16).[4]

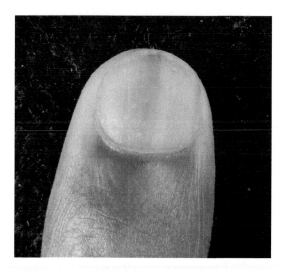

Figure 10.14 Rosenau's depressions in diabetes mellitus.

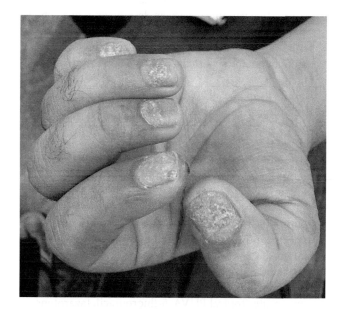

Figure 10.16 Nail surface is rough and appears as "sand-blasted" in trachyonychia.

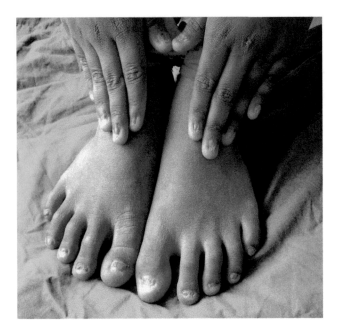

Figure 10.17 Twenty-nail dystrophy: atrophy and scarring of all the nails and also partial loss of a few of the nails.

- It can be idiopathic, familial, congenital, or acquired.
- Hazelrigg et al. observed trachyonychia in all 20 nails in children and defined it as "twenty-nail dystrophy" (Figure 10.17). In acquired form, it is a manifestation of alopecia areata, psoriasis, and lichen planus. Recently, it has been described in ichthyosis vulgaris, IgA deficiency, eczema, and vitiligo.[1]
- However, isolated nail abnormality is the most common presentation.
- "Twenty-nail dystrophy" is clinically characterized by loss of shiny surface of plate and appears as a sandpaper texture. Two variants have been described. In one, whole nail becomes rough and gives the appearance of sandpaper and in the other type, plate surface retains its shiny nature but many superficial punctate depressions are noted.[1]
- Despite its name, all 20 nails are not necessarily affected and uniformly involved. Besides roughness, thinning, splitting at free edge, and distal chipping are other clinical features of "twenty-nail dystrophy."
- Histopathology demonstrates psoriatic or lichen planus pathology, especially in longitudinal nail biopsies.
- Trachyonychia or twenty-nail dystrophy is a benign condition. In children, spontaneous resolution is expected; however, in adults it may take chronic course.
- **Treatment:** This nail plate abnormality is treated with corticosteroids either by topical, intramatricial, or systemic route. Topical PUVA, 5-fluorouracil, tazarotene, may be of some help.[1] Emollient and systemic biotin reduces the nail fragility.[11]

ONYCHOSCHIZIA

- **Synonym:** Lamellar nail dystrophy
- **Introduction:** It is splitting of nail plate at the free edge in fingers and toes.[4]
- Nail is formed in layers analogous to skin layers and, in this condition, it is split horizontally into layers (Figure 10.18).[4]
- Exogenous factors contribute to this defect. Repeated soaking of nails in water followed by drying is attributed. Hence, it is commonly seen in those who are involved in such occupational activity. Up to 27%–35% of adult women are affected by onychoschizia due to repeated watering and followed by drying of fingernails (Figure 10.19). However, mere occupation

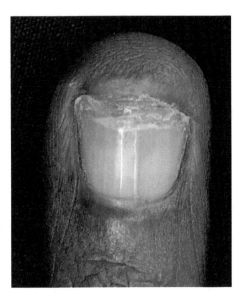

Figure 10.18 Horizontal split at the free edge in onychoschizia.

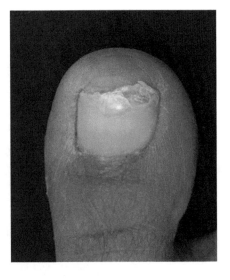

Figure 10.19 Transverse split extending to the proximal portion of nail plate in onychoschizia.

is not contributory; it is also observed in lichen planus, psoriasis, polycythemia Vera, impaired peripheral circulation, ageing and Darier's disease, and HIV infection.[1]

- Onychoschizia along with dyspareunia may be first clue for the recurrences of malignant glucagonoma.[12]
- Splits are also reported in retinoid therapy.[13]
- Clinically it is characterized by splitting of nail plate at the free edges. It may be localized or full length of free edge may be involved.
- Electron microscopy reveals horizontal separation of nail plate, which may, sometimes, extend up to proximal nail fold. It also demonstrates individual cells lying in the empty spaces. These observations indicate lamellar splitting in onychoschizia occurs between the cell layers.[2]
- These findings are proved in vitro by Wallis et al. by exposing the nails to water followed by dehydrating them. Hence, onychoschizia results from repeated watering followed by drying. Organic solvents, detergents, and acidic or basic solutions are also contributory.[14]
- **Treatment:** It consists of retaining of hydration by gloves and emollient nail creams. Application of hydrophilic petrolatum cream to the wet nails will reverse the clinical changes.

ONYCHOMADESIS

- **Introduction:** It is spontaneous separation of nail plate from the nail bed in its proximal portion.
- It implies limited lesion affecting the proximal part of matrix. It results from temporary cessation of growth of nail lasting for more than 2 weeks.[1]
- Initially small cleavage appears under the proximal portion of the nail. This forms a shallow ulcer that does not involve the deeper layers. When injury is taken off, nail regrows over again distally.
- In latent onychomadesis, nail plate demonstrates transverse split because of complete inhibition of nail growth for 1–2 weeks.
- It is seen in severe bullous disorders, drug reactions (Figure 10.20), and severe psychological stress.
- It may be idiopathic or familial.[15]
- Sometimes total loss of nail is observed due to destruction of matrix following trauma and lichen planus (Figure 10.21).[2]

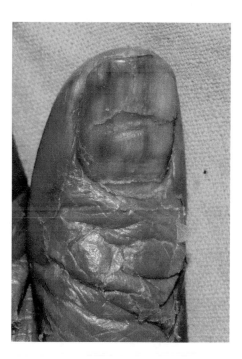

Figure 10.20 Onychomedesis showing transverse split with new growth proximally.

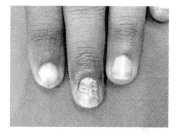

Figure 10.21 Onychomedesis affecting single digit in lichen planus.

PTERYGIUM

- **Introduction:** The term pterygium is derived from the Greek word pterygion meaning wing.[1]
- Two types are described. One is dorsal (pterygium unguis) and the other one is ventral (pterygium inversus unguis).
- **Dorsal pterygium:** It is characterized by linear fibrotic scar tissue extending from proximal nail fold on to the surface of nail bed. Usually nail plate divides into two halves due to severe and deep fissure leaving behind

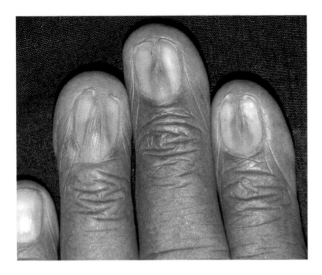

Figure 10.22 Fibrous tissue dividing nail plate into two halves in pterygium in early stage.

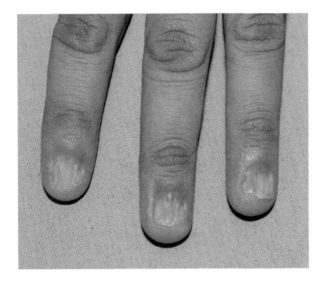

Figure 10.23 Pterygium with total loss of nail plate in late stage of lichen planus.

remnants of nail plate (Figure 10.22). Occasionally, whole nail plate is lost (Figure 10.23).

- It indicates severe nail disease and is due to destruction of nail matrix. Since matrix does not produce nail plate, epithelium of proximal fold attaches itself to the nail bed epithelium directly and both grow distally together. This results in "wing-like" scar tissue on the nail bed.[4]
- Classically it is seen in lichen planus and characterized by the scarring of part of or whole nail plate. Extent of scar depends on the involvement of nail matrix. Localized destruction of matrix produces linear scar tissue in the initial stages at proximal nail fold. Later it spreads to the nail bed in wing like pattern as the nail tissue grows distally. This causes deep fissure on the nail plate making it thin, which ultimately becomes divided into two parts. When complete matrix is affected, total loss of nail plate with permanent atrophy of nail is seen.[2]

- It is specific finding in lichen planus and hallmark of severe disease. However, it is also observed in other conditions such as onychotillomania, scarring trauma, radiotherapy, dyskeratosis congenita, leprosy, peripheral vascular disease, severe bullous disorders, and neuropathic damage.[16] It can be congenital.[2]
- **Ventral pterygium:** When nail bed epithelium extends distally in the under surface of the nail, it forms a tissue dislocating hyponychium and obscuring distal groove. It is called ventral pterygium. Causes include trauma, systemic sclerosis, lupus erythematosus, infections, and familial subungual pterygium.[4]
- **Treatment:** Early stage of pterygium due to lichen planus is treated with oral steroids to halt the progression. Late pterygium is very difficult to manage since atrophy and scarring would have been settled.

LUCENCY

- Nail is normally transparent and lucid in the texture.
- Its natural texture is affected by alterations in the cellular and intercellular arrangement.
- Trauma, disease conditions, chemotherapy, or poison produce parakeratotic nail cells, resulting in loss of nail lucency. Other causes include chronic eczema (Figure 10.24), congenital keratoderma of palms (Figure 10.25) and soles, and occupational hazard due to repeated contact with cement (Figure 10.26).[4]

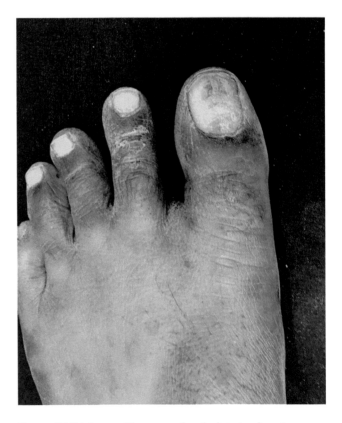

Figure 10.24 Loss of lucency of nail plate in chronic eczema.

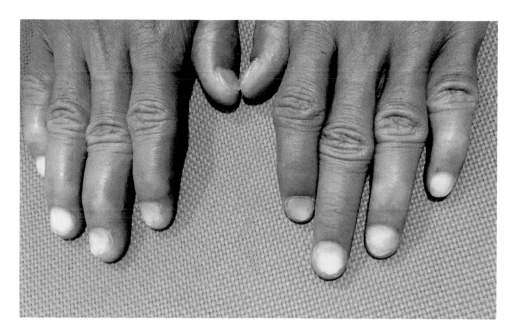

Figure 10.25 Congenital keratoderma showing loss of lucency along with koilonychia.

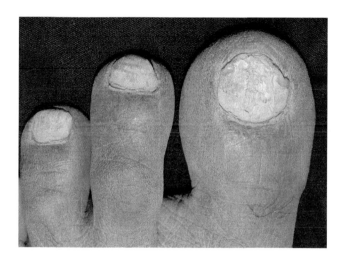

Figure 10.26 Opacity of all the toenails due to repeated contact with cement in mason. Crumbling of nail plate is seen.

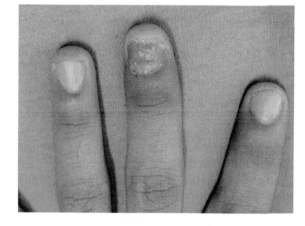

Figure 10.27 Psoriasis showing thickening of nail plate with surface erosions.

- Keratinocyte fiber disorganization is observed by electron microscopy. Treatment of underlying causes brings lucency of nail plate back.

NAIL PLATE THICKENING

- The nail plate gains thickness as it grows distally.
- Thick nails suggest a long intermediate matrix.[2]
- The vascular supply, subungual hyperkeratosis, and drugs influence the nail thickening.
- Subungual hyperkeratosis due to onychomycosis, pachyonychia congenita, pityriasis rubra pilaris, or psoriasis (Figures 10.27 through 10.29) also results in nail plate thickening.

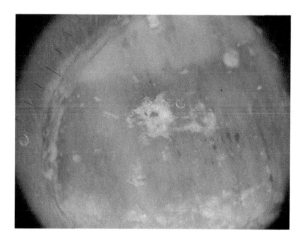

Figure 10.28 Dermoscopic image of Figure 10.27 shows white scale and areas with splinter hemorrhages.

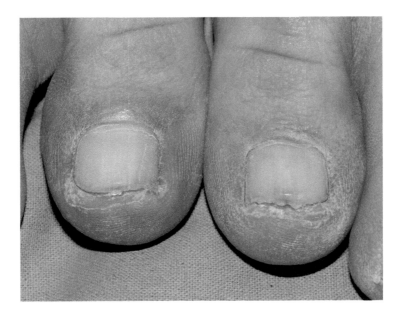

Figure 10.29 Nail plate is thickened in both big toenails in psoriasis.

NAIL PLATE THINNING

- Nail plate thinning is defined as thickness of nail plate less than 0.5 mm.
- Such nails are called soft nails, hapalonychia, or egg shell nails.
- They break easily or split at free edge of nail plate.
- They are seen in leprosy, hemiplegia, occupational contact with chemicals, and lichen planus. In lichen planus, uniform thinning is due to atrophy of proximal nail matrix and is referred to as "angel wing" deformity (Figures 10.30 and 10.31).[1]
- Treatment includes painting the nails with 5% aluminum chloride in propylene glycol. Iron supplements help thin nails even in the absence of iron deficiency.
- Biotin 5–10 mg daily might be helpful in some cases.

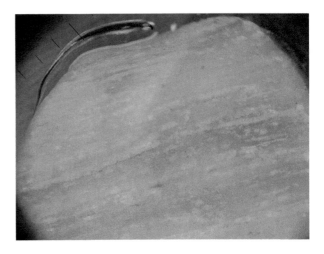

Figure 10.31 Dermoscopy of Figure 10.31 shows longitudinal ridging in a regular pattern indicating thin nails.

BRITTLE NAILS

- Changes in the nail consistency result in brittle nails (Figure 10.32). It depends on factors like health of the nails with variations in the water content and keratin constituents.[2]
- Less water content in the nails make them brittle. Low lipid levels in the nails are also contributory.
- Local causes include damage by alkalis, solvents, sugar solutions, and hot water. Soaking the nails in soap water or varnish removers ends up in drying the nails. This method is commonly carried out by manicurists. Dermatological diseases like eczema, lichen planus, and onychomycosis (Figure 10.33) affecting nails locally present with brittle nails.

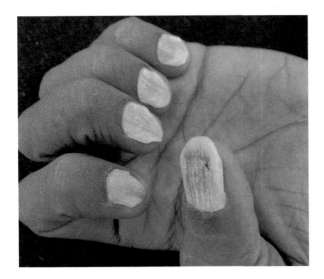

Figure 10.30 "Angel-wing" deformity due to whole-nail plate thinning in lichen planus.

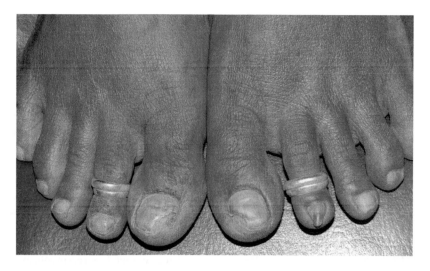

Figure 10.32 Brittle nail resulting in partial loss at free edge in toenails.

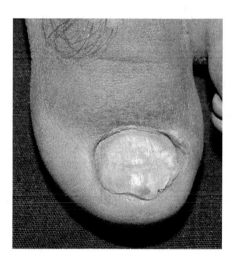

Figure 10.33 Onychomycosis resulting in brittling of nail plate due to invasion by fungus.

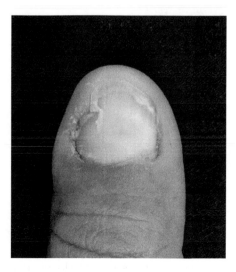

Figure 10.34 Longitudinal split extending from free as a result of brittle nails in vitamin deficiency.

- Anemia; deficiency of vitamins A, C, B$_6$ (Figure 10.34); and impairment of peripheral nervous system are the general causes for brittle nails.

CURVATURE ABNORMALITIES

Koilonychia

- **Introduction:** It is common nail dystrophy in which dorsal surface of nail plate becomes flat or truly concave. It is derived from Greek word *koilos* meaning hollow.
- Pathogenesis of koilonychia is not known but it is suggested that anoxia and atrophy of distal matrix are contributory.[1]
- Healthy infants may have toenail koilonychia, which will become normal in due course.
- Two types of koilonychia are described. One is acquired and the other is familial or idiopathic (Figure 10.35).
- In familial form, it is a component of LEOPARD syndrome, monilethrix, and nail–patella syndrome.
- Koilonychia has been noted in a single family in four consecutive generations.[17]
- Iron deficiency is the most common cause of acquired koilonychia (Figure 10.36).[18]
- It may develop before clinical or laboratory signs of anemia manifest. Hemochromatosis, polycythemia vera, malnutrition, and pellagra are other causes of koilonychia.
- **Clinical features:** Koilonychia is the converse of clubbing. It is more appreciated when viewed from the side. When a drop of water is put on the surface, it will not fall off. It should be noted that nails in koilonychia are brittle. It is commonly seen in fingernails rather than toenails.
- Dermatological diseases like lichen planus, psoriasis, lichen striatus, keratoderma (Figure 10.25), Darier's disease, and acanthosis nigricans can also result in koilonychia. Occupational toenail koilonychia is observed in rickshaw pullers in northern India.
- Treatment includes correction of iron deficiency anemia and management of underlying causes.

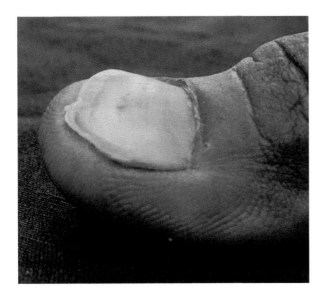

Figure 10.35 Spoon-shaped nail plate in koilonychia due to increased concavity of nail plate.

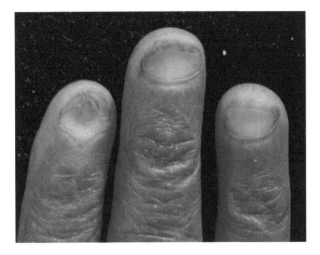

Figure 10.36 Koilonychia in iron deficiency anemia in this patient.

Clubbing

- **Synonyms:** Hippocrates fingers, acropachy.
- **Introduction:** Trousseau first called the condition clubbing of nails, and it was originally described by Hippocrates. Clubbing is the most common clinical sign in nails. There are increased transverse and longitudinal curvatures of nail plate along with hypertrophy of soft tissue of nail pulp.[1]
- **Etiopathogenesis:** Increased blood flow to nail unit vasculature is contributory rather than vessel hyperplasia, although MRI implicates hypervascularity. Microvascular infarcts resulting from platelet aggregation and altered vagal tone also contribute to clubbing.
- Mutations in HPGD and SLCO2A1 genes have been linked to clubbing in primary hypertrophic osteoarthropathy (pachydermoperiosteosis).[4]

- It can be hereditary or acquired. In hereditary form, autosomal dominant with variable penetrance is believed to be responsible.[19]
- Clubbing is also a feature of thyroid acropachy, which is characterized by clubbing of fingers and toe with thickening and fibrosis of subcutaneous tissues.
- Unilateral clubbing (Box 10.1) is seen in arterial aneurysms, arteriovenous fistulae, and local injury.[1]
- Clinical changes are present in nails and fingertips. Nails bulge along both the longitudinal and the transverse axis. Changes are prominent in radial three digits. Tissues around terminal phalanx become hypertrophied and appear as "drum sticks" (Figure 10.37).
- It is insidious in onset, and sometimes abrupt clubbing can be seen lung carcinoma.
- Three geometric assessments exist: Lovibond's, Curth's angles, and Schamroth's window.[4]
- Lovibond's angle is found at the junction between the nail plate and proximal nail fold. Normally it is less than 160°. It is altered to more than 180° in clubbing.
- Angle at the distal interphalangeal joint is called as Curth's angle and is normally 180°. It is lessened to 160° in clubbing.
- Schamroth's window is formed when dorsal aspects of fingers opposite hands are opposed. In clubbing this window is closed.
- Clubbing should be differentiated from pseudoclubbing, wherein over-curvature of transverse and longitudinal axis is present. However, Lovibond's angle is normal. It is usually seen in short and dystrophic distal phalanx.
- Management includes differentiation of etiological factors for clubbing and treatment of underlying causes (Table 10.6).[1,2]

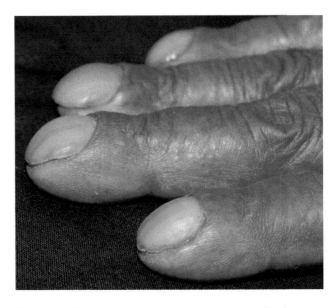

Figure 10.37 Increased transverse and longitudinal curvature of nail plate resulting in drum stick appearance in clubbing.

Table 10.6 Causes of bilateral clubbing[1,2]

Cardiovascular disorders	Aortic aneurysms
	Congenital/acquired cardiovascular disease
Broncho-pulmonary conditions	Intrathoracic neoplasms
	Chronic intrathoracic suppurative disorders
	Fibrosing alveolitis
Gastrointestinal disorders	Hepatic disorders
	Multiple polyposis, ulcerative colitis, cystic fibrosis, malignancy
	Bacillary dysentery, amoebic dysentery
Hematological	Chronic meth-hemoglobinemia, polycythemia, thalassemia, chronic myeloid leukemia
Endocrine	Graves's disease, POEMS syndrome
Hereditary clubbing	
Drugs	Hypervitaminosis A, heroin abuse, laxative abuse, heavy metal poisoning, Angiotensin II receptor blocker
Miscellaneous	Malnutrition, alcoholism, HIV infection, Syringomylea, SLE

BOX 10.1: Causes of unilateral clubbing[1]

- Idiopathic
- Arterial aneurysms
- Arteriovenous fistula
- Hemiplegia
- Raynaud's syndrome
- Pancoast tumor
- Subluxation of shoulder
- Pancoast tumor
- Median nerve injury
- Sarcoidosis
- Nail pulp infections
- Local injury

LEUCONYCHIA

Introduction: White nails are the most common variant of nail discoloration or dyschromia. It is divided into three types.[2]

1. **True leuconychia:** It results from the nail matrix involvement in which nail plate appears white and opaque.
   - This is because of structural modifications of nail matrix. Due to defective keratinization, there is persistence of nuclei with trapping of air, which gives opacity or white discoloration to the nail plate.
   - It can be congenital, acquired, or idiopathic. Congenital form is due to genetic defect in the chromosome 12q13.[20]
   - Congenital leuconychia is seen in palmoplantar keratoderma, pili torti, LEOPARD syndrome, congenital hyperparathyroidism, and keratosis pilaris.
   - Acquired leuconychia is rare and partial involvement is common. Mees' lines are transverse white lines. In Darier's, longitudinal leuconychia is observed.

- Total leuconychia appears milky, ivory, chalky, or porcelain in color. Growth is accelerated in true leuconychia.
- It may be complete (total) (Figure 10.38) or partial (subtotal).
- Partial is again divided into transverse, punctate, variegate, and longitudinal.[4]
- Transverse leuconychia presents as 1–2 mm white lines on the nail plate. It is due to micro trauma, arsenic poisoning, and rejection of allograft.[2]
- Interestingly, white lines occur at the same level in each nail.
- Punctate leuconychia appears as white spots of 1–3 mm size either single or multiple. They can be seen without any detectable cause. They are referred to as fortune or gift spots by the patients (Figure 10.39).[1]
- Variegate leuconychia presents as multiple irregular, thread-like streaks run across the nail plate.

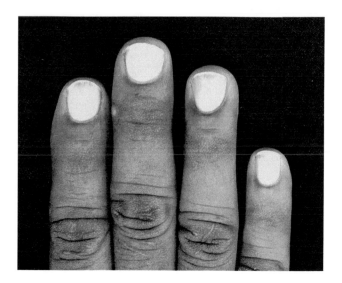

Figure 10.38 Total true leuconychia involving all the nails with complete whitening.

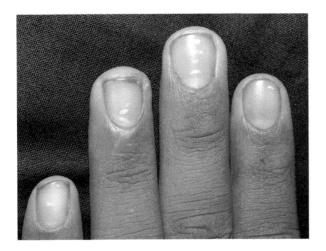

Figure 10.39 Multiple white spots are seen in many nails in punctate variant of true leuconychia.

2. **Apparent leuconychia:** Whitening of nail plate is because of abnormal subungual tissues.
   - Changes in the nail bed structure give rise to whitish discoloration of nail plate. It should be noted that nail matrix and nail plate are absolutely normal unlike true leuconychia. Pallor of nail bed due to anemia and vascular impairment are also responsible for apparent leuconychia.[1]
   - Terry's nails, half-and-half nails, Muehrck's nails, and macrolunula in leprosy are the examples of apparent leuconychia (Figure 10.40).[1]
   - Terry's nail describes a nail with proximal white and distal normal color of nail plate. It is seen in cirrhosis.
   - Half-and-half nails are seen in uremic patients in whom proximal white and distal brownish discoloration is noted.
   - Muehrck's nails are seen in hypoalbuminemia as paired bands of white lines. Pink line lies between the white lines. Correction of the condition reverses the sign.[4]

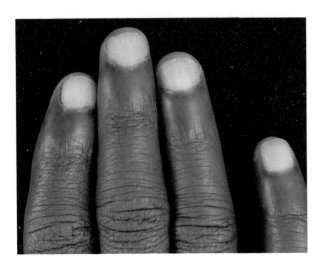

Figure 10.40 Apparent leuconychia in leprosy due to impaired vasculature to the nail bed.

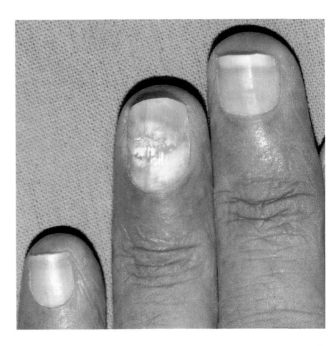

Figure 10.41 Pseudoleuconychia due to white colonies of fungus in onychomycosis.

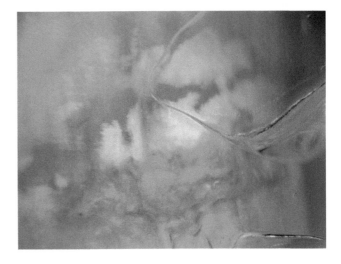

Figure 10.42 Dermoscopy of Figure 10.41 shows white areas in the nail plate.

3. **Pseudoleuconychia:** It is whitening of nail plate and nail bed due to the external origin. Onychomycosis (Figures 10.41 and 10.42) or granulation of keratin material results in pseudoleuconychia.[21]

Treatment: No specific treatment is available for leuconychia except for attending to the underlying cause.

LONGITUDINAL MELANONYCHIA

- **Introduction:** Longitudinal melanonychia is appearance of linear streaks or bands of pigmentation on the nail (Figure 10.43). Nail melanocytes are quiescent and generally

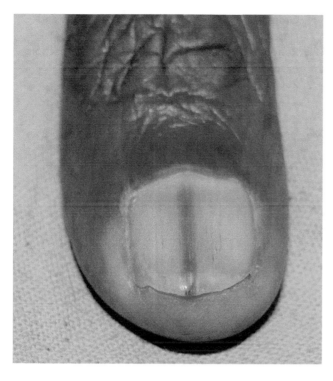

Figure 10.43 Longitudinal melanonychia showing linear streaks of pigmentation.

do not produce melanin. Hence, pigmentation of nail should arouse a warning and should be critically evaluated.[1]

- Melanonychia is due to melanocyte activation or hyperplasia.
- Many factors produce melanonychia, but malignant melanoma is very important to consider and should be ruled out.
- Several clinical signs including Hutchinson's sign are used to identify malignant melanoma affecting nail unit. Periungual pigmentation including proximal nail fold is called Hutchinson's sign.
- It should be differentiated from the pseudo-Hutchinson's sign, where pigmentation of periungual tissue occurs due to other conditions.[1]
- Dermoscopy picks early pigmentation of proximal nail fold and is referred to as "micro-Hutchinson's sign."[22]

For more details, refer chapter on chromonychia (chapter 11).

KEY POINTS

Considering that nails play an important role as a symptom of internal systemic diseases, nail plate displays numerous changes ranging from thinning to total loss of nail plate. A keen observation of nails would serve as a good diagnostic tool in clinical practice. Nail plate can give very important clues in diagnosing many dermatological and systemic conditions and hence we can say cutaneous examination is incomplete without a look at nail unit in general and nail plate in particular.

REFERENCES

1. Puri KJPS. Nail and its disorders. In: Sacchidan S, Inamadar AC, Oberai C (Editors). *IADVL Textbook of Dermatology*, 4th ed. Mumbai, India: Bhalani Publishing House; 2015. pp. 1588–1647.
2. Baran R, Dawber RPR. Physical signs. In: Baran R, Dawber RPR (Editors). *Diseases of Nails and Their Management*, 2nd ed. Oxford, UK: Blackwell Scientific Publications; 1994. pp. 35–80.
3. Heller J. Dystrophia unguium mediana canaliformis. *Dermatol Z* 1928; 51: 416–419.
4. de Berker DAR, Richert B, Baran R. Acquired disorders of nail and nail unit. In: Griffiths C, Barker J, Bleiker T, Chalmers R, Creamer D (Editors). *Rook's Textbook of Dermatology*, 9th ed. Oxford, UK: Wiley Blackwell; 2016. pp. 95.1–95.65.
5. Baran R. Hanek E, Richert B. Pincer nails: Definition and surgical treatment. *Dermatol Surg* 2001; 27: 261–266.
6. Zaias N. Psoriasis of the nail unit. *Dermatol Clin* 1984; 2: 49–505.
7. Yung A, Johnson P, Goodfield MJD. Isotretinoin-induced elkonyxis. *Br J Dermatol* 2005; 153: 669–670.
8. Ganor S. Diseases sometimes associated with psoriasis II: Alopecia areata. *Dermatologica* 1977; 154: 338.
9. Green RA, Scher RK. Nail changes associated with diabetes mellitus. *J Am Acad Dermatol* 1987; 16: 1015–1021.
10. Alkiewicz J. Trachyonychie. *Ann Dermatol Syphil* 1950; 10: 136.
11. Tosti A, Peluso AM, Piraccini BM. Nail diseases in children. In: James WD, Cockrell CJ, Dzubow LM, Paller AS, Yancy KB (Editors), *Advances in Dermatology*, Vol. 13. St. Luis, MO: Mosby; 1998. pp. 353–372.
12. Chao SC, Lee JY. Brittle nails and dyspareunia as first clues to the recurrences of malignant glucogonoma. *Br J Dermatol* 2002; 146: 1071–1074.
13. Baran R. Retinoids and the nails. *J Dermatol Treat* 1990; 1: 151–154.
14. Wallis MS, Bowen WR, Guin JR. Pathogenesis of onychoschizia (lamellar splitting). *J Am Acad Dermatol* 1991; 24: 44–48.
15. Mehra A, Murphy RJ, Wilson BB. Idiopathic familial onychomedesis. *J Am Acad Dermatol* 2000; 43: 349–350.
16. Boyd AS, Neldner KH. Lichen planus. *J Am Acad Dermatol* 1991; 25: 593–619.
17. Prathap P, Asokan N. Familial koilonychia. *Ind J Dermatol* 2010; 55(4): 406–407.
18. Hogan GR, Jones B. The relationship of koilonychia and iron deficiency in infants. *J Pediatr* 1970; 77: 1054.

19. Stone OJ. Spoon nails and clubbing: Significance and mechanisms. *Cutis* 1975; 16: 235–241.
20. Norgett EE, Wolf F, Balme B et al. Hereditary white nails: A genetic and structural study. *Br J Dermatol* 2004; 151: 65–72.
21. Grossman M, Scher RK. Leuconychia: Review and classification. *Int J Dermatol* 1990; 29: 535–541.
22. Ronger S, Touzet S, Ligeron C et al. Dermatoscopic examination of nail pigmentation. *Arch Dermatol* 2002; 138: 1327–1333.

11

Chromonychia

MICHELA STARACE, AURORA ALESSANDRINI, AND BIANCA MARIA PIRACCINI

INTRODUCTION

Normally, the nail plate is transparent, but it appears pink because of the underlying color of the vascularized nail bed. At the distal level, the nail plates separate from the underlying tissues of the hyponychium, and therefore free margin has a white color.

Nail color alterations (chromonychia) have a wide variety of presentations.

Chromonychia can be caused by the deposit of a pigment on the nail plate (exogenous pigmentation), by a pigmentation of the nail bed, or by production of the pigment from the nail matrix. In some cases, the diagnosis is clinical, but more often other investigations, such as dermoscopy or mycology, may help in identifying the cause, allowing an accurate diagnosis.

Exogenous versus endogenous chromonychia

The first step of evaluation of chromonychia is determining whether chromonychia is exogenous or endogenous. Exogenous chromonychia may be seen after occupational or other exposure to dyes (e.g., silver nitrate, potassium permanganate; Figure 11.1) and decorative use of henna. The proximal margin of nail dyschromia in such cases follows the curve of proximal nail folds (Figure 11.2a). On the other hand, the proximal margin of chromonychia of endogenous origin parallels lunula (Figure 11.2b).

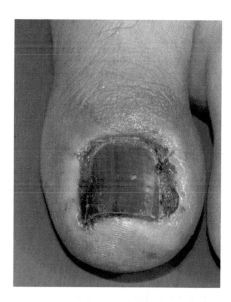

Figure 11.1 Exogenous pigmentation due to potassium permanganate staining. (Courtesy of Piyush Kumar.)

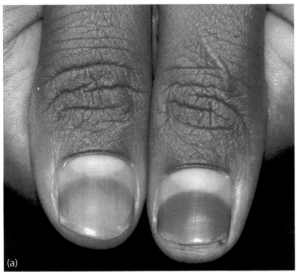

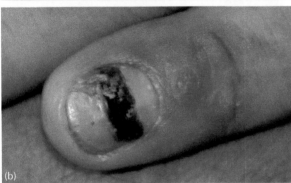

Figure 11.2 **(a)** Exogenous pigmentation due to henna. Note the proximal margin of pigmentation follows the shape of proximal nail fold. (Courtesy of Piyush Kumar.) **(b)** Endogenous pigmentation due to subungual hematoma. Note the proximal margin of pigmentation follows the shape of lunula. (Courtesy of Piyush Kumar.)

LEUKONYCHIA

Leukonychia is the most common chromatic abnormality of the nail, characterized by white discoloration of a part of the nail plate or the complete nail plate, and can be divided into three different types: true leukonychia, apparent leukonychia, and pseudoleukonychia.

- **True leukonychia** results from altered keratinization of the distal nail matrix. Parakeratotic nuclei are retained in nail plate and thus the nail appears opaque and white in color owing to the diffraction of light by parakeratotic cells (Figure 11.3). True leukonychia may also develop secondary to repetitive trauma to the matrix resulting in the formation of white bands/spots. True leukonychia moves distally as the nail grows.[1]

    Clinically, true leukonychia is sub-divided into punctate, transverse, longitudinal, and total types, and is summarized in Table 11.1.
- In **apparent leukonychia**, the white discoloration has its origin in the nail bed with subungual tissues'

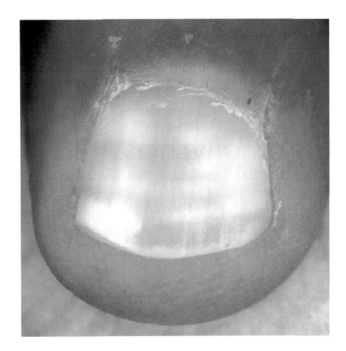

Figure 11.3 True leukonychia

Table 11.1 Types of true leukonychia

Clinical type	Causes
Punctate	Idiopathic, trauma, psoriasis
Transverse	Trauma, heavy metal poisoning (e.g. Mees' lines), chemotherapy
Longitudinal	Multiple bands (with alternating bands of erythronychia)—Darier disease, Hailey–Hailey disease
	Single band—Onychopapilloma[2]
Total	Mostly congenital

Source: Baran, R. and Perrin, C., *Br. J. Dermatol.*, 133, 267–269, 1995.

involvement. True and apparent leukonychia may be differentiated clinically by diascopy. The whitish discoloration disappears (or fades) with pressure in cases of apparent leukonychia, but not in true leukonychia. The phenomenon is observed because of changes in the nail bed vasculature on pressure, visible through the translucent nail plate. Also, apparent leukonychia is not modified by nail growth. Apparent leukonychia has been commonly described in the following clinical scenario:

a. **Terry's nails** are commonly observed in patients with liver cirrhosis, where the whole nail appears white, except a 1–2 mm pink to brown distal band, and the lunula may or may not be visible (Figure 11.4). This finding has been observed in chronic congestive heart failure and in cases of adult-onset diabetes mellitus too.

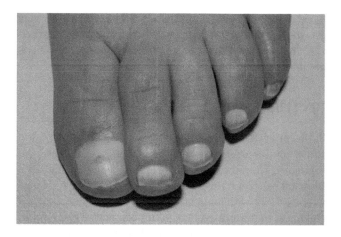

Figure 11.4 Clinical picture of Terry's nails.

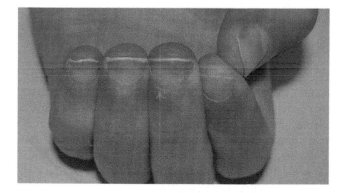

Figure 11.5 Clinical picture of half-and-half nails.

b. **Half and half nails (Lindsay's nails)** are observed in hemodialysis patients, where there is a definite border between the proximal area (opaque white) and the distal area (pink or reddish brown) occupying 20%–60% of nail bed (Figure 11.5). Distal reddish brown pigmentation does not fade with pressure. Though it has diagnostic value, it does not correlate with degree of renal impairment or with blood urea nitrogen or creatinine levels.

c. **Muehrcke's lines** are present as multiple transverse whitish bands, parallel to the lunula. This change is commonly seen after chemotherapy and in chronic hypoalbuminemia of less than 2 mg/dl (seen in nephrotic syndrome, glomerulonephritis, liver disease, and malnutrition), and is commonly found on the second, third, and fourth fingernails. Thumb nail involvement is rare. The lines tend to resolve with correction of hypoalbuminemia.

- **Pseudoleukonychia** has an external origin. The term pseudoleukonychia is used when the matrix or nail bed is not responsible for the nail plate alteration, for example in onychomycosis or in keratin granulations due to nail varnish. In particular, in proximal subungual onychomycosis (PSO) a white discoloration below the nail plate in the lunula area is present, while the remaining nail plate is normal. In white superficial onychomycosis (WSO), a nail plate with several small white to yellow opaque and friable patches is present. Dermoscopy shows single or multiple opaque white irregular spots of the nail plate surface (Figure 11.6). These alterations depend on the modality of colonization of fungi, and mycological examination is required.

Utility of dermoscopy in leukonychia

Dermoscopy, like diascopy, allows distinguishing true leukonychia from apparent leukonychia and pseudoleukonychia. During dermoscopy, the white areas appear within the nail plate in true leukonychia (and in pseudoleukonychia), while in apparent leukonychia, white spots appear underneath the nail plate. In true leukonychia, dermoscopy usually shows one or more white dots or transverse bands inside the plate, with a normally smooth and transparent nail plate surface. In transverse leukonychia, the white lines run parallel to the lunula and the space separating each transverse band indicates the intervals between traumatic events. Application of the gel does not change the white appearance.

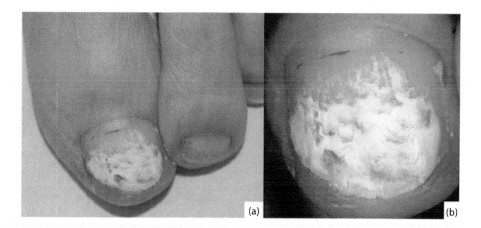

(a) (b)

Figure 11.6 Clinical picture (a) and dermoscopy (b) of white superficial onychomycosis.

GREEN NAILS

A green discoloration of the nail plate associated with onycholysis or chronic paronychia can be caused by *Pseudomonas aeruginosa* infection, where this Gram-negative bacterium colonizes the subungual space or the dorsal nail plate, producing the yellow-green pigment pyocyanin.[3,4]

It affects healthy people whose hands are constantly exposed to water, soaps, and detergents or are subject to mechanical trauma, especially in the elderly.

The color of pigmentation may vary from pale green to very dark green to black nail pigmentation to the naked eye and a melanic pigmentation has to be excluded, especially when this coloration appears as a longitudinal arrangement along the lateral side of the nail plate (Figure 11.7).

The great adherence of the color to the nail plate is due to production of an irregular nail plate surface. Onychoscopy shows the yellow-green color of the discoloration and its localization. In green nails associated with chronic paronychia, the green color is adherent to the nail surface in close proximity with the proximal nail fold, which is edematous and without the cuticle. The discoloration involves the lateral nail and is more evident proximally; it does not have a longitudinal shape and is associated with an irregular nail plate surface. Scraping the nail plate with a curette removes the pigment.

In green nails due to onycholysis, dermoscopy permits observing the border of the subungual pigmentation where the color typically fades into pale green at the margin of the detachment.

The differential diagnosis includes chemical exposure to solutions containing pyocyanin or pyoverdine.[5] After clipping away of the detached nail plate, a pale green-yellow pigmentation is evident on the bottom of the nail plate and on the nail bed: the clinical history and examination may also suggest the presence of paronychia and onycholysis.

Management includes cutting the onycholytic nail plate and topical antiseptics.

ERYTHRONYCHIA

The term erythronychia describes a red nail discoloration with round or irregular shape or with a longitudinal band originating from the lunula and running along the nail until the distal nail plate. The corresponding nail plate may be normal or present with longitudinal fissures and a distal subungual mass. In most cases, benign tumors may be responsible.

Red spots on the lunulae (mottled lunulae) are considered to be non-specific manifestations of nail matrix psoriasis, as they can also be present in other diseases, such as nail lichen planus and eczema.

Onychopapilloma

The term was proposed by Baran and Perrin in 2000[6] and indicates a benign tumor that arises from the distal matrix/proximal nail bed, inducing a band of longitudinal erythronychia. The distal nail plate may show a fissure and a subungual filiform hyperkeratotic mass underneath the nail plate in the area corresponding to the visible longitudinal band. An evident subungual mass with onycholysis can be a sign of onychopapilloma of bigger size.

Dermoscopy is useful for the diagnosis, showing a longitudinal red band, starting from the lunula and reaching to the distal margin, often associated with splinter hemorrhages (Figure 11.8).

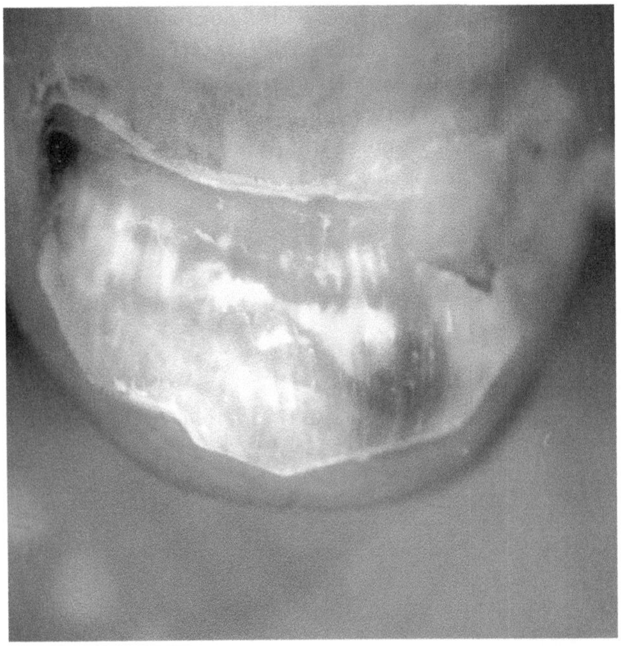

Figure 11.7 Onychoscopy of Pseudomonas aeruginosa colonization in a great toenail.

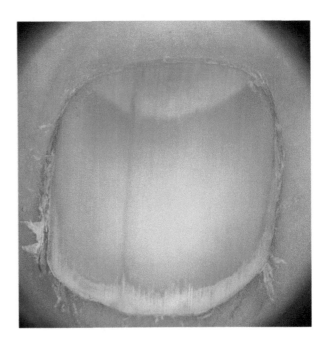

Figure 11.8 Onychoscopy of erythronychia due to onychopapilloma.

In particular, the width of the band is small and demarcation with surrounding uninvolved nail plate is sharp and parallel; moreover, the subungual hyperkeratosis is extremely limited, so that the patient notes it because of the occurrence of bleeding while cutting off the nail distal edge.

Dermoscopic features of onychopapilloma have been recently described by Tosti et al.[2]: they observed that, dermoscopically, the distal edge showed a keratotic subungual mass in correspondence to the streak in all cases, and that splinter hemorrhages could be the only onychoscopy sign.

Dermoscopy allows the differentiation from onychomatricoma, where the honeycomb aspect at the distal part of the nail plate is diagnostic.

Glomus tumor

Glomus tumor is an uncommon tumor of the neuromyoarterial glomus bodies located in the nail bed dermis. It is a painful benign nail tumor, occurring most commonly in the subungual area of the first and second fingernails. The classic triad of symptoms that typically exceed clinical signs includes intense, paroxysmal pain, pinpoint tenderness; cold sensitivity; and irradiation of pain along the same arm.[7]

When visible, this tumor is a red-purple subungual mass, while bigger masses may be associated with onycholysis, nail plate thinning, and fissuring.

However, in most cases, this tumor is not visible clinically, due to its small dimensions and deeper position, or may appear as an erythematous area suggestive of vascular abnormalities.

Dermoscopy with gel can be very useful to have a better visualization of the mass: the tumor appears as a deep red-purple discolored area, with blurred borders or as a band of longitudinal erythronychia that does not usually reach the distal margin.[8] The intensity of the red contrasts with the pale pink color of the surrounding nail bed and with the white color of the lunula.[9]

Nail plate dermoscopy can show the presence of vascular structures, too, evident as small red ramified vessels.

A new tool for the diagnosis of glomus tumor is the "pink glow" sign visible in UV light, where a pinkish glow suggests the vascular nature of the tumor.[10] Intraoperative onychoscopy of the nail matrix and bed after nail plate removal aids in tumor localization and in the visualization of the vascular pattern of the lesion, which appears as ramified telangiectasias over a blue background.[11] This method helps in the delimitation of surgical margins. Nail bed intraoperative onychoscopy may also show residual macroscopic tumor foci.

MRI permits detection of the subungual lesion, which can also be seen by ultrasound if bigger than 3 mm in diameter. Surgical removal is the only option.

Darier's disease

Darier's disease is an autosomal dominant genodermatosis with high penetrance characterized by dark keratotic papules on the skin, located mainly over the seborrheic sites of the body, mucous membrane lesions, and nail changes.[12]

The nail changes can occur in absence of cutaneous disease and typically involves 2–3 fingernails, causing a longitudinal erythronychia.[13]

Dermoscopy shows alternate red and white streaks that may be associated with nail plate thinning. Splinter hemorrhages may be visible, associated with distal splitting of the nail plate that may be more or less marked, especially along the red bands.

YELLOW DISCOLORATION

Onychomycosis

Onychomycosis is the most common infective disease affecting nail. It is frequent in the toenails of elderly, where it can reach a prevalence of 40%. In most of the cases onychomycosis is caused by dermatophytes, *Trichophyton rubrum* or *Trichophyton interdigitale*. Non-dermatophyte molds (NDM) like *Scopulariopsis brevicaulis*, *Fusarium solani* or *Fusarium oxysporum*, *Aspergillus* sp., and *Acremonium* sp. are responsible for 15% of cases; *Candida* nail infection is rarer and occurs only when predisposing factors like immunosuppression and diabetes are present. Clinical diagnosis of onychomycosis always requires laboratory confirmation. In onychomycosis, a nail discoloration is typical; in particular, in distal subungual onychomycosis fungi reach the nail plate through the hyponychium, invading the undersurface of the nail unit plate spreading proximally, and the nail plate appears yellow-white, in association with onycholysis and subungual hyperkeratosis.

Dermoscopy shows these yellow longitudinal striae in the onycholytic nail plate and an overall appearance of the affected nail plate in bands of fading colors resembling aurora borealis (Aurora borealis pattern) (Figure 11.9).[14]

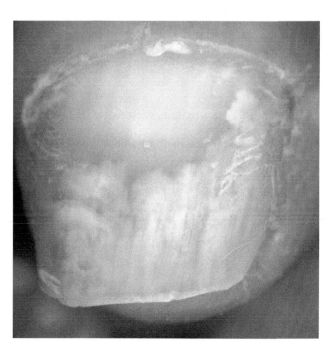

Figure 11.9 Onychoscopy of distal subungual onychomycosis.

Another possible manifestation is dermatophytoma, where there is a subungual accumulation of hyphae and scales, and it appears as a yellow-orange round area under the nail plate, connected distally with a longitudinal streak corresponding to onycholysis. Dermoscopy can be useful for diagnosis, showing a round yellow-orange patch in the mid nail bed, connected by a thin narrow channel to the distal edge of the nail plate.[15]

Treatment depends on clinical type, number of involved nails, and severity of the infection.

Yellow nail syndrome

The yellow nail syndrome (YNS) is a rare disorder, characterized by the triad: *yellow nails, respiratory problems,* and *lymphedema.*[15]

These features are not always present together and the diagnosis can be done when two of them are present and even with nail changes alone. Pleuropulmonary symptoms and lymphedema usually precede the onset of nail signs by 3–5 years. The patient is typically an adult.

Usually all 20 nails are involved and they manifest a yellowish discoloration, together with arrest or reduced nail growth, nail plate thickening, lack of cuticles, increased transverse curvature, and onycholysis (Figure 11.10). An ultrasound

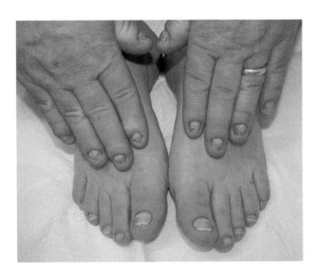

Figure 11.10 Clinical picture of yellow nail syndrome.

examination of lower limbs and chest X-ray are recommended. YNS may occasionally be paraneoplastic. Vitamin E orally has been used as a treatment modality.

BROWN-BLACK DISCOLORATION

Splinter hemorrhages

Splinter hemorrhages are frequently due to trauma, but may also be seen in nail psoriasis, onychomycosis, or nail tumors, i.e., onychopapilloma. They may also be seen in systemic disorders like subacute bacterial endocarditis or autoimmune connective tissue disorders like systemic lupus erythematosus and dermatomyositis.

They correspond to hemorrhages of capillaries of the nail bed, which run longitudinally in rows of the dermal papillae and clinically appear as one or more longitudinal red-to-brown striae, deep red in color and a few millimeters in length located in the distal nail plate.

Dermoscopy with gel enhances visualization of the longitudinal orientation of the red lines (Figure 11.11). No specific treatment is needed.

Subungual hematoma

Subungual hematoma is the most common cause of brown-black pigmentation.

There are two types of hematoma, acute and chronic. In the first case, the diagnosis is very easy, because the clinical history of a trauma explains the origin of the pigmentation, while chronic types are caused by repetitive microtrauma that the patient often does not realize.

Dermoscopy better defines the features of a hematoma: the round shape and its homogeneous pigmentation, without the longitudinal lines that characterize melanonychia. The color of hematoma depends on the time from the occurrence of the trauma. A recent hematoma is located deep under the plate and appears red-purple to black in color, with round margins at the proximal edge and with a streaked and filamentous distal end (Figure 11.12).[16] One or several red-black small round spots representing smaller blood extravasations may be present. Older lesions are different because they are more superficial, located in the ventral nail

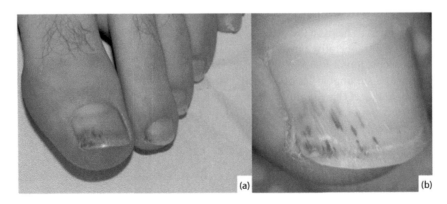

Figure 11.11 Clinical picture (a) and dermoscopy (b) of splinter hemorrhages of great toenail.

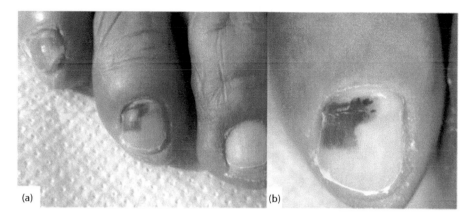

Figure 11.12 Clinical picture **(a)** and dermoscopy **(b)** of subungual hematoma.

plate, and roundish, red-brown in color, often surrounded by small multiple blood globules of paler color or splinter hemorrhages globules. No treatment is required.

Fungal melanonychia

Fungal melanonychia is caused by *Trichophyton rubrum*-variant melanoid or by other non-dermatophyte fungi. The nail is characterized by subungual hyperkeratosis with yellow and brown scales and brown or black irregular bands, better seen with dermoscopy[17] (Figure 11.13). Mycology is mandatory for diagnosis, and treatment includes topical or systemic antifungals.

Melanonychia

The term melanonychia describes a black-brown pigmentation of the nail due to the presence of melanin within the nail plate. Usually it appears as a longitudinal band that starts from the proximal margin extending to the distal margin of the nail, following the growth of the nail, or involves the whole of the nail plate.

When a patient presents with melanonychia, the diagnostic approach is

- To establish if the pigment is melanin or not
- To determine if the development of melanonychia is due to an activation or proliferation of matrix melanocytes
- To distinguish if this manifestation is benign or malignant

A melanic pigmentation is a brown-black longitudinal band within the nail plate, while exogenous pigmentation includes different substances that adhere to the nail plate and does not usually have a longitudinal appearance, such as a subungual hematoma or *Pseudomonas* infection.

Another very useful clinical clue includes the number of involved digits—if more than one digit is involved, the first thought should be melanocytic activation, like in drug-induced melanonychia, which appears with a grey background of the band with thin greyish regular and parallel lines, and borders (Figure 11.14). When only one digit is involved by melanonychia, a proliferative process has to be considered and it is necessary to understand whether it is benign or malignant.

The age of the patient is crucial: nail matrix nevi are typically seen in childhood, while nail melanoma in children is extremely rare.[18]

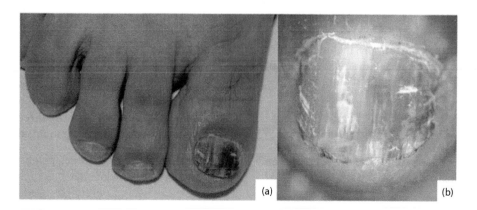

Figure 11.13 Clinical picture **(a)** and dermoscopy **(b)** of fungal melanonychia.

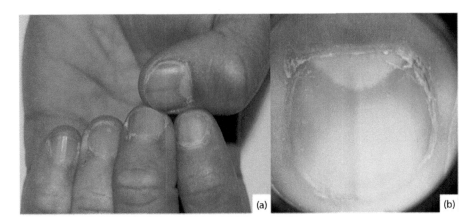

Figure 11.14 Clinical picture (a) and dermoscopy (b) of melanocytic activation due to onychophagia.

MELANONYCHIA IN CHILDREN

Melanonychia in children requires a different approach, because dermoscopic features observed in adult nail apparatus melanoma are generally observed in benign pediatric cases.

Nail matrix nevi may be present at birth or may occur later on, more frequently in the thumb. Dermoscopic patterns that suggest a nevus are the presence of a brown background with longitudinal brown-to-black regular and parallel lines with regular spacing and thickness and, more important in children, black dots due to pigment accumulation in the nail plate. These dots are black in color, with a regular size and shape (less than 0.1 mm), irregularly distributed along the lines, and sometimes forming a shallow pit at the periphery. At other times, it is possible to find them within the pigmented lines often interrupting the lines. In most young patients, the dots will disappear over time. Dermoscopic patterns that may suggest a melanoma in children are a rapid evolution of brown background with longitudinal, brown-to-black lines with irregular color, spacing, and thickness and ending abruptly. However, these features can also be seen in longitudinal melanonychia in children and their specificity in youth is very low.[19]

MELANONYCHIA IN ADULTS

In adulthood, the clinical ABCDEF rule for nail pigmentation[20] should always be associated with dermoscopy for diagnostic accuracy (Table 11.2). Dermoscopic features suggestive of nail melanoma include a brown-to-black background of the band with longitudinal lines irregular in their thickness, spacing, color, or parallelism[21] (Figure 11.15).

However, this rule is not always reliable, as it is possible to find lines that are irregular in width or color also in benign lesions. The conditions where dermoscopy is not performable are thickened nails, blurred borders of the lesions, and a nail plate totally black.[22]

Table 11.2 The ABCDEF of subungual melanoma

Acronym	Feature	Description
A	Age peak	50–70y
B	Band	Nail band
	Brown-black pigment	Pigmentation
	Breadth	>3 mm
	Border	Irregular/blurred
C	Change	Rapid increase in size/ growth rate of nail band
	Lack of change	Failure of nail dystrophy to improve despite adequate treatment
D	Digit involved	Thumb > index finger
	Dominant hand	Single digit > multiple digits
E	Extension	Extension of pigment involving proximal or lateral nail fold (Hutchinson's sign) or free edge of nail plate
F	Family or personal history	Of previous melanoma or dysplastic nevus syndrome

A recent study demonstrated a strong association between clinical and dermoscopic findings in nail band pigmentation, helping to distinguish if the band is benign or malignant. The authors identify **three important dermoscopic patterns** that could help in this distinction:

1. The width of the band, which involves more than 2\3 of the nail plate in melanoma

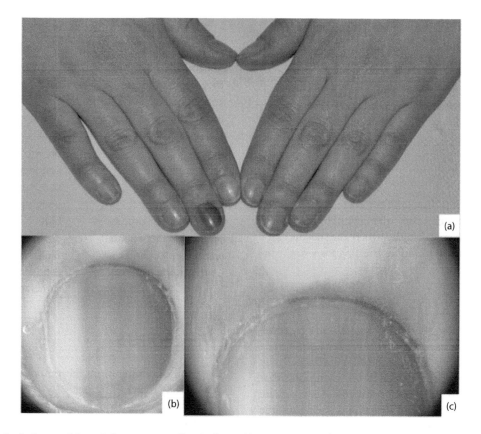

Figure 11.15 Clinical picture (a) and dermoscopy (b–c) of acral lentiginous melanoma.

2. The presence of grey to black color
3. The presence of nail dystrophy that increases three times the risk of detecting a nail melanoma[23]

Dermoscopy of the hyponychium and periungual tissues permits discovering the micro-Hutchinson's sign, a periungual pigmentation seen with dermoscope but not with naked eye that corresponds to the initial radial growth of melanoma into adjacent tissue. The micro Hutchinson's sign could be associated with a band of melanonychia or with amelanotic melanoma, characterized by the lack of melanin pigment.

A recent study[24] created an algorithm to indicate, step by step, the correct way to follow an adult patient with suspected nail apparatus melanoma. In case of longitudinal melanonychia, first of all, we have to look at the nail plate and the periungual tissue for any pigmentation visible by the naked eye and then with dermoscopy. If there is pigmentation, the diagnosis of melanoma is highly suggestive and a biopsy is mandatory. Without periungual pigmentation the aspect of the pigmented band can direct the diagnosis. The most frequent aspect of nail apparatus melanoma is an irregular line pattern with brown-to-black background. Nail plate changes, indicative of nail matrix damage, are also suggestive for a malignancy. In cases

of a nail bed nodule with ulceration, its association with Hutchinson's sign is diagnostic for invasive nail melanoma. The use of a dermoscope may detect micro Hutchinson's sign and the irregular vascular structures with atypical vessels. Considering the limitations and issues with reliability of dermoscopic findings, one should keep the threshold for biopsy low as the gold standard for a definitive diagnosis of nail pigmentation is histopathology.[25]

CHROMONYCHIA IN SYSTEMIC DISORDERS AND DRUGS[26,27]

Systemic disorders

Many systemic disorders can cause nail color modifications and these signs can be very useful for the clinician. The nails provide a long, sustained, historical record of profound temporary abnormalities of the control of skin pigment, which otherwise might pass unnoticed. Color is also affected by the state of the skin vessels, various intravascular factors such as anemia, carbon monoxide poisoning, and methemoglobinemia.

When the cause is exogenous, such as occupational derived agents or topical application of therapeutic agents, the nail discoloration follows the shape of the proximal nail

Table 11.3 Some dermatological disorders affecting nail color

Systemic disorder	Color change
Cronkhite–Canada syndrome	grey/black
Laugier–Hunziker syndrome	brown
Lupus erythematosus	reddish
Pityriasis rubra pilaris	dark
Reiter syndrome	psoriasis-like
Kawasaki disease	orange-brown

folds; otherwise, if the discoloration corresponds to the shape of the lunula, systemic disorders might be suspected.

The important systemic disorder, where the specific color modification of the nail is useful for the diagnosis, are summarized in Table 11.3.

Drugs[28]

The nails are frequently altered by systemic drugs, especially by some categories, such as anti-cancer agents, retinoids, and antiretrovirals. Drug-induced nail changes may sometimes be severe and be associated with symptoms that require the patient to interrupt treatment. An adequate knowledge of adverse effects of drugs and their possible preventive and therapeutic measures may help to increase patient compliance to therapy. Drug-induced nail changes usually involve several or all the 20 nails and appear in temporal correlation with drug intake (Figure 11.16). They are usually dose-related and reversible after drug discontinuation. Severity of symptoms is also related to individual sensitivity to the drug, as the same dose of an agent can produce different degrees of nail changes in the different patients. The typical nail color alteration due to drugs is melanonychia. The main drugs are listed in Table 11.4.

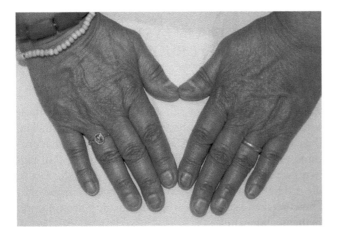

Figure 11.16 Clinical picture of Muehrcke's lines and melanocytic activation due to chemotherapy agents in a woman with breast cancer.

Table 11.4 Drug-induced color alterations

Drug	Color alterations
Anticonvulsant drugs	Ochre-brown
Tricyclic antidepressants	Leuconychia
Rotigotine	Green
Tetracycline	Yellow
Minocycline	Blue
Clofazimine	Brown
Lamivudine	Longitudinal melanonychia
Zidovudine	Longitudinal melanonychia
Antifungal agents	Longitudinal melanonychia
Cardiovascular drugs	Blue
Anticoagulants agents	Red
Antimalarial agents	Bluish-brown
Chemotherapeutic agents	Diffuse and longitudinal melanonychia

KEY POINTS

- Nail color alterations (chromonychia) have a wide variety of presentations.
- Chromonychia can be caused by the deposit of a pigment on the nail plate, by a pigmentation of the nail bed, or by production of the pigment from the nail matrix.
- The diagnosis is clinical, but dermoscopy or mycology may help identify the cause.
- Color such as red, yellow, or green are a typical sign of benign lesions, while brown-black discoloration could be a clinical presentation of malignant lesions.
- Nail color abnormalities could be an expression of nail diseases or systemic disorders.

REFERENCES

1. Baran R, Perrin C. Transverse leukonychia of toenails due to repeated microtrauma. *Br J Dermatol* 1995; 133: 267–269.
2. Tosti A, Schneider SL, Ramirez-Quizon MN, Zaiac M, Miteva M. Clinical, dermoscopic, and pathologic features of onychopapilloma: A review of 47 cases. *J Am Acad Dermatol* 2016; 74(3): 521–526.
3. Chiriac A, Brzezinski P, Foia L, Marincu I. Chloronychia: Green nail syndrome caused by Pseudomonas aeruginosa in elderly persons. *Clin Interv Aging* 2015; 10: 265–267.
4. Maes M, Richert B, de la Brassinne M. Green nail syndrome or chloro-nychia. *Rev Med Liege* 2002; 57: 233–235.

5. Leung LK, Harding J. A chemical mixer with dark-green nails. *BMJ Case Rep* 2015; 2015: bcr2014209203.

6. Baran R, Perrin C. Longitudinal erythronychia with distal subungual keratosis: Onychopapilloma of the nail bed and Bowen's disease. *Br J Dermatol* 2000; 143: 132–135.

7. Kallis P, Miteva M, Patel T, Zaiac M, Tosti A. Onychomatricoma with concomitant subungual glomus tumor. *Skin Appendage Disord* 2015; 1(1): 14–17.

8. Maehara Lde S, Ohe EM, *Enokihara* MY, Michalany NS, Yamada S, Hirata SH. Diagnosis of glomus tumor by nail bed and matrix dermoscopy. *An Bras Dermatol* 2010; 85: 236–238.

9. de Berker D. Erythronychia. *Dermatol Ther* 2012; 25: 603–611.

10. Thatte SS, Chikhalkar SB, Khopkar US. "Pink glow": A new sign for the diagnosis of glomus tumor on ultraviolet light dermoscopy. *Indian Dermatol Online J* 2015; 6(Suppl 1): S21–S23.

11. Rai AK. Role of intraoperative dermoscopy in excision of nail unit glomus tumor. *Indian Dermatol Online* 2016; 7(5): 448–450.

12. Suryawanshi H, Dhobley A, Sharma A, Kumar P. Darier disease: A rare genodermatosis. *J Oral Maxillofac Pathol* 2017; 21(2): 321.

13. Cohen PR. Longitudinal erythronychia: Individual or multiple linear red bands of the nail plate: A review of clinical features and associated conditions. *Am J Clin Dermatol* 2011; 12(4): 217–231.

14. Piraccini BM, Balestri R, Starace M, Rech G. Nail digital dermoscopy (onychoscopy) in the diagnosis of onychomycosis. *J Eur Acad Dermatol Venereol* 2013; 27(4): 509–513.

15. Jesùs-Silva MA, Fernandez-Martinez R, Roldan-Marin R, Arenas R. Dermoscopic patterns in patients with a clinical diagnosis of onychomycosis-result of a prospective study including data of potassium hydroxide (KHO) and culture examination. *Dermatol Pract Concept* 2015; 5(2): 39–44.

16. Lencastre A, Lamas A, Sà D, Tosti A. Onychoscopy. *Clin Dermatol* 2013; 31(5): 587–593.

17. Wang YJ, Sun PL. Fungal melanonychia caused by Trichophyton rubrum and the value of dermoscopy. *Cutis* 2014; 94(3): E5–E6.

18. Murata Y, Kumano K. Dots and lines: A dermoscopic sign of regression of longitudinal melanonychia in children. *Cutis* 2012; 90: 293–296.

19. Iorizzo M, Tosti A, Di Chiacchio N, Hirata SH, Misciali C, Michalany N, Domiguez J, Toussaint S. Nail melanoma in children: Differential diagnosis and management. *Dermatol Surg* 2008; 34: 974–978.

20. Levit EK, Kagen MH, Scher RK, Grossman M, Altman E. The ABC rule for clinical detection of subungual melanoma. *J Am Acad Dermatol* 2000; 42: 269–274.

21. Thomas L, Dalle S. Dermoscopy provides useful information for the management of melanonychia striata. *Dermatol Ther* 2007; 20: 3–10.

22. Piraccini BM, Dika E, Fanti PA. Nail disorders: Practical tips for diagnosis and treatment. *Dermatol Clin* 2015; 33: 185–195.

23. Benati E, Ribero S, Longo C, Piana S, Puig S, Carrera C, Cicero F et al. Clinical and dermoscopic clues to differentiate pigmented nail bands: An international dermoscopy society study. *J Eur Acad Dermatol Venereol* 2017; 31(4): 732–736.

24. Starace M, Dika E, Fanti PA, Patrizi A, Misciali C, Alessandrini A, Bruni F, Piraccini BM. Nail apparatus melanoma: dermoscopic and histopathologic correlations on a series of 23 patients from a single centre. *J Eur Acad Dermatol Venereol* 2018; 32(1): 164–173.

25. Ruben BS. Pigmented lesions of the nail unit: Clinical and histopathology features. *Semin Cutan Med Surg* 2010; 29: 148–158.

26. Holzberg M. The nail in systemic disease. In: Baran R, de Berker DAR, Holzberg M, Thomas L, editors. *Baran & Dawber's Diseases of the Nails and Their Management*, 4th ed. Oxford, UK: Wiley and Blackwell; 2012. pp. 315–391.

27. Piraccini BM. *Nail disorders: A Practical Guide to Diagnosis and Management*. Springer, Milan, Italy, 2014.

28. Baran R, Fouilloux B, Robert C. Drug-induced nail changes. In: Baran R, de Berker DAR, Holzberg M, Thomas L, editors. *Baran & Dawber's Diseases of the Nails and Their Management*, 4th ed. Oxford, UK: Wiley and Blackwell; 2012. pp. 413–435.

12

Ingrown nail

AZZAM ALKHALIFAH AND BERTRAND RICHERT

INTRODUCTION

Nail problems are a common motive for consultation in dermatology, with ingrown nail being a very frequent reason. Ingrown nail, also called onychocryptosis (from Greek: *onyx* = nail, *kryptos* = hidden), is the impingement of the nail plate into the surrounding soft tissue, usually the lateral nail fold. All age groups can be affected by this multifactorial condition. It is painful with inflammatory, swollen, and sometimes, oozing periungual tissue. While patient's quality of life is largely affected, medical treatments are often tried with limited curative efficacy. Surgical treatment is the most effective treatment with a diversity of techniques and results. Different medical and surgical techniques will be exposed in this chapter. The choice of the approach depends on the skills of the physician and the clinical presentation.

EPIDEMIOLOGY

Ingrown nail is by far the most commonly encountered nail complaint. The exact percentage is difficult to determine as ingrown nails can be treated by internists, surgeons, podiatrists, dermatologists, or even with home remedies. It affects principally toenails, mostly the big toe.

A study in Washington showed that 20% of patients presenting to a general practitioner with a foot problem have an ingrown nail. In Dutch general practice, the prevalence of ingrown nails is of 54/10,000 registered cases each year[1], while in the UK, there are more than 10,000 new cases per year[2]. All age groups can be affected, but it appears that there is a first peak between 15–24 years old, more boys than girls, and a second peak in elderly, mostly in women[1].

In the literature, there are few epidemiologic studies of this under-estimated problem. More studies are needed to determine the impact on the quality of life of patients and the cost for the health system.

ETIOPATHOGENESIS

Ingrown nail is a nail impinged in the surrounding soft tissues. The most controversial question is: which, from the plate and the soft tissues, is the origin of the problem? Should we work on the nail or on the periungual tissues? There is no universal answer. In some cases, the nail is problematic, while in others the cause is the hypertrophic surrounding tissue, and sometimes it can be both. Best management is a case-by-case analysis followed by an adapted treatment.

The pain and inflammation that usually accompany ingrown nails can be caused by any of the following:

- Epidermal breakage of periungual tissues by the nail plate (widened or over-curved nail, hypertrophic soft tissues, tight shoes, or other causes).

- Epidermal penetration by a laterodistal spur caused by improper nail clipping (by clipping the nail too short, which may leave the most lateral part, creating the spur).
- Pinching of the sub-ungual tissues by a pincer nail is a cause of pain. In some cases, the constant traction of the distal nail bed by the pincer nail may result in a traction osteophyte, which is an extremely tender condition, even to bedsheet contact.
- Secondary infection of the epidermal break may occur, but remain rare. Most physicians wrongly consider the swelling and the redness as a result from infection, while it is only acute inflammation.

Risk factors of ingrowing toenails

- Some experts believe that thinner nails are at more risk, but this remains unproven.
- Anatomical abnormalities of toes with the subsequent abnormal position and friction may predispose to the development of ingrowing nails (hallux valgus, hallux erectus, Morton's toe).
- Osteoarthritis in older people promotes pincer nails. Radiographs and MRI have shown that a widening of the base of the distal phalanx in osteoarthritis results in widening and flattening of the matrix and the proximal part of the nail plate. As a result, a transverse over-curvature of the distal part of the plate develops.
- Many experts suggest familial predisposition. The cause is not proven to be genetic; it may be simply behavioral (i.e., improper cutting of the nails).
- Repetitive traumas on the nail's free border against the tip of the shoe during running or some sports (e.g., tennis).
- Diabetes (insensitive foot, impaired vision so inadequate nail care).
- Obesity and chronic lower limb edema (thyroid, cardiac, and renal disorders).
- Improper nail cutting:
  - Teenagers: Hyperhidrosis, enhanced by sneakers, cause skin and nail softening. Teenagers tend to play with and tear off their softened nails, causing laterodistal nail spicules that may pierce the skin.
  - Individuals with more transverse curvature and wider nails may clip their nails too short and leave a spur in the lateral edge that, in time, pierces the skin of the lateral groove.
  - Inadequate nail care in elderly (impaired vision, reduced mobility).

QUALITY OF LIFE

Ingrown nail is a benign condition but often strongly alters patients' quality of life:

1. Pain may be severe. Daily activities (walking, running, playing), work, footwear, and even sleeping are impaired. Continuous oozing may also occur, needing renewed dressings.

2. Secondary infection increases pain and oozing and may progress to cellulitis or subcutaneous collections if not treated.
3. In the long term, fibrosis and hypertrophy of lateral folds may develop.

CLINICAL FEATURES, CLASSIFICATION, AND SEVERITY INDEX

Depending on the location of the ingrown nail, the following classification may be proposed[3].

Lateral ingrowing nail

1. **Lateral ingrowing nail without modification of the curvature of the plate**

- **Trapezoidal nail:** In this congenital condition, the nail plate appears narrow proximally and widens distally. The nail plate itself is not narrower proximally but is covered by the junction proximal-lateral nail fold, which is too medial (Figure 12.1). Trapezoidal nail rarely gets ingrown.
- **Juvenile ingrowing toenail:** This is the most common type of ingrowing nails. It affects mainly adolescents and is precipitated by improper trimming (short and oblique cut of the laterodistal corner of the nail or tearing off softened nails), which may leave a spicule that grows and penetrates the skin of the lateral groove (Figure 12.2). In addition, the lateral border of the nail tends to crumble due to constant humidity, resulting in lateral indentations. The saw-like effect of these indentations on the lateral fold results in inflammation and granulation tissue.
- **Hypertrophic soft tissues in teenagers and adults:** Chronic ingrowing is responsible for chronic inflammation, which may lead progressively to hypertrophy of soft tissues. This hypertrophy is different from granulation tissue as it consists mainly of fibrous tissue. It is very variable in size, and oozing is common as well as evil-smelling. Amazingly, pain is not intense (Figure 12.3).

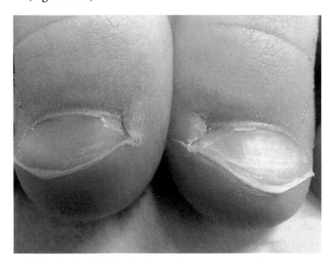

Figure 12.1 Trapezoidal nail.

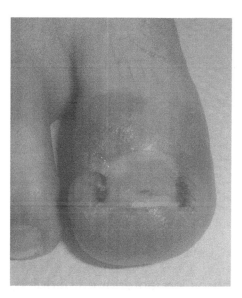

Figure 12.2 Ingrowing nail, juvenile type.

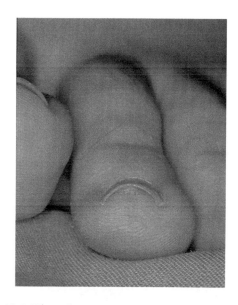

Figure 12.4 Tile nail.

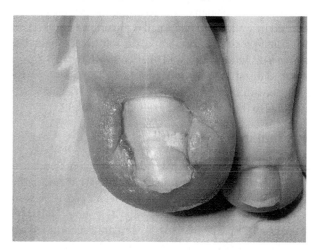

Figure 12.3 Ingrowing nail with hypertrophic soft tissue.

2. **Lateral ingrowing with modification of the curvature of the plate**

- **Tile nail (more common in young people):** A transverse over-curvature of the whole plate that keeps the same width distally and proximally (lateral edges remain parallel). It is milder and less symptomatic than the other types (Figure 12.4).
- **Plicated nail (more common in elderly):** The transverse curvature of the nail plate is normal except at one or both of its lateral margins, where it bends at 90° forming a right angle (Figure 12.5). This condition is usually asymptomatic unless pressure is applied on the nail (mainly by shoes) inducing a conflict between the angled nail and the soft tissues.
- **Pincer nail (more frequent in adults on toes):** A transversally over-curved nail pinching the nail bed. The transverse curvature is increasing towards the distal part of the nail in a conical manner. The distal over-curvature raises, creating traction on the nail bed and the bone (by the fibers fixing the nail unit to the tip

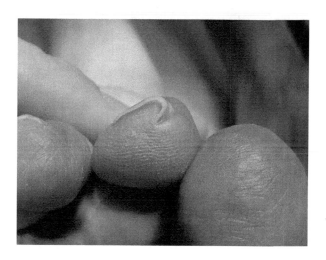

Figure 12.5 Plicated nail.

of the phalanx). This traction may result in a traction osteophyte, which can be seen on radiographs. The pain is variable and not related to the curvature degree; a mild increase in the curvature can produce severe pain. Bed sheet pain is a typical sign of pincer nails. Pincer nails have two origins:

- Hereditary form (positive family history): Symmetric with a lateral deviation of the big toenail and a medial deviation of the lesser ones (Figure 12.6).
- Acquired form: An asymmetric affection (Figure 12.7). On toenails, it is mainly caused by chronic improper footwear but also by osteoarthritis, psoriasis, onychomycosis, subungual tumors, trauma, etc. On fingernails, pincer nails can be caused by osteoarthritis or drug intake[4]. The causes of pain in pincer nails are the pinched nail bed (lateral-pressure pain) or the traction hyperostosis (upper-pressure pain).

- **Circumferential nail**: The extremely curved pincer nail where the two lateral edges of the nail plate join distally to form a tube-like nail that may be filled with keratin (Figure 12.8). This form is surprisingly not painful by itself, but it impairs the footwear as shoes may produce a painful pressure on the thickened nail.

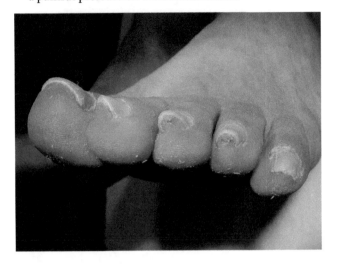

Figure 12.6 Pincer nail, hereditary form.

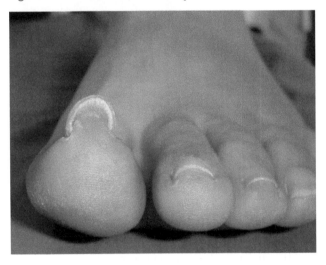

Figure 12.7 Pincer nail, acquired form.

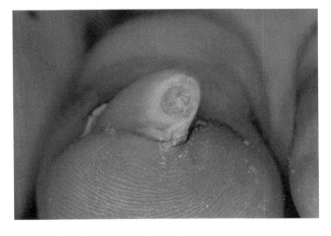

Figure 12.8 Circumferential nail.

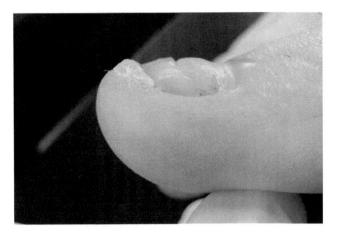

Figure 12.9 Distal ingrowing.

Distal ingrowing (anterior embedding) nail

The nail plate normally applies pressure on the nail bed and the distal part of the phalanx, counteracting the plantar pressure produced by walking. When a nail is missing or cut too short, this counterpressure is lost, and distal soft tissues mound up forming a distal wall. This wall interferes with the nail growth leading to distal ingrowing (Figure 12.9). The condition may aggravate with distal wall hyperkeratosis or a traction osteophyte (due to the traction of the raised distal pulp).

Proximal ingrowing nail

Retronychia (a term given by de Berker and Rendall in 1999): The condition is characterized by a triad associating the arrest of nail growth, xanthonychia, and proximal paronychia (Figure 12.10). It mainly affects young adults, but all age groups can be affected. It is mainly seen in women (>80%) and mostly on great toenails (>90%)[5]. Probably due to trauma from footwear, the nail is pushed back and raised proximally, so the proximal margin is detached from the nail matrix. A new nail grows beneath the old one pushing it

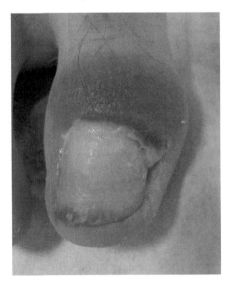

Figure 12.10 Retronychia.

upwards but gets stuck again distally then a third nail plate may grow beneath it and so on. Being lifted and irritated by the stacked sharp nails, the proximal nail fold gets inflamed giving rise to a proximal paronychia. Sometimes, granulation tissue develops under the proximal nail fold. Shortening of the nail bed is another clinical sign of retronychia.

Laterodistal ingrowing nail

- **Harpoon nail**
  A variant of ingrowing nails in which a lateral spur penetrates the lateral groove distally and may emerge distally forming a fistula (Figure 12.11). The latter may be inflammatory in its acute phase or epithelialized, non-inflammatory in the chronic phase[6].
- **Hypertrophic laterodistal lip in infants**
  A hypertrophic lip that covers the nail laterally or distally, mostly on the big toe (Figure 12.12). It can be congenital or develop shortly thereafter. The child refuses to wear shoes due to pain. Spontaneous remission may happen[7].

Severity index

Several severity indexes have been published (Heifetz, Frost, Mozena, Martinez, Kline). Heifetz index is the favored index of the authors because it helps to decide for the best treatment: conservative for stage 1, definitive narrowing of the nail for stage 2, and debulking of the hypertrophic soft tissues for stage 3[8].

Heifetz Stages	Clinical signs
I	Slight erythema and swelling of the nail grooves (Figure 12.13a)
II	Acute infection and suppuration (Figure 12.13b)
III	Chronic infection, granulation tissue in the nail grooves, and hypertrophy of the surrounding tissues (Figure 12.13c)

DIFFERENTIAL DIAGNOSIS

Ingrowing nail is an easy-to-diagnose condition. However, when facing oozing granulation tissues, neoplastic and infectious disorders should always be ruled out. The clinician should always send the granulation tissue for histology.

Tumors: Squamous cell carcinoma in-situ (Bowen disease) and amelanotic melanoma can present as granulation

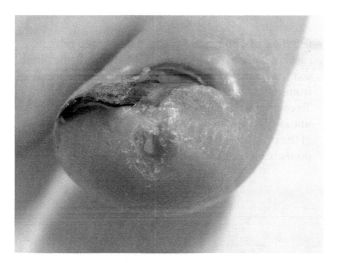

Figure 12.11 Harpoon nail.

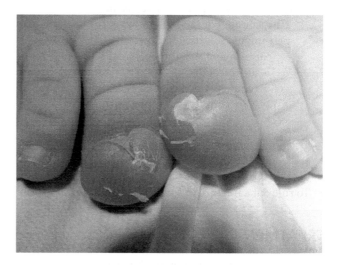

Figure 12.12 Voluminous hypertrophic fold in an infant.

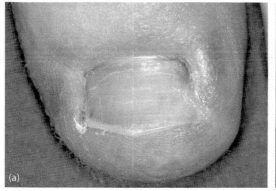
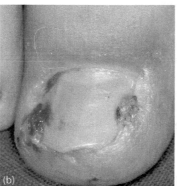
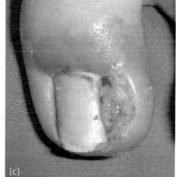

Figure 12.13 **(a)** Heifetz stage 1; **(b)** Heifetz stage 2; **(c)** Heifetz stage 3.

tissue with oozing. They should be ruled out when facing an atypical presentation of ingrown nails, in an adult especially if there is nail plate destruction.

Granulation tissue may resemble pyogenic granuloma (PG), but they are not the same. PG is a circumscribed lesion made of benign lobular proliferation of capillaries.

Infections: Acute bacterial or viral paronychia is erythematous, swollen, and painful. Infective paronychia is acute and usually accompanied by vesicular (viral) or pustular (bacterial) lesions with a nail of regular width.

INVESTIGATIONS

- **Onychoscopy** has a limited value in ingrowing nails as the diagnosis is obvious clinically. It may be helpful in rare cases when we suspect a neoplastic differential diagnosis (squamous cell carcinoma, melanoma).
- **Bacteriologic** swab for direct examination, culture, and antibiogram is indicated before starting the antibiotic therapy for secondarily infected ingrowing nail.
- **Imaging** may be helpful in some instances:
  - **Ultrasound**: For the exploration of the nail unit and peri-ungual soft tissues. Especially for:
    - Suspicion of sub-cutaneous collection in case of acute infection
    - To confirm the diagnosis of retronychia
  - **X-rays**: To assess the bony phalanx:

- Traction hyperostosis in pincer nails and anterior embedding
- Osteoarthritis in elderly patients with pincer nail
- To rule out a fracture in a post-traumatic painful nail

TREATMENT

The definitive treatment of ingrowing nails is surgical. For mild cases (Heifetz 1), non-surgical conservative methods can improve or even treat the condition.

Conservative treatment

Advantages
- Easy, non-invasive
- No complications or risks
- Performed at home or in the office

Disadvantages
- Need compliance for weeks/months
- Slow efficacy
- High rate of failure and recurrence

Indications
- Heifetz 1
- When the cause is transitory (nail loss, improper clipping, nail fracture)
- When patient refuses surgery
- Patient with uncontrolled diabetes or vascular impairment
- Infants or children with nails not yet completely developed

Techniques (or Methods)
1. *Compression/massage*
   It is used in mild cases in newborns or after nail loss. Continuous compression or daily massage is performed with hydrating, antimicrobial, or corticosteroid creams to spread nail folds away from the plate.
2. *Taping*
   This method is used in Heifetz 1, distal or lateral ingrowing, or when the cause is transitory. An adhesive tape is secured on the border of the affected fold, which is pulled down and away from the nail in an oblique and proximal direction over the pulp of the toe (Figure 12.14). If adhesion is impaired, by hyperhidrosis or oozing, acetone, and a medical adhesive liquid may be added. The tape should be kept 24/7 and changed when adhesion or tension is released. The procedure is continued until complete resolution.
3. *False nails*
   (acrylic nails, preformed plastic nails, or nail gels): In cases of nail loss (accidental or post-surgical), the distal soft tissues may heap up from the plantar pressure from walking and shoes, leading to distal embedding. To counteract this pressure, false nails may be applied, until full regrowth of the nail. However, detachment of the prosthesis is common from the excessive plantar pressure on the great toenail.

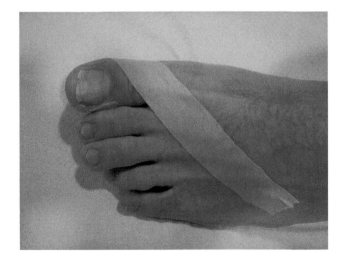

Figure 12.14 Taping for a transitory ingrowing induced from cutting the distal lateral corner. The tape pulls away the offending nail plate alleviating the pain. This procedure has to be performed until the nail plate has regrown completely.

4. *Dental thread/cotton*

These are easy, inexpensive methods to treat mild cases with transitory cause. A piece of cotton or a dental thread is inserted under the nail to separate it from the nail fold. The process is painful the first days and should be repeated every day with adding a bit more of cotton each time; then, when completely painless, the cotton is fixed with acrylic or cyanoacrylate glue for one week. Cotton nail cast and rolled cotton padding are newly reported techniques with good, rapid results. A piece of cotton, after being introduced between the nail plate and periungual tissue, is fixed immediately with cyanoacrylate. The advantage is that they do not need to be repeated every day[9,10].

5. *Orthonyxia (nail brace)*

is indicated for ingrowing nails due to transverse over-curvature. Two types of braces are available, adhesive or hooked, and both seek to lift the lateral edges of the nail plate progressively. Adhesive braces are made of a thin strip of composite material glued to the nail plate. The hooked one, less used nowadays, is a dental wire, which is applied over the nail plate and curves to be hooked under the lateral edges of the over-curved nail. The position of the brace is modified monthly and removed when the aspect of the nail returns to normal. Recently, shape memory braces, made of titanium or copper-aluminum-manganese, have been developed. Those different braces relieve the pain within days and flatten the nail plate progressively. However, they do not treat the cause and recurrence is the rule.

6. *Nail tube splinting (sleeve technique)*

A plastic gutter, similar to vinyl intravenous drip infusion tube, is used to surround the lateral edge of the nail and separate it from the nail fold. Acute and chronic ingrowing nails, even with granulation tissue, can be treated by this method with good results, especially if the cause is transitory (e.g., nail spicule). Under digital nerve block, the laterodistal nail is elevated to expose the offending part of the lateral plate. The plastic gutter is incised longitudinally and slipped in the fold around the lateral edge of the nail plate. The gutter is secured with an adhesive tape or better with an acrylic resin or even with absorbable sutures. Pain is usually relieved in a week, but the gutter should be kept in place a few months until the lateral edge of the nail has grown over the tip of the toe.

Surgical treatment

As explained before, the cause of ingrowing nails may be the nail, surrounding soft tissues, or both. So, the treatment should focus on narrowing the nail plate, debulking the soft tissues, or sometimes on both. Each approach can be done by different procedures, but, as there are no well-conducted comparative trials in the literature, there is no single best procedure for all patients. It should be a case-by-case analysis. Surgeons should perform the technique they have mastered and which is best adapted to correct the cause of

ingrowing. Of course, risks, postoperative morbidity, and cosmetic result should be considered.

NAIL PLATE NARROWING TECHNIQUES

a. *Chemical cauterization of one or both lateral horns of the matrix*

This is an easy technique with a very high success rate, that should be known by all dermatologists. It is indicated for acute ingrowing (Heifetz 1-2) with or without granulation tissue and for pincer and plicated nails. Chemical cautery with phenol 88% has been performed for more than 70 years. Compared to other surgical procedures, it is the most effective technique in terms of success rate, morbidity, and recurrence as per a recent review in Cochrane Library[2]. In the largest studies, its success rate is shown to be at least 95%[11]. Phenol has three interesting effects. It destroys tissues (by coagulating proteins) and disinfects the surgical field (by killing all germs) with an anesthetic effect for several weeks (by demyelinating nerve ends)[8].

After a digital nerve block, a tourniquet is applied. Any granulation tissue is removed with a curette to expose the offending part of the nail. To assess the adequate width of lateral nail strip to be removed, the lateral fold is pressed gently against the nail plate; the part of plate covered by the fold should be removed. Using an elevator, the dorsal surface of the nail plate is separated from the proximal nail fold; then, the ventral part is separated from the nail bed and matrix (lateral horn). The nail strip is then split with nail nippers or scissors up to its most proximal extremity. After removing the strip and drying the area, phenol is applied with the elevator, a cotton swab, a urethral swab, or a nasopharyngeal swab for 2–4 minutes (Figure 12.15a–e). The tourniquet should prevent any single blood drop, which may alter the efficacy of the cauterant. The surgeon should take care to avoid any lateral onycholysis, which may allow sliding of the cauterant with extra cauterization of the matrix resulting in excessive permanent narrowing of the plate. For this reason, nail nippers are preferred over other tools that may produce an onycholysis of the preserved nail while cutting.

A histologic study on cadavers demonstrated that phenol needs 4 minutes to destroy the nail matrix until the basal layer[12]. The curettage of the matrix does not increase the success rate but increases the risk of periostitis[11]. Phenolization of the matrix is safe in diabetic patients and children.

Other matrix cauterants include sodium hydroxide 10%[13], which is applied for 1 minute, and trichloroacetic acid 100%[14], both with similar success rates and quick healing.

b. *Wedge excision*

This procedure is the surgeon's favored one. Several variants of wedge excisions exist (Winograd's, Frost's, Suppan's, and Emmert's procedures). They are all, in different ways, are aimed at surgically removing a lateral strip of nail, its bed, and the lateral horn of the matrix (Figure 12.16a and b). The toughest part is

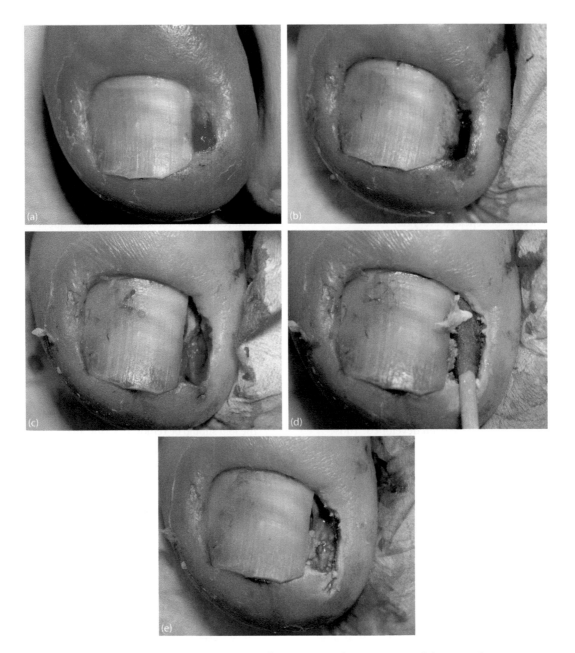

Figure 12.15 (a) Ingrowing nail with granulation tissue. Before surgery; (b) Curettage of the granulation tissue exposes the spur responsible for the ingrowing; (c) Avulsion of a lateral strip of nail, the new distal edge being at the free edge; (d) Chemical cautery of the lateral matrix of the nail and corresponding nail bed; (e) Immediate post op.

to fully remove the lateral horns of the matrix, which strongly adheres to the periosteum and may extend to half of the lateral aspect of the great toe. These procedures should not be recommended anymore as, in unskilled hands, they lead to frequent complications, including infections in 20% of cases, lateral deviation, spicule formation (very common), and inclusion nail[11].

c. *Lasers*

The lateral nail strip is removed, surgically or with CO_2 laser in cutting mode, then the proximal nail fold is incised and reclined. The exposed matrix and lateral horn are then vaporized with the CO_2 laser. The advantage is its hemostatic effect, but the procedure needs an experienced and skilled laser surgeon[11]. The success rate has never been shown to be superior to chemical cautery.

d. *Radiosurgery*

Here, the destruction of the lateral horn is done by a radio wave technique. The advantage of the radiosurgery is that the heat is generated in the tissue itself while the electrode remains cold, giving a precise effect and preventing the destruction of surrounding tissues[15].

e. *Curettage of lateral horns*

This procedure should not be performed as the removal is always incomplete, leading to spicule formation and inclusion cysts. If performed aggressively, it is associated with periostitis and even osteitis.

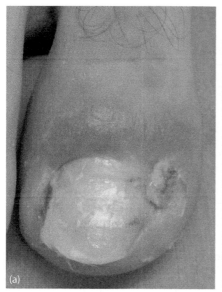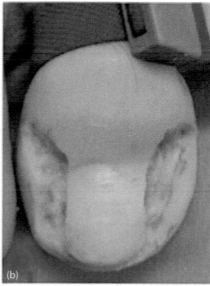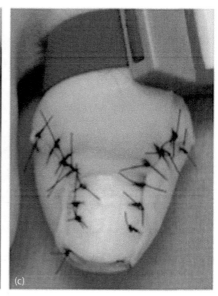

Figure 12.16 WEDGE EXCISION. (a) Ingrowing nail pre-operatively; (b) Two lateral incisions, lazy S type, remove the plate, the bed, and the corresponding lateral horns of the matrix. This corresponds indeed to two wide lateral longitudinal biopsies; (c) Immediate post op. (Courtesy N di Chiacchio, Brazil.)

SOFT TISSUE DEBULKING

a. *Howard–Dubois procedure*

First described by Howard in 1893, then reintroduced by Dubois in 1974 to become a popular procedure of soft tissue debulking[16]. It consists of removing a horizontal crescent of soft tissues at the tip of the toe, parallel to the distal edge of the nail and 5 mm below the distal groove (Figure 12.17a–c). It is the technique of choice for distal embedding, and also indicated for hypertrophic lateral folds. Some authors proposed unilateral variants of the technique for hypertrophic lateral fold[11].

b. *Vandenbos procedure*

Procedure was first described in 1959 by Vandenbos and Bowers then slightly modified recently by Chapeskie and Kovac[17]. Severe hypertrophy of the lateral folds is the best indication. It consists of a wide excision of the whole lateral fold up to the proximal nail fold and reaching the tip of the toe, leaving the most distal part of the pulp (Figure 12.18a and b). The wound is then left for secondary intention healing. The nail plate and matrix are left untouched. Hemostasis can be obtained by gentle electrocautery or a running lock suture. In a series of 124 patients (212 surgical sites), the Vandenbos procedure had a cure rate of 100%. A median follow-up time of 8 years showed excellent cosmetic results without any recurrence[17]. Patients should be informed of the long healing time (up to 8 weeks).

c. *Super-U procedure*

This is a U-shaped debulking technique developed by Peres Rosa, a Brazilian dermatologist[18]. It is similar to the Vandenbos procedure but the proximal fold is not involved and the median part of the toe tip is removed (Figure 12.19a–c). Success rates are similar to the Vandenbos'.

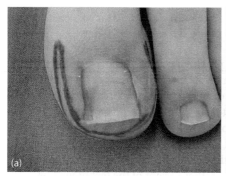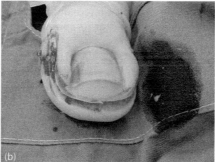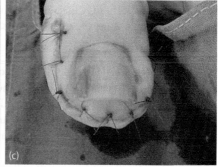

Figure 12.17 DUBOIS' PROCEDURE. (a) Ingrowing nail, chronic type with hypertrophic lateral folds. See the drawing of the incisions; (b) Excision of a crescent of soft tissue down to the bone; (c) Suturing the defect immediately expands the folds and fully exposes the nail plate.

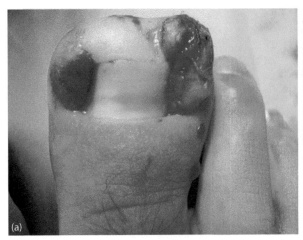
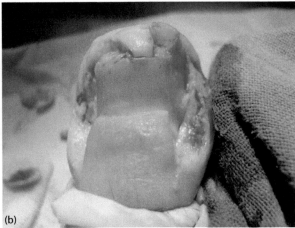

Figure 12.18 VANDENBOS' PROCEDURE. **(a)** Huge hypertrophic granulation tissue, on both side of the great toenail; **(b)** Wide removal of the lateral fold, leaving the hyponychium in place. The defect is left for secondary intention.

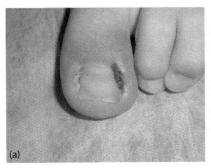
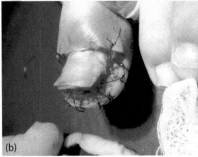
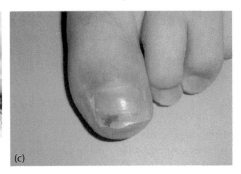

Figure 12.19 SUPER-U PROCEDURE. **(a)** Ingrowing nail with chronic swelling of the lateral nail folds (Collivao Perez Rosa, Brazil); **(b)** Removal en bloc, in a U-shape, of the lateral and distal folds (Courtesy Perez Rosa, Brazil); **(c)** After secondary intention healing. (Courtesy Perez Rosa, Brazil.)

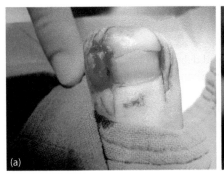
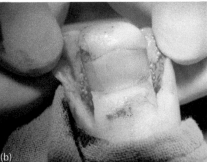
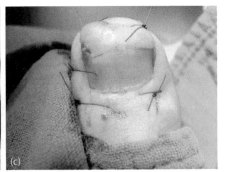

Figure 12.20 NOEL' PROCEDURE. **(a)** Prominent hypertrophic lateral folds. Pre-operative aspect; **(b)** After vertical excision of two wedges of soft tissue reaching the pulp; **(c)** After re-approximation of the defect.

d. *Noël's procedure*

It consists in a vertical wedge excision of the lateral fold down to the pulp (Figure 12.20a–c). The medial incision line skims to the lateral edge of the nail plate and the bone. The excision should be deep enough to remove large amount of soft tissues[19]. Simple interrupted sutures are enough to close the defect.

e. *Tweedie and Ranger's transposition flap*

This transposition flap is performed to lower a lateral hypertrophic lip. The procedure is easy to perform with a high success rate (>90%). The scalpel is inserted vertically in the proximal part of the lateral sulcus to have it reappear 1 cm below in the lateral aspect of the toe. The blade is pushed distally until the two incisions join at the distal tip of the toe, freeing a flap with a proximal pedicle. The lower part of the flap is trimmed to allow a lower transposition of the flap. After suturing the flap, a small upper defect is then left to heal by secondary intention[20] (Figure 12.21). Another variant of the technique was described by Bose, by cutting away the proximal part of the flap, leaving the whole area to heal by a second intention, which is, in fact, a unilateral super-U[21].

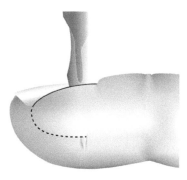

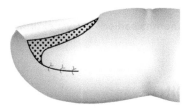

Figure 12.21 Tweedie and Ranger flap for hypertrophic lateral lip.

AVULSION

This is not a curative procedure of ingrowing nail, except in retronychia. As the distal adhesion of the plate to its bed, a proximal approach is recommended to avoid hurting the distal bed.

DEROOFING

It has a single indication, harpoon nails. Like in fistulas, a probe is inserted in the fistula, and a scalpel removes the roof. This allows visualization of the harpoon and its cure by chemical cautery[6] (Figure 12.22a and b).

COMPLICATIONS AND PROGNOSIS

It is important to know the complications, to prevent and to deal with them. If a complication happens, the patient should feel reassured by the doctor's care and his management.

1. *Postoperative pain*
   As the fingertips are one of the most innervated parts of the body, severe pain is expected after nail surgery, including continuous pain, pulsatile pain (due to blood flow), or even an allodynia, which is a severe pain upon touch. Pain can be minimized by the injection of long-acting anesthetics (bupivacaine or ropivacaine), pain-killers, bulky non-tight dressing the first days to protect from traumas, and keeping the limb elevated for at least 48 hours to prevent swelling. Pain is very uncommon with chemical cautery, but may occur with surgeries of soft tissue debulking.

2. *Postoperative bleeding*
   A common complication of this highly vascularized area, especially with wide debulking. Ordinary hemostatic measures can be used for mild-moderate bleeding (35% aluminum chloride, alginate dressing) but electrocoagulation should be avoided. In case of severe postoperative bleeding, injecting 0.5 cc of the anesthetic (or normal saline) around the digital artery (as a wing block) will act as a volumetric tourniquet until clotting occurs[8]. Of course, a bulky dressing and elevating the limb are to be respected for at least 48 hours. Blood thinners should never be stopped as it has been shown that this increases the risk of cerebrovascular complications.

3. *Post-operative dysesthesia*
   Nerves might be affected by the anesthetic or the surgery leading to post-operative, long-lasting numbness, tingling, or loss of sensation. In a recent study, 47% of patients reported a post-operative sensory disturbance, but 70% of them improved 6–12 months later[22].

4. *Infection*
   Antiseptic measures should be respected for nail surgery. The most important risk factor is lack of hygiene and inadequate homecare. Patients with poor hygiene are asked to scrub their digits twice daily during the two days preceding the surgery. For patients with limited mobility, a relative or a home nurse is to be considered for the post-operative care. If infection occurs, a bacterial swab is done and an empirical antibiotic against staphylococcus is started, then adapted later.

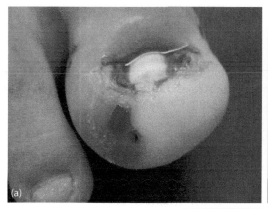
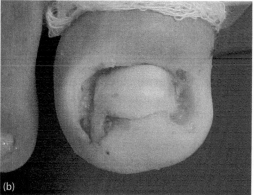

Figure 12.22 (a) Harpoon nail; (b) Deroofing exposes the spur harpooning the lateral fold.

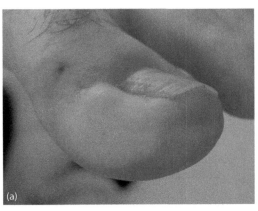
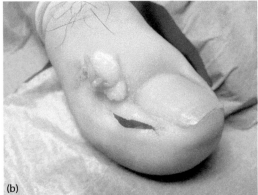

Figure 12.23 **(a)** Implantation cyst following a successful Dubois' procedure 6 months earlier; **(b)** Cyst extirpated.

Antibiotic prophylaxis should be prescribed for prevention of endocarditis, infection of joint prosthesis, or if the surgery involves the bone.

5. *Necrosis*

Mostly in patients with altered vascularization. Causes include extended use of tourniquet, too tight stitches, excess volume infiltration, or from administration of lidocaine with epinephrine in patients with altered blood supply (safe in healthy people but not needed as tourniquet assures a bloodless field).

6. *Recurrence*

A common complication, due to improper technique or no (or only partial) destruction of the lateral matrix. Surgeons should be aware that the presence of blood during the chemical cautery is a common cause of recurrence as the cauterant will coagulate blood proteins instead of matrix proteins.

7. *Implantation cyst*

The implantation of epidermal cells into deeper layers may rarely happen, leading to formation of a cyst months later. This has been reported after Zadik surgery (Figure 12.23a and b)[23].

8. *Reflex sympathetic dystrophy*

A rare but serious mysterious complication reported with bony fractures and very exceptionally with nail surgery[24]. The syndrome has three phases, acute (hours–days), dystrophic (3–6 months), and atrophic (9 months post-surgery). The acute phase consists of a triad of sensory (continuous pain, allodynia, hyperalgesia), autonomic (vasospasms, hypo- or hyperhidrosis), and motor symptoms (tremor, weakness). The dystrophic phase is characterized by a thin glossy skin with hypo/hypertrichosis and nails may be affected. The atrophic phase consists a skin and muscular atrophy with or without joint contractures. This syndrome affects more women around 50 years old and mostly on fingers. Asking the patient to mobilize the digit two days after surgery might be a preventive measure. Early recognition and multidisciplinary management are necessary.

KEY POINTS

- Ingrowing nail is a frequent problem affecting the quality of life of a lot of patients.
- All age groups and both sexes can be affected.
- The causative part may be the nail, surrounding soft tissues, or both.
- Types are lateral, distal, laterodistal, or proximal ingrowing with many subtypes.
- Conservative treatment is considered for minor cases with transitory cause.
- Surgical treatment is mandatory for cases with permanent cause.
- Two main types of surgery are available, definitive narrowing of the nail or debulking of soft tissues.
- Several procedures are described for each type. There is no single best procedure. The procedure with the highest success rate should be chosen depending on the surgeon skills and on the clinical features of each case.

REFERENCES

1. Eekhof JA, Van Wijk B, Knuistingh Neven A, van der Wouden JC. Interventions for ingrowing toenails. *Cochrane Database Syst Rev.* 2012;4:CD001541. doi:10.1002/14651858. CD001541.pub3.

2. Rounding C, Bloomfield S. Surgical treatments for ingrowing toenails. *Cochrane Database Syst Rev.* 2005;2:CD001541. Review. Update in: *Cochrane Database Syst Rev.* 2012;4:CD001541.

3. Baran R. Ingrown nails. *Ann Dermatol Venereol.* 1987;114(12):1597–1604.

4. Failla V, Richert BJ, Nikkels AF. Pincer nails associated with pamidronate. *Clin Exp Dermatol.* 2011;36(3):305–306. doi:10.1111/j.1365-2230.2010.03919.x.

5. De Berker DA, Richert B, Duhard E, Piraccini BM, André J, Baran R. Retronychia: Proximal ingrowing of the nail plate. *J Am Acad Dermatol.* 2008;58(6):978–983. doi:10.1016/j.jaad.2008.01.013.

6. Richert B, Caucanas M, DiChiacchio N. Surgical approach to harpoon nail: A new variant of ingrowing toenail. *Dermatol Surg.* 2014;40(6):700–701. doi:10.1111/dsu.0000000000000023.

7. Piraccini BM, Parente GL, Varotti E, Tosti A. Congenital hypertrophy of the lateral nail folds of the hallux: Clinical features and follow-up of seven cases. *Pediatr Dermatol.* 2000;17(5):348–351.

8. Richert B, Chiacchio ND, Caucanas M, Chiacchio NGD. *Management of Ingrowing Nails: Treatment Scenarios and Practical Tips.* Cham, Switzerland: Springer, 2016.

9. Gutiérrez-Mendoza D, DeAnda-Juárez M, Ávalos VF, Martínez GR, Domínguez-Cherit J. "Cotton nail cast": A simple solution for mild and painful lateral and distal nail embedding. *Dermatol Surg.* 2015;41(3):411–414. doi:10.1097/DSS.0000000000000294.

10. d'Almeida LF, Nakamura R. Onychocryptosis treatment pearls: The "rolled cotton padding" maneuver and the "artificial resin nail" technique. *Dermatol Surg.* 2016;42(3):434–436. doi:10.1097/DSS.0000000000000616.

11. Richert B. Surgical management of ingrown toenails: An update overdue. *Dermatol Ther.* 2012;25(6):498–509. doi:10.1111/j.1529 8019.2012.01511.x.

12. Boberg JS, Frederiksen MS, Harton FM. Scientific analysis of phenol nail surgery. *J Am Podiatr Med Assoc.* 2002;92(10):575–579.

13. Bostanci S, Kocyigit P, Gürgey E. Comparison of phenol and sodium hydroxide chemical matricectomies for the treatment of ingrowing toenails. *Dermatol Surg.* 2007;33(6):680–685.

14. Kim SH, Ko HC, Oh CK, Kwon KS, Kim MB. Trichloroacetic acid matricectomy in the treatment of ingrowing toenails. *Dermatol Surg.* 2009;35(6):973–979. doi:10.1111/j.1524-4725.2009.01165.x.

15. Hettinger DF, Valinsky MS, Nuccio G, Lim R. Nail matrixectomies using radio wave technique. *J Am Podiatr Med Assoc.* 1991;81(6):317–321.

16. Dubois JP. Treatment of ingrown nails. *Nouv Presse Med.* 1974;3(31):1938–1940.

17. Chapeskie H, Kovac JR. Case series: Soft-tissue nail-fold excision: A definitive treatment for ingrown toenails. *Can J Surg.* 2010;53(4):282–286.

18. Rosa IP, DiChiacchio N, DiChiacchio NG, Caetano L. "Super u": A technique for the treatment of ingrown nail. *Dermatol Surg.* 2015;41(5):652–653. doi:10.1097/DSS.0000000000000351.

19. Noël B. Surgical treatment of ingrown toenail without matricectomy. *Dermatol Surg.* 2008;34(1):79–83.

20. Tweedie JH, Ranger I. A simple procedure with nail preservation for ingrowing toe-nails. *Arch Emerg Med.* 1985;2(3):149–154.

21. Bose B. A technique for excision of nail fold for ingrowing toenail. *Surg Gynecol Obstet.* 1971;132(3):511–512.

22. Walsh ML, Shipley DV, de Berker DA. Survey of patients' experiences after nail surgery. *Clin Exp Dermatol.* 2009;34(5):e154–e156. doi:10.1111/j.1365-2230.2008.03073.x.

23. Vanhooteghem O, Henrijean A, André J, Richert B, De La Brassinne M. Ingrown nails: A complication of surgery for an in-growing toe-nail using the Zadik procedure. *Ann Dermatol Venereol.* 2006;133(12):1009–1010.

24. Guerrero-González GA, DiChiacchio NG, D'Apparecida Machado-Filho C, DiChiacchio N. Complex regional pain syndrome after nail surgery. *Dermatol Surg.* 2016;42(9):1116–1118. doi:10.1097/DSS.0000000000000776.

Inflammatory Nail Diseases

13

Nail psoriasis

CHANDER GROVER AND SUBUHI KAUL

INTRODUCTION

Psoriasis is a chronic dermatologic disorder, affecting 0.19%–3.15% of the general population, reported prevalence being as high as 4.8% in some studies.[1,2] Nail involvement is a common accompaniment in psoriasis, often existing with skin lesions; however, isolated nail psoriasis is seen in approximately 5%–10% of psoriasis.[3,4] Varying evidence of nail psoriasis is present in up to one-half of patients with any clinical variant of psoriasis; hence, should be actively looked for.[2] The presence of psoriatic arthritis is often associated with more frequent and severe nail disease. Nail involvement in patients with psoriatic arthritis has been found to be as high as 87%.[5] In fact, it is a predictor for associated arthritis due to the intimate micro-anatomical relationship between the nail unit and the musculoskeletal system.[6] This suggests that nail disease is an important aspect of psoriasis with distinctive sequelae, necessitating special management strategies.

Although skin lesions are considered to represent psoriasis, arthritis and nail involvement are equally important manifestations. Despite frequent involvement of the nail unit in psoriasis, it is often overlooked and its impact on patient's quality of life is under estimated. This disregard often ensures that, for the patient, the deformity turns into a disability.

EPIDEMIOLOGY

Nail psoriasis is reflective of skin disease more often than not, following similar patterns. Psoriasis affects all ages, having a bimodal age distribution (initial peak in the second decade and then the fifth decade). Both sexes are equally affected, even though the onset is slightly earlier in females.[2] Psoriasis affects the joints in nearly one-third of cases and nail involvement is seen in up to 78.3% of these.[7] The predisposition to develop nail manifestations increases with the disease duration, reaching a lifetime occurrence of 80%–90%.[5] The disease typically runs a relapsing and remitting course with variable severity and prognosis, which may not be well correlated with the severity of the skin disease or that of the joint.

ETIOPATHOGENESIS

In recent years, our understanding of the pathophysiology of psoriasis has undergone a major shift, from a keratinocyte hyperproliferation model to an immune dysfunction process. Nevertheless, the etio-pathogenesis remains incompletely understood with a complex interplay of **genetic, immune dysregulation,** and **environmental** factors being considered responsible for the manifestations.

Genetic factors

It is postulated that there are two pathogenetically distinct forms of psoriasis:

- **Type I**, early onset disease, which has strong hereditary predisposition, Human Leucocyte Antigen (HLA) associations and a more severe course.
- **Type II**, late onset disease, which tends to be sporadic, HLA independent, and a usually milder course.

The bimodal peak of onset in psoriasis supports this supposition,[2] giving credence to the importance of genetic factors in initiation of psoriasis. Additionally, concordance rate is higher in monozygotic twins (70%) than in dizygotic twins (20%).[8] However, the genetics of psoriasis are quite complex with more than 30 single-nucleotide polymorphisms (SNPs) known to contribute to the disease risk.[8]

Immunologic factors

Psoriasis shows interplay of both the innate and adaptive immune systems with epidermal cells responding to resultant stimuli (Figure 13.1). The immune pathways being activated in psoriasis are the amplified constitutive or inducible immune pathways, present normally in human skin.

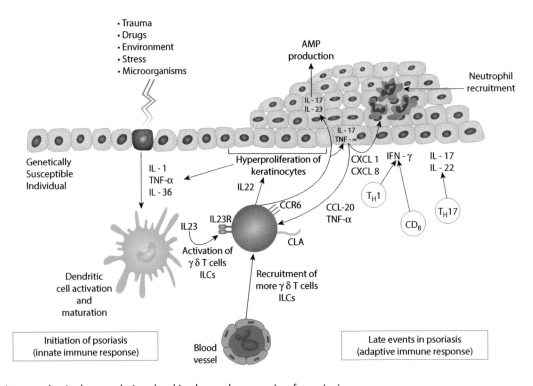

Figure 13.1 Immunological cascade involved in the pathogenesis of psoriasis.

These include the epidermal keratinocytes, which are key participants in the innate immunity, inducing and switching off classes of T cells, recruited to the skin. The key components of the immune mediation of psoriasis are:

T CELLS IN PSORIASIS

Psoriasis is considered a Th1-dominant disease, due to an increase in cytokines of the Th1 pathway viz. interferon gamma (IFN-γ), IL-2, and interleukin 12(IL-12) in the psoriatic plaques. The increased IL-2 from the activated T-cells and IL-12 from Langerhans cells upregulate the genes' coding for transcription of cytokines like IFN-γ, TNF-α (tumor necrosis factor), and IL-2, responsible for further differentiation.[3]

The increased dermal T-lymphocytes are a mixture of CD4+ and CD8+ cells, with CD4+ predominance. Most T cells in skin lesions are memory cells that express cutaneous lymphocyte antigen (CLA). Recently, γδ T cells have been found to be the IL-17-producing cells in psoriasis. IL-17 is now considered a key cytokine in the formation of the psoriatic phenotype and many of the genes induced by this cytokine in keratinocytes are highly expressed in psoriasis lesions, including chemokines and antimicrobial peptides (AMPs). IL-17 induces IL-19 and IL-36γ in psoriasis lesions, which may then lead to proliferative responses in keratinocytes. IL-20 and IL-22 have similar trophic effects on the epidermis.[8,9]

INNATE IMMUNITY IN PSORIASIS

Natural killer (NK) cells play an important role in psoriasis pathogenesis by releasing cytokines such as IFN-γ, TNF, and IL-22. NKT cells are a heterogeneous group of innate cells sharing some features of both NK cells and T cells. CD1d, an invariant stimulator of NKT cells, is abundantly expressed in psoriatic epidermis.[8] In psoriasis lesions, abundant IL-23 is available from dendritic cells and macrophages. It is required for the expansion and survival of T cells that produce IL-17. Langerhans cells (immature dendritic cells) are also found in abundance in skin lesions of psoriasis.[9,10]

KERATINOCYTES IN PSORIASIS

The main cell type expressing IL-17 receptor in psoriasis is the keratinocyte. Keratinocytes respond by upregulating mRNAs for a range of inflammatory products. Collectively, the cytokines IL-17, IFN-γ, IL-22, and TNF cause keratinocyte proliferation, chemokine, cytokine, and AMP production. This becomes a self-amplifying loop, as these products act back on the dendritic cells, T cells, and neutrophils to perpetuate the cutaneous inflammatory process.[8–10] The increased vascularity that is a prominent and constant feature of psoriasis is due to increased angiogenesis driven primarily by vascular endothelial growth factor (VEGF) secreted by activated keratinocytes.[8] For a comprehensive description of the complex pathogenesis of psoriasis the reader is referred to detailed texts on the subject.[8–11]

Environmental factors

A number of environmental factors like trauma, infections, drugs, seasonal variation, hormonal factors, and psychological stress have been associated with psoriasis and are implicated in the initiation of disease process as well as exacerbation of pre-existing disease. An example of Koebner response in nail psoriasis is the more frequent involvement of the dominant hand index and thumb.[12]

Factors inducing nail psoriasis

Due to its close association with the enthesis of the distal interphalangeal joint (DIP), it has been suggested that the nail is an appendage of the musculoskeletal system rather than the skin. With magnetic resonance imaging (MRI), it has been demonstrated that the extensor tendon is almost continuous distally with the nail unit and a network of collateral ligaments anchor the lateral margins. This explains the frequency of nail involvement in patients with psoriatic arthritis, who usually have clinical or subclinical inflammation of the DIP joint.[6,12]

Nevertheless, varying manifestations of nail psoriasis ensue; their pathogenesis, depending on the site involved, is elaborated below.

CLINICAL FEATURES

Fingernails are more commonly involved in psoriasis. Simultaneous involvement of fingernails and toenails is reported in 82% of patients; while 18% present with isolated fingernail involvement.[7] A variety of nail changes can be observed in psoriasis depending on the site of the nail unit affected by the disease process (Table 13.1).

Classically, nail psoriasis presents as pitting, onycholysis, subungual hyperkeratosis, nail bed discoloration, and onychodystrophy. Other nail manifestations include the diagnostic salmon patch/oil drop, leukonychia, splinter hemorrhages, red spots in the lunula, and crumbling of nail plate.[2,3]

Several studies have reported pitting to be the most common sign (seen in 80%–90% of patients at some point in their life). This is closely followed by onycholysis.[5] The majority of the lesions of nail psoriasis result from matrix and/or nail bed involvement. The type of nail lesion and an understanding of structure involved in the production of that defect guide us in choosing an appropriate targeted therapy, thus maximizing therapeutic efficacy and minimizing side effects.

Nail matrix involvement

This results in manifestations involving the nail plate (surface or the entire depth). Pitting, transverse grooves, nail plate thickening, crumbling, red spots in lunula, leukonychia, and splitting suggest matrix disease.

Table 13.1 Phenotypes of nail psoriasis

Site of involvement	Nail matrix	Nail bed	Nail fold
Clinical features	Pitting	Onycholysis	Paronychia
	Beau's lines	Oil spot/salmon patch	Acropustulosis
	Leukonychia	Subungual hyperkeratosis	Psoriatic plaque
	Red spot in lunula	Splinter hemorrhage	Glomerular dilation of capillaries (only dermatoscopy)
	Crumbling	Discoloration	Nail fold capillaroscopic abnormalities
	Onychomadesis		
	Longitudinal striations		
	Trachyonychia		

Source: Burns, T. et al., Rook's Textbook of Dermatology, 8th ed., John Wiley & Sons, Singapore, 23–26, 2010.

NAIL PITTING

It is the most common manifestation of nail psoriasis involving fingernails more frequently than toenails (Figure 13.2).[5,13] Pits are punctate depressions in the nail plate produced by dysfunction of proximal matrix, which leaves behind parakeratotic cells persisting within the newly formed nail plate. With subsequent nail plate growth and exposure to the environment, the poorly adherent parakeratotic cells slough off of the nail plate surface, leaving behind depression and scaling. A deep pit indicates involvement of intermediate and ventral matrix as well, whereas the length of a pit points to period of time the matrix was affected by disease.

The pits in psoriasis are usually irregular and shallow but can involve the entire depth of the plate to leave a full-thickness defect known as elkonyxis. Extensive pitting causing surface irregularities gives the appearance of trachyonychia (Figure 13.3).[2] It is generally accepted that a patient with greater than 20 fingernail pits is suggestive of psoriasis as the etiology whereas greater than 60 pits per person is unlikely to be found in the absence of psoriasis.[4]

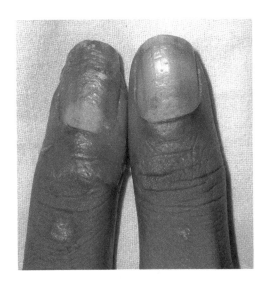

Figure 13.2 Extensive pitting in a case of nail psoriasis.

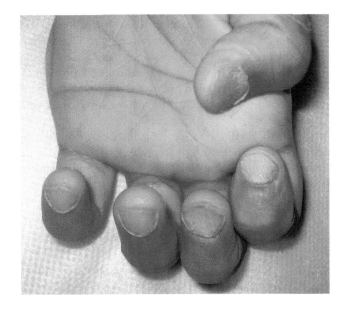

Figure 13.3 A patient with cutaneous psoriasis presenting with trachyonychia involving multiple nails.

TRANSVERSE GROOVES (BEAU'S LINES)

When psoriatic lesion affects a wider area of nail matrix, it results in the formation of transverse grooves (Figure 13.4). These Beau's lines tend to be irregular and incomplete and are again a common finding in psoriatic nails.

RED SPOT IN LUNULA

Erythematous spots in lunula can also arise due to involvement of intermediate and ventral nail matrices.[14] This is the visible part of the matrix, seen through the nail plate.

LEUKONYCHIA

Psoriatic involvement of intermediate and ventral matrices leads to persistence of parakeratotic foci within the substance of the nail plate, giving it a white appearance (Figure 13.5). According to electron microscopy studies conducted by McGonagle et al., clear vacuoles have been demonstrated in the leukonychic part of the nail; a role of lipid vacuoles is also possible.[11]

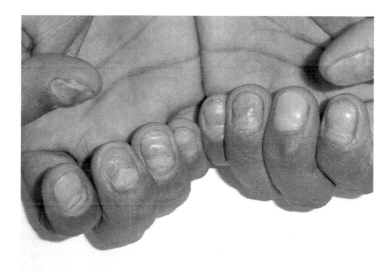

Figure 13.4 Beau's lines in a case with nail psoriasis.

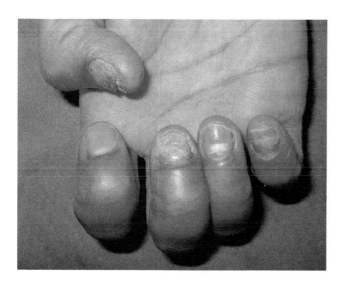

Figure 13.5 Leukonychia involving the ring fingernail in a patient with nail psoriasis.

NAIL PLATE CRUMBLING

Crumbling of the nail plate is a sequel of extensive and prolonged involvement of the entire nail matrix by the disease process (Figure 13.6).[2]

NAIL SPLITTING

Involvement of the distal matrix, where the deeper layers of the nail plate are produced, can lead to splitting of the nail plate structure. This is more commonly seen in lichen planus (LP) than psoriasis.

Nail bed lesions

Involvement of the nail bed with the psoriatic process is less common than the matrix disease. The manifestations include the following:

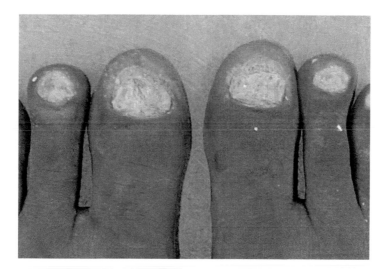

Figure 13.6 Extensive nail disease leads to total dystrophy of nail plate and crumbling.

ONYCHOLYSIS

This is distal separation of the nail plate from the nail bed involving the hyponychium (Figure 13.7). The resultant disruption of the onychocorneal band allows air to enter, giving a whitish opaque appearance to the detached nail plate. Psoriatic onycholysis characteristically has an erythematous border (Figure 13.8).[15] Some studies report it to be the most common psoriatic nail change, with toenails being more commonly affected than fingernails.[16–18]

"OIL SPOT"/"SALMON PATCH"

These represent focal nail bed psoriasis patch characterized by an orange area surrounded by a yellowish-brown margin beneath the paler pink, normal nail plate (Figure 13.9).

NAIL PLATE DISCOLORATION

There are multiple factors contributing to nail plate discoloration in psoriasis. Yellow discoloration commonly occurs due to nail thickening and subungual hyperkeratosis, and it is more common in the toenails (Figure 13.10). Infection is another important cause of discoloration. This can occur with *Candida* spp. as well as *Pseudomonas* invasion (green discoloration). Onychomycosis (OM) can simultaneously involve psoriatic nails, leading to variable color patterns (Figure 13.11).[2]

SUBUNGUAL HYPERKERATOSIS

Impaired desquamation and consequent collection of cells underneath the nail plate are responsible for subungual hyperkeratosis. In psoriasis, this is silvery white and

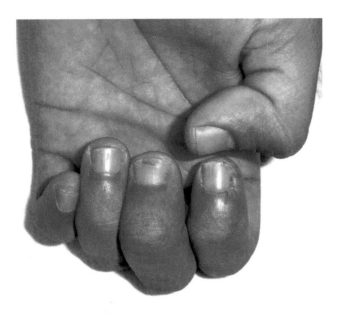

Figure 13.7 Psoriatic onycholysis involving multiple nails.

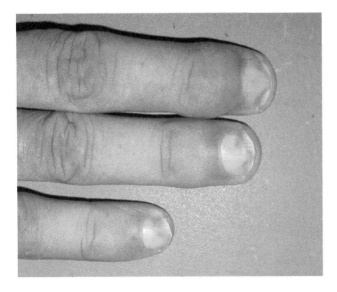

Figure 13.8 Characteristic erythematous border of the distal onycholysis, strongly suggesting psoriasis as a cause.

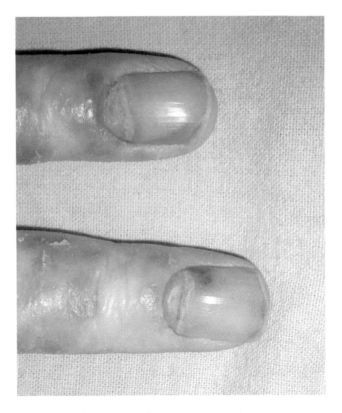

Figure 13.9 Salmon patch seen as an erythematous patch in the nail bed.

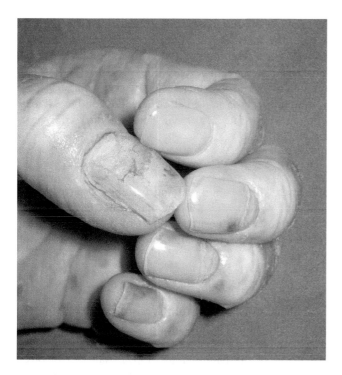

Figure 13.10 Yellow discoloration of multiple nails in psoriasis.

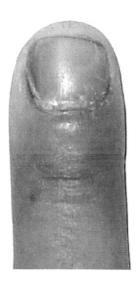

Figure 13.11 Onychomycosis co-existing with psoriasis with characteristic color changes.

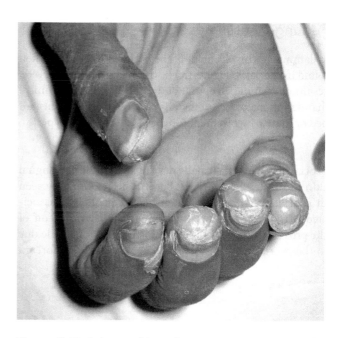

Figure 13.12 Subungual hyperkeratosis in a psoriatic nail.

SPLINTER HEMORRHAGES

These are linearly arranged hemorrhages of the nail bed, usually 2 or 3 mm long, more common at the distal end of the nail (Figure 13.13). They reflect the rupture of delicate capillaries of the nail bed vessels with subsequent tracking of extravasated blood along the longitudinal furrows.[2]

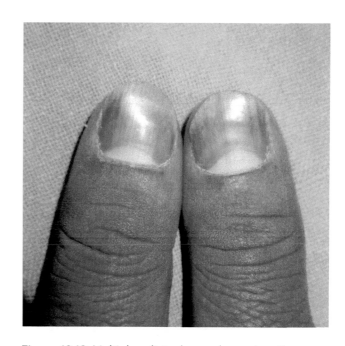

Figure 13.13 Multiple splinter hemorrhages in nail psoriasis.

compact, not easily scraped off, as in OM (Figure 13.12). The subungual hyperkeratosis can lift off the plate so as to cause discomfort or pain during daily activity. It has also been observed to be the most common abnormality in a study.[7]

Periungual tissue psoriasis

Inflammatory involvement of the periungual tissue is often found in psoriasis (Figure 13.14). This may at times be severe, resulting even in disruption of the nail matrix. The clinical manifestations of periungual disease (with or without nail bed or matrix involvement) can be of the following types.

SUBACUTE OR CHRONIC PSORIATIC PARONYCHIA

Psoriatic paronychia usually develops when the periungual skin is affected by psoriasis, but it is also commonly seen in psoriatic arthritis with nail involvement. It is associated with inflammation, thickening, and rounding off of the proximal nail fold, associated with a loss of cuticle due to the psoriatic process (Figure 13.15). This allows foreign material like dirt, microorganisms, or allergenic substances to enter the space beneath the nail fold; the resultant nail plate becoming thin, rough, or irregular. Episodes of acute inflammation may intervene. The proximal and/or lateral nail folds may also be affected by erythematous, scaly plaques of psoriasis as seen elsewhere. Loss of the nail may follow, with scaling of the nail bed or a deep transverse furrow.[2]

ACROPUSTULOSIS

Characterized by subungual and periungual pustules and destructive pustulation of the nail unit (Figure 13.16), acropustulosis may occur as a part of pustular psoriasis, palmoplantar pustulosis, and acrodermatitis continua of Hallopeau.

ACRODERMATITIS CONTINUA OF HALLOPEAU

It is a distinctive form of localized pustular psoriasis involving the nail unit. The pustules first appear on the distal extremities of the phalanges and are more common in the first finger of the hand (Figure 13.17). Nail bed involvement may follow and result in nail dystrophy, anonychia, or osteolysis of the distal phalanx. Resorptive osteolysis of fingers or toes may also occur.[4] The nail plate may be lifted off by sterile pustules in the nail bed and matrix, destroying it completely. Usually, there is erythema and discomfort at digital end.[2,14]

PARAKERATOSIS PUSTULOSA

This is an eczematoid eruption that predominantly affects children. Earlier it was believed to be a manifestation of nail psoriasis. Contrary to the name, pustules are rare and the condition is characterized by scaly patches affecting the skin surrounding the nail plate of the first two fingers and the great toes.[19]

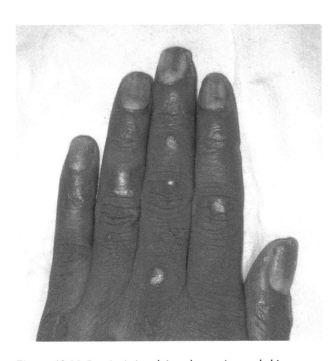

Figure 13.14 Psoriasis involving the periungual skin.

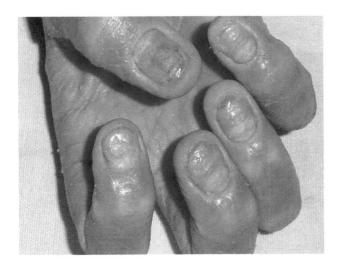

Figure 13.15 Chronic paronychia in a nail psoriasis.

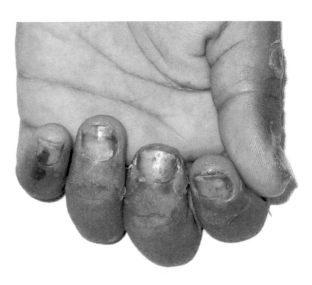

Figure 13.16 Acropustulosis seen as multiple pustular and erosive lesions in a patient with nail psoriasis.

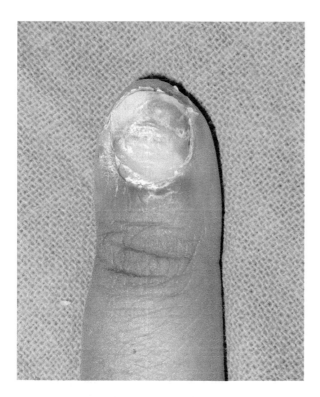

Figure 13.17 Acrodermatitis continua of Hallopeau.

Psoriatic onycho-pachydermo periostitis

It is a lately described rare variant of psoriatic arthritis, characterized by psoriatic onychodystrophy, onycholysis, soft tissue thickening over distal phalanx, and periosteal reaction with absence of DIP involvement.[2] Psoriatic onycho-pachydermo periostitis may involve nails of any finger or toe; however, great toes are involved in most reported literature.[20]

DIFFERENTIAL DIAGNOSIS

Confirming a diagnosis of nail psoriasis purely on clinical grounds can be quite challenging because of numerous overlaps with other nail dystrophies. Common differentials to be considered include:

- **Onychomycosis (OM)**: Some of the nail changes of psoriasis, especially subungual hyperkeratosis and onycholysis, are in common with OM. However, the subungual hyperkeratosis in OM is usually friable in comparison with that of psoriasis (compact hyperkeratosis) and is often accompanied by white/brown/black nail plate discoloration. The important clinical differentiating points between psoriasis and OM have been summarized in Table 13.2. OM and nail psoriasis are also known to co-exist and were reported to be 47% in an Indian study.[4] This highlights the importance of ruling out concomitant fungal infection prior to treatment. The salient features of OM in psoriatic nails have been summarized in Box 13.1.
- **Lichen Planus**: Thinning, onychorrhexis, and crumbling are also seen in LP. However, longitudinal melanonychia, pterygium formation, and subsequent nail loss are characteristics of LP that aid in distinguishing the two.
- **Alopecia areata**: Extensive pitting is frequently seen in alopecia areata, the presence of which can precede the onset of hair loss, thus presenting a diagnostic dilemma. Nonetheless, pitting in alopecia areata is fine and geometric "scotch-plaid" versus the coarse, irregular pitting of psoriasis.
- **Traumatic nail dystrophy**: Isolated onycholysis of the nails is most commonly traumatic or idiopathic in origin. It can be differentiated from psoriasis by the absence of characteristic proximal erythematous border.

Table 13.2 Diagnostic pointers helpful to differentiate between nail psoriasis and onychomycosis

	Nail psoriasis	Onychomycosis
Clinical features	Distal onycholysis with erythematous proximal border	Distal onycholysis without erythematous border. The border may be jagged proximally
	Pitting present	Pitting not found
	Fingernails affected more commonly	Toenails more commonly involved
	Several nails involved	One or a few nails affected
	May be associated with arthritis or cutaneous lesions of psoriasis	May be associated with Tinea corporis or manuum
Investigations	KOH nail and fungal culture mostly negative	KOH and fungal culture may be positive
	Histopathology shows nail bed epithelial hyperplasia and hypergranulosis	No granular layer
	PAS stain will be negative	PAS stain shows fungal elements

Source: Burns, T. et al., *Rook's Textbook of Dermatology*, 8th ed., John Wiley & Sons, Singapore, 23–26, 2010; Dogra, A. and Arora, A.K., *Indian J. Dermatol.*, 59, 319–333, 2014.

BOX 13.1: Onychomycosis (OM) affecting a psoriatic nail—important considerations[21–24]

- Though studies show conflicting data, the prevalence of OM in psoriatic patients appears to be increased when compared with control groups and literature on healthy populations.
- OM appears to be more common in psoriatic nails with morphological changes in nail plate.
- Though there is no conclusive data, candida and non-dermatophyte molds are considered more frequent invading agents as compared to dermatophytes.
- Some studies have documented higher prevalence of dermatophytes in OM of the toenails in psoriatic patients. These studies also reported yeast to be the most common pathogen of OM of the fingernails in these patients.
- Apart from the physical breach due to nail psoriasis, systemic treatment of immunosuppressive drugs like methotrexate and cyclosporine, and anti-TNFα therapy (especially infliximab) are believed to be predisposing factors for OM in psoriatic nails.
- Fungal invasion might aggravate nail psoriasis through Koebner phenomenon. Hence, simultaneous treatment of co-existing OM is desirable.
- Terbinafine has been reported to aggravate psoriasis and, hence, needs to be avoided for treatment of OM in psoriatic patients.
- As mentioned earlier, yeasts and non-dermatophyte molds appear to be more common invading agents, itraconazole is considered preferred antifungal drug. However, response to treatment is poor as compared to the general population.

HISTOPATHOLOGY OF NAIL PSORIASIS

Histopathology of even the normal nail is different from that of skin; correspondingly, nail psoriasis histopathology is also different from that of skin psoriasis. There are further variations according to the clinical focus of involvement within the nail unit. Histopathological features of nail psoriasis similar to those of skin psoriasis include presence of neutrophilic infiltrate, hyperkeratosis with parakeratosis, spongiosis, serum-like exudates within the horny layer, hypogranulosis, epithelial hyperplasia or psoriasiform hyperplasia of nail bed epithelium, and dilated capillaries in the papillary dermis. However, changes distinctive to the nail unit include the finding that nail matrix and bed epithelium (which normally do not have a granular layer) develop a granular layer, whereas the hyponychium, which normally has a granular layer, loses it when involved in psoriasis.[2]

The nail plate structure may show transverse splits and pits, lined with parakeratotic cells originating from the

Table 13.3 Hanno's criteria for histopathological diagnosis of nail psoriasis [a,b]

Major criterion	Minor criteria
The presence of neutrophils in the nail bed epithelium and in adherent parakeratotic fragments of the nail plate.	1. The presence of hyperkeratosis with parakeratosis 2. Serum-like proteinaceous exudates within the horny layer 3. Focal changes in the granular layer 4. Psoriasiform hyperplasia of the nail bed epithelium 5. Dilated sub-epithelial blood vessels

Source: Grover, C. et al., *Br. J. Dermatol.*, 153, 1153–1158, 2005; Hanno, R. et al., *J. Am. Acad. Dermatol.*, 14, 803–809, 1986.
[a] A diagnosis requires the presence of one major or two minor criteria.
[b] PAS negativity is an additional criterion proposed by Grover et al.

most proximal part of the matrix, or the ventral aspect of the proximal nail fold.[2] Wherever the nail plate is lost, the nail bed may form a false nail composed of compacted hyperkeratosis.

Subungual hyperkeratosis is characterized by mounds of parakeratotic keratinocytes beneath the nail plate. Neutrophils infiltrate throughout these mounds, even forming Munro microabscesses.[2,25] Amorphous material (interpreted as glycoproteins) may accumulate within these keratotic masses. Nail bed epidermis develops acanthosis, and elongation of rete ridges are present.[25] This is best interpreted in horizontal sections. There is dilatation and tortuosity of the capillaries in the dermal papillae, another characteristic feature of nail psoriasis. A histopathological diagnosis of nail psoriasis is based on diagnostic criteria proposed by Hanno et al. (Table 13.3).[26]

Several histopathologic findings are shared by OM and psoriasis (including the presence of neutrophil collections and serum crusts); Grover et al. proposed that it is primarily the presence or absence of fungal elements (spores and hyphae) on PAS-stained sections that allow these two to be differentiated; hence, PAS negativity should be an additional diagnostic criteria.[17] However, considering frequent co-existing OM in a psoriatic nail, positive PAS staining does not exclude the diagnosis of nail psoriasis.

INVESTIGATIONS

Diagnosis of nail psoriasis can be made easily in a patient with concomitant skin psoriasis. Close examination with a hand-lens can help appreciate the changes in a greater detail. However, in cases of isolated nail psoriasis (5%–10% of cases) and in patients presenting with a diagnostic conundrum to a dermatologist the use of other diagnostic techniques is mandated. The important diagnostic techniques include the following.

Dermoscopy[4,27]

Dermoscopy of nail (onychoscopy) is a rapid, non-invasive, and inexpensive test that can be used as a diagnostic aid in nail psoriasis. Although it mostly enhances the appearance of already visible features, onychoscopy does bring into focus findings that are otherwise not readily visible, thus helping avoid nail biopsies. Dermoscopic signs of nail psoriasis are as follows:

- Pits – irregular depressions on the nail plate surface with a peripheral whitish halo suggestive of scaling (Figure 13.18)
- Onycholysis – opaque nail plate that is either homogenously white or comprises multiple longitudinal striations. The proximal border of onycholysis is not jagged (unlike OM) and has an erythematous area composed of reddish globules, surrounded by whitish halo (Figure 13.19)

- Salmon patches – irregular reddish to orange areas in the nail bed, which vary in both size and shape (Figure 13.20)
- Splinter hemorrhages- linear red-brown, black, or purplish streaks that run longitudinally (Figure 13.21)
- Blood vessels – dilated tortuous and irregularly distributed capillaries seen in the proximal nail fold, distal nail bed, and hyponychium (Figures 13.22 and 13.23)

Videodermoscopy[4]

Video dermoscopy is a modification of dermoscopy, wherein a video camera with high magnification lenses (10x to 1000x) is used. The main advantage of this technique is that it enables the storage of images on a computer and allows visualization on a screen.

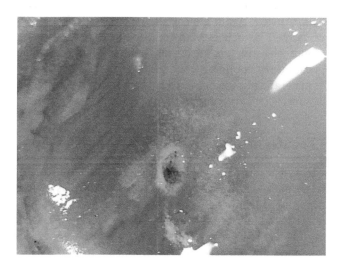

Figure 13.18 Characteristic pit of nail psoriasis as seen on onychoscopy (50x).

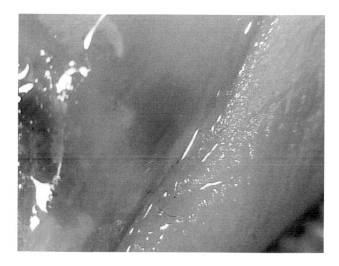

Figure 13.20 Salmon patch visualized in the nail bed (70x).

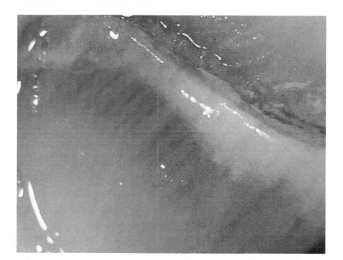

Figure 13.19 Psoriatic onycholysis with characteristic erythematous border (50x).

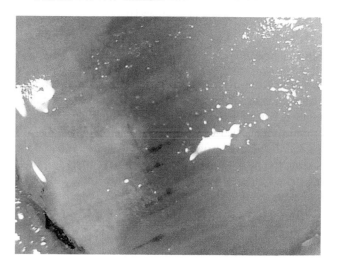

Figure 13.21 Multiple, linear splinter hemorrhages involving the distal part of the nail bed (50x).

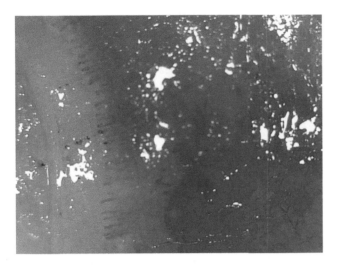

Figure 13.22 Multiple dilated capillaries involving the proximal nail fold with a prominent subpapillary plexus (100x).

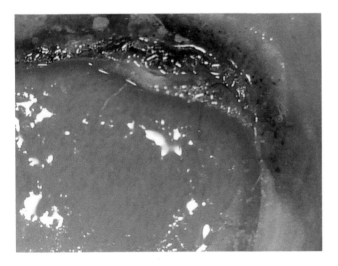

Figure 13.23 Dilated glomerular capillaries involving the hyponychium in a patient with psoriatic onycholysis and compact subungual hyperkeratosis (100x).

Nail biopsy[28,29]

A biopsy from a representative site can show diagnostic histopathological changes. Nail biopsy can then be taken as an excision biopsy or a punch biopsy. Histopathology of nail psoriasis varies according to the site of the disease (as detailed above). Confirmation of diagnosis is based on finding a combination of features that have been proposed in various studies. Hanno's criteria with the addition of PAS stain should help in an unambiguous diagnosis of nail psoriasis.

Capillaroscopy[4]

The capillary density, as observed with periungual capillaroscopy, is decreased in psoriasis patients with psoriasis and even lower in those with nail psoriasis. A vascular area and coiled capillary loops in the nail fold are other features appreciated.

Ultrasound[4]

A high-frequency probe and high-resolution ultrasound machine are required for visualization of the skin and nail unit. In psoriatic onychopathy, nail plate may have loss of definition or hyperechoic parts. In advanced disease, wavy thickened plate morphology may be appreciable. An increased blood flow in the nail bed can be seen with power Doppler technique.

Optical coherence tomography[30,31]

The principle of optical coherence tomography (OCT) is that reflected infrared light intensity varies with the position of the reflecting structures; this is measured and a 3-D image is constructed. Aydin et al recently compared ultrasound versus OCT in nail psoriasis and found OCT to provide a more objective and detailed assessment. Leukonychia appears as regular linear white stripes in the middle third of the plate, and pits were observed to be wavy irregularities in the superficial part of the plate.

ASSESSMENT OF NAIL PSORIASIS

Scoring systems for evaluation of nail psoriasis are essential for both gauging the initial severity of disease as well as the response achieved by various treatments. For cutaneous psoriasis, the Psoriasis Area and Severity Index (PASI) is the most widely accepted system for assessment of severity. It does not, however, cover nail involvement. Thus, the need for a separate system led to the development of several scoring systems. All the indices score the absence or presence of characteristic features of nail psoriasis.[32] Some of the commonly used indices are detailed below and their salient features are tabulated (Table 13.4).

Nail psoriasis severity index (Tables 13.5 and 13.6)

Nail Psoriasis Severity Index (NAPSI), initially described by Rich and Scher, is an objective and reproducible tool for estimating the severity of psoriatic nail involvement. It is the most commonly used index, mainly used to measure the efficacy of therapeutic interventions. NAPSI considers the site affected by the disease process. Assessment of each individual nail needs to be calculated. Of the eight features of nail psoriasis identified for the purpose of NAPSI, four involve the matrix (pitting, leukonychia, red spots in the lunula, nail plate crumbling) and four involve the nail bed (onycholysis, splinter hemorrhages, subungual hyperkeratosis, oil spot/salmon patch).

Table 13.4 Salient features of common nail scoring systems

	NAPSI	Target NAPSI	NAPPA	Baran's	N-Nail
Features scored	Pits, red spot, leuko, crumbling, onycholysis, SHk, Spl hg, oil spot	Same as NAPSI	Same as NAPSI, only four nails assessed	Pits, onycholysis, SHk, Beau's lines	Onycholysis, pits, crumbling, Beau's lines, SHk
Advantage	Used in clinical trials	Only the most severely affected nail scored	Focuses on quality of life	Best reflects clinical severity	Best reflects clinical severity
Disadvantage	Time consuming, leukonychia and red spots in lunula are non-specific for psoriasis	May not be representative of the overall treatment response	Questionnaire based, may not be practical in a clinic setting	Caliper required to measure SHk	Not validated yet

Source: Klaassen, K.M.G. et al., *J. Am. Acad. Dermatol.*, 70, 1061–1066, 2014; Baran, R.L., *Br. J. Dermatol.*, 150, 568–569, 2004. NAPSI—Nail Psoriasis Severity Index; NAPPA—Nail Assessment in Psoriasis and Psoriatic Arthritis; N-Nail—Nijmegen Nail Psoriasis Activity Index tool; SHk—Subungual hyperkeratosis; leuko—leukonychia; spl hge—splinter hemorrhages.

Table 13.5 Features to be recorded in NAPSI

Nail matrix features	Nail bed features
Pitting	Onycholysis
Crumbling	Oil spot/salmon patch
Leukonychia	Subungual hyperkeratosis
Red spot in lunula	Splinter hemorrhage

Source: Rich, P., and Scher, R.K., *J. Am. Acad. Dermatol.*, 49, 206–212, 2003.

Table 13.6 Scoring

Scoring of a single nail[a]	Total score range
0 = absence of findings	Single nail = 0–8
1 = present in 1/4 quadrants	All fingernails = 0–80
2 = present in 2/4 quadrants	All toenails = 0–80
3 = present in 3/4 quadrants	All nails = 0–160
4 = present in 4/4 quadrants	

Source: Rich, P., and Scher, R.K., *J. Am. Acad. Dermatol.*, 49, 206–212, 2003.

[a] Scoring is done for nail matrix and nail bed findings in each quadrant.

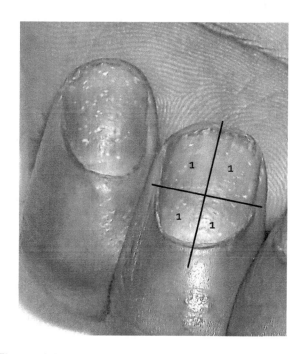

Figure 13.24 How to calculate NAPSI (Nail Area Psoriasis Severity Index).

For the purpose of calculating NAPSI, the nail is divided into four imaginary quadrants, and presence of features of nail matrix or nail bed involvement is assessed in each quadrant (Figure 13.24). The total score ranges from 0 to 8 for each nail and the sum of scores on all nails provides a severity index ranging from 0–80 or 0–160, if the toenails are included.[33]

The NAPSI has been questioned by many authors. van der Velden et al. suggested that leukonychia was present in 65% of the control population and could be therefore a questionable feature of nail psoriasis. NAPSI also does not consider the number of pits or red spots per quadrant, or the size of oil spots or thickness of subungual hyperkeratosis. This limits its utility in assessing improvement with treatment. Nail crumbling gets the same score as a pit, even though it is considerably more severe. Pustular psoriasis and psoriatic arthritis are not given any weightage in NAPSI. Despite its limitations, NAPSI is still the most widely used method to evaluate nail psoriasis.[33]

Modified NAPSI[34] (Table 13.7)

The modified NAPSI (mNAPSI) again involves assessment of four quadrants of a chosen nail, where parameters in each quadrant are assessed separately according to severity (0 = unaffected, 1 = mild, 2 = moderate, and 3 = severe). The overall score for the chosen nail ranges from 0 to 96. Overall, mNAPSI was found to have excellent inter-observer reliability, making it a valuable tool for scoring nail psoriasis.

Target NAPSI[35]

"Target nail" is chosen as the nail most severely affected at baseline. Every feature for this nail is graded, with a maximum possible score of 8 per quadrant and 32 per nail. Throughout the course of the study, this nail is assessed, even though it may no longer remain the most severely affected.

Nail assessment in psoriasis and psoriatic arthritis[36]

The Nail Assessment in Psoriasis and Psoriatic Arthritis (NAPPA) scoring system consists of three parts that holistically assess the severity of nail psoriasis.

1. **NAPPA-QoL** (quality of life) is a questionnaire that assesses a patient's quality of life. The questions focus on the intensity of complaints during the last week and are rated on a 5-point scale (scored 0–4).
2. **NAPPA-PBI** (patient benefit index) is also a patient questionnaire comprised of two parts. The first part is answered before treatment initiation. It is called Patient Needs Questionnaire (PNQ), in which patients rate 24 treatment goals on a 5-option scale. The second includes the same items but is completed by the patients either during or after treatment.
3. **NAPPA-CLIN** (clinical severity) is a brief version of NAPSI that involves assessment of only four digits rather than all 20.

The three-component NAPPA tool is a valid, reliable, and practical instrument to assess patient-relevant nail psoriasis outcomes.

Baran's scoring system[37] (Table 13.8)

Baran devised a numeric system that categorizes clinical features according to the site of the pathology. The clinician is required to grade the severity of each clinical sign and

Table 13.7 Modified NAPSI

Score	Pits	Nail plate crumbling	Onycholysis and/or oil-drop dyschromia[a]
0	None	Absent	Absent
1	1–10	1%–25% of nail	1%–10% of nail
2	11–49	26%–50% of nail	11%–30% of nail
3	≥50	>50% of nail	>30% of nail
		Red spots in lunula	
0 if absent		Nail bed hyperkeratosis	
1 if present		Leukonychia	
		Splinter hemorrhages	

Source: Cassell, S.E. et al., *J. Rheumatol.*, 34, 123–129, 2007.
a Onycholysis and oil spot are calculated together.

Table 13.8 Baran's scoring system

Score	No. of pits	Beau's lines	Subungual hyperkeratosis[a]	Onycholysis (%)[b]
1 (slight)	<10	1 groove	<2	<25
2 (moderate)	10–20	2–3 grooves	2–3	25–50
3 (severe)	>20	>3 grooves	>3	>50

Source: Baran, R.L., *Br. J. Dermatol.*, 150, 568–569, 2004.
a Subungual hyperkeratosis is measured with a caliper.
b Onycholysis, leukonychia, trachyonychia, and oily spots are graded separately in the same manner. The nail is divided into eight equal portions (each portion constitutes 12.5% of the whole nail).

then sum up the final score. Nail signs originating from the proximal matrix (pits, Beau's lines, onychomadesis, and nail loss), intermediate matrix (leukonychia), subungual tissues distal to the lunula (hyperkeratosis, onycholysis, splinter hemorrhages, oil spots), or involving the whole nail unit are considered. However, splinter hemorrhages are excluded from this grading, as are onychomadesis and nail loss.

Cannavo et al.[38]

This scoring system evaluates five signs of fingernail psoriasis viz. onycholysis, pitting, oil spot, hyperkeratosis, and nail plate crumbling. It was initially developed to assess response to treatment with topical cyclosporine. The severity of each feature was graded from 0 (absent) to 3 (severe). Additionally, patients were asked to assess their disease severity, quality of life impairment, and treatment efficacy. This system is qualitative, quick, and practical.

Nijmegen nail psoriasis activity index tool (Table 13.9)[32]

The Nijmegen Nail Psoriasis Activity Index (N-NAIL) tool was recently developed to address the need for a scoring system that adequately reflects disease severity and allows assessment of treatment response. It is a complex scoring system detailed in Table 13.9.

Nail psoriasis quality of life questionnaire-based assessment

Considering the significant impact of nail disease on psychosocial make-up of the patients, an objective and convenient tool in the form of a questionnaire has been developed to evaluate the impact on patients' quality of life. The Nail Psoriasis Quality of Life (NPQ10) assessment, published in 2010, contains 10 items that assess the location of nail lesions, the degree of pain, and the frequency with which it leads to irritability, negative moods, and difficulty in performing daily tasks, such as putting on shoes, getting dressed, driving, and conducting domestic activities.[39]

TREATMENT OF NAIL PSORIASIS

Nail disfigurement in psoriasis is a significant source of pain and social embarrassment for the affected patients. A vast majority of psoriasis patients with nail involvement (90%) find the cosmetic appearance of their nails distressing, forcing them to hide their hands or shy away from social or business interactions.[40] Moreover, it leads to impairment of daily activities like nail-trimming problems, discomfort wearing shoes, ability to pick up small objects, etc., thus adversely affecting household chores as well as employment. De Jong reported that 93% of patients consider nail psoriasis as a major cosmetic issue, 51.8% report pain during daily activities, and 48% experience occupation-related problems. Overall, treatment is rated as disappointing with only 19.3% showing marked improvement post-treatment.[41] Also, it takes a long time, sometimes 4–6 months, to show appreciable clinical improvement.

Prior to commencing therapy, thorough patient counseling and education is required. The possibility of disease recurrence and need for prolonged treatment must be emphasized. General measures that would benefit patients are presented in Table 13.10. The treatment of nail psoriasis is considered challenging and there are several topical, oral, and injectable medications available for its management (Table 13.11). In 2015, best practice recommendations were proposed by the National Psoriasis Foundation for

Table 13.9 N-NAIL score

Feature	Score[a]			
	0	1	2	3
Oil spot/onycholysis	Absent	0%–25%	25%–50%	>50%
Pitting	Absent	Mild	Moderate	Severe
Crumbling	Absent	Mild	Moderate	Severe
Beau's lines	Absent	1 line	2 lines	3 lines
Subungual hyperkeratosis	Absent	1 mm	2 mm	≥3 mm

Source: Klaassen, K.M.G. et al., J. Am. Acad. Dermatol., 70, 1061–1066, 2014.
[a] All 10 fingernails are scored for all five features; End score is the sum of all 10 nails. The higher the score, the more severe the nail psoriasis.

Table 13.10 General measures for all patients with nail psoriasis

Measure taken	Benefit
Nails should be kept short	Prevents exacerbation of onycholysis
Avoidance of manicures/pedicures/excessive trauma	Prevention of disease exacerbation by trauma induced Koebner phenomenon
Generous use of emollients	Protects cuticle
Avoidance of contact with irritants, like detergents	Prevents paronychia, exacerbation of onycholysis

Source: Dogra, A. and Arora, A.K., Indian J. Dermatol., 59, 319–333, 2014.

Table 13.11 Treatment options for nail psoriasis

Topical	Systemic	Intralesional	Physical
Clobetasol 0.05%, 1%, 8% nail lacquer	Methotrexate	Triamcinolone acetonide 0.1% 5 mg/mL	595 nm pulse dye laser
Calcipotriol ointment 50 μg/g	Cyclosporine	Methotrexate 2.5 mg (nail bed or proximal nail fold)	Photodynamic therapy
Combination of calcipotriol and betamethasone ointment	Acitretin		Grenz rays
Tazarotene 0.1% gel	Apremilast		Electron beam
Tacrolimus 0.1% ointment	TNF alpha inhibitors (adalimumab, infliximab, golimumab)		Superficial radiotherapy
CsA[a] 70% in maize oil	IL-12/23 inhibitors (Ustekinumab)		
Apremilast nail lacquer	IL-17 inhibitors (Secukinumab, Ixekizumab)		
Hyaluronic acid and chondroitin sulphates	Tofacitinib (phase III trial)		
Anthralin (0.4% initially, increased to 2%)			
5-Fluorouracil cream 1%			
Indigo naturalis 0.1–0.2 mg/mL			

Source: Crowley, J.J. et al., *JAMA Dermatol.*, 151, 87, 2015; de Vries, A.C.Q. et al., Interventions for nail psoriasis, in Spuls, P.I. (Ed.)., *Cochrane Database of Systematic Reviews*, John Wiley & Sons, Chichester, UK, p. CD007633, 2013; Grover, C. et al., *Clin. Exp. Dermatol.*, 42, 420–423, 2017; Arango-Duque, L.C. et al., *Actas Dermosifiliogr*, 108, 140–144, 2017; Kushwaha, A.S. et al., *AAPS PharmSciTech*, 18, 2949–2956, 2017; Merola, J.F. et al., *J. Am. Acad. Dermatol.*, 77, 79–87, 2017; Grover, C. et al., *J. Dermatol.*, 32, 963–968, 2005; Pasch, M.C., *Drugs*, 76, 675–705, 2016.

[a] CsA: Cyclosporine A.

nail psoriasis in four clinical scenarios[42] (Table 13.12). The safety of the chosen drugs in special situations like pregnancy, children, lactation, elderly age groups, etc. needs to be decided on a case-to-case basis.

There is evidence of differential effects of treatments on nail disease manifestations depending on the component of the nail unit involved. Methotrexate was found comparatively more efficacious in improving matrix disease whereas systemic cyclosporine (CsA) improved bed disease more effectively.[42]

Nail matrix: For nail matrix pathology, topical preparations need to be applied over the proximal nail fold. **Pitting** was most responsive to topical CsA, followed by tazarotene, clobetasol, hyaluronic acid with chondroitin sulphate, and infliximab. **Crumbling** of nail plate improved with topical cyclosporine and infliximab, whereas there was no change with tazarotene and worsening with topical calcipotriol. **Red spots** in lunula were completely cleared by infliximab but unaffected by calcipotriol. Clearance of **leukonychia** was seen with infliximab, whereas both tazarotene and calcipotriol failed to show improvement in this feature.[43]

Nail bed: For nail bed disease, topical preparations can be applied over nail plate (lacquer form) or hyponychium and lateral nail fold area. Careful clipping of onycholytic nail allows better access to the diseased area. **Onycholysis** is reported to improve with topical CsA, hyaluronic acid with chondroitin sulphate, tazarotene, clobetasol, and infliximab, while topical calcipotriol is reported to not produce any change. **Subungual hyperkeratosis** responds to topical CsA, infliximab, tazarotene, clobetasol, 5-fluorouracil, calcipotriol, betamethasone-salicylic acid combination, and hyaluronic acid with chondroitin sulphate. **Splinter hemorrhages** have been seen to be responsive to infliximab.

Table 13.12 Evidence-based treatment recommendations for nail psoriasis

Clinical scenario	Recommended treatment
Isolated nail psoriasis • 3 out of 10 nails • Onycholysis, distal hyperkeratosis, pitting • Treatment naïve	1. Topical high-potency corticosteroids 2. Combination of topical calcipotriol with high potency corticosteroids 3. Intralesional corticosteroids
Nail psoriasis refractory to topical therapy • 5 out of 10 nails involved • Moderate to severe pain	1. Adalimumab 2. Etanercept 3. Intralesional corticosteroids 4. Ustekinumab 5. Methotrexate 6. Acitretin (In descending order of preference)
Psoriasis of skin and nails • >8% BSA[a] involved • 5 out of 10 nails with severe nail dystrophy • Moderate to severe pain	1. Adalimumab 2. Etanercept 3. Ustekinumab 4. Methotrexate 5. Acitretin 6. Infliximab 7. Apremilast
Psoriasis affecting skin, nails, joints • Psoriatic arthritis • >8% BSA[a] involved • 5 out of 10 nails with severe nail dystrophy	1. Adalimumab 2. Etanercept 3. Ustekinumab 4. Infliximab 5. Methotrexate 6. Apremilast 7. Golimumab (In descending order of preference)

Source: Crowley, J.J. et al., JAMA Dermatol., 151, 87, 2015.
[a] BSA: Body surface area.

Salmon patches/oil drops have been shown to clear with tazarotene, clobetasol, infliximab, CsA, 5-fluorouracil, and calcipotriol with/without betamethasone.[43]

A recent Cochrane review concluded that the most effective treatments for nail psoriasis were infliximab, golimumab, superficial radiotherapy, electron beam, and grenz rays; however, as these modalities may cause serious adverse effects they are not used unless the patient has concomitant extensive cutaneous psoriasis or arthritis or a major decline in daily activity or psychosocial well-being.[43]

CONCLUSION

Nail psoriasis is a major cause of disfigured nails. Considering the high prevalence of nail involvement in psoriatics, the number of patients diagnosed is high. The disease is more than a cosmetic disfigurement as it points towards a possible underlying enthesitis and psoriatic arthritis. Nail psoriasis presents with myriad manifestations, making it a confusing diagnosis at times. The use of onychoscopy and nail histopathology can help confirm the diagnosis.

Just as the clinical manifestations are numerous, so are the treatment options available. The challenge lies in being able to individualize treatment options depending on various patient-specific, disease-specific, and nail-specific considerations.

REFERENCES

1. Kurd SK, Gelfand JM. The prevalence of previously diagnosed and undiagnosed psoriasis in US adults: Results from NHANES 2003-2004. *J Am Acad Dermatol* 2009;60(2):218–224.
2. Burns T, Breathnach S, Cox N, Griffiths C. *Rook's Textbook of Dermatology*, 8th ed. Singapore: John Wiley & Sons; 2010. pp. 23–26.
3. Jiaravuthisan MM, Sasseville D, Vender RB, Murphy F, Muhn CY. Psoriasis of the nail: Anatomy, pathology, clinical presentation, and a review of the literature on therapy. *J Am Acad Dermatol* 2007;57:1–27.

4. Dogra A, Arora AK. Nail psoriasis: The journey so far. *Indian J Dermatol* 2014;59(4):319–333.

5. Tan EST, Chong WS, Tey HL. Nail psoriasis: A review. *Am J Clin Dermatol* 2012;13(6):375–388.

6. Langenbruch A, Radtke MA, Krensel M, Jacobi A, Reich MAK. Nail involvement as a predictor of concomitant psoriatic arthritis in patients with psoriasis. *Br J Dermatol* 2014;171(5):1123–1128.

7. Salomon J, Szepietowski JC, Proniewicz A. Psoriatic nails: A prospective clinical study. *J Cutan Med Surg* 2003;7:317–321.

8. Lowes MA, Suárez-Fariñas M, Krueger JG. Immunology of psoriasis. *Annu Rev Immunol* 2014;32:227–255.

9. Krueger JG, Bowcock A. Psoriasis pathophysiology: Current concepts of pathogenesis. *Ann Rheum Dis* 2005;64(Suppl 2):ii30–i36.

10. Mudigonda P, Mudigonda T, Feneran AN, Alamdari HS, Sandoval L, Feldman SR. Interleukin-23 and interleukin-17: Importance in pathogenesis and therapy of psoriasis. *Dermatol Online J* 2012;18(10):1.

11. McGonagle D, Palmou Fontana N, Tan AL, Benjamin M. Nailing down the genetic and immunological basis for psoriatic disease. *Dermatology* 2010;221(suppl 1):15–22.

12. McGonagle D, Tan AL, Benjamin M. The nail as a musculoskeletal appendage–Implications for an improved understanding of the link between psoriasis and arthritis. *Dermatology* 2009;218(2):97–102.

13. Zaias N. Psoriasis of the nail. A clinical-pathologic study. *Arch Dermatol* 1969;99(5):567–579.

14. Schons KRR, Knob CF, Murussi N, Beber AAC, Neumaier W, Monticielo OA. Nail psoriasis: A review of the literature. *An Bras Dermatol* 2014;89:312–317.

15. Bolognia JL, Jorizzo JL, Schaffer JV. *Dermatology*, 3rd ed. Beijing, China: Elsevier Saunders; 2012. pp. 1136–1137.

16. Brazzelli V, Carugno A, Alborghetti A, Grasso V, Cananzi R, Fornara L et al. Prevalence, severity and clinical features of psoriasis in fingernails and toenails in adult patients: Italian experience. *J Eur Acad Dermatol Venereol* 2012;26(11):1354–1359.

17. Grover C, Reddy BSN, Chaturvedi KU. Diagnosis of nail psoriasis: Importance of biopsy and histopathology. *Br J Dermatol* 2005;153:1153–1158.

18. Van der Velden HMJ, Klaassen KMG, Van de Kerkhof PCM, Pasch MC. Fingernail psoriasis reconsidered: A case-control study. *J Am Acad Dermatol* 2013;69(2):245–252.

19. Pandhi D, Chowdhry S, Grover C, Reddy BS. Parakeratosis pustulosa: A distinct but less familiar disease. *Indian J Dermatol Venereol Leprol* 2003;69(1):48–50.

20. Vasudevan B, Verma R, Pragasam V, Dabbas D. Unilateral psoriatic onychopachydermo-periostitis. *Indian J Dermatol Venereol Leprol* 2012;78(4):499–501.

21. Klaassen KM, Dulak MG, van de Kerkhof PC, Pasch MC. The prevalence of onychomycosis in psoriatic patients: A systematic review. *J Eur Acad Dermatol Venereol* 2014;28(5):533–541.

22. Rigopoulos D, Papanagiotou V, Daniel R 3rd, Piraccini BM. Onychomycosis in patients with nail psoriasis: A point to point discussion. *Mycoses* 2017;60(1):6–10.

23. Zisova L, Valtchev V, Sotiriou E, Gospodinov D, Mateev G. Onychomycosis in patients with psoriasis—A multicentre study. *Mycoses* 2012;55(2):143–147.

24. Shemer A, Trau H, Davidovici B, Grunwald MH, Amichai B. Onychomycosis in psoriatic patients—Rationalization of systemic treatment. *Mycoses* 2010;53(4):340–343.

25. Elder DE. *Lever's Histopathology of the Skin*, 10th ed. Beijing, China: Wolters Kluwer; 2009. pp. 3070–3086.

26. Hanno R, Mathes BM, Krull EA. Longitudinal nail biopsy in evaluation of acquired nail dystrophies. *J Am Acad Dermatol* 1986;14:803–809.

27. Grover C, Jakhar D. Onychoscopy: A practical guide. *Indian J Dermatol Venereol Leprol* 2017;83(5):536.

28. Grover C, Nanda S, Reddy BSN, Chaturvedi KU. Nail biopsy: Assessment of indications and outcome. *Dermatol Surg* 2005;31(2):190–194.

29. Grover C, Reddy BS, Chaturvedi U. Role of nail biopsy as a diagnostic tool. *Indian J Dermatol Venereol Leprol* 2012;78(3):290.

30. Aydin SZ, Ash Z, Del Galdo F, Marzo-Ortega H, Wakefield RJ, Emery P et al. Optical coherence tomography: A new tool to assess nail disease in psoriasis? *Dermatology* 2011;222(4):311–313.

31. Aydin SZ, Castillo-Gallego C, Ash ZR, Abignano G, Marzo-Ortega H, Wittmann M et al. Potential use of optical coherence tomography and high-frequency ultrasound for the assessment of nail disease in psoriasis and psoriatic arthritis. *Dermatology* 2013;227(1):45–51.

32. Klaassen KMG, Van de Kerkhof PCM, Bastiaens MT, Plusjé LGJM, Baran RL, Pasch MC. Scoring nail psoriasis. *J Am Acad Dermatol* 2014;70(6):1061–1066.

33. Rich P, Scher RK. Nail psoriasis severity index: A useful tool for evaluation of nail psoriasis. *J Am Acad Dermatol* 2003;49:206–212.

34. Cassell SE, Bieber JD, Rich P, Tutuncu ZN, Lee SJ, Kalunian KC et al. The modified Nail Psoriasis Severity Index: Validation of an instrument to assess psoriatic nail involvement in patients with psoriatic arthritis. *J Rheumatol* 2007;34(1):123–129.

35. Parrish CA, Sobera JO, Elewski BE. Modification of the nail psoriasis severity index. *J Am Acad Dermatol* 2005;53(4):745–746.

36. Augustin M, Blome C, Costanzo A, Dauden E, Ferrandiz C, Girolomoni G et al. Nail Assessment in Psoriasis and Psoriatic Arthritis (NAPPA):

Development and validation of a tool for assessment of nail psoriasis outcomes. *Br J Dermatol* 2014;170(3):591–598.

37. Baran RL. A nail psoriasis severity index. *Br J Dermatol* 2004;150(3):568–569.

38. Cannavò SP, Guarneri F, Vaccaro M, Borgia F, Guarneri B. Treatment of psoriatic nails with topical cyclosporin: A prospective, randomized placebo-controlled study. *Dermatology* 2003;206(2):153–156.

39. Ortonne JP, Baran R, Corvest M, Schmitt C, Voisard JJ, Taieb C. Development and validation of nail psoriasis quality of life scale (NPQ10). *J Eur Acad Dermatology Venereol* 2010;24:22–27.

40. Baran R. The burden of nail psoriasis: An introduction. *Dermatology* 2010;221(suppl 1):1–5.

41. de Jong EM, Seegers BA, Gulinck MK, Boezeman JB, van de Kerkhof PC. Psoriasis of the nails associated with disability in a large number of patients: Results of a recent interview with 1,728 patients. *Dermatology* 1996;193(4):300–303.

42. Crowley JJ, Weinberg JM, Wu JJ, Robertson AD, Van Voorhees AS. National psoriasis foundation. Treatment of nail psoriasis. *JAMA Dermatol* 2015;151(1):87.

43. de Vries ACQ, Bogaards NA, Hooft L, Velema M, Pasch M, Lebwohl M et al. Interventions for nail psoriasis. In: Spuls PI (Ed.). *Cochrane Database of Systematic Reviews*. Chichester, UK: John Wiley & Sons; 2013. p. CD007633.

44. Grover C, Daulatabad D, Singal A. Role of nail bed methotrexate injections in isolated nail psoriasis: Conventional drug via an unconventional route. *Clin Exp Dermatol* 2017;42(4):420–423.

45. Arango-Duque LC, Roncero-Riesco M, Usero Bárcena T, Palacios Álvarez I, Fernández López E. Treatment of nail psoriasis with Pulse Dye Laser plus calcipotriol betametasona gel vs. Nd: YAG plus calcipotriol betamethasone gel: An intrapatient left-to-right controlled study. *Actas Dermosifiliogr* 2017;108(2):140–144.

46. Kushwaha AS, Repka MA, Narasimha Murthy S. A novel apremilast nail lacquer formulation for the treatment of nail psoriasis. *AAPS PharmSciTech* 2017;18(8):2949–2956.

47. Merola JF, Elewski B, Tatulych S, Lan S, Tallman A, Kaur M. Efficacy of tofacitinib for the treatment of nail psoriasis: Two 52-week, randomized, controlled phase 3 studies in patients with moderate-to-severe plaque psoriasis. *J Am Acad Dermatol* 2017;77(1):79–87.

48. Grover C, Bansal S, Nanda S, Reddy BS. Efficacy of triamcinolone acetonide in various acquired nail dystrophies. *J Dermatol* 2005;32(12):963–968.

49. Pasch MC. Nail psoriasis: A review of treatment options. *Drugs* 2016;76(6):675–705.

14

Nail lichen planus

IFFAT HASSAN, MOHAMMAD ABID KEEN, AND YASMEEN JABEEN BHAT

INTRODUCTION

Lichen planus (LP) is an inflammatory dermatitis of idiopathic origin that can involve the skin, mucous membranes, hair, and nails. Nail lichen planus (NLP) usually presents in association with cutaneous, mucosal, or scalp lesions but may be the sole manifestation of the disease. It may involve the nail matrix, proximal and lateral nail folds, nail bed, and/or the hyponychium. Nail signs of LP may not be pathognomonic since similar changes may be caused by traumatic or other inflammatory dermatoses.

EPIDEMIOLOGY

Nail involvement may occur in 1%–10% cases of LP, mostly in the setting of widespread cutaneous disease.[1] NLP may occur at any age, but is most common in the fifth and sixth decades. In one of the studies, about 50% of the patients with NLP were between 50 and 70 years of age.[2] Tosti et al.[3] reported that 11% of patients with NLP were children and postulated that NLP in children is underestimated due to lack of skin and mucosal lesions, which makes clinical diagnosis difficult. Likewise, Kanwar and De suggested that the general hesitation of dermatologists to perform nail biopsies on children may be another reason for underdiagnosis of the disease in this age group.[4] Fingernails are more commonly involved than toenails.[5]

ETIOPATHOGENESIS (BOX 14.1)

The etiology and pathogenesis of NLP remain unclear. An autoimmune reaction in which CD8+T lymphocytes attack

---

BOX 14.1: Etiopathogenesis: Salient points

- T-cell-mediated autoimmune disease
- Involvement of T helper and T cytotoxic lymphocytes, natural killer (NK) cells, and dendritic cells
- T-cell activation central to the pathogenesis of LP
- Cytotoxic T-cell infiltration into the epithelium result in apoptotic basal keratinocytes
- Role of CXCR3- and CCR5-mediated signaling pathways

---

basal keratinocytes leading to apoptosis of the cells has been favored. Various potential triggers, e.g., viral or bacterial antigens, metal ions, drugs, or physical factors, could initiate the autoimmune process.[6] Nonetheless, the role of the individual trigger factors is controversial.

CLINICAL FEATURES

NLP can present with very diverse morphological patterns and is characterized by thinning, longitudinal ridging, and distal splitting of the nail plate[7] (Figure 14.1) (Box 14.2). Although mild NLP is usually asymptomatic, deformation of the fingernails is cosmetically distressing. Failure to treat NLP results in nail loss or permanent nail dystrophy in some cases. Therefore, the condition should be treated effectively in its early stage.

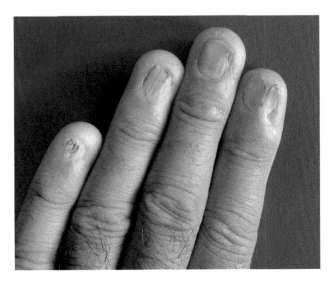

Figure 14.1 Thinning, longitudinal ridging, and distal splitting of the nail plate.

Table 14.1 Nail changes as per nail component involvement

Nail component involvement	Resultant changes
Nail matrix involvement	• Longitudinal ridging • Trachyonychia • Pterygium • Irregular nail pitting • Onychorrhexis • Crumbling • Fragmentation of the nail plate
Nail bed involvement	• Violaceous lines or papules visible through nail plate • Subungual hyperkeratosis • Onycholysis
Nail fold changes	• Lateral pterygium (hypertrophic lesions involving proximal and lateral nail folds)
Hyponychial changes	• Subungual tumorous keratotic growth (onychopapilloma)

BOX 14.2: Clinical patterns of NLP

- Thinning of the nail plates
- Longitudinal ridging
- Pterygium unguis
- Trachyonychia
- Onycholysis
- Onychorrhexis
- Koilonychia
- Subungual hyperkeratosis
- Chromonychia
- Onychomadesis

A myriad of nail changes can be observed depending on the site and severity of involvement of different components of nail (Table 14.1). These can be classified into:

1. Nail matrix involvement
2. Nail bed involvement
3. Nail fold changes
4. Hyponychial changes

Characteristic nail lesions of LP include dorsal pterygium and trachyonychia. An early change in the existing nail plate is the "pup tent" (Figure 14.2) appearance of the distal normal nail plate where the nail plate separates from the nail bed and is lifted up, with the lateral edges sloping when the nail is seen end-on. A pterygium (Figure 14.3) develops through adhesion of eponychium and matrix leading first to a split nail and later to possible complete loss of the nail plate. Trachyonychia is characterized by marked roughness of the nail plate, loss of transparency, and often by a gray discoloration. If the destruction of nail matrix

is very extensive, along with the involvement of nail bed and the cuticle, there is a permanent and total loss of the nail plate, which is replaced by scar tissue (onychoatrophy) (Figures 14.4 and 14.5). Furthermore, erosive NLP may rarely occur with painful erosions and consequent scarring. Less frequent signs of NLP described by Tosti et al[8,9] include erythematous patches of the lunula, melanonychia, splinter hemorrhages, koilonychia, and yellow nail syndrome-like changes.

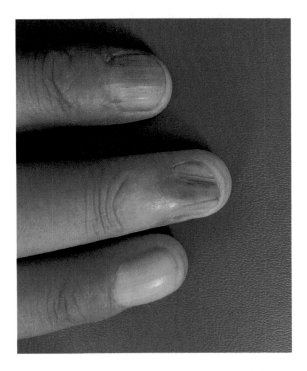

Figure 14.2 Pup tent sign in a patient with nail lichen planus.

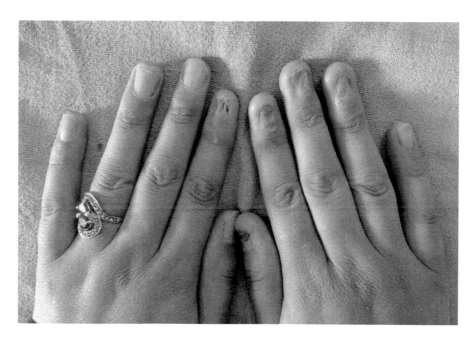

Figure 14.3 Nail lichen planus with pterygium formation.

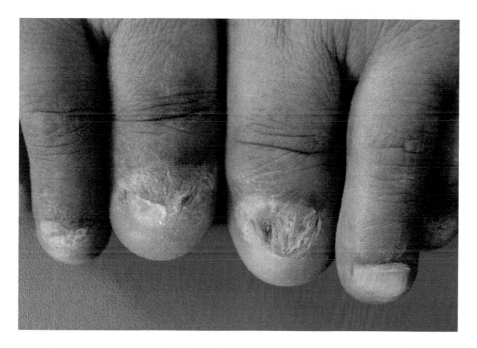

Figure 14.4 Onychoatrophy in a patient with nail lichen planus.

Nail lesions can precede the appearance of LP on the rest of the skin or on the mucous membranes or develop in a delayed fashion. Different nails in the same individual may show different morphologic changes and with varying degrees of severity.

Trachyonychia and twenty-nail dystrophy

Trachyonychia is characterized by brittle, thin nails, with excessive longitudinal ridging. It is histologically characterized by spongiosis and exocytosis of inflammatory cells into the nail epithelia; typical features of LP or psoriasis can also be detected. The term "twenty-nail dystrophy" (TND) is used to describe trachyonychia involving all twenty nails.[10,11] Nails become lusterless with diffuse ridging and in severe cases develop a sand paper-like surface.[12] Trachyonychia may be idiopathic or may be associated with various cutaneous or systemic disorders such as alopecia areata,[13] vitiligo,[14] or atopic dermatitis.[15] Trachyonychia is seen in 10% of patients affected by NLP in which NLP is most often isolated.[16] A 51-year-old man with TND produced by LP with positive reaction to nickel and gold on

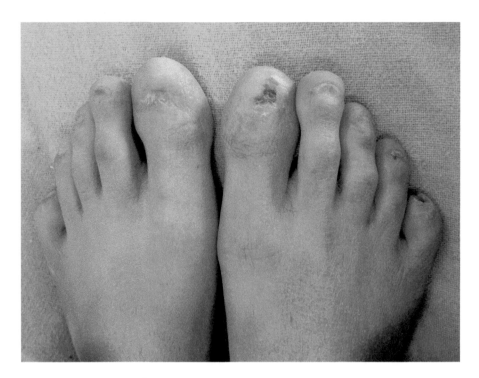

Figure 14.5 Onychoatrophy in nail lichen planus.

patch testing has been reported.[17] Since trachyonychia is a disease of the nail matrix, a nail matrix punch or a longitudinal nail biopsy is required for a pathological diagnosis.[18] The histopathologic features associated with trachyonychia include spongiosis and exocytosis of the inflammatory cells into the nail epithelia. Typical histopathological findings of psoriasis or LP might be seen in trachyonychia caused by these disorders.[18]

DIFFERENTIAL DIAGNOSIS OF NAIL LICHEN PLANUS

When nail changes occur in a patient with LP of the skin, the diagnosis of NLP becomes relatively easy. However, when the disease is limited to the nails, accurate diagnosis might be difficult. Furthermore, LP can lead to permanent scarring, so early diagnosis becomes very crucial. Features differentiating NLP from other conditions are tabulated in Table 14.2.

DIAGNOSIS

NLP can be diagnosed by clinical examination, nail dermatoscopy (onychoscopy), and biopsy for histopathological examination.

Onychoscopy

Histopathology in many occasions is not enough to come to a conclusive diagnosis. Dermatoscopy, a complementary tool, has proven to be useful in its diagnosis, management, and prognosis. Early manifestations seen on dermoscopy include pitting of the nail matrix and trachyonychia,

Table 14.2 Differential diagnosis of nail lichen planus

Nail psoriasis	• Irregular and deeper pits • Pits are variable in depth and shape • Accompanying skin lesion • Histopathology can establish the diagnosis
Trachyonychia	• Lusterless nails • Histology may differentiate it from nail lichen planus
Yellow nail syndrome	• Rough, thickened nails, with dark yellow discoloration • Over-curvature of nails, slow growth • Associated pleural effusion and/or bronchiectasis
Systemic amyloidosis	• Uniformly thinned, brittle nails • Longitudinal ridging (onychorrhexis) with distal split
Other conditions	• Dystrophy and onychoatrophy following SJS, sequel of severe bacterial infection or trauma to nail matrix, genetic causes, peripheral vascular impairment, aging and radiodermatitis

while advanced disease often shows chromonychia, lamina fragmentation, onycholysis, and splinter hemorrhage[19] (Figures 14.6 through 14.8). Dermoscopy of the dorsal pterygium (Figures 14.9 and 14.10) shows that it is formed by skin and continues with the skin of the proximal nail fold. The color is pink-red with elongated capillaries in early lesions, while it is white in longstanding lesions, due to

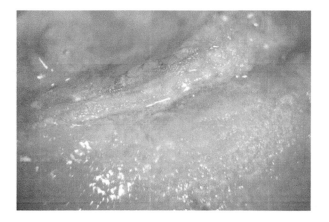

Figure 14.6 Dermoscopy showing nail plate thinning and subungual hyperkeratosis with no capillary changes in hyponychium, unlike psoriasis.

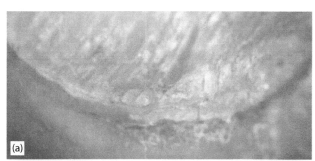

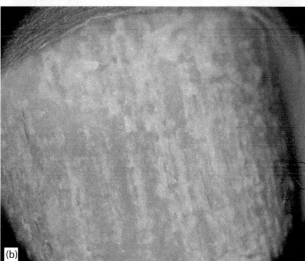

Figure 14.7 (a) Longitudinal fissures, fragmentation, fragility, and thinning of nail plate on dermoscopy. (b) Nail plate thinning and longitudinal ridging on dermoscopy (courtesy of Prof. Archana Singal)

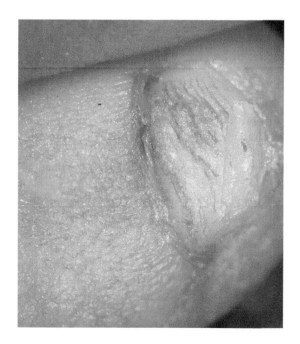

Figure 14.8 Rough nail plate, transverse ridging on dermoscopy.

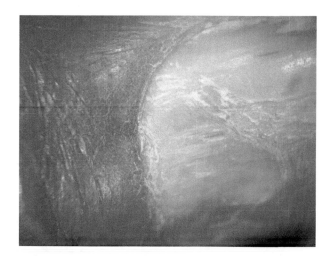

Figure 14.9 Dermoscopy showing early pterygium.

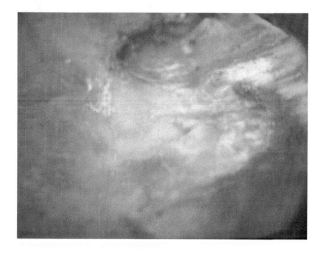

Figure 14.10 Dermoscopy showing late pterygium.

BOX 14.3: Dermoscopy of nail lichen planus: Salient features

- Early manifestations include pitting of the nail matrix and trachyonychia.
- Advanced disease shows chromonychia, lamina fragmentation, onycholysis, and splinter hemorrhage.
- Trachyonychia reveals nail plate showing multiple fine and superficial longitudinal fissures.
- It is also useful for the follow-up of cases.

fibrosis.[20] Onychoscopy in trachyonychia reveals nail plate showing multiple fine and superficial longitudinal fissures covered by thin scales.[20] Not much work has been done on onychoscopy of NLP. Dermoscopic features of NLP in various studies are tabulated in Box 14.3.

Dermoscopy is useful for the follow up of NLP, as it allows observation of the proximal nail plate, where LP emerges from the nail fold; it shows the regrowing nail plate and permits evaluating the response to therapy at an early stage.[20] Dermoscopic features of NLP have been tabulated in Table 14.3.

Histopathology

LP in the nail shares many histologic features with its counterpart in LP of the skin: hyperkeratosis, hypergranulosis, irregular epidermal hyperplasia, a lichenoid infiltrate with the formation of Civatte bodies, vacuolar degeneration of the basement membrane, and pigmentary incontinence (Figures 14.11a–c). However, the nail can present certain additional features, such as parakeratosis and serous exudates. Besides, lymphocytes predominate in the infiltrate with a few macrophages, eosinophils, and plasma cells. An infiltrate primarily of plasma cells has been described.[22] Salient histopathogical features of NLP are tabulated in Table 14.4.

Table 14.3 Dermoscopic pattern of nail lichen planus in various studies

Nakamura R et al.[19]	Dermatoscopic photographic data of 11 patients having 79 nails affected with nail lichen planus were analyzed. Nail matrix features seen were trachyonychia (in 40.6% cases), pitting (34.2%), pterygium (21.5%), and red lunula (3.8%). Nail bed features highlighted were chromonychia (55.7% cases), nail fragmentation (50.6%), splinter hemorrhages (35.4%), onycholysis (27.8%), and subungual keratosis (7.5%). It was concluded that nail bed features and converging longitudinal streaks are suggestive of aggressive characteristics, indicating a poor prognosis and possibly a poor response to therapy.[18]
Friedman et al.[21]	The authors reported chromonychia, subungual hyperkeratosis, and onycholysis and nail plate destruction as being the onychoscopic features of nail lichen planus.

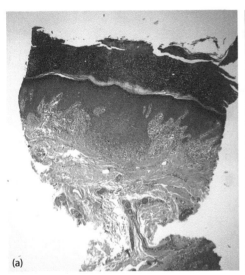
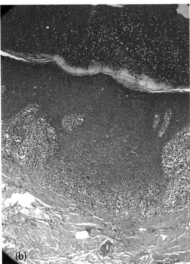
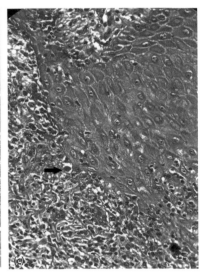

Figure 14.11 (a) Acanthosis, focal hypergranulosis, and band-like infiltration in the upper dermis (H&E x 40). (Courtesy of Dr. Piyush Kumar.) (b) Extensive basal layer damage, lymphocytic exocytosis and lymphohistiocytic infiltration obscuring the dermoepidermal junction (H&E x 100). (Courtesy of Dr. Piyush Kumar.) (c) Higher magnification. Note Civatte body (arrow) (H&E x 400). (Courtesy of Dr. Piyush Kumar.)

Table 14.4 Histopathological features of nail lichen planus

Nail unit	Histopathological feature
Nail plate	• Compact orthokeratosis, focal parakeratosis, serum crusts
Nail bed epithelium	• Diffuse hypergranulosis, colloid bodies (rare), saw tooth acanthosis, eosinophilia of keratinocytes
Nail matrix	• Similar changes as seen in nail bed epithelium
Hyponychium	• May have hyperkeratosis
Nail matrix and bed dermis	• Lichenoid infiltrate, marked fibrosis in papillary and reticular dermis

TREATMENT

Treatment of NLP is difficult and disappointing. Treatment depends on the stage and severity of nail damage (Table 14.5). Topical corticosteroid therapy is commonly considered as a first-line treatment for NLP, although it is usually ineffective. If more than three nails are involved, systemic corticosteroids (oral prednisone and intramuscular triamcinolone acetonide) are considered as a first-line treatment; however, prolonged or repeated use of systemic corticosteroids may cause considerable side effects.[23] Intralesional steroid injections have also been seen to be efficacious in treating NLP.[24] For involvement of up to three nails, intralesional steroid injections can be considered, but such injections are very painful and relapses are common.[25] Topical tacrolimus has been seen to be effective in treating NLP and was found to be more effective than topical corticosteroids.[26] Patients not responding to corticosteroids can be treated with second line medications like antimalarials,[27] retinoids like acitretin,[28] or alitretinoin[29] and cyclosporine.[30] Etanercept has been found to be an effective treatment modality for LP limited particularly to the nails.[31] Severe cases with permanent damage to the nail matrix that has resulted in scarring and pterygium formation can only be treated with surgery.

Table 14.5 Treatment of nail lichen planus

Number of digits involved	Treatment options and level of evidence
Fewer than three	Intralesional steroids (level of evidence IA)
More than three	Oral prednisolone (level of evidence 1B) Intramuscular triamcinolone acetonide (level of evidence 2B) Topical tacrolimus (level of evidence 1A) Acitretin, alitretinoin, cyclosporine, and etanercept in resistant cases (level of evidence 2B)

There are two methods to repair a split nail depending on the width of the cicatricial pterygium: excision with a meticulous repair or free matrix graft.[32]

KEY POINTS

- Nail involvement is a common manifestation of disseminated LP. Isolated nail involvement too is known and may pose a diagnostic challenge.
- Affected nails present with longitudinal ridges, pitting, onychorrhexis, distal splitting, and pterygium formation.
- Biopsy shows classical histopathological features of LP.
- Dermoscopy may aid in evaluation of disease progress and prognosis.
- Differential diagnosis includes nail psoriasis, onychomycosis, and nail-manifested alopecia areata.
- Untreated cases progress to anonychia, so diagnosis and prompt treatment is important.
- Treatment options include topical, systemic, and intralesional steroids as well as topical tacrolimus, retinoids, and antimalarials.
- Increased awareness of this nail disorder will result in a more frequent diagnosis and better understanding of the disorder.

REFERENCES

1. Zaias N. The nail in lichen planus. *Arch Dermatol* 1970; 101: 264–271.
2. Goettmann S, Zaraa I, Moulonguet I. Nail lichen planus: Epidemiological, clinical, pathological, therapeutic and prognosis study of 67 cases. *J Eur Acad Dermatol Venereol* 2012; 26: 1304–1309.
3. Tosti A, Piraccini BM, Cambiaghi S, Jorizzo M. Nail lichen planus in children. Clinical features, response to treatment, and long-term follow-up. *Arch Dermatol* 2001; 137: 1027–1032.
4. Kanwar AJ, De D. Lichen planus in childhood: Report of 100 cases. *Clin Exp Dermatol* 2010; 35: 257–262.
5. Tosti A, Piraccini BM, Cambiaghi S, Jorizzo M. *Color Atlas of Nails*. Berlin, Germany: Springer; 2010. Nail Lichen Planusin; pp. 83–85.
6. Lehman JS, Tollefson MM, Gibson LE. Lichen planus. *Int J Dermatol* 2009; 48: 682–694.
7. Boyd AS, Neldner KH. Lichen planus. *J Am Acad Dermatol* 1991; 25: 593–619.
8. Tosti A, Peluso AM, Fanti PA, Piraccini BM. Nail lichen planus: Clinical and pathologic study of twenty-four patients. *J Am Acad Dermatol* 1993; 28: 724–730.
9. Tosti A, Piraccini BM, Cameli N. Nail changes in lichen planus may resemble those of yellow nail syndrome. *Br J Dermatol* 2000; 142: 848–849.

10. Tosti A, Bardazzi F, Piraccini BM, Fanti PA. Idiopathic trachyonychia (twenty-nail dystrophy): A pathological study of 23 patients. *Br J Dermatol* 1994; 131: 866–872.

11. Taniguchi S, Kutsuna H, Tani Y, Kawahira K, Hamada T. Twenty-nail dystrophy (trachyonychia) caused by lichen planus in a patient with alopecia universalis and ichthyosis vulgaris. *J Am Acad Dermatol* 1995; 33: 903–905.

12. Sakata S, Howard A, Tosti A, Sinclair R. Follow up of 12 patients with trachyonychia. *Australas J Dermatol* 2006; 47: 166–168.

13. Tosti A, Fanti PA, Morelli R, Bardazzi F. Trachyonychia associated with alopecia areata: A clinical and pathologic study. *J Am Acad Dermatol* 1991; 25: 266–270.

14. Peloro TM, Pride HB. Twenty-nail dystrophy and vitiligo: A rare association. *J Am Acad Dermatol* 1999; 40: 488–490.

15. Scher RK, Fischbein R, Ackerman AB. Twenty-nail dystrophy: A variant of lichen planus. *Arch Dermatol* 1978; 114: 612–613.

16. Peluso AM, Tosti A, Piraccini BM, Cameli N. Lichen planus limited to the nails in childhood: Case report and literature review. *Pediatr Dermatol* 1993; 10: 36–39.

17. Yokozeki H, Nuyama S, Nishioka K. Twenty-nail dystrophy (trachyonychia) caused by lichen planus in a patient with gold allergy. *Br J Dermatol* 2005; 152: 1089–1091.

18. Gordon KA, Vega JM, Tosti A. Trachyonychia: A comprehensive review. *Indian J Dermatol Venereol Leprol* 2011; 77: 640–645.

19. Nakamura R, Broce AA, Palencia DP, Ortiz NI, Leverone A. Dermatoscopy of nail lichen planus. *Int J Dermatol* 2013; 52: 684–687.

20. Alessandrini A, Starace M, Piraccini BM. Dermoscopy in the evaluation of nail disorders. *Skin Appendage Disord* 2017; 3: 70–82.

21. Friedman P, Sabban EC, Marcucci C, Peralta R, Cabo H. Dermoscopic findings in different clinical variants of lichen planus. Is dermoscopy useful? *Dermatol Pract Concept* 2015; 5: 51–55.

22. Hall R, Wartman D, Jellinek K, Robinson-Bostom L, Telang G. Lichen planus of the nail matrix with predominant plasma cell infiltrate. *J Cutan Pathol* 2008; 35 (Suppl 1): 14–16.

23. Evans AV, Roest MA, Fletcher CL, Lister R, Hay RJ. Isolated lichen planus of the toenails treated with oral prednisolone. *Clin Exp Dermatol* 2001; 26: 412–414.

24. Brauns B, Stahl M, Schon MP, Zutt M. Intralesional steroid injection alleviates nail lichen planus. *Int J Dermatol* 2011; 50: 626–627.

25. Alsenaid A, Eder I, Ruzicka T, Braun-Falco M, Wolf R. Successful treatment of nail lichen planus with alitretinoin: Report of 2 cases and review of the literature. *Dermatology* 2014; 229: 293–296.

26. Ujiie H, Shibaki A, Akiyama M, Shimizu H. Successful treatment of nail lichen planus with topical tacrolimus. *Acta Derm Venereol* 2010; 90: 218–219.

27. Mostafa WZ. Lichen planus of the nail: Treatment with antimalarials. *J Am Acad Dermatol* 1989; 20: 289–290.

28. Piraccini BM, Saccani E, Starace M, Balestri R, Tosti A. Nail lichen planus: Response to treatment and long-term follow-up. *Eur J Dermatol* 2010; 20: 489–496.

29. Pinter A, Patzold S, Kaufmann R. Lichen planus of nails-successful treatment with alitretinoin. *J Dtsch Dermatol Ges* 2011; 9: 1033–1034.

30. Florian B, Angelika J, Ernst SR. Successful treatment of palmoplantar nail lichen planus with cyclosporine. *J Dtsch Dermatol Ges* 2014; 12: 724–725.

31. Irla N, Schneiter T, Haneke E, Yawalkar N. Nail lichen planus: Successful treatment with etanercept. *Case Rep Dermatol* 2010; 2: 173–176.

32. Haneke E. Advanced nail surgery. *J Cutan Aesthet Surg* 2011; 4: 167–175.

15

Trachyonychia

ARCHANA SINGAL AND M. N. KAYARKATTE

DEFINITION AND NOMENCLATURE

"Trachyonychia" is derived from the Greek word *trakos* meaning rough and *onyx* meaning nail.[1] The original French term was "sand-blasted nails," as the appearance was likened to the nails being rubbed with sand paper. Trachyonychia is used to describe thin, brittle nails with excessive longitudinal ridging. The term trachyonychia was first introduced by Alkiewicz in 1950. Its acquired idiopathic version was later termed as twenty-nail dystrophy (TND) by Hazelrigg et al. in 1977.[2] However, the term twenty-nail dystrophy is misleading because in trachyonychia any number of nails can be affected and the nail changes can be of varying severity in different nails. There have been debates to abandon the term TND as it does not provide any information about the etiology. Moreover, the term TND lacks specificity as many conditions can lead to dystrophy of all 20 nails apart from trachyonychia.[3,4]

INTRODUCTION

Trachyonychia is a non-scarring disorder of the nail unit that most commonly presents with rough, longitudinally ridged nails (opaque trachyonychia) or less frequently, uniform, opalescent nails with pits (shiny trachyonychia).[5]

EPIDEMIOLOGY

Incidence and prevalence: Exact incidence of trachyonychia is not known as it is believed to be under-reported. It was estimated to constitute 1.5% of the population consulting for nail disorders in a cohort.[6]

The most common association of trachyonychia is with alopecia areata and trachyonychia is estimated to affect 3.65% of cases of alopecia areata.[3]

Age and sex: Trachyonychia can affect patients of all ages. It was initially thought to occur exclusively in children but adult cases have been described frequently. Children are more likely to get affected and the maximum incidence has been observed in the age group of 3–12 years.[1] There is no sex predilection and both male and females are equally affected. However, one study revealed female preponderance in childhood trachyonychia as compared to male preponderance in adult onset one.[7]

Genetics: Genetics play a very minor role, with an autosomal dominant mode of transmission. Trachyonychia has been reported in a Sicilian family and in monozygotic twins.[8,9] However, these may possibly be due to its association with alopecia areata, which may affect twins and several members of a family.

PATHOPHYSIOLOGY

Nail plate changes in trachyonychia result from the inflammatory activity occurring in the nail matrix, predominantly in the proximal nail matrix and the ventral part of the proximal nail fold (PNF). Accordingly, clinical changes are seen in the dorsal nail plate. It has been hypothesized that there is considerable variation in the severity of inflammatory activity within the nail matrix. This non-uniform inflammation along the nail matrix leads to sandpaper nails as it is more constant or as shiny trachyonychia where there are interspersed periods of normal nail matrix function.[10]

CLINICAL FEATURES AND VARIANTS

Trachyonychia is a morphological entity characterized by roughness with excessive longitudinal ridging. The disease can involve a single nail to all the twenty nails. Fingernails are more commonly affected than the toenails.[5] The nail plate may be thickened or thinned. Cuticles may also be thickened and ragged.[5]

The two different subtypes of trachyonychia were first described by Baran, based on clinical appearance and severity (Table 15.1).[5,11]

- Opaque trachyonychia, the more severe type, is characterized by rough nails with longitudinal ridges that appear to have been rubbed by sandpaper (Figures 15.1 through 15.3).
- The less severe type, shiny trachyonychia, is characterized by shiny, opalescent nails with numerous pits (Figures 15.4 and 15.5).
- The combination of both features presenting as a mixed variant is also reported, which may show superficial scaling of the nail plate, hyperkeratosis of the cuticles, koilonychia, and onychoschizia.

Table 15.1 Variants of trachyonychia

Features	Opaque nails	Shiny nails
Frequency	More commonly seen	Less frequent Higher association with alopecia areata
Appearance	• Rough nails that appear to have been rubbed by sandpaper. • Nails are brittle, thin, and rough with excessive longitudinal ridging due to fine superficial striations found in a parallel pattern. • Koilonychia may be present.	• Shiny, opalescent nails with numerous pits. • Nails retain their luster, presenting with superficial ridging and multiple small geometric pits. • Koilonychia may be present.
Pathophysiology	Remittent, waxing, and waning inflammatory insult to the nail matrix that never ceases	Intermittent, focal, and regularly recurrent inflammatory insult to the matrix that is separated by periods of normal matrix function
Prognosis	More severe clinical course	Less severe course

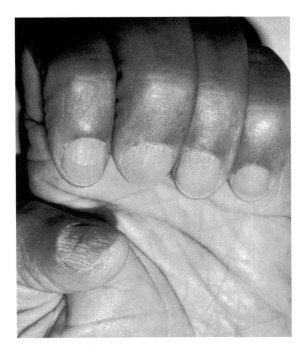

Figure 15.1 Opaque trachyonychia in an adult male; nails have longitudinal ridging.

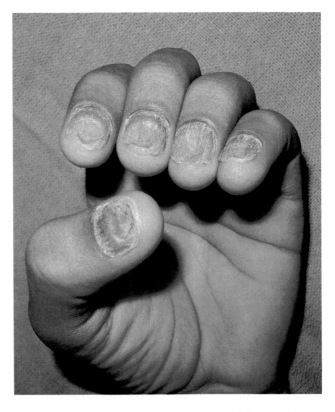

Figure 15.2 Opaque trachyonychia in a child; note the associated koilonychias and ragged cuticle.

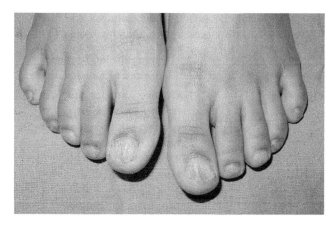

Figure 15.3 Opaque trachyonychia involving all toenails.

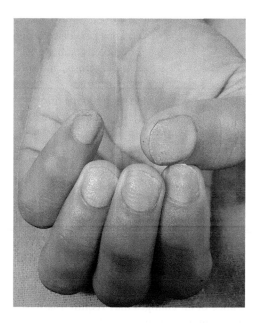

Figure 15.4 Shiny trachyonychia with multiple closely set small pits on the nail surface that reflect light.

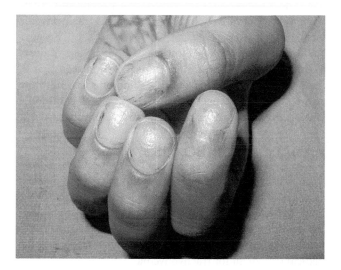

Figure 15.5 Shiny trachyonychia in a patient with alopecia areata (ophiatic variant).

ASSOCIATIONS

Trachyonychia can be idiopathic or a manifestation of a heterogenous group of disorders. Alopecia areata is the only condition that is so frequently associated with trachyonychia (most commonly the shiny type) that it is mandatory to look for alopecia areata in all cases.[6]

Various associations have been enumerated in Table 15.2.

DIAGNOSIS

Diagnosis of trachyonychia is mainly clinical and does not necessitate laboratory workup. However, a standard evaluation protocol should be followed in all patients.

1. A detailed personal and family history is to be obtained for skin and systemic diseases.
2. Examination of skin, hair, and mucosae is warranted to identify associated alopecia areata or skin and mucosal signs of psoriasis and lichen planus.
3. Keeping other causes of nail dystrophy in mind, a nail clipping must be taken in all cases, which is a non-invasive procedure. The nail clipping should be subjected to direct microscopic examination in KOH (to look for fungal elements as onychomycosis is a close differential diagnosis) and histopathology (with PAS staining) for clues to other underlying pathology. For example, histological changes of nail psoriasis may be present in a patient diagnosed clinically as idiopathic trachyonychia.

Table 15.2 Reported dermatologic and non-dermatologic diseases associated with trachyonychia

Dermatologic diseases	Non-dermatologic diseases
• Alopecia areata	• Immunoglobulin A deficiency
• Lichen planus	• Balanced translocation 46, XX
• Vitiligo	
• Psoriasis	• Immune thrombocytopenic purpura
• Ichthyosis vulgaris	• Autoimmune hemolytic anemia
• Atopic dermatitis	
• Incontinentia pigmenti	
• Pemphigus	• Amyloidosis
• Congenital cutaneous candidiasis	• Sarcoidosis
• Knuckle pads	• Reflex sympathetic dystrophy
• Hereditary punctate palmoplantar keratoderma	• Down syndrome
• Hay–Wells syndrome	
• Darier's disease	
• Judo nails	

Source: Haber, J.S. et al., *Skin Appendage Disord.*, 2, 109–115, 2017.

HISTOPATHOLOGY

Histopathological confirmation of disease is generally not recommended to confirm the diagnosis of trachyonychia or to delineate the underlying specific diagnosis. However, nail biopsy has a role in severe and recalcitrant cases or when the clinical diagnosis is ambiguous. Longitudinal nail unit biopsy is preferred as multiple anatomic areas of nail unit may be screened.

Wilkinson et al. were the first to evaluate histopathological features in cases of idiopathic trachyonychia and described distinctive histological feature of focal spongiotic inflammation of the nail matrix.[12] Based on this finding, the authors proposed that idiopathic trachyonychia may be a subgroup of endogenous eczema limited to the nail matrix. In another study of 23 patients with idiopathic trachyonychia (TND), spongiotic changes were observed in 19 patients, psoriasiform features in three patients, and features of lichen planus in one patient. None of their patients developed any skin lesion in the 2-year follow-up period.[13] Trachyonychia due to nail lichen planus has been reported to occur in patients with alopecia areata, suggesting that these two diseases can occur simultaneously.[14] Grover et al. evaluated the utility of longitudinal nail biopsy in 32 patients of TND, of which 21 (65.3%) had concomitant skin disease. Spongiotic histology was seen in only 48% cases. Significant side effects in the form of secondary infection (12%), scarring and secondary dystrophy of nail unit (28%), and reduction in total nail width (43%) were encountered. Therefore, a careful assessment of risk-benefit ratio must be made before performing the procedure.[15]

DIFFERENTIAL DIAGNOSIS

The term trachyonychia has been incorrectly applied to conditions that can cause widespread nail dystrophy of all 20 nails such as inflammatory and systemic diseases, ectodermal disorders, and infections (Table 15.3).

Diagnosis of trachyonychia is based on a specific morphology and the mere presence of fissures and splitting is not consistent with this diagnosis.[5]

Table 15.3 Differential diagnosis and their key features for distinguishing from trachyonychia

Conditions	Distinguishing features from trachyonychia
Onychomycosis	Chromonychia, onycholysis, subungual hyperkeratosis.
Alopecia areata	Often difficult to make a distinction, as the geometric, superficial pitting is similar to that in the shiny trachyonychia variety.

(Continued)

Table 15.3 (*Continued*) Differential diagnosis and their key features for distinguishing from trachyonychia

Conditions	Distinguishing features from trachyonychia
Brittle nails	Nails have some longitudinal ridging and superficial splitting but do not exhibit the typical roughness and excessive ridging as seen in trachyonychia.
Lichen planus	Nails exhibit longitudinal fissures and pterygium, which are not seen in trachyonychia. Melanonychia can be present.
Psoriasis	Nails exhibit pitting, oil spots, and nail bed discoloration, onycholysis, subungual hyperkeratosis, and splinter hemorrhages.
Senile nails	Mild longitudinal ridging that does not usually involve the entire nail plate as in trachyonychia.

DISEASE COURSE AND PROGNOSIS

Trachyonychia never produces nail scarring, even if it is seen in association with lichen planus. Therefore, it is considered a benign condition. Most of the patients with trachyonychia improve spontaneously with time, though the disappearance of all changes may require many years. The prognosis and management of trachyonychia is not related to the underlying disease that is responsible for the nail abnormalities. For example, trachyonychia due to lichen planus does not produce scarring or nail atrophy and can be managed conservatively in the same way as trachyonychia due to other causes.

Though prognosis does not depend on the age of onset and the number of nails affected, it has been seen that in those with childhood onset with symptoms lasting more than 6 years, spontaneous improvement is less common.[16] Also, trachyonychia does not predispose to onychomycosis.

MANAGEMENT (BOX 15.1)

Trachyonychia per se is not harmful to the patient but nail lesions tend to affect the quality of life adversely. Therefore, many patients request treatment. In addition to counselling, various topical and systemic treatment modalities have been used. However, there is no single evidence-based medical treatment for trachyonychia.

BOX 15.1: Treatment options for trachonychia

- **Conservative**
  - Counseling
  - Emollients
  - Nail paint (camouflage)
- **Topicals**
  - Potent steroid – under occlusion
  - Calcipotriol + Betamethasone
  - Tazarotene
  - 5-Fluorouracil (5-FU)
- **Systemic therapy**
  - Acitretin
  - Cyclosporine
  - Oral mini-pulse with betamethasone
  - Chloroquine
- **Intramatricial**
  - Inj Triamcinolone
- **PUVA therapy**
- **Nail plate dressings**

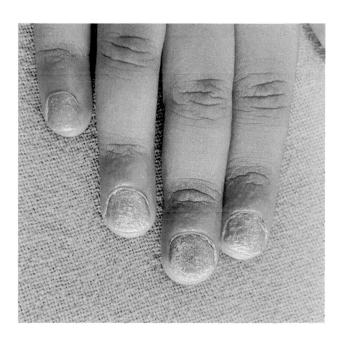

Figure 15.6 Pre-treatment picture of trachyonychia in a 6-year-old girl.

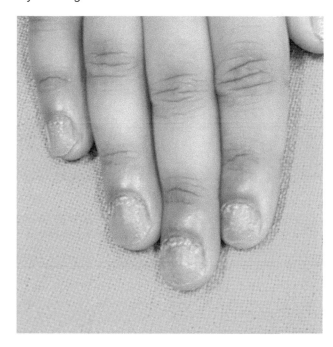

Figure 15.7 Significant improvement 6 months after application of emollients.

Conservative approach

Trachyonychia is mainly a cosmetic concern. It is non-scarring, with complete spontaneous regression reported in 50% of the patients in 6 years with average disease duration of 42 months.[16] Hence, assurance to the patients with a wait-and-watch policy may be advocated especially in children, where invasive procedures are difficult and side effects of the systemic therapy need to be avoided. Children are known to have a shorter disease course as compared to adults.

Evaluation of the underlying associations and alleviation of the cause is essential, e.g., trachyonychia caused by lichen planus in a patient with gold allergy has been reported that improved on removing the cause.[17] An emollient may be advised to improve the nail surface texture in opaque trachyonychia (Figures 15.6 and 15.7) and nail polish to improve appearance in shiny trachyonychia.[6]

Topical therapy

Topical therapy is a safe, painless, non-invasive, effective, and convenient method of treating trachyonychia, especially in children.

- Among these, potent topical steroids are preferred. The paper tape occlusion method of potent steroids is highly encouraged due to efficient permeation to the nail matrix through the PNF.[18]
- Other topical options include calcipotriol/betamethasone dipropionate ointment applied once daily to PNF for 6 months,[19] tazarotene gel,[20] and 5% 5-fluorouracil.[21]

Procedure-based options

- Intralesional injections of triamcinolone into the PNF and nail matrix at a dose of 2.5–10 mg have shown results as early as 4 weeks.[22]
- Topical psoralen UVA has shown modest success in a few case reports.[23,24]

Nail plate dressings

Ultrathin adhesive layer with lactic acid, silicon dioxide, aluminum acetylacetonate, vinyl co-polymer, and azelaic acid have been used once a week. Significant improvement was noted at 3 months and near-complete resolution at 6 months.

Systemic therapy

Systemic treatments include biotin 2.5 mg/day, cyclosporine (2–3.5 mg/kg/day), retinoids, systemic corticosteroids in the form of weekly oral mini-pulse.[25–28] Recently JAK-STAT inhibitor like tofacitinib citrate has been tried.[29]

In trachyonychia due to psoriasis, acitretin and cyclosporin are effective options. Since trachyonychia is primarily a cosmetic concern, the systemic treatment should be considered keeping in mind the risk factors and patient preference.[5]

The treatment algorithm is given in Figure 15.8.

Various treatment modalities have been summarized in Table 15.4.[30]

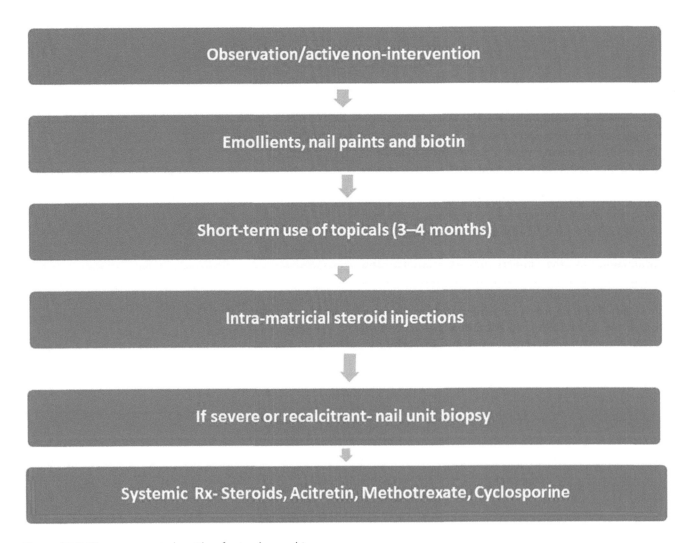

Figure 15.8 The treatment algorithm for trachyonychia.

Table 15.4 Summary of treatment for trachonychia

Treatment (Ref)	Author	Dose	Treatment duration	Outcome
Topical Steroids[18]	Sakiyam et al.	Overnight under occlusion	6 months	Nail plate features became less conspicuous
Intramatricial Triamcinolone[22,31]	Sammam et al., Grover et al.	2.5 mg per dose	Bimonthly for 4 months	Relapse, painful, proximal nail fold, need long-term compliance (effective in four children)
Oral Betamethasone weekly pulse[28]	Mittal et al.	4 mg	Mini pulse therapy (2 consecutive days every week for 2 months)	Shown to be effective. Usually fewer side effects vs. the daily dose of corticosteroids over weeks and months
Topical Tazarotene[20]	Soda et al.	0.10%	Nightly for 3 months	Required two courses, with side effects of peeling, erythema on proximal nail fold (showed improvement in one patient with alopecia areata)
Oral Acitretin[27]	Kolbach-Rengifo et al.	0.3 mg/kg	Daily for 3 months	Psoriatic trachyonychia (improvement in roughness, ridging, pitting, subungual hyperkeratosis)
Cyclosporine A[26]	Lee et al.	3 mg/kg/day	Daily for 2.5 months	Psoriatic trachyonychia (successful in 5 patients)
PUVA[23]	Halkier-Sorensen et al.	0.7–1.4 J/cm^2	Three times a week for 7 months	All treated nails showed significant improvement
5-fluorouracil[21]	Schissel et al.	5%	6 months	Psoriatic trachyonychia; periungual irritation limits its use
Oral Griseofulvin/ steroid[32]	Sehgal et al.	10mg/kg	6 months	LP trachyonychia
Oral Biotin[25]	Mohrenschlanger et al.	20 mg	Daily	Primary biliary cirrhosis patient Partial resolution
Topical Petrolatum[33]	Kumar et al.	Not known	Not known	Partial resolution seen

KEY POINTS

- Trachyonychia refers to a morphologic entity of the nail unit characterized by rough lusterless nails with excessive longitudinal ridging.
- It is more commonly seen in pediatric populations.
- Two clinical forms exist: Opaque trachyonychia is the more severe type and is characterized by rough sand-blasted nails. The less severe shiny trachyonychia is characterized by shiny, opalescent nails with numerous pits.
- Diagnosis is mainly clinical. A nail unit biopsy is not advocated. Histology when performed shows spongiosis inflammation of the matrix in idiopathic trachyonychia.
- Prognosis is excellent as it is a non-scarring process. Nail changes in trachyonychia are self-limiting. Spontaneous regression is expected in >50% cases in a few years.
- A conservative approach is hence the best approach.
- Various topical and systemic treatments have been tried in severe cases and when the patient requests treatment.

REFERENCES

1. Scheinfeld NS. Trachyonychia: A case report and review of manifestations, associations, and treatments. *Cutis* 2003;71:299–302.
2. Hazelrigg DE. Twenty-nail dystrophy of childhood. *Arch Dermatol* 1977;113:73.
3. Tosti A, Bardazzi F, Piraccini BM, Fanti PA. Idiopathic trachyonychia (twenty-nail dystrophy): A pathological study of 23 patients. *Br J Dermatol* 1994;131:866–872.
4. Baran R, Dawber R. TND of childhood: A misnamed syndrome. *Cutis* 1987;39:481–482.
5. Jacobsen AA, Tosti A. Trachyonychia and twenty-nail dystrophy: A comprehensive review and discussion of diagnostic accuracy. *Skin Appendage Disord* 2016;2:7–13.
6. Tosti A, Piraccini BM, Iorizzo M. Trachyonychia and related disorders: Evaluation and treatment plans. *Dermatol Ther* 2002;15:121–125.
7. Lee YB, Cheon MS, Park HJ, Cho BK. Clinical study of twenty-nail dystrophy in Korea. *Int J Dermatol* 2012;51:677–681.
8. Balci S, Kanra G, Aypar E, Son YA. Twenty-nail dystrophy in a mother and her 7-year-old daughter associated with balanced translocation 46, XX, t(6q13;10p13). *Clin Dysmorphol* 2002;11:171–173.

9. Pavone L, Li Volti S, Guarneri B, La Rosa M, Sorge G, Incorpora G et al. Hereditary twenty-nail dystrophy in a Sicilian family. *J Med Genet* 1982;19:337–340.

10. Gordon KA, Vega JM, Tosti A. Trachyonychia: A comprehensive review. *Indian J Dermatol Venereol Leprol* 2011;77:640–645.

11. Haber JS, Chairatchaneeboon M, Rubin AI. Trachyonychia: Review and update on clinical aspects, histology, and therapy. *Skin Appendage Disord* 2017;2:109–115.

12. Wilkinson JD, Dawber RPR, Bowers RP, Fleming K. Twenty-nail dystrophy of childhood. Case report and histopathological findings. *Br J Dermatol* 1979;100:217–221.

13. Tosti A, Bardazzi F, Piraccini BM, Fanti PA. Idiopathic trachyonychia (twenty-nail dystrophy): A pathological study of 23 patients. *Br J Dermatol* 1994;131:866–872.

14. Tosti A, Fanti PA, Morelli R, Bardazzi F. Trachyonychia associated with alopecia areata: A clinical and pathologic study. *J Am Acad Dermatol* 1991;25:266–270.

15. Grover C, Khandpur S, Reddy BSN, Chaturvedi KU. Longitudinal nail biopsy: Utility in 20-nail dystrophy. *Dermatol Surg* 2003;29:1125–1129.

16. Sakata S, Howard A, Tosti A, Sinclair R. Follow up of 12 patients with trachyonychia. *Australas J Dermatol* 2006;47:166–168.

17. Yokozeki H, Niiyama S, Nishioka K. Twenty-nail dystrophy (trachyonychia) caused by lichen planus in a patient with gold allergy. *Br J Dermatol* 2005;152:1087–1089.

18. Sakiyama T, Chaya A, Shimizu T, Ebihara T, Saito M. Spongiotic trachyonychia treated with topical corticosteroids using the paper tape occlusion method. *Skin Appendage Disord* 2016;2:49–51.

19. Park J-M, Cho H-H, Kim W-J, Mun J-H, Song M, Kim H-S et al. Efficacy and safety of calcipotriol/betamethasone dipropionate ointment for the treatment of trachyonychia: An open-label study. *Ann Dermatol* 2015;27:371–375.

20. Soda R, Diluvio L, Bianchi L, Chimenti S. Treatment of trachyonychia with tazarotene. *Clin Exp Dermatol* 2005;30:301–302.

21. Schissel DJ, Elston DM. Topical 5-fluorouracil treatment for psoriatic trachyonychia. *Cutis* 1998;62:27–28.

22. Grover C, Bansal S, Nanda S, Reddy BSN. Efficacy of triamcinolone acetonide in various acquired nail dystrophies. *J Dermatol* 2005;32:963–968.

23. Halkier-Sørensen L, Cramers M, Kragballe K. Twenty-nail dystrophy treated with topical PUVA. *Acta Derm Venereol* 1990;70:510–511.

24. Arias-Santiago S, Fernández-Pugnaire MA, Husein El-Ahmed H, Girón-Prieto MS, Naranjo Sintes R. Niño de 9 años con traquioniquia: Buena respuesta al tratamiento con apósitos ungueales. *An Pediatr* 2009;71:476–477.

25. Möhrenschlager M, Schmidt T, Ring J, Abeck D. Recalcitrant trachyonychia of childhood–Response to daily oral biotin supplementation: Report of two cases. *J Dermatolog Treat* 2000;11:113–115.

26. Lee YB, Cheon MS, Eun YS, Cho BK, Park YG, Park HJ. Cyclosporin administration improves clinical manifestations and quality of life in patients with 20-nail dystrophy: Case series and survey study. *J Dermatol* 2012;39:1064–1065.

27. Kolbach-Rengifo M, Navajas-Galimany L, Araneda-Castiglioni D, Reyes-Vivanco C. Efficacy of acitretin and topical clobetasol in trachyonychia involving all twenty nails. *Indian J Dermatol Venereol Leprol* 2016;82:732.

28. Mittal R, Khaitan BK, Sirka CS. Trachyonychia treated with oral mini pulse therapy. *Indian J Dermatol Venereol Leprol* 2001;67:202–203.

29. Ferreira SB, Scheinberg M, Steiner D, Steiner T, Bedin GL, Ferreira RB. Remarkable improvement of nail changes in alopecia areata universalis with 10 months of treatment with tofacitinib: A case report. *Case Rep Dermatol* 2016;8:262–266.

30. Tongdee E, Shareef S, Favreau T, Touloei K. A case of twenty nail dystrophy and review of treatment options. *J Am Osteopath* 2016;36:43–46.

31. Samman PD. Trachyonychia (rough nails). *Br J Dermatol* 1979;101:701–705.

32. Sehgal VN, Abraham GJS, Malik GB. Griseofulvin therapy in lichen planus: A double blind controlled trial. *Brit J Dermatol* 1972;87:383–385.

33. Kumar MG, Ciliberto H, Bayliss SJ. Long-term follow-up of pediatric trachyonychia. *Pediatr Dermatol* 2015;32:198–200.

PART 5

Infective Nail Diseases

16

Dermatophytic onychomycosis

MALCOLM PINTO AND MANJUNATH M. SHENOY

INTRODUCTION

Onychomycosis (OM) is a common fungal infection of the nail unit that gradually leads to dystrophic changes of the nail plate and nail bed. OM may be caused by the dermatophytes, non-dermatophytic molds (NDM), and yeast. Dermatophytic OM, also referred to as tinea unguium (TU), is the most common form of OM.

EPIDEMIOLOGY

The estimated frequency of OM is 8%–14% based on surveys of adults seeking treatment at primary care or dermatology offices in the United States and Canada. This increases with age and may be as high as 50% among individuals older than 70 years.[1] Dermatophytes appear to be the most common agent causing fingernail infection but toenail diseases may be caused by a non-dermatophytic molds in many instances. In a clinico-mycological study from India of 100 consecutive patients of KOH and culture-positive dermatophyte toenail OM, males were more commonly affected; Distal lateral subungual onychomycosis (DLSO) was the most common clinical variant and *Trichophyton interdigitale* was the most common etiological fungus implicated.[2] Pediatric OM is a growing public health concern all over the world. OM was found to be more prevalent in children aged ≥10 years, those with ≥3 siblings, unemployed fathers, living in the rural area, and wearing rubber shoes.[3]

ETIOPATHOGENESIS

Predisposing factors

- Hot and humid climate, smoking, peripheral vascular disease, psoriasis, hereditary palmoplantar keratoderma, immunosuppression, repeated trauma to the nail, and occlusive foot wear.
- Genetic predisposition to DLSO by *Trichophyton rubrum* is known.[4]
- Sex predilection: Males are affected more frequently as compared to females possibly due to more frequent nail damage resulting from sports and leisure activities amongst male adolescents.
- Children: Positive association with Down syndrome, fungal infection on other body parts, premature birth and perinatal hypoxia, and HIV infection in other family members.
- OM involving toenails is about seven times more common than that of fingernails. TU of toenails is more frequent possibly due to a three times slower growth rate. First and second toe are most often affected as they are more susceptible to trauma and pressure from footwear.

Agents

Dermatophytes cause the majority of the infections of fingernails and toenails. Various species causing infections include:

- *Trichophyton rubrum*
- *Trichophyton mentagrophytes* var. *interdigitale* (*Trichophyton interdigitale*)
- *Epidermophyton floccosum*
- *Microsporum* species[5]

Pathogenesis

Dermatophytes possess keratolytic, proteolytic, and lipolytic activities that enable them to invade the skin, nail, and hair. Ventral and middle layers of the nail plate are mostly affected as the keratin in this region is comparatively soft and in close proximity to the underlying living cells. Approximately 30% of patients with ringworm infection elsewhere on the body tend to acquire TU.[6]

Classification

The clinical classification of OM has been summarized in Table 16.1.

1. Primary OM: Clinical presentation results due to invasion by the fungus.
2. Secondary OM: Fungal infection of nails previously afflicted with some other non-infective nail pathology.

Table 16.1 Clinical classification of onychomycosis

Clinical type	Clinical features
1. Distal lateral subungual onychomycosis (DLSO)	Hyperkeratosis and range of dyschromias including melanonychia, onycholysis (which may be sole abnormality), and longitudinal streaking in mid or lateral nail plate regions
2. Superficial onychomycosis (white or black)	1. Patchy or transverse (more common presentation) 2. Originating from beneath proximal nail fold 3. With deep penetration: fungi invade from superficial to deep aspects of nail plate
3. Endonyx onychomycosis (EO)	Involvement of the inner surface of nail plate without inflammation of the nail bed, onycholysis, or subungual hyperkeratosis
4. Proximal subungual onychomycosis (PSO)	1. Patchy 2. Striate (transverse or longitudinal) 3. Secondary to paronychia
5. Mixed pattern onychomycosis (MPO)	Combination of different clinical patterns in the same nail or in the different nails. • DLSO plus SO • SWO plus PSO • DLSO plus PSO
6. Total dystrophic onychomycosis (TDO)	This may occur as secondary change to advanced states of other patterns of nail plate invasion; alternatively, it may occur as primary change where it is associated either with disease with severe immunodeficiency, e.g., HIV/AIDS, or in chronic mucocutaneous candidosis.
7. Secondary onychomycosis	Fungal nail plate invasion may occur secondary to other nail pathologies where clinical changes are dominated by morphologic features of underlying disease.

Source: Hay, R.J., and Baran, R., *J. Am. Acad Dermatol.*, 65, 1219–1227, 2011.

Clinical types

1. Distal Lateral Subungual Onychomycosis: This type of OM, also known as nail bed dermatophytosis, is the most common clinical type of OM.
   The most common dermatophyte species causing DLSO is *Trichophyton rubrum* followed by *T. Mentagrophytes var. interdigitale, T. Tonsurans,* and *Epidermophyton floccosum.*

   DLSO is characterized by the interrelated features of subungual hyperkeratosis, onycholysis, and paronychia. The nail plate gets first affected from the under and lateral edges and then spreads proximally along the nail bed. Clinically, there are discrete foci of onycholysis in the distal/lateral part and subungual hyperkeratosis accompanied by nail discoloration. With progress of infection, opaque streaks develop in the nail plate. Spikes refer to the hyperkeratotic yellow-colored thickened band of nail that progress proximally towards the matrix (Figures 16.1 through 16.3).

   Dermatophytoma: It refers to the thick mass of fungal hyphae and necrotic keratin between nail plate and nail bed. This often requires surgical excision as these dormant fungal elements in dermatophytoma are known to form a biofilm restricting the penetration of antifungal drugs leading to persistence of infection.

   "One hand two feet" tinea syndrome: Distinct clinical pattern in DLSO caused by *T. rubrum* in which the fungus spreads from the plantar and palmar surface of feet and hands. OM in this condition is often preceded by a traumatic event and the dominant hand involved in scratching the feet or picking the nails is often affected (Figure 16.4).[7]

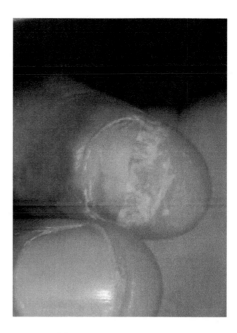

Figure 16.2 Distal lateral subungual onychomycosis with dermatophytoma.

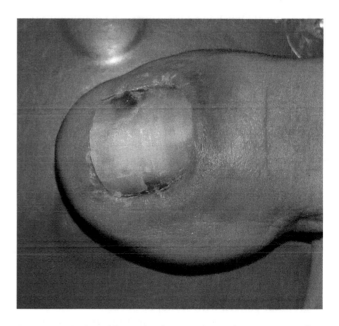

Figure 16.3 Distal lateral subungual onychomycosis with paronychia.

Chronic dermatophytosis syndrome: This entity caused by *T. mentagrophytes* var. *interdigitale* in susceptible hosts is characterized by DLSO of the toenails, tinea pedis, and tinea cruris. It generally presents in the sixth decade of life as minute plantar vesicles of size 1mm containing a large number of hyphae that gradually dry up, leaving a keratinous collarette and thick skin of the soles. Later on, other sites, especially the nail beds, become infected, leading to DLSO. A small subgroup of patients may present with moccasin-type of severe tinea pedis.

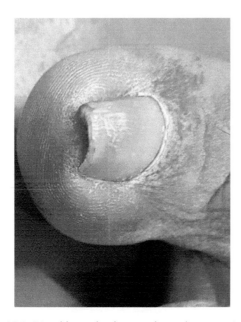

Figure 16.1 Distal lateral subungual onychomycosis with pincer nail.

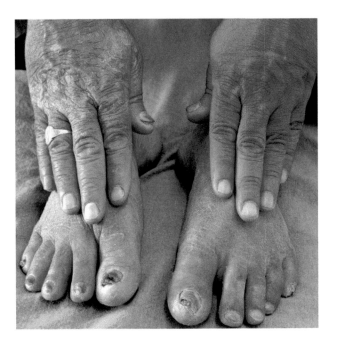

Figure 16.4 Two feet-one hand syndrome. (courtesy: Dr. Piyush Kumar.)

2. Superficial Onychomycosis: Superficial onychomycosis (SO) is a rare, distinctive pattern of OM in which the upper surface of the nail plate is the primary site of invasion. Superficial white OM (SWO) mainly involves toenails and *T. mentagrophytes* var. *interdigitale* is responsible for more than 90% of cases. Clinically, there is presence of small, well-delineated opaque white islands on the dorsal nail plate that coalesce, resulting in a rough, soft, crumbly chalky white appearance to the entire nail surface—hence, the term leukonychia trichophytica. SWO usually affects a single toenail and may show a diffuse involvement of the nail both in width and depth. *T. mentagrophytes* var. *interdigitale* infections present with rather pruritic, vesicular eruption affecting the plantar arch and sides of the foot and heel accompanied by SWO.[5] Superficial black onychomycosis (SBO) due to *Neoscytalidium dimidiatum* on dermoscopy reveals a granular pattern with scalloped border.

3. Endonyx onychomycosis: In this type, the fungus penetrates the nail plate with milky white patches without subungual hyperkeratosis or onycholysis and has been described with *T. soudanense* and *T. violaceum*.

4. Proximal Subungual Onychomycosis: Proximal subungual onychomycosis (PSO) affects the fingernails and toenails. *T. rubrum, T. mentagrophytes, T. schoenleinii, T. tonsurans,* and *T. megninii* have been implicated. The infection starts from the stratum corneum on the ventral aspect of the proximal nail fold, migrates to the underlying matrix, and then spreads distally under the nail plate. Subungual hyperkeratosis, transverse leukonychia, onychomadesis, and destruction of the proximal nail plate take place. Periungual inflammation associated with purulent discharge is not uncommon. Patients with AIDS may present with a rapidly progressive form of PSO that occurs when the CD 4 count falls to less than 450 cells/mm³ (Figures 16.5 and 16.6).

5. Total dystrophic onychomycosis: Total dystrophic onychomycosis (TDO) represents the most advanced form where infection progresses to total destruction of the entire nail including the nail plate, nail bed, and matrix. The nail crumbles leaving behind a thickened abnormal dystrophic nail bed retaining keratotic nail debris (Figure 16.7).

6. Mixed pattern onychomycosis: Different clinical patterns of the nail plate infection may be encountered in the same patient in different nails as well as in the single nail. Co-occurrence of PSO and SO or DLSO and SO is commonly seen.

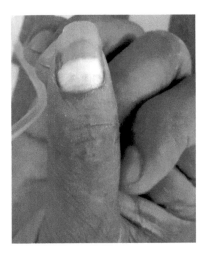

Figure 16.5 Proximal subungual onychomycosis and Tinea mannum in patient with HIV infection.

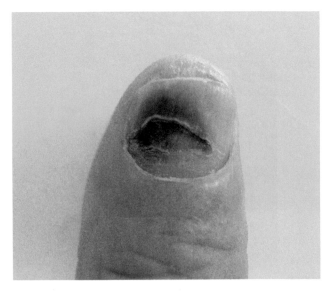

Figure 16.6 Proximal subungual onychomycosis.

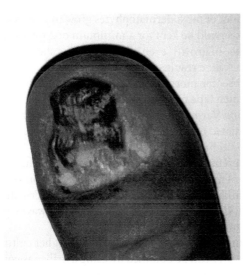

Figure 16.7 Total dystrophic onychomycosis.

Grading of onychomycosis

Clinical grading of the severity of onychomycotic nail disease is necessary for clinical trial inclusion criteria, for guiding choice of treatment, and for the prediction of therapeutic outcome.

1. Onychomycosis Severity Index (OSI) score[8]
   OSI Score is obtained by multiplying the score for the area of involvement (range, 0–5) by the score for the proximity of disease to the matrix (range, 1–5). Ten points are added for the presence of a longitudinal streak or a patch (dermatophytoma) or for greater than 2 mm of subungual hyperkeratosis. Following is the grading of OM severity based on the points:

Mild OM: 1–5
Moderate OM: 6–15
Severe OM: 16–35

2. Scoring Clinical Index for Onychomycosis (SCIO index)
3. Onychomycosis Area Severity Index Score (OASIS)

Differential diagnosis

The common clinical differential diagnoses are discussed in (Table 16.2).

Table 16.2 Differential diagnosis of onychomycosis

Disease	Features
Psoriasis	Presence of pitting and oil drop sign. Fingernails more commonly affected and associated arthritis may be present
Reiter's syndrome	Reddish-brown hue of the nail bed
Pityriasis rubra pilaris	Splinter hemorrhages, longitudinal ridging, and moderate thickening of nail bed

(Continued)

Table 16.2 (*Continued*) Differential diagnosis of onychomycosis

Disease	Features
Darier's disease	Longitudinal leuko- or erythronychia terminating in a distal "V"-shaped notch
Lichen planus	Ridging, roughened nail plate, thinning of nail plate, pterygium
Chronic eczema	Pitting with transverse ridging and furrows, adjacent skin usually involved
Pachyonychia congenita	Discoloration, tubular, hard and barrel shaped nail plate projecting upwards
Norwegian scabies	Large collection of scales in nail bed, digital pulp, and proximal nail fold
Asymmetric gait nail unit syndrome (Chapter 37)	Onycholysis, subungual hyperkeratosis, nail plate surface changes, typical nail plate alteration, distal toe skin hyperkeratosis
Keratin granulations (Chapter 35)	A harmless cosmetic problem mimicking superficial white onychomycosis, crumbling of the nail plate with whitish discoloration

DIAGNOSIS OF TINEA UNGUIUM

Accuracy of clinical diagnosis in OM is low Clinical predictors of a diagnosis of OM:

- History of tinea pedis in last year
- Scaling on soles
- White crumbly patches on nail
- Nail discoloration[9]

Clinical appearance caused by different fungal species is usually indistinguishable and laboratory diagnosis in such cases is essential (Tables 16.3 and 16.4).

Table 16.3 Steps of specimen collection

- Topical for 2 weeks and systemic antifungal drugs for 4 weeks are withheld.
- Fingernails and toenails are sampled separately and associated tinea pedis or mannum should also be scraped. Entire nail unit should be thoroughly cleaned with alcohol to remove contaminants.
- Using a nail clipper, affected nail bed should be exposed by removing the onycholytic nail plate and the hyperkeratotic nail bed is scraped with a solid or disposable scalpel or curette.
- Outermost debris should be discarded and sampling of distal nail plate should be avoided as it frequently contains contaminants that may obscure the growth of pathogenic fungi.
- Site of the nail with high yield of viable hyphae: Advancing edge closest to the cuticle.
- Transport of sample: Sterile container or a black paper.
- Processing of the specimen: Carried out within a week.

Table 16.4 Sites for sample collection

Type of OM	Sample collection site
DLSO	Nail bed and underside of the nail plate from the advancing edge as proximal to the cuticle as possible
PSO	Deeper portion of nail plate and proximal nail bed as close to the lunula as possible; paring the superficial normal surface of the nail plate is desirable.
SWO	Surface scrapings or shavings from the friable areas of leukonychia discarding the outmost surface and collecting the deeper white debris
Endonyx	Nail clipping

Source: Singal, A., and Khanna, D., Indian J. Dermatol. Venereol. Leprol., 77, 659–672, 2011.

DIAGNOSTIC TECHNIQUES

Direct microscopy

- Specimen for microscopy can be mounted in a solution of 10%–30% KOH or NaOH mixed with 5% glycerol or DMSO, warmed to emulsify lipids and hasten clearing.[11]
- Slide should be examined first under 10x and then under 40x lens magnification for fungal hyphae or arthrospores or yeast forms. Direct microscopy establishes presence or absence of fungi but cannot identify the specific pathogen or differentiate viable from nonviable fungi.
- Counter-stains: Chlorazol black, Chicago Sky blue, or Parker's blue-black ink can be used to increase the sensitivity and specificity.
- Calcofluor white (CW): Fluorescent whitening agent that stains chitin in the fungal cell wall can also be used but it requires a fluorescent microscope. CW was found to have a sensitivity of 92% and specificity of 95% in one study.
- Phase contrast microscopy: Helps to differentiate between types of hyphae or arthroconidia.

Culture

- Culture is essential for ascertaining the exact etiologic fungus.
- Different types of media used for culturing nail specimens include:
  - Primary medium containing cycloheximide that inhibits the growth of NDMs and bacteria, e.g., dermatophyte test media (DTM), Sabouraud peptone-glucose agar (Emmon's modification).
  - Secondary media like Sabouraud glucose agar (SGA) and Potato dextrose agar (PDA) that are free of cycloheximide and allow isolation of NDMs. Chloramphenicol and gentamicin may be added to SGA or PDA to eliminate bacterial contamination from nonsterile sites.

- Colonies of most dermatophytes grow in 2 weeks. All plates should be kept for a minimum of 2 weeks and absence of growth even after 3–6 weeks should be taken as a negative result.
- Microscopic morphology is studied by utilizing teased or Scotch tape preparations in lactophenol cotton blue (LPCB). Various species of Trichophyton can be differentiated by biochemical tests such as urease and hair perforation tests.
- Interpretation: Growth on both types of media is indicative of a dermatophyte while growth only on cycloheximide free media is suggestive of non-dermatophytic mold. If a dermatophyte is isolated, it is always considered to be the likely pathogen.
- Culture yield in OM is generally low. Higher culture sensitivity can be obtained by using a driller as compared to curettage and by proper selection of the site for sampling.[12]

Histopathology

- Histopathology of nail specimens using periodic acid Schiff (PAS) stain is very useful for diagnosis of OM.
- Indication:
  a. Repeatedly negative KOH mount and culture in patients with high clinical suspicion
  b. Differentiating from onychodystrophy caused by psoriasis and lichen planus
  c. To distinguish whether a fungus is invasive or a colonizer
- Presence of hyphae in the nail plate confirms the pathologic role of fungus and is considered to be diagnostic for OM (Figure 16.8).
- Histological sections may be improvised using a chitin-softening solution containing mercuric chloride, chromic acid, acetic acid, and 95% alcohol.
- PAS staining: Single method with the highest sensitivity in terms of detection of fungal elements (hyphae) in nail

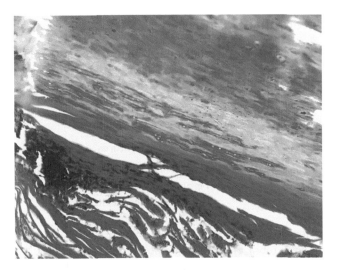

Figure 16.8 Nail plate showing hyphae (H&E x 400). (Courtesy of Dr. Piyush Kumar.)

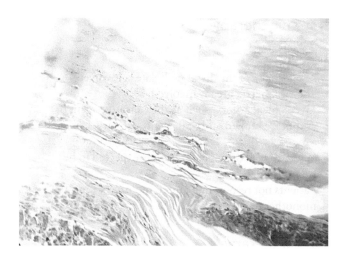

Figure 16.9 Periodic acid-Schiff stain showing fungal elements (PAS x 400). (Courtesy of Dr. Piyush Kumar.)

Table 16.5 Sensitivity and specificity of diagnostic modalities in onychomycosis

Method of detection	Sensitivity	Specificity
KOH Mount	50%–60%	86.4%
Fungal culture	25%–80%	100%
Calcofluor white staining	92%	95%
Histopathology using PAS stain	90%	High (regarded as gold standard)
PCR	93.3%	100%

Source: Grover, C., and Khurana, A., *Indian J. Dermatol. Venereol. Leprol.,* 78, 263–270, 2012; Shenoy, M.M. et al., *Indian J. Dermatol. Venereol. Leprol.,* 74, 226–229, 2008; Li, X.F. et al., *Eur. J. Dermatol.,* 21, 37–42, 2011.

specimens (Figure 16.9). PAS stains glycogen and mucoproteins in the fungal cell wall. In one study, PAS was found to be more sensitive than KOH preparation and culture alone (92% vs. 80% or 59%, respectively) and PAS staining plus culture had the best sensitivity overall (Table 16.5).[13]

- Grocott Methenamine silver stain provides greater contrast between the fungus and the surroundings.
- Limitations: Unlike culture, histopathology cannot differentiate between viable or nonviable organisms, nor does it help to identify the particular pathogen as both dermatophytes and molds produce hyphae and large, thick-walled arthrospores.

Onychoscopy[17]

Onychoscopy is dermatoscopic examination of nail unit and its components, namely, the proximal nail fold, lateral nail fold, hyponychium, nail plate, and bed. Longitudinal striae and jagged edges with other features such as intermittent spiked pattern (Figure 16.10), chromonychia, and distal irregular termination on onychoscopy are the findings that supplement the clinical diagnosis of DLSO.

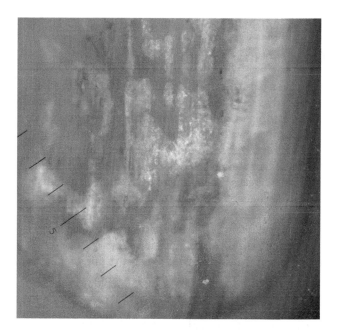

Figure 16.10 Onychoscopy showing onycholysis with longitudinal streaks and jagged spikes. (courtesy: Dr. Shekhar Neema.)

Newer modalities of diagnosis

Other less frequently used tests to diagnose onychomycosis include:

- Immunohistochemistry and dual-flow cytometry: These techniques are useful to identify mixed infections and allow for quantification of the fungal load in the nail plate.
- DNA-based methods: PCR-RFLP assays, double-round PCR, real-time PCR, and PCR direct sequencing have been used recently for detecting fungi.
- Triplex PCR: Very high sensitivity and specificity and can differentiate between dermatophyte, candida, and molds.
- Confocal laser scanning microscopy: This modality is comparable to PAS and is superior to KOH; however, their use is currently limited by their cost and complicated technique.[18]
- Optic coherence tomography: This is a reliable, convenient, noninvasive technique used to visualize fungal elements *in vivo* based on measurement of reflected infrared light intensity as a function of position. Several areas in the nail can be screened at once making it possible to detect persisting hyphae during systemic or topical treatment. High cost and limited availability currently prevent widespread use of this technique.
- Matrix-assisted laser desorption/ionization time-of-flight mass spectrometry and phase contrast hard X-ray microscopy are other techniques under evaluation.

TREATMENT

Considerations in treatment

- OM is a cosmetically disfiguring and debilitating disease adversely affecting the self-esteem of the patients and leading to depression. Apart from the pain and difficulty in walking, it carries the risk of cellulitis in elderly and diabetic foot in predisposed patients.
- Efficacy assessment are often based on final evaluation at 48–52 weeks, whereas it takes around 4–6 months and 12–18 months for a diseased finger- and toenail to be replaced, respectively.
- In the treatment of OM, the desired endpoints are mycological cure and clinical recovery.
- Mycological cure is defined as negative microscopy and culture. Clinical cure is defined as a nail without any clinical signs of OM whereas complete cure is defined as having both mycological and clinical cure.
- Clearance of the nail plate is defined either by clinical cure with 100% clearance of signs or clinical success with a residual affected nail area less than 10% with restoration of normal nail growth (at least 4 or 5 mm in 6 months) and no signs of onycholysis, hyperkeratosis, paronychia, discoloration, or fragility.
- An ideal antifungal drug would be one with broad spectrum of activity, favorable nail kinetics, economic, with good long-term cure rates, limited drug-drug interactions, and minimal or no side effects.[10]

Treatment options

Medical:

1. Topical
2. Systemic
3. Combination of topical and systemic

Laser
Light therapy
Surgical

MEDICAL

Topical therapy

Indications:

- Distal subungual onychomycosis (DSO) affecting <50% of the nail without matrix area involvement, without the presence of yellow streaks along the lateral margin of the nail and without dermatophytoma.
- A few (three or four) nails are infected.
- SWO restricted to the dorsum of nail plate.
- Melanonychia is absent.
- Thin, fast growing nails in children.
- Maintenance after a course of oral therapy is required as prophylaxis in patients at risk of recurrence.

Systemic therapy

Indications:

- At least 50% of the distal nail plate is involved.
- The nail matrix area is involved.
- Mycological criteria such as the causative agent or agents are known and oral agents can target specific fungi.
- When topical drug penetration is expected to be suboptimal.
- Patients not responding after 6 months of topical monotherapy.

Topical therapy

Advantages:

1. Direct application of medication to the affected area decreases the potential for serious adverse events such as drug toxicity and interactions.
2. Topical preparations ensure nail penetration within a few hours of treatment.
3. Pediatric OM responds better to topical therapy than adult disease.
4. Penetration of topical drugs is faster than oral drugs when used with optimum vehicle such as a lacquer.
   - Lacquers: Specialized transungual drug delivery systems (TUDDS) that produce a non-water-soluble film following application and evaporation of solvent that remains in contact with the nail for extended period of time. TUDDS provides high concentration gradient of the drug essential for maximal penetration.
5. The two main drugs that have been used topically are ciclopirox and amorolfine.

CICLOPIROX

- Hydroxypyridone derivative with fungicidal action against dermatophytes.
- Mechanism: It acts as a chelating agent and inhibits several iron- and aluminum-dependent mitochondrial enzymes and mitochondrial electron transport processes leading to reduced synthesis of proteins and nucleic acids.
- Rapid penetration into the mycotic nail keratin ensures escalation of the 8% concentration of ciclopirox in nail lacquer to 34.8% on application.
- Method of application: Applied to the nail as a coat daily over and above the previous applications. The layer of the lacquer is removed once weekly.
- Duration: Treatment needs to be continued for 48 weeks for an effective response.
- Mycological cure rates ranging from 46%–85% were reported in a metanalysis.[19]
- Side effect profile: It is generally well-tolerated with few adverse effects such as periungual erythema, transient irritation, and burning and itching of nail bed or adjacent skin.

AMOROLFINE

- Morpholine derivative with fungicidal and fungistatic effect against dermatophytes.
- Mechanism: It affects membrane fluidity by inhibiting two important enzymes—14 α reductase and delta 7–8 isomerase—in ergosterol biosynthesis.
- Concentration of amorolfine increases from 5% to 27% with solvent evaporation.
- Nail lacquer formulation helps in preventing reinfection and helps to increase nail hydration by semi-occlusion, thus limiting the formation and persistence of drug resistance fungal spores.
- Frequency of application: Amorolfine nail lacquer (ANL) is applied once or twice per week for 6–12 months.
- Clinical cure rates in the range of 38%–54% have been reported with amorolfine.[20]
- Side effect profile: Local irritation, onycholysis, contact dermatitis, and bluish or yellowish nail discoloration.

NEWER TOPICALS IN ONYCHOMYCOSIS

- **Luliconazole:** Recent data reveal that 10% luliconazole solution has very low systemic absorption and excellent local tolerability.
- **Efinaconazole:** Efinaconazole is a newer topical triazole antifungal that has been approved by the U.S. Food and Drug Administration (FDA) in June 2014 for the treatment of mild to moderate toenail OM. Complete cure rates were higher in mild OM patients treated with once daily 10% Efinaconazole topical solution.[21]
- **Tavaborole:** It is a new-class, boron-based, pharmaceutical approved in July 2014 by the FDA for the treatment of OM of the toenails due to the dermatophytes *T. rubrum* and *T. mentagrophytes*.
  - Tavaborole represents a new class of protein synthesis inhibitors that exhibit antifungal properties and is available as a 10% solution.
  - Tavaborole is a highly specific fungal protein synthesis inhibitor that targets fungal cytoplasmic leucyl-transfer ribonucleic acid (tRNA) synthetase (LeuRS), an aminoacyl-tRNA synthetase (AARS).

Systemic therapy

- Systemic therapy forms the cornerstone of treatment of TU.
- Systemic therapy, however, carries the drawback of high cost, low levels in nails due to decreased peripheral circulation, and drug interactions in elderly population.
- Oral antifungals used to treat TU include griseofulvin; azoles including ketoconazole, itraconazole, and fluconazole; and allylamine terbinafine.

GRISEOFULVIN

- Source: Penicillium species such as *P. Griseofulvum*.
- Mechanism: It acts by blocking the formation of mitotic spindle and is effective only against dermatophytes.

- The need for prolonged administration results in poor compliance.
- Mycological cure rates in fingernail infections are around 70%, while in toenail OM, reported efficacy is only 30%–40%.
- The adult dose is 500 mg to 1 gm given for 6–9 months in fingernail infection and 12–18 months in toenail infection. Dosage of Griseofulvin for the micronized form and ultramicrosized form are 15–20 mg/kg/day and 10–15 mg/kg/day, respectively.
- Absorption is increased with ultra-micronized or micronized particle form and with fatty food.
- It is contraindicated in pregnancy, lupus erythematosus, hepatocellular failure, and acute intermittent porphyria.

Azole antifungals

KETOCONAZOLE

- It is an imidazole derivative that acts by blocking the cytochrome P-450 enzyme used in the conversion of lanosterol to ergosterol in the formation of fungal cell membrane.
- Blockage of human cytochrome P-450-dependent adrenal androgen bio-synthesis may result in gynecomastia, especially at higher doses above 600 mg daily. Drug-induced hepatitis has been reported rarely.
- Daily recommended dose is 200–400 mg/day administered with meals for 6–12 months.
- Ketoconazole is not recommended for routine use in OM in view of its significant adverse effects, especially liver injury, and availability of more efficacious and safer options.

FLUCONAZOLE

- Water-soluble drug that possibly aids in rapid penetration into the nail plate with detectable levels at 48 hours. It persists in cured nails in high concentrations 3–6 months after the end of treatment.
- Oral bioavailability is high and not dependent on gastric ph, presence of food, antacids, or H2 receptor antagonists.
- It is not generally recommended as first-line therapy because of limited data concerning its use in monotherapy for dermatophyte OM.
- A recent review evaluating seven studies using fluconazole treatment for OM found mycological cure rates ranging from 36% to 100% for placebo-controlled studies. However, the cure rates were lower (31%) when compared with terbinafine (75%) and itraconazole (61%).[22]
- Hepatic side effects are lesser as compared to other congeners.
- Fluconazole inhibits both CYP3A4 and CYP2C9 and close monitoring is required when prescribing drugs metabolized by these enzymes with narrow therapeutic

index. Drug interactions are fewer with fluconazole especially when administered once weekly.

- Doses between 150 to 450 mg weekly for 6 months were clinically and mycologically effective as well as safe and well tolerated.[23]

ITRACONAZOLE

- Triazole antifungal with mechanism of action similar to ketoconazole, though it binds more specifically to fungal cytochrome P-450.
- It is a highly lipophilic drug with the oral bioavailability being maximum when taken with a full meal and is enhanced by acidic conditions.
- Itraconazole is incorporated into the nail through both nail matrix and nail bed and is detectable in the nail as early as 7 days after starting therapy and persists for up to 6–9 months following discontinuation of therapy.
- Monitoring for hepatic functions is recommended in patients with pre-existing derangement, those receiving continuous therapy for >1 month and with concomitant use of other hepatotoxic drugs and in those who have experienced liver toxicity with other drugs.
- It is contraindicated in patients with congestive cardiac failure due to increased risk of negative inotropic effects.
- Due to its ability to prolong the QT interval and increase the risk of arrhythmia, drugs like cisapride, pimozide, and quinidine are contraindicated for co-administration.
- Itraconazole is given as a 200 mg dose once daily for 3 months or preferably as pulse regime with 200 mg twice daily for 1 week each month. Two such pulses are given for fingernail OM and three for toenail disease.
- Intermittent therapy was shown to have equal mycological and higher clinical cure rates in a multicentric double-blind randomized trial comparing the continuous and daily regimen.[24]

Allylamine

TERBINAFINE

- Terbinafine, an allyamine, inhibits the fungal squalene epoxidase, leading to accumulation of squalene and deficiency of ergosterol.
- Terbinafine is well-absorbed orally with more than 70% bioavailability. It is widely distributed in various body tissues including the nail matrix.
- It is keratinophilic and detectable in the nail within 24 hours after initiating therapy and up to 90 days after stopping treatment.
- It is FDA-approved as a continuous treatment with dose of 250 mg daily for 6 weeks for fingernail OM and 12 weeks for toenail OM (Figure 16.11a–c).
- The LION study demonstrated superiority of terbinafine in terms of long-term mycological and clinical cure and lower risk of recurrence than itraconazole.[25]
- Gupta et al. and Sikder et al. found intermittent terbinafine regime consisting of two courses of terbinafine 250 mg daily given for 4 weeks with an interval of 4 weeks without terbinafine to be more efficacious than pulse itraconazole for treatment of toenail OM.[26,27]
- Yadav et al. suggested that Terbinafine in pulse dosing is as effective as continuous dosing and cost effective in the treatment of dermatophyte toenail OM.[28]

NEWER SYSTEMIC ANTIFUNGAL DRUGS

- Gupta et al. evaluated the role of ravuconazole in the treatment of DLSO. Mycological cure was seen in 59% of subjects in the 200 mg/day group, which was significantly higher than the rates found in the other groups. Headache was the most common adverse effect noted.[29]
- Posaconazole pulse therapy (oral suspension of 400 mg twice daily, taken with a meal on the first 5 days of each

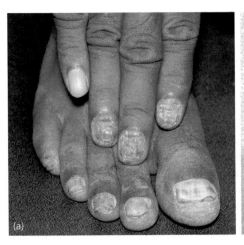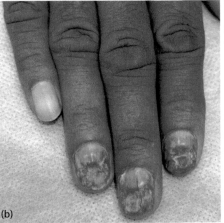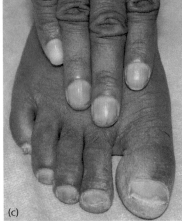

Figure 16.11 **(a)** Distal lateral subungual onychomycosis of toenails with total dystrophic onychomycosis of fingernails; **(b)** Improvement in fingernails after 1 month of continuous terbinafine treatment (250 mg daily); **(c)** Clinical cure of fingernails onychomycosis with significant improvement in toenails after 5 months of continuous terbinafine treatment. (Courtesy of Dr. Piyush Kumar.)

Table 16.6 Side effects associated with systemic antifungal drugs

Name of drug	Side effects
Griseofulvin	Headache, Gastrointestinal (GI) side-effects, and occasionally allergic reactions such as urticaria.
Ketoconozole	Gastric intolerance, hepatitis, gynecomastia, raised liver enzymes.
Fluconazole	Headache, skin rash, GI complaints, erythroderma, Toxic epidermal necrolysis (TEN) and thrombocytopenia, insomnia.
Itraconazole	Headache, GI symptoms, asymptomatic abnormalities of liver function, morbilliform rash, constipation, gastritis, pruritus, urticaria, thrombocytopenia, rhabdomyolysis, congestive cardiac failure, pulmonary edema
Terbinafine	GI, asymptomatic liver enzyme abnormalities, hepatitis, pruritus, urticaria and eczema, morbilliform rash, Acute generalised exanthematous pustulosis, TEN, Stevens–Johnson syndrome, pancytopenia, agranulocytosis and thrombocytopenia, Sub-acute cutaneous lupus erythematosus and systemic lupus erythematosus, bullous pemphigoid, and autoimmune hepatitis

month, repeated for 3 months) has been reported to produce partial response.

- Pramiconazole is a new addition to the family of triazole agents. It is absorbed rapidly and has a long half-life making once-daily dosing feasible. In pre-clinical studies, it has shown similar/superior activity to ketoconazole and itraconazole.

ADVERSE EFFECTS

The adverse effects of commonly used systemic antifungals have been summarized in Table 16.6

LASERS AND LIGHT-BASED THERAPIES

Laser therapy is becoming increasingly popular as a treatment modality in OM. The proposed mechanism of action of lasers in the treatment of OM remains unclear. Laser systems in near infra-red spectrum (780–3000 nm wavelength) exert their effect by direct heating of the target tissues. By using the pulsed beam mode, these lasers deliver "selective photo thermolysis" delivering of a short burst of laser light energy into the target tissue causing a rapid elevation in temperature into the defined target area. In the laboratory, eradication of the common dermatophyte *Trichophyton rubrum* has been demonstrated using pulsed laser technology.

Table 16.7 Device-based therapies in onychomycosis

Laser devices	Long-pulsed Nd-YAG, short-pulsed Nd-YAG, Q-switched Nd-YAG, near-infrared diode, titanium sapphire laser
Photodynamic therapy	5-aminolevulinic acid (ALA), methyl amino levulinate (MAL), Sylsens B (non-heme porphyrin)
Drug delivery systems	Iontophoresis (terbinafine), ultrasound (terbinafine, ciclopirox)

They all have been reviewed in the Table 16.1. These may circumvent the adverse effects of systemic therapies (Table 16.7).[30]

MODIFICATIONS OF CONVENTIONAL THERAPY

Combination therapy

- Clinical success rates are 35%–50% and 25%–40% for terbinafine monotherapy and itraconazole monotherapy, respectively. The relapse rate even in the best clinical trials is at least 25%. This has necessitated the use of combination therapy in an attempt to improve the cure rate and reduce relapse.
- Advantages: Combination of different treatment modalities may be synergistic with drugs acting at different levels. This may allow reduction in oral dosing and shorten the total duration of therapy and drug toxicity resulting in increased patient tolerance and compliance while improving efficacy and reducing relapse.
- Combination of amorolfine with itraconazole was shown to be more efficacious than itraconazole alone (87% vs. 46%).[31]
- Combination regimes can be administered sequentially or in parallel. In parallel treatment, both oral and topical drugs are given simultaneously and are used in patients likely to fail therapy. Sequential therapy involves administration of oral drug alone for a period of time followed by topical drug and is recommended for patients showing a poor response to treatment such as positive microscopy after 3–6 months of treatment.

Supplementary therapy

- Supplementary therapy involves microscopic examination and culture at 24 weeks or 6 months following start of therapy and extended administration of oral antifungal (4 weeks of daily terbinafine or another pulse of itraconazole) in patients with positive culture.
- Proposed rationale: Window of opportunity for booster therapy until 6–9 months from start of therapy, during which residual drug concentration can still be detected within the nail and a short burst of extra therapy during this time may be just sufficient to produce cure especially in patients who were likely to fail therapy.

Sequential therapy

- Sequential therapy combines the use of two oral antifungals working at two different pathways in ergosterol metabolism.
- In this therapy, patients were given two pulses of itraconazole followed by one or two pulses of terbinafine. The results were compared with patients receiving three to four pulses of terbinafine alone. Complete cure was seen in 52% versus 32% of patients, respectively.[10]
- Itraconazole is administered before terbinafine because the former is barely detectable in plasma 10–14 days after completing a pulse, thus limiting the cumulative hepatotoxicity and drug interactions of terbinafine and itraconazole.

BATT and BOAT

- The boosted oral antifungal treatment (BOAT) therapy was designed to target dormant chlamydospores and arthroconidia within the nail plate in order to produce sensitive hyphae that are less refractory to treatment with antifungals. This was performed by securing a piece of Sabouraud dextrose agar to the affected nail plate for 48 hours following the weekly pulse of itraconazole.
- A pilot study suggested that this protocol improved the mycological cure rate in comparison to conventional treatments (>90%).[10]
- A similar approach is boosted antifungal topical treatment (BATT), which was designed to improve the therapeutic efficacy of ANL.
- These therapies, however, carry the risk of over stimulation and systemic spread of fungi that are not susceptible to the antifungal agent and are therefore not yet widely accepted.

Surgical intervention

- Partial removal of the nail can be the most effective option in cases of lateral nail plate involvement or in patients with onycholytic pockets or dermatophytoma.
- Surgical methods can be used to remove part (debridement) or all (avulsion) of the nail plate. Such methods usually should be combined with oral and/or topical treatments and should not be used alone.
- Nails can be removed using a carbon dioxide laser.
- Surgical distal removal is a painful procedure and carries the risk of infection and abnormal nail regrowth (distal nail embedding), which is frequent. Nail plate removal should be accompanied by debridement of subungual debris from the nail bed or grooves.
- Malay et al. found combination of debridement and nail lacquer application (76.74% rate mycological cure) to be more effective than debridement alone.[32]
- Chemical nail avulsion involving application of keratolytic chemicals, such as 40% urea to the affected nail,

resulting in chemical onycholysis, can also be employed. Chemical removal should be reserved for patients with very thick nails and for patients unable to tolerate mechanical removal.
- Mechanical nail abrasion using sandpaper fraises or a high-speed hand piece at the beginning of treatment with antifungal nail lacquer decreases the critical fungal mass and aids the penetration of the topical agent into the deepest nail layers.

Relapse

- OM relapse is defined as the reappearance of the same infection, which could be due to either reinfection or recurrence.
- Recurrence is defined as the return of the disease within 1 year of therapy completion. Reinfection implies contracting the infection again after having achieved cure, usually after a period of 1 year.
- Therapeutic failure can occur due to lack of diagnostic accuracy, inappropriate choice of antifungal or mode of delivery, presence of dormant conidia as in dermatophytoma, sequestrated mycelium pockets or resistant fungal species, or lack of consistent penetration.

Drug resistance

- Terbinafine is the most effective and potent drug against dermatophytes. Resistance to terbinafine, though rare, has been reported.
- Resistance to azole antifungals is more widely known.[33]
- Organisms resistant to one group are usually sensitive to the antifungals from other groups, possibly suggesting a target specific mechanism of resistance.
- Antifungal susceptibility testing may be undertaken in patients showing poor or unsatisfactory response to the treatment. However, drug resistance is not the only cause of poor response. The moon factors responsible for poor clinical response and measures to correct them have been summarized in Table 16.8.

SPECIAL POPULATIONS

Pregnancy and lactation

- Itraconazole and fluconazole: Category C
- Terbinafine: Category B
- Use of systemic drugs should be avoided in pregnancy
- Topical therapies: Mainstay of therapy
- All oral antifungals are excreted in breast milk and hence contraindicated in lactating mothers[34]

Children

- Screen for concomitant tinea capitis and pedis.
- Screen for cutaneous mycoses in the parents/siblings.
- Griseofulvin: Only licensed antifungal for use in children with OM with a recommended dose for age groups

Table 16.8 Poor prognostic factors and strategies to manage them

Poor prognostic factor	Strategy
Areas of nail involvement >50% Subungual hyperkeratosis >2 mm Significant lateral disease	Consider appropriate oral therapy as first line, possibly in combination with topical. Surgical debridement or partial nail avulsion may be added if inadequate response.
Dermatophytoma	Early consideration for surgical excision followed by combination therapy
Positive culture at 24 weeks	Consider supplemental therapy Consider BOOST and BATT
Age >65 years Poor nail growth	Ensure bioavailability and compliance Monitor/assess for any possible drug interaction Consider sequential therapy
TDO with matrix involvement Patients with immunosuppression Diminished peripheral circulation Genetic predisposition Males	Consider combination (sequential/supplementary) therapy Educate and counsel regarding nail care Ensure treatment of affected contacts

Table 16.9 Weight-wise dosage of terbinafine and itraconazole in children

Weight (kg)	Dose of terbinafine (mg/day)	Dose of itraconazole (mg)
>40	250	200 mg/day
20–40	125	100 mg/day
<20	62.5	5 mg/kg/day

of 1 month and above of 10 mg/kg daily (micronized and ultra-micronized preparation).

- Terbinafine and itraconazole have been safely used in treatment of OM with favorable outcome and the former is approved for treatment of tinea capitis in children above 4 years of age (Table 16.9).[35]

Elderly

- Factors leading to increased incidence and poor response to treatment in elderly
  a. Poor peripheral circulation
  b. Diabetes
  c. Repeated nail trauma
  d. Longer exposure to pathogenic fungi
  e. Suboptimal immune function
  f. Inactivity or inability to cut toenails or maintain good/standard foot care
- Management of TU may include no therapy, palliative treatment with mechanical or chemical debridement, topical antifungal therapy, oral antifungal agents, or a combination of treatment modalities.
- Terbinafine is considered the drug of choice due to greater mycological cure rates, less serious and fewer drug interactions, and a lower cost than continuous itraconazole therapy.[36]
- Nail lacquers in the elderly:

a. Advantage: Monotherapy for patients with SWO or in combination with systemic antifungal therapy for patients with recurrence. Patients receiving multiple concomitant medications due to risk of possible interactions can safely be started on nail lacquer.
b. Disadvantage: Frequency of application, periodic routine debridement of affected nails, and long duration of therapy.

Diabetics

- Diabetics are reported to be 2.5–2.8 times more likely to have OM than the control population and the risk is further increased in male patients.
- The combination of ischemia, sensory neuropathy, and direct adverse effects on host defense mechanisms render these patients especially vulnerable to foot infections.
- Topical preparations: Preferable but carry the drawback of prolonged treatment and cumbersome application due to comorbid obesity and advanced age.
- Foot care interventions including nail drilling in combination with topical therapies have been shown to be effective in the treatment of OM in diabetics.
- Terbinafine forms the first line of treatment due to its relatively low risk of drug-drug interactions and proven efficacy in this population.

CONCLUSION

Fluorescent microscopy using CW and confocal laser scanning microscopy may play in the future an important role in the diagnosis of OM. Topical tavaborole, efinaconazole, and luliconazole are the recent additions to the therapy. Systemic therapy has been stranded at the pulse antifungal therapy and new regimes have not been widely accepted. Device-based therapies are gaining popularity.

REFERENCES

1. Gupta AK, Jain HC, Lynde CW, Macdonald P, Cooper EA, Summerbell RC. Prevalence and epidemiology of onychomycosis in patients visiting physicians' offices: A multicenter Canadian survey of 15,000 patients. *J Am Acad Dermatol* 2000; 43(2Pt 1): 244–248.

2. Yadav P, Singal A, Pandhi D, Das S. Clinico-mycological study of dermatophyte toenail onychomycosis in New Delhi, India. *Indian J Dermatol* 2015; 60: 153–158.

3. Gulgun M, Balci E, Karaoglu A et al. Prevalence and risk factors of onychomycosis in primary school children living in rural and urban areas in Central Anatolia of Turkey. *Indian J Dermatol Venereol Leprol* 2013; 79: 777–782.

4. Zaias N, Tosti A, Rebell G et al. Autosomal dominant pattern of distal subungual onychomycosis caused by Trichophyton rubrum. *J Am Acad Dermatol* 1996; 34: 302–304.

5. Hay RJ, Baran R. Onychomycosis: A proposed revision of the clinical classification. *J Am Acad Dermatol* 2011; 65: 1219–1227.

6. Rashid A, Scott E, Richardson MD. Early events in the invasion of the human nail plate by Trichophyton mentagrophytes. *Br J Dermatol* 1995; 133: 932–940.

7. Sobera JO, Elewski BE. Onychomycosis. In: Scher RK, Daniel CR, editors. *Nails: Diagnosis, Therapy, Surgery.* 3rd ed. Philadelphia, PA: Elsevier Saunders; 2005. pp. 123–131.

8. Carney C, Tosti A, Daniel R et al. A new classification system for grading the severity of onychomycosis: Onychomycosis Severity Index. *Arch Dermatol* 2011; 147(11): 1277–1282.

9. Fletcher CL, Hay RJ, Smeeton NC. Onychomycosis: The development of a clinical diagnostic aid for toenail disease. Part I. Establishing discriminating historical and clinical features. *Br J Dermatol* 2004; 150: 701–705.

10. Singal A, Khanna D. Onychomycosis diagnosis and treatment. *Indian J Dermatol Venereol Leprol* 2011; 77: 659–672.

11. Kaur R, Kashyap B, Bhalla P. Onychomycosis-epidemiology, diagnosis and management. *Indian J Med Microbiol* 2008; 26: 108–116.

12. Shemer A, Trau H, Davidovici B, Grunwald MH, Amichai B. Collection of fungi samples from nails: Comparative study of curettage and drilling techniques. *J Eur Acad Dermatol Venereol* 2008; 22: 182–185.

13. Weinberg JM, Koestenblatt EK, Tutrone WD, Tishler HR, Najarian L. Comparison of diagnostic methods in the evaluation of onychomycosis. *J Am Acad Dermatol* 2003; 49: 193–197.

14. Grover C, Khurana A. Onychomycosis: Newer insights in pathogenesis and diagnosis. *Indian J Dermatol Venereol Leprol* 2012; 78(3): 263–270.

15. Shenoy MM, Teerthanath S, Karnaker VK, Girisha BS, Krishna Prasad MS, Pinto J. Comparison of potassium hydroxide mount and mycological culture with histopathologic examination using periodic acid-Schiff staining of the nail clippings in the diagnosis of onychomycosis. *Indian J Dermatol Venereol Leprol* 2008; 74: 226–229.

16. Li XF, Tian W, Wang H et al. Direct detection and differentiation of causative fungi of onychomycosis by multiplex polymerase chain reaction-based assay. *Eur J Dermatol* 2011; 21: 37–42.

17. Nargis T, Pinto M, Shenoy MM, Hegde S. Dermoscopic features of distal lateral subungual onychomycosis. *Indian Dermatol Online J* 2018; 9(1): 16–19.

18. Cinotti E, Fouilloux B, Perrot JL, Labeille B, Douchet C, Cambazard F. Confocal microscopy for healthy and pathological nail. *Eur Acad Dermatol Venereol* 2014; 28: 853–858.

19. Gupta AK, Schouten JR, Lynch LE. Ciclopirox nail lacquer 8% for the treatment of onychomycosis: A Canadian perspective. *Skin Therapy Lett* 2005; 10: 1–3.

20. Lauharanta J. Comparative efficacy and safety of amorolfine nail lacquer 2% versus 5% once weekly. *Clin Exp Dermatol* 1992; 17 Suppl 1: 41–43.

21. Rodriguez DA. Efinaconazole topical solution, 10%, for the treatment of mild and moderate toenail onychomycosis. *J Clin Aesthet Dermatol* 2014; 8: 24–29.

22. Brown SJ. Efficacy of fluconazole for the treatment of onychomycosis. *Ann Pharmacother* 2009; 43: 1684–1691.

23. Scher RK, Breneman D, Rich P et al. Once-weekly fluconazole (150, 300, or 450 mg) in the treatment of distal subungual onychomycosis of the toenail. *J Am Acad Dermatol* 1998; 38(6 Pt 2): S77–S86.

24. Havu V, Brandt H, Heikkilä H et al. A double-blind, randomized study comparing itraconazole pulse therapy with continuous dosing for the treatment of toenail onychomycosis. *Br J Dermatol* 1997; 136: 230–234.

25. Sigurgeirsson B, Billstein S, Rantanen T et al. L.I.O.N. Study: Efficacy and tolerability of continuous terbinafine (Lamisil) compared to intermittent itraconazole in the treatment of toenail onychomycosis. Lamisil vs. Itraconazole in Onychomycosis. *Br J Dermatol* 1999; 141 Suppl 56: 5–14.

26. Gupta AK, Lynch LE, Kogan N, Cooper EA. The use of an intermittent terbinafine regimen for the treatment of dermatophyte toenail onychomycosis. *J EurAcad Dermatol Venereol* 2009; 23: 256–262.

27. Sikder AU, Mamun SA, Chowdhury AH, Khan RM, Hoque MM. Study of oral itraconazole and terbinafine pulse therapy in onychomycosis. *Mymensingh Med J* 2006; 15: 71–80.

28. Yadav P, Singal A, Pandhi D, Das S. Comparative efficacy of continuous and pulse dose terbinafine regimes in toenail dermatophytosis: A randomized double-blind trial. *Indian J Dermatol Venereol Leprol* 2015; 81: 363–369.

29. Gupta AK, Leonardi C, Stoltz RR, Pierce PF, Conetta B. Ravuconazole onychomycosis group. A phase I/II randomized, double-blind, placebo-controlled, dose ranging study evaluating the efficacy, safety and pharmacokinetics of ravuconazole in the treatment of onychomycosis. *JEADV* 2005; 19: 437–443.

30. Gupta A, Simpson F. Device-based therapies for onychomycosis treatment. *Skin Therapy Lett* 2012; 17: 4–9.

31. Lecha M. Amorolfine and itraconazole combination for severe toenail onychomycosis: Results of an open randomized trial in Spain. *Br J Dermatol* 2001; 145 Suppl 60: 21–26.

32. Malay DS, Yi S, Borowsky P, Downey MS, Mlodzienski AJ. Efficacy of debridement alone versus debridement combined with topical antifungal nail lacquer for the treatment of pedal onychomycosis: A randomized, controlled trial. *J Foot Ankle Surg* 2009; 48: 294–308.

33. Mendez-Tovar LJ, Manzano-Gayosso P, Velásquez-Hernández V et al. Resistance to azolic compounds in clinical Trichophyton spp. strains. *Rev Iberoam Micol* 2007; 24: 320–331.

34. Baran R, Hay RJ, Garduno JI. Review of antifungal therapy, part II: Treatment rationale, including specific patient populations. *J Dermatolog Treat* 2008; 19: 168–175.

35. Ginter-Hanselmayer G, Weger W, Smolle J. Onychomycosis: A new emerging infectious disease in childhood population and adolescents. Report on treatment experience with terbinafine and itraconazole in 36 patients. *J Eur Acad Dermatol Venereol* 2008; 22: 470–475.

36. Gupta AK, Konnikov N, Lynde CW. Single-blind, randomized, prospective study on terbinafine and itraconazole for treatment of dermatophyte toenail onychomycosis in the elderly. *J Am Acad Dermatol* 2001; 44: 479–484.

17

Non-dermatophytic onychomycosis

AVNER SHEMER

INTRODUCTION

Onychomycosis is a fungal infection of the toenails and/or fingernails that causes discoloration, thickening, and separation from the nail bed. Onychomycosis accounts for 50%–60% of all nail disorders, occurring in 10% of the general population.[1–3] This fungal nail infection is mostly caused by dermatophytes and yeast, while non-dermatophyte molds (NDMs) account for approximately 10% of onychomycosis infections worldwide.[4,5] NDM onychomycosis comprises a diagnostic challenge given that NDMs more often are innocuous contaminators of the nails and laboratory. Thus, diagnostic criteria have been suggested when identifying NDM as an etiologic agent.[4] Systemic treatment with oral azoles including Itraconazole and Fluconazole and oral allylamines represented by terbinafine is the common therapy. While efficacy rates have been established for these drugs for yeast and dermatophyte onychomycosis,[6] there is a paucity of data and contradictory results regarding the treatment of NDM onychomycosis.

EPIDEMIOLOGY

Onychomycosis is the most common nail infection, occurring in 10% of the adult population, increasing with age, and is more prevalent in males.[5,7,8] NDM is considered a less common onychomycosis agent, with prevalence ranging from 1.45% to 17.5%, according to different diagnostic methods and geographic locations.[9] A 2015 population-based review testing culture-proven toenails discovered NDM prevalent in 0.37% of the population.[10] Common NDM involved in onychomycosis include *Scopulariopsis brevicaulis, Fusarium* spp., *Aspergillus* spp., *Acremonium, Scytalidium,*[4] and *Hendersonula toruloidea.*[11] In South America, *Fusarium* spp. may be the most prevalent cause for NDM onychomycosis. In European countries *Scopulariopsis brevicaulis, Aspergillus, Acremonium,* and *Fusarium* are the most prevalent causes.[4]

ETIOPATHOGENESIS

NDM mostly invade toenails; fingernail onychomycosis caused by NDM is extremely rare.[1] The prevalent NDM are *Scopulariopsis brevicaulis, Fusarium* spp., *Aspergillus* spp., *Acremonium* spp., *Scytalidium* spp., and *Hendersonula toruloidea.* The infecting fungus invades the affected nails through either the hyponychium, proximal nail fold, or superficial outer layer of the nail plate. Each penetration site yields a different clinical presentation. From the initial penetration site, the infecting agent spreads and contaminates the remaining parts of the nail. Infected nails can contaminate other healthy nails in the same individual or other healthy individuals. Onychomycosis can cause discoloration of the nail plate, thickening, subungual hyperkeratosis, leukonychia, onycholysis (separation of nail plate from its bed), total nail dystrophy, paronychia, and pitting. Although NDM is isolated in onychomycosis cases, caution should be taken when establishing a diagnosis due to their role as innocuous contaminators of the nails and feet. To establish a diagnosis repeated cultures demonstrating the same NDM and excluding other infecting agents are needed.[4,11,12]

CLINICAL FEATURES AND SUBTYPES

Onychomycosis can cause discoloration of the nail plate, thickening, subungual hyperkeratosis, leukonychia, separation of nail plate from its bed, total nail dystrophy, paronychia, and pitting.[3]

Onychomycosis can be divided into seven different subtypes, according to mode of infection and fungal port of entry to the nail plate.[13]

The seven subtypes are the following:

1. **Distal lateral subungual onychomycosis (DLSO)** is the most common onychomycosis subtype. The invasion of the nail plate by the fungus begins with the hyponychium. From there the infecting fungus migrates proximally on the ventral part of the nail plate and over the nail bed towards the proximal nail fold.[13] Focal parakeratosis and subungual hyperkeratosis due to the inflammation caused by the fungus lead to onycholysis (separation between the nail plate and the nail bed) and thickening of the subungual area. DLSO may appear in variable clinical presentation. Usually the infected nail plate becomes thickened and opaque with a yellowish-brown color.[14] DLSO caused by NDM (Figures 17.1 and 17.2) has an appearance similar to that caused by dermatophytes, but it is often associated with periungual inflammation. In the case of *Acremonium* spp. DLSO, typically one or two thin longitudinal streaks are located in the middle portion of the nail plate.[4]

2. **Superficial onychomycosis (SO)** is divided into two categories: superficial white onychomycosis (SWO) and superficial black onychomycosis (SBO). SWO occurs when the infecting fungus invades the superficial outer layer of the nail plate. The clinical presentation is of patchy opaque white islands, which may coalesce and cover all or most of the nail plate as the infection persists. The nail becomes rough, soft, and crumbly. SWO occurs primarily in the toenail. *Fusarium, Aspergillus, Acremonium,* and *Scytalidium* could cause SWO. In SBO the discoloration is black and could be a result of *Scytalidium dimidiatum* infection.[11]

3. **Proximal subungual onychomycosis (PSO)** occurs when the infecting fungi invade the proximal nail fold and spread distally between the nail plate and the nail bed. The clinical presentation is of proximal onycholysis and subungual hyperkeratosis with a destruction of the proximal nail plate. In the case of mold PSO, *Fusarium* spp. is the most common pathogen. PSO associated with NDM involves proximal plate discoloration and may cause periungual inflammation.[4]

4. **Endonyx onychomycosis (EO)** involves the interior nail plate, without any nail bed involvement. Typical findings include nail splitting and discoloration, without subungual hyperkeratosis appearance. EO is usually associated with *Trichophyton soudanense* infection, but can be caused by other organisms such *as Trichophyton violaceum.*[15]

5. **Total dystrophic onychomycosis (TDO)** is the most advanced form of any subtype and is often an end-stage manifestation of PSO or DLSO. This subtype is characterized by complete nail plate destruction and presents as a thickened, keratotic debris-covered, opaque, yellow-brown-colored nail (Figures 17.3 and 17.4).

6. **Mixed pattern onychomycosis** combines one or more of the above subtypes. The most common mixed pattern onychomycosis presentation is SWO with either PSO or DLSO.[16]

7. **Secondary onychomycosis** is secondary to nail deformity such as trauma, psoriasis,[13] or other reasons such as cosmetic nail procedures.[17]

A systematic review by Gupta et al. in 2012 found 151 confirmed cases of NDM onychomycosis involving DLSO, SWO, and PSO. NDM onychomycosis was not found in other disease subtypes such as EO or TDO.[4] In the case of DLSO, four major agents were identified: *Scopulariopsis brevicaulis* (30.7%), *Aspergillus* (26.1%), *Acremonium* (17.0%), and *Fusarium* (14.8%); in SWO, *Acremonium* (44.7%), *Fusarium* (27.7%), and *Aspergillus* (25.5%); in PSO, *Scopulariopsis brevicaulis* (62.5%) and *Aspergillus* (37.5%) were identified.

A fungal infection of the toenails might also be subclinical (without a clinical manifestation). The normal-appearing nail plate may act as a reservoir for infectious dermatophyte and non-dermatophyte organisms. Once unimpeded by the immune-system, these organisms are inclined to proliferate to produce clinically apparent disease.[18]

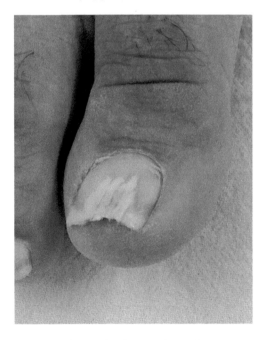

Figure 17.1 Distal lateral subungual onychomycosis caused by *Fusarium* spp.–initial stage. (Courtesy of Prof. Archana Singal.)

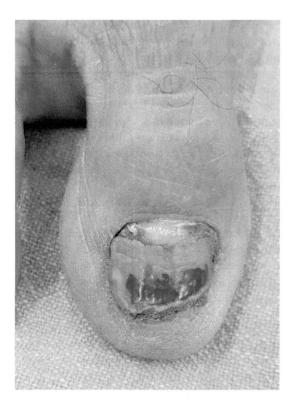

Figure 17.2 Distal lateral subungual onychomycosis caused by non-dermatophytic mold (species identification could not be done). (Courtesy of Prof. Archana Singal.)

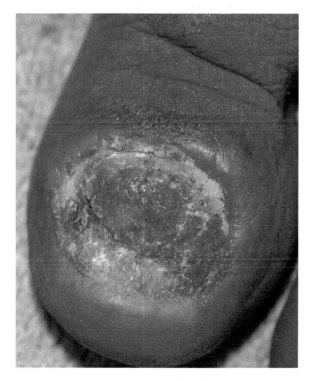

Figure 17.3 Total dystrophic onychomycosis caused by *Fusarium* spp. (Courtesy of Dr Soumyajit Roychoudhury, Consultant Dermatologist, Behrampore, West Bengal, India.)

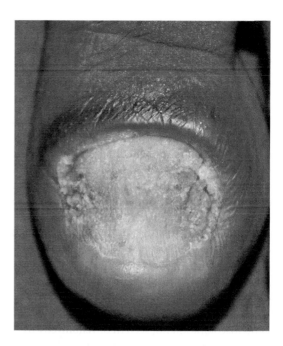

Figure 17.4 Post treatment image after 12 weeks of voriconazole. (Courtesy of Dr Soumyajit Roychoudhury, Consultant Dermatologist, Behrampore, West Bengal.)

DIFFERENTIAL DIAGNOSIS

Only 50% of nail problems are caused by onychomycosis, but other non-fungal etiologies may mimic the clinical presentation of onychomycosis. Although the clinical appearance and patient history can help differentiate onychomycosis from non-fungal etiologies, a definitive diagnosis is made by both direct microscopy and mycological culture. Predisposing factors such as diabetes mellitus, older age, immunosuppression, and nail trauma as well as a history of tinea pedis point to onychomycosis.[14] Clinical presentation of subungual hyperkeratosis, yellow-brown discoloration, and onycholysis are likely the result of a fungal infection but could also be the result of infectious agents, skin disorders, and chronic nail trauma. Some of these conditions are as follows:

Infectious conditions:

1. Chronic paronychia—chronic inflammation of the proximal paronychium caused by *Streptococcus*, *Staphylococcus*, or *Candida*. Clinical presentation may include changes in nail shape, color, or texture. There is often loss of the cuticle and separation of the nail fold from the nail plate. Other findings may include cross striations and nail growth disorders.[15]

Skin disorders:

1. Chronic dermatitis—Included in this group are contact dermatitis and atopic dermatitis. In the case of contact dermatitis, accumulation of a sensitizing substance occurs under the nail and may cause subungual dermatitis and

onycholysis. Periungual tissue inflammation can lead to acute or chronic onychodystrophy.[15]

2. Lichen planus—Fingernails are usually affected in the disease; however, in some cases the toenails might be involved. Yellowish-brown color, distal grooves or notches, onycholysis, subungual hyperkeratosis, and trachyonychia are among the nonspecific findings that might resemble onychomycosis. The characteristic findings in the nails are longitudinal grooves, longitudinal fissures, and progressive thinning of the nail plate.[15]

3. Psoriasis—Subungual hyperkeratosis and onycholysis are common findings of both onychomycosis and nail psoriasis. However, additional clinical features may help differentiate the two. In 80%–90% of individuals psoriasis usually involves other skin sites or joint arthritis; however, in 5% of the cases it may involve only the nails.[15,19] Clinical features that support nail psoriasis include fine pitting on the nail surface and oil drop discoloration (irregular areas of yellow or pink discoloration not seen in onychomycosis). Onychomycosis may coexist with nail psoriasis and is found in higher prevalence in psoriasis patients.[14,20] Shemer et al. have shown lower response rates to systemic Itraconazole in treatment of onychomycosis in psoriasis patients than in the general population.[20]

Trauma:

1. Footwear—onycholysis, subungual keratosis of the nail bed, nail plate abnormalities, paronychia, and even plate detachment due to friction of the toenails (especially the big toe) against the shoe

2. Cosmetic manipulation—may lead to paronychia caused by infection with *S. aureus* and *Pseudomonas* spp.[15]

DIAGNOSIS

The presentation of dystrophic nails in a clinical examination should alert the clinician to the possibility of onychomycosis, but a definitive diagnosis is made by both direct microscopy and mycological culture. The technique of specimen collection is imperative for a correct laboratory diagnosis. The sample must be collected according to the subtype of onychomycosis.

In the case of DLSO, the specimen should be obtained with a curette or a drill from the subungual area under the nail plate and the nail bed. When using a curette, collection of nail material from the most proximal site of the affected nail leads to the best results in the detection of onychomycosis and improves the culture sensitivity.[21,22] The drilling technique was found to be statistically better than curettage. Vertical drilling from the proximal part of the affected nail was found to be the best procedure for nail sampling.[22]

In SWO, the specimen should be scraped from the upper superficial nail plate with a number 10 or 15 scalpel blade. In PSO, the specimen is taken from the proximal subungual area with a curette, scalpel blade number 15, or by drilling.[13]

After obtaining the sample, a direct smear is performed as a screening test followed by a mycological culture with and without cycloheximide in order to identify the mycologic pathogen. Direct microscopy can provide clues about the pathogen's identity, but it cannot differentiate among pathogens, nor can it demonstrate viability.[16] In order to confirm the diagnosis of onychomycosis, viability of the fungal agent must be proven by a mycological culture.

Direct microscopy serves as a screening test for the presence of fungal elements. The specimen is placed in a 5%–20% KOH solution. The KOH dissolves the keratin leaving the fungal cell intact to be mounted on a slide. The mounted specimen can be mixed with 40% dimethyl sulfide to help dissolve the keratin. Heating the slide (1 h at 54°C) causes dissolution and lipid emulsification. The slide is examined under ×40 magnification.[7,14] A chitin-specific Chlorazol Black E can be used in order to accentuate to hyphae.[14] Parker blue-black permanent ink, lactophenol Cotton Blue (LPCB) (Figure 17.5), or fluorescent agents can also be added to enhance visualization.[4] The possibility of false negative result occurs at a rate of 5%–15%. The fungal elements visualized could help differentiate between dermatophyte, yeast, and mold and should match the mycological culture.[14]

After the clinical examination and direct microscopy, a culture will confirm the diagnosis of onychomycosis and identify the infecting microorganism. The specimen is placed on two different media. The first medium is used to test for dermatophyte in the specimen—a dermatophyte test medium or Sabouraud dextrose agar with supplementary antibiotics to inhibit bacterial growth and cycloheximide to inhibit NDM. The second medium contains supplementary antibiotics but

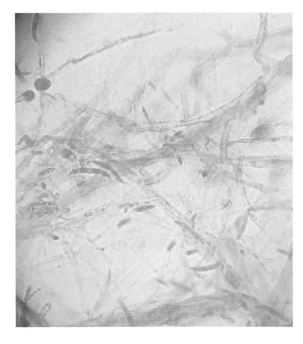

Figure 17.5 Lactophenol Cotton Blue (LPCB) wet mount showing *Fusarium macroconidia* and *microconidia*, isolated from case in Figure 17.3. (Courtesy of Dr Soumyajit Roychoudhury, Consultant Dermatologist, Behrampore, West Bengal, India.)

is a cycloheximide-free medium, allowing NDM to overgrow the slower-growing yeast and dermatophyte. The two media are grown for a period of 7 days to 6 weeks at 25°C–37°C. If growth occurs on both media the infecting agent is most likely a dermatophyte; if growth occurs only on the cycloheximide-free medium, the infective agent might be a mold.[14]

Although demonstrating viability, the culture cannot distinguish causative agents from contaminants.[4] This is especially the case with NDM, which are more often innocuous contaminators of the feet and nails. Dermatophyte exclusion criteria published by Walshe and English in 1966[23] still hold today. All dermatophyte isolates should be considered pathogens. All other isolated organisms are likely contaminants and need to be further investigated.[4,14] Direct microscopy result consistent with dermatophyte isolation is sufficient for a diagnosis. However, in the case of NDM more criteria should be met. Gupta identified six major diagnostic criteria routinely used in the literature and suggested using at least three of the six to rule out contamination.[4] The six major criteria being direct microscopy, isolation in culture, repeated isolation in culture, inoculum counting, failure to isolate a dermatophyte in culture, and histology.

Successive NDM isolations increase the probability that the isolated mold is the causative agent. Consistent isolations reduce the likelihood of a dermatophyte false negative result. If the fungal pathogen is a dermatophyte it will most probably grow in the successive cultures. If the isolated NDM is a contaminant rather than a true pathogen it is less likely to be consistently isolated[4,14] (Figures 17.6 through 17.9).

Mycological culture demonstrates viability but is time consuming and may be associated with false negative result.[24] Histologic examination of the nail using periodic acid-Schiff staining can provide results within 24 hours and was found to be more sensitive than KOH or culture alone.[24,25] Moreover, histology is the only method of diagnosis that can demonstrate nail invasion. However, histology cannot differentiate dermatophytes from NDMs, as it cannot identify the pathogenic fungus.

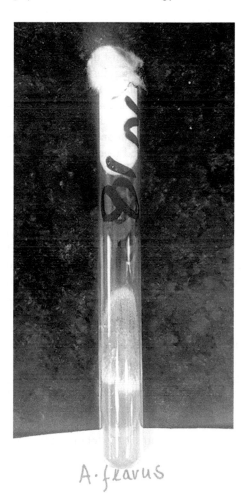

Figure 17.6 Yellow-green colonies of *Aspergillus flavus* can be seen. (Courtesy of Prof. Archana Singal.)

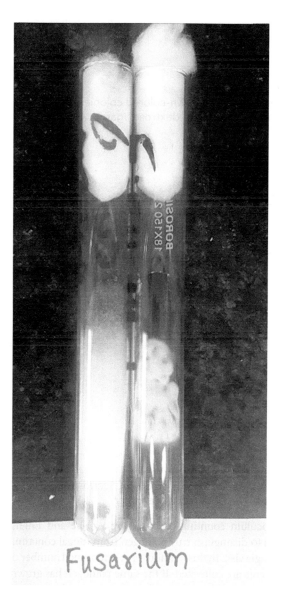

Figure 17.7 White-colored colony with velvety surface colony of *Fusarium* on PDA. (Courtesy of Prof. Archana Singal.)

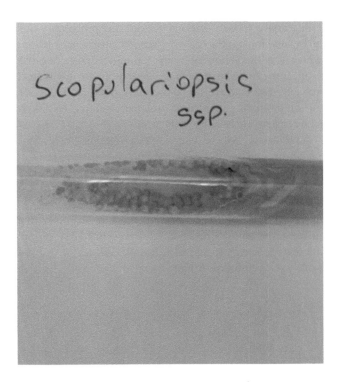

Figure 17.8 Light brown-colored colonies of *Scopulariopsis* potato dextrose agar.

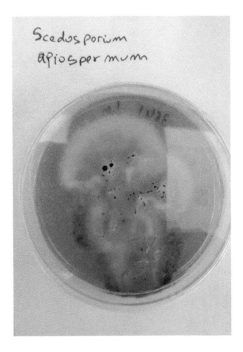

Figure 17.9 Smoky gray colony of *Scedosporium apiospermum* on potato dextrose agar.

Inoculum counting proposed by Walshe and English[23,26] aimed to distinguish true pathogen from fungal contaminants in a single visit. In this method, a predetermined number of nail fragments are cultivated. If the same pathogen has grown in a predefined number of inocula, it is presumably the causative pathogen. Walshe and English's criteria were a minimum of five inocula out of 20, together with compatible direct microscopy and no dermatophyte isolation in culture. Gupta has shown

that four inocula out of 15 (corresponding with 5 out of 20) was only predictive of NMD onychomycosis 23.3% of the time, and 89.7% for counts of 15 of 15.[27] Shemer et al. suggested that three nail samples from the affected nail, taken during a second visit, would suffice in diagnosing NDM onychomycosis.[11]

TREATMENT

Onychomycosis treatment's aim is to eradicate the causative organism and retrieve normal appearance. Therapeutic options include antifungal medications (systemic and topical), which are the therapy cornerstone, and physical intervention (laser treatment, surgery, and photodynamic therapy), which are less commonly in use. Data regarding the different therapies' efficacy against onychomycosis caused by NDM is limited. Topical antifungal treatment (Tavaborole, Ciclopirox, Efinaconazole, and Amorolfine) has shown some action against NDM, but efficiency as antifungal monotherapy is still undetermined and known to have limited nail plate penetrance.[28,29]

Systemic therapy is the gold standard for all types of onychomycosis. The older antimycotic drugs Griseofulvin and ketoconazole have been replaced by the newer more effective triazoles and allylamines. Griseofulvin has limited efficacy against dermatophytes and is not effective against molds and yeasts.[13,14] Ketoconazole was the first orally active imidazole with broad spectrum effect against dermatophytes as well as against NDMs and yeast. The drug must be consumed until total cure, meaning the affected nail has fully regrown. Side effects such as vomiting, headaches, abdominal pain, pruritus, and fever have been reported. Hepatotoxicity in a 1:10,000 reported incident ratio is the most significant side effect.[14] Due to the long-term consumption period together with significant side effects, this agent was of limited use in treating onychomycosis.

Itraconazole, a triazole, is a broad-spectrum antimycotic drug effective against dermatophytes, NDM, and yeasts. It was approved for the treatment of onychomycosis in 1995. Itraconazole interferes with ergosterol synthesis by inhibiting lanosterol 14α-demethylase. Ergosterol is a crucial component of fungal cell membrane. Itraconazole rapidly penetrates the nail plate and can be detected in the distal nail plate within seven days from treatment onset. The rapid distribution to the nail plate indicates diffusion through the nail bed. Itraconazole levels in the nails can be detected as much as six months after cessation of treatment.[30]

A continuous regimen of 200 mg/day Itraconazole for 3 months and a pulse regimen of 400 mg/day for 1 week, monthly for 3–4 months, are approved by the U.S. Food and Drug Administration (FDA). Total drug exposure (AUC) for pulse therapy after 3 months is 40% of that in the continuous regimen (743 and 1785 μg/h/mL, respectively). Besides its reduced cost, reduced total exposure in pulse therapy improves its safety profile in comparison to continuous dosing.[30] Efficacy in treating dermatophyte onychomycosis is well established in both continuous and pulse therapy with Itraconazole (Figures 17.10 and 17.11).

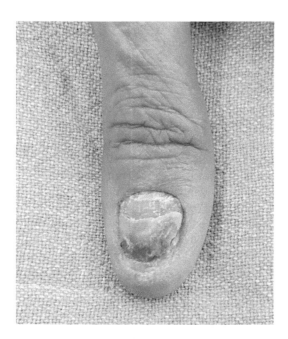

Figure 17.10 Distal lateral subungual onychomycosis caused by *Fusarium* spp. (Courtesy of Prof. Archana Singal.)

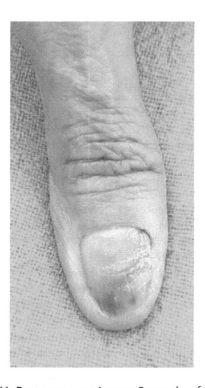

Figure 17.11 Post-treatment image: 3 months after treatment with Itraconazole. (Courtesy of Prof. Archana Singal.)

Terbinafine, the main representative of the allylamine class, was approved for the treatment of onychomycosis in 1991 in the United Kingdom. Terbinafine is highly effective against dermatophytes and some yeasts, but has low efficacy against NDM.[13] Terbinafine is both fungicidal and fungistatic.

Terbinafine interferes with ergosterol synthesis by inhibiting squalene epoxidase, an enzyme that catalyzes the conversion of squalene to squalene epoxide. This inhibition results in the accumulation of squalene in the cell cytoplasm and the deficiency in ergosterol. Terbinafine owe its fungicidal activity to squalene accumulation, which leads to lipid droplets within the cytoplasm, disruption of the cells' homeostasis, and the release of lytic enzymes, while its fungistatic activity is a result of ergosterol deficiency. Terbinafine is incorporated in the nail plate through the nail bed and nail matrix.[30] Terbinafine levels in the nail can be detected for six months after cessation of therapy.[14] The acceptable dosage for onychomycosis is 250 mg a day for 3–4 months.

Several studies have compared the efficacy of both continuous and pulse therapy using Itraconazole with that of a continuous terbinafine regimen in the treatment of dermatophyte onychomycosis.[31-34] Continuous terbinafine therapy was found to have superior cure rates in comparison to continuous and pulse therapy with Itraconazole. However, there is a paucity of data regarding the treatment of NDM. Several studies have shown Itraconazole to have the higher efficacy. A prospective study of 15 patients comparing the efficacy of intermittent Itraconazole with continuous terbinafine showed superior cure rates favoring Itraconazole.[35] In a similar study done in Sri Lanka, Itraconazole also had better cure rates against NDM. After three pulse treatments for toenails and two for fingernails, Itraconazole showed a 9.2% cure rate compared to 2.0% with terbinafine. After 12 months of treatment, cure rates were 65.1% and 54.64% for Itraconazole and terbinafine, respectively.[36] A systematic review by Gupta et al.[4] found evidence for the efficacy of Itraconazole pulse treatment and daily terbinafine in treating *Scopulariopsis brevicaulis* (24 of 32 and 12 of 14 complete cures, respectively). In the case of *Aspergillus* spp., terbinafine pulse treatment provided complete cure in 30 of 34 cases, pulse Itraconazole in 3 of 3, and daily Itraconazole in 4 of 7. Daily Itraconazole was ineffective in the treatment of *Acremonium* spp. (0 of 3 cases).

COMPLICATIONS AND PROGNOSIS

Onychomycosis could result in contamination of other healthy patients, and infected nails could contaminate other healthy nails in the same patient. Although onychomycosis is fundamentally a cosmetic problem, in immunocompromised patients periungual inflammation could potentially cause cellulitis.

Bad prognostic factors for the total cure of antifungal agents can be divided into four subgroups:[13] nail characteristics, patient characteristics, laboratory characteristics, and antifungal agent characteristics.

Nail characteristics

1. Thickened nail plate higher than 2 mm
2. Slow growth of nail plate

3. Involvement of more than 75% of the nail plate/bed
4. Nail matrix involvement
5. Longitudinal spike/streak
6. Lateral nail disease
7. Severe onycholysis
8. High nail severity index

Patient characteristics

1. Immuno-compromised individuals
2. Family history of onychomycosis
3. Poor hygiene
4. Older age
5. Down syndrome
6. Severe onychomycosis
7. Poor compliance
8. Poor vascularization
9. Diabetes mellitus
10. Severe tinea pedis
11. Recurrent nail trauma

Laboratory characteristics

1. False negative result due to cycloheximide in the fungal culture media that prevents NDM or yeasts growth
2. Misidentification of the fungus in the culture
3. Technical laboratory mistakes

Antifungal agents

1. Incorrect dosage
2. Drug interactions
3. Shorter period of treatment than needed
4. Incorrect antifungal agent (e.g., Griseofulvin for the treatment of NDM)
5. Poor bioavailability

Nail characteristics can predict good or poor response to treatment. Carney et al.[36] suggested the Onychomycosis Severity Index (OSI) score. OSI is a system that defines the severity of onychomycosis. It is obtained by multiplying the score for the area of involvement (range 0–5) by the score for the proximity of disease to the matrix (range 1–5). Ten points are added for the presence of a longitudinal streak or a patch (dermatophytoma) or for greater than 2 mm of subungual hyperkeratosis. Mild onychomycosis corresponds to a score of 1–5, moderate 6–15, and severe 16–35.

Another system for evaluating onychomycosis severity is the Investigator's Global Assessment (IGA), which assesses the overall severity of onychomycosis on the target toenail according to the percent of nail involvement according to the following scale:

0 = 0% nail involvement
1 = 0% to ≤10% nail involvement
2 = 10% to ≤25% nail involvement
3 = 25% to ≤50% nail involvement
4 = 50% to ≤75% nail involvement
5 = 75% nail involvement

KEY POINTS

- The clinical presentation of NDM onychomycosis cannot be distinguished from that of dermatophyte onychomycosis. Thus, NDM cannot be diagnosed based on clinical presentation alone.
- Since NDMs are more often innocuous contaminants of the hands and feet, NDM culture result does not necessarily indicate a true pathogen. Dermatophyte exclusion criteria and successive isolation of the same pathogen coincide with onychomycosis clinical presentation.
- Systemic treatment with either Itraconazole or terbinafine is the common treatment. There is a paucity of data and contradicting evidence regarding the efficacy of Itraconazole and of terbinafine for the treatment of NDM onychomycosis. Without clear evidence of which drug has the higher efficacy, either drug could be administered for NDM onychomycosis and can be replaced by the other in case of absence of response to treatment.

REFERENCES

1. Gupta AK, Jain HC, Lynde CW, Macdonald P, Cooper EA, Summerbell RC. Prevalence and epidemiology of onychomycosis in patients visiting physicians' offices: A multicenter Canadian survey of 15,000 patients. *J Am Acad Dermatol* 2000;43:244–248.
2. Thomas J, Jacobson GA, Narkowicz CK, Peterson GM, Burnet H, Sharpe C. Toenail onychomycosis: An important global disease burden. *J Clin Pharm Ther* 2010;35(5):497–519.
3. Narain U, Bajaj AK. Onychomycosis: Role of non dermatophytes. *Int J Adv Med* 2016;3(3):643–647.
4. Gupta AK, Drummond-Main C, Cooper EA, Brintnell W, Piraccini BM, Tosti A. Systematic review of nondermatophyte mold onychomycosis: Diagnosis, clinical types, epidemiology, and treatment. *J Am Acad Dermatol* 2012;66(3):494–502.
5. Gupta AK, Ryder JE, Summerbell RC. The diagnosis of nondermatophyte mold onychomycosis. *Int J Dermatol* 2003;42:272.
6. Gupta AK, Ryder JE, Johnson AM. Cumulative meta-analysis of systemic antifungal agents for the treatment of onychomycosis. *Br J Dermatol* 2004;150(3):537–544.
7. Westerberg DP, Voyack MJ. Onychomycosis: Current trends in diagnosis and treatment. *Am Fam Physician* 2013;88(11):762–770.

8. Sigurgeirsson B, Steingrimsson O. Risk factors associated with onychomycosis. *J Eur Acad Dermatol Venereol* 2004;18:48–51.

9. Tosti A, Piraccini BM, Lorenzi S. Onychomycosis caused by non dermatophytic molds: Clinical features and response to treatment of 59 cases. *J Am Acad Dermatol* 2000;42:217–224.

10. Gupta AK, Daigle D, Foley KA. The prevalence of culture-confirmed toenail onychomycosis in at-risk patient populations. *J Eur Acad Dermatol Venereol* 2015;29:1039–1044.

11. Shemer A, Davidovici B, Grunwald MH, Trau H, Amichai B. New criteria for the laboratory diagnosis of nondermatophyte moulds in onychomycosis. *Br J Dermatol* 2009;160:37–39.

12. Gupta AK. Treatment of dermatophyte toenail onychomycosis in the United States. A pharmacoeconomic analysis. *J Am Podiatr Med Assoc* 2002;92:272–286.

13. Shemer, A. Update: Medical treatment of onychomycosis. *Dermatol Ther* 2012;25:582–593.

14. Elewski BE. Onychomycosis: Pathogenesis, diagnosis, and management. *Clin Microbiol Rev* 1998;11(3):415–429.

15. Allevato MA. Diseases mimicking onychomycosis. *Clin Dermatol* 2010;28(2):164–177.

16. Elewski BE. Large scale epidemiological study of causal agents of onychomycosis: Mycological findings from the multicenter onychomycosis study of terbinafine. *Arch Dermatol* 1997;133:1317–1318.

17. Dyląg M, Flisowaska E, Bielecki P, Koziol-Galczyńska M, Jasińska W. Secondary onychomycosis development after cosmetic procedure-case report. *J Clin Med Exp* 2017;1:37–45.

18. Shemer A, Gupta AK, Farhi R, Daigle D, Amichai B. When is onychomycosis? A cross-sectional study of fungi in normal-appearing nails. *Br J Dermatol* 2015;172(2):380–383.

19. Brodell RT, Elewski BE. Superficial fungal infections: Errors to avoid in diagnosis and treatment. *Postgrad Med* 1997;101:279–287.

20. Shemer A, Tru H, Davidovici B, Grunwald MH, Amichai B. Onychomycosis in psoriatic patients: Rationalization of systemic treatment. *Mycoses* 2010;53(4):340–343.

21. Shemer A, Trau H, Davidovici B, Grunwald MH, Amichai B. Nail sampling in onychomycosis: Comparative study of curettage from three sites of the infected nail. *J Dtsch Dermatol Ges* 2007;5(12):1108–1111.

22. Shemer A, Davidovici B, Grunwald MH, Trau H, Amichai B. Comparative study of nail sampling techniques in onychomycosis. *J Dermatol* 2009;36(7):410–414.

23. Walshe MM, English MP. Fungi in nails. *Br J Dermatol* 1966;78:198–207.

24. Weinberg JM, Koestenblatt EK, Tutrone WD, Tischler HR, Najarian L. Comparison of diagnostic methods in the evaluation of onychomycosis. *J Am Acad Dermatol* 2003;49(2):193–197.

25. Wilsmann-Theis D, Sareika F, Bieber T, Schmid-Wendtner MH, Wenzel J. New reasons for histopathological nail-clipping examination in the diagnosis of onychomycosis. *J Eur Acad Dermatol Venereol* 2011;25(2):235–237.

26. English MP. Nails and fungi. *Br J Dermatol* 1976;94:697–701.

27. Gupta AK, Cooper EA, MacDonald P, Summerbell RC. Utility of inoculum counting (Walshe and English criteria) in clinical diagnosis of onychomycosis caused by nondermatophytic filamentous fungi. *J Clin Microbiol* 2001;39:2115–2121.

28. Gupta AK, Cooper EA. Update in antifungal therapy of dermatophytosis. *Mycopathologia* 2008;166:353–367.

29. Jo Siu WJ, Tatsumi Y, Senda H, Pillai R, Nakamura T, Sone D, Fotherfill A. Comparison of in vitro antifungal activities of efinaconazole and currently available antifungal agents against a variety of pathogenic fungi associated with onychomycosis. *Antimicrob Agents Chemother* 2013;57:1610–1616.

30. De Doncker P. Pharmacokinetics of orally administered antifungals in onychomycosis. *Int J Dermatol* 1999;38(Suppl 2):20–27.

31. Sigurgeirsson B, Billstein S, Rantanen T, Ruzicka T, di Fonzo E, Vermeer BJ, Goodfield MJ, Evans EG. L.I.O.N. Study: Efficacy and tolerability of continuous terbinafine (Lamisil) compared to intermittent itraconazole in the treatment of toenail onychomycosis. Lamisil vs. Itraconazole in onychomycosis. *Br J Dermatol* 1999;141(Suppl 56):5–14.

32. De Backer M, De Keyser P, De Vroey C, Lesaffre E. A 12-week treatment for dermatophyte toe onychomycosis: Terbinafine 250 mg/day vs. itraconazole 200 mg/day—A double-blind comparative trial. *Br J Dermatol* 1996;134(Suppl 46):16–17.

33. Bräutigam M, Nolting S, Schopf RE, Weidinger B. Randomised double blind comparison of terbinafine and itraconazole for treatment of toenail tinea infection. *BMJ* 1995;311:919–922.

34. Gupta AK, Greurek-Novak T, Konnikov N, Lynde CW, Hofstader S, Summerbell RC. Itraconazole and terbinafine treatment of some nondermatophyte molds causing onychomycosis of the toes and a review of the literature. *J Cutan Med Surg* 2001;5:206–210.

35. Ranawaka RR, Nagahawatte A, Gunasekara TA, Weerakoon HS, de Silva SH. Randomized, double-blind, comparative study on efficacy and safety of itraconazole pulse therapy and terbinafine pulse therapy on nondermatophyte mold onychomycosis: A study with 90 patients. *J Dermatolog Treat* 2016;27(4):364–372.

36. Carney C, Tosti A, Daniel R, Scher R, Rich P, DeCoster J, Elewski B. A new classification system for grading the severity of onychomycosis: Onychomycosis severity index. *Arch Dermatol* 2011;147(11):1277–1282.

18

Infections and infestations of nail unit

VINEET RELHAN AND VIKRANT CHOUBEY

INTRODUCTION

Bacterial and viral infections together form a sizable proportion of nail unit infections in most outpatient dermatology clinics. Nail units that have been damaged from previous trauma or any pre-existing dermatoses are particularly prone to certain infections. The intrinsic morphology and microscopic structure of the nail unit makes it relatively resistant to various types of infections. However, owing to the lack of an extensive circulatory system in certain parts of the nail unit, and thus a relative inaccessibility of the immune system to these parts, the body is unable to eradicate the causative microbes from the nail once the infection sets in. Therefore, a thorough understanding of the nail unit structure as well as etiopathogenesis of various bacterial and viral infections is necessary for appropriate management. As awareness for most nail infections is low, they often tend to go unnoticed and hence untreated, leading to significant physical and psychological morbidity.

Various bacterial and viral infections, and parasitic infestations affecting the nail unit have been listed in Box 18.1.

BACTERIAL INFECTIONS

Acute paronychia

Introduction: Acute paronychia usually results from local trauma to the nail folds from an ingrown nail, nail biting, thorn prick, or from certain procedures like manicure leading to pushing back of the cuticle.

BOX 18.1: Bacterial and viral infections affecting the nail unit

BACTERIAL INFECTIONS

Acute paronychia
Gonorrhea
Syphilis
Leprosy
Mycobacterium marinum
Mycobacterium tuberculosis
Diphtheria

VIRAL INFECTIONS

Herpes simplex
Herpes zoster
Hand, foot, and mouth disease
Orf
Human papillomavirus
Chikungunya
HIV

PARASITIC INFESTATIONS

Scabies
Tungiasis
Pediculosis
Subungual myiasis

Table 18.1 Acute paronychia compared to chronic paronychia

	Acute paronychia	Chronic paronychia
Clinical features	Erythema Swelling Raised local temperature Often pustules and abscess Fluctuance	Boggy swelling Erythema (less than acute paronychia)
Involved microbes	*S. aureus* *S. pyogenes* Rarely other bacteria	*Candida albicans* Rarely bacteria
Risk factors	Trauma Nail spa Finger sucking Nail biting	Wet work Irritant exposure (Homemakers, Housecleaners)
Management	Wet soaks Antibiotics Drainage	Avoidance of wet work and irritant exposure Topical steroid, tacrolimus Antifungals

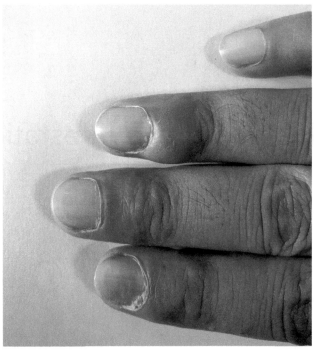

Figure 18.1 Acute paronychia. Erythema and swelling of the proximal nail fold of the ring finger. Traumatic retraction of the cuticle secondary to manicure can be spotted.

Trauma results in disruption of barrier function between the nail folds and cuticle and enables bacterial inoculation of the nail unit. Superimposed acute paronychia also occurs frequently in nail units damaged by chronic paronychia; the differentiation between both the entities is important (Table 18.1). Rarely, acute paronychia occurs as a manifestation of other disorders affecting the digits, such as pemphigus vulgaris.[1]

Etiology: Acute paronychia is most commonly caused by *Staphylococcal aureus*. Other organisms that may be involved include *Streptococcus pyogenes*, *Pseudomonas aeruginosa*, *coliforms*, and *Proteus vulgaris*.[2-4] In patients with exposure to oral flora, other anaerobic Gram-negative bacteria may also be involved.

Clinical Features: Acute paronychia typically involves a single nail. It presents as rapid onset erythema, edema, and tenderness of the lateral or proximal nail folds, 2–5 days after the initial event, usually trauma (Figure 18.1). Sometimes there is accumulation of purulent material under the nail folds, as may be evident from the drainage of pus on application of pressure. At times, frank pustules may be formed similar to a bullous pyoderma. If untreated, a subungual abscess may form that is extremely painful. This may become a part of a "collar stud" abscess that may communicate with deeper necrotic tissue via a sinus. As a consequence of such deep-seated infection in proximity to the nail matrix, transient or permanent dystrophy of the nail plate may occur. Pus formation can proximally separate the nail from its underlying attachment, causing elevation of the nail plate. Recurrent acute paronychia may evolve into chronic paronychia.

Complications: Complications of acute paronychia may include subungual abscess, cellulites of hand, and osteomyelitis. Recurrent or untreated acute paronychia may lead to nail plate dystrophy. Acquired periungual fibrokeratoma has also been reported.[5]

TREATMENT

Medical management

A course of oral penicillinase-resistant antibiotics should be started in all patients with superficial infections in addition to warm water soaks. Pseudomonal infection of the nail unit requires use of systemic fluoroquinolones. Topical ciprofloxacin, gentamicin, silver sulfadiazine, nadifloxacin, bacitracin, polymyxin B, sodium hypochlorite, and acetic acid have all been tried successfully.

Surgical management

If paronychia does not resolve despite best medical treatment, surgical intervention may be indicated to provide instant pain relief. Also, if an abscess has developed, incision and drainage must be performed. Surgical debridement may also be required in case of fulminant infection.

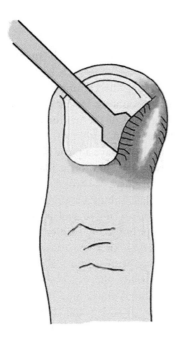

Figure 18.2 No incision technique.

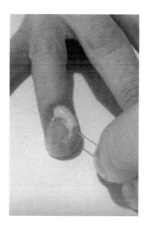

Figure 18.3 Simple incision technique.

No incision technique: Less advanced paronychial abscesses can be drained simply by gently elevating the eponychial fold from the nail by using a nail spatula or elevator (Figure 18.2). This separation is performed at the junction of the perionychium and the eponychium and extends proximally enough to permit visualization of the proximal nail edge. Then, the proximal third of the nail can be excised with scissors and the pus evacuated.

The wound should be well irrigated with isotonic sodium chloride solution, and plain gauze packing should be inserted under the fold to keep the cavity open and allow drainage. The patient should receive oral antibiotics for 5–7 days. The packing is removed after 2 days, and warm sodium chloride solution soaks are begun.

Simple incision technique: The simplest and often least painful incision can be made without anesthesia, using only an 18-gauge needle. The technique is performed as follows (Figure 18.3).

- The needle is positioned with bevel up and laid horizontally on the nail surface; it is inserted at the lateral nail fold where it meets the nail itself, at the point of maximum fluctuance.
- The skin of the nail fold is lifted, releasing pus from the paronychia cavity.
- A gentle side-to-side motion may then be used to increase the size of the incision made by the needle, improving drainage. This procedure is generally painless as the area incised is made up mostly of necrotic tissue.
- Gentle pressure can be placed on the external skin to express the remaining pus.

- The cavity can then be irrigated with saline.
- A small piece of 1/4-in gauze can be inserted into the paronychia cavity for continued drainage. The wound is subsequently covered with a sterile bandage.

Single-incision and double-incision techniques: If the paronychia is more advanced, it may need to be incised and drained. A digital anesthetic block is usually necessary. If an anesthetic agent is used, it should consist of 1% lidocaine. If the paronychia involves only one lateral fold of the finger, a single longitudinal incision should be placed with either a no. 11 or no. 15 blade directed away from the nail fold to prevent proximal injury and a subsequent nail growth abnormality (Figure 18.4). If both lateral folds of the finger are involved, incisions may be made on both sides of the nail, extending proximally to the base of the nail. The next steps are as follows:

- After the single or double incision is made, the entire eponychial fold is elevated to expose the base of the nail and drain the pus.
- The proximal third of the nail is removed.
- After the abscess is drained, the pocket should be well irrigated with isotonic sodium chloride solution, packed with plain packing, and dressed.
- The patient should receive oral antibiotics for 5–7 days.
- The dressing and packing are removed in approximately 2 days, and the affected finger is treated with warm soaks for 10–15 minutes, 3–4 times per day.

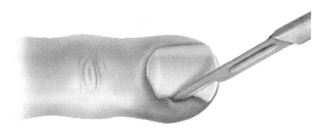

Figure 18.4 Surgical drainage for acute paronychia. The scalpel is advanced between the nail fold and nail plate to elevate the nail fold.

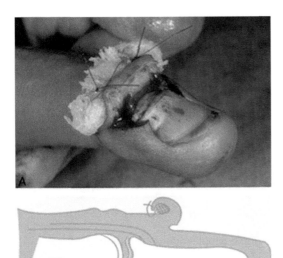

Figure 18.5 Swiss roll technique.

Swiss Roll Technique: The infection may continue under the eponychial fold and involve the opposite nail fold as a *runaround* abscess. In these patients, the Swiss roll technique described by Pabari et al. can be performed (Figure 18.5).[6]

- Nail fold elevated by making an incision on either side using no. 15 scalpel blade.
- Elevated nail fold is reflected proximally over a non-adherent dressing that is rolled like a Swiss roll and secured to the skin with two anchoring non-absorbable sutures.
- A simple dressing of the finger is done.
- After 48 hours, dressing is opened and wound cleaned. In severe chronic infections dressing may be kept for 7 days.
- Nail fold is allowed to fall back to its original position and it heals by secondary intention.

Gonorrhea

The hallmark of disseminated gonococcemia is the appearance of skin lesions. The most common skin lesions are vesicopustules, present juxta-articularly over the extensor surfaces of hands and toes as well as around the nails. Hemorrhagic bullae may also occur. Primary extra-genital cutaneous gonorrhea may present with a fingertip abscess extending under the nail plate.[7] A gram stain of the fluid obtained from the vesiculopustular lesions should be performed in suspected cases and followed by a culture if required. Histopathology shows intraepidermal spongiform pustules and leukocytoclastic vasculitis.

Syphilis

Syphilis can lead to nail unit involvement in varied forms (Table 18.2).

Fingers are among the common sites of primary extra-genital syphilis, accounting for 14% of the cases.[8] A chancre over the free edge of the nail or one of the lateral nail folds has been reported. Unlike other sites, these chancres are usually painful and have a more chronic course. Painless unilateral, epitrochlear, and/or axillary lymphadenopathy ensues. Nail involvement in secondary syphilis may include changes on nail plate, subungual tissue, periungual tissue, or finger pulp. Various forms of nail plate changes described include but are not limited to brittleness with a tendency to splitting and fissuring otherwise known as "onyxis craquelé," onycholysis, pitting with a linear arrangement of the pits from the root forwards, elkonyxis in and around the lunula, Beau's lines, onychogryphosis, and onychomadesis. The nail plate may become dull, dry, and thickened with a distinct line of demarcation between the affected proximal part and the unaffected distal portion that retain polish and color, but a wedge-shaped thickening of the free edge has been described. Dark brown pigmentation of the nail may occur, which may present as diffuse discoloration of the entire nail plate or as longitudinal streaks. The very rare amber-colored nail plates resembling false nails were considered by Degos

Table 18.2 Nail unit involvement in syphilis

Stage of Syphilis	Involved part of nail unit	Lesion
Primary	Periunguam	Chancre
Secondary	Nail plate	Thinning
		Thickening
		Dull dry nails
		Discoloration
		Fissuring
		Splitting
		Onycholysis
		Elkonyxis
		Pitting
		Beau's lines
		Onychogryphosis
		Onychomadesis
		Anonychia
	Nail bed	Subungual papules
		Subungual hyperpigmentation
	Periunguium	Paronychia
		Erythematous scaly plaques
		Ulceration
Tertiary	Nail plate	Anonychia
	Periunguium	Gumma

to be a characteristic change of late syphilis. Subungual papular lesions may appear later, which heal gradually, leaving behind hyperpigmentation. A pea-to-bean-sized patch appears under the normally transparent nail. At first the patch is intensely red, later yellow. The nail plate becomes thinned and fractured at this spot. In the moist forms, several nails may be affected, but often only one is involved. The lesion begins as paronychia followed by separation of proximal and lateral nail folds from the nail plate, allowing discharge of the entrapped inflammatory debris.[9] This results in a discharging horseshoe-shaped ulcer. If untreated, the nail later blackens and is shed, exposing an unhealthy-looking ulcer on the nail bed with permanent anonychia. Erythematous scaly plaques involving the paronychium have also been reported.[10] Syphilitic paronychia may also occur in congenital syphilis. The differential diagnosis includes acute septic paronychia, which is generally more painful, and chronic paronychia.

Tertiary syphilis very rarely affects the nail apparatus as gummata, which results in secondary necrosis with permanent nail loss when the matrix has been destroyed.

The disease is treated as per the usual recommendations that are followed in accordance with the stage of the disease.

Leprosy

Nail involvement in leprosy has been observed in up to 64% of patients.[11] Nail changes in leprosy can be caused by multiple factors including neuropathy, vascular impairment, infections, etc. (Table 18.3).

Table 18.3 Nail changes associated with leprosy

Mechanism	Lesions
Neuropathy, trauma	Subungual hemorrhage
	Melanonychia
	Onycholysis
	Onychauxis
	Brachyonychia/racket nails
	Onychogryphosis/claw nails
	Dorsal pterygium
	Onychoheterotopia/ectopic nails
	Anonychia
Vascular Insufficiency	Longitudinal ridging
	Longitudinal splitting
	Onychauxis
	Dorsal pterygium
	Thinning of nail plate
	Thickening of nail plate
Infections	Bacterial
	Fungal
Other causes	Pseudomacrolunula
	Leukonychia
	Terry nails

Trophic changes are responsible for grayish discoloration and loss of delineation from the rest of the subungual area, leading to what is known as a pseudo macrolunula. Nail changes in tuberculoid and lepromatous patients are similar, despite wide differences in pathology. Factors only associated with lepromatous disease are invasion of the bones of the terminal phalanges by lepromatous granulomas and endarteritis occurring during type-2 lepra reactions. These may result in multiple Beau's lines and dorsal pterygium. The phalanges develop osteolysis and there is progressive telescoping of the digital bones. When deformities such as a "preacher's hand" occur, claw nails and other unusual appearances are produced. Dystrophic changes may occur in the nails, with progressive destruction, leaving small fragments at the corner of the nail bed, or ventral pterygium.[12] Painless abscesses may occur periungually with destruction of the nails. This appears more often in the upper than lower limbs. Walking barefoot, the sitting position normally assumed and the type of footwear all produce anatomical and physiological changes in the feet and legs. They may lead to pathological processes or modify those that pre- or coexist (Figures 18.6 through 18.8).

In one study, 300 leprosy patients were recruited to study the pattern and frequency of nail changes. The most common nail change was longitudinal melanonychia, which is caused when repeated trauma occurs, leading to activation of melanocytes.[11] In an Egyptian study including 115 leprosy patients and 60 patients with diabetic peripheral neuropathy, a similar incidence of nail changes was detected in both multibacillary and paucibacillary patients (86%). Flag sign (alternating horizontal bands of whitish and pinkish discoloration of the nail) has also been described.

Mycobacterium marinum infection

Mycobacterium marinum infection may present in fish-tank or aquarium cleaners and in individuals who frequently obtain pedicures, initially as paronychia or as granulomatous papules, nodules, plaques, or ulceration. Abscess formation has been reported as well. A break in the skin is necessary for inoculation. A history of trauma while working in tanks may be obtained in some patients, following which symptoms manifest after a varied incubation period of 5–270 days (average 21 days).[13] Diagnosis is often missed and a history of occupational exposure gives an important clue. Diagnosis can be best made by molecular methods. Culture may yield the mycobacterium in about half the cases.[14] Histopathological examination shows a mixed infiltrate of neutrophils with lymphocytes as well as foreign body giant cells, with granulomas. Treatment usually comprises a combination of cotrimoxazole, rifampicin, tetracyclines, or clarithromycin.

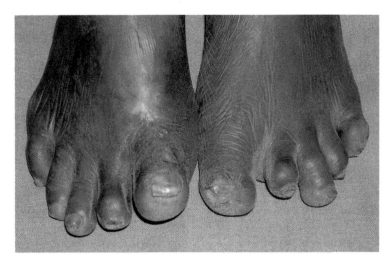

Figure 18.6 Dystrophic nail in case of lepromatous leprosy.

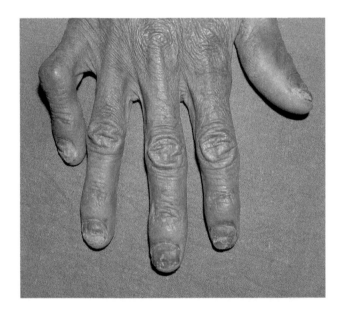

Figure 18.7 Leukonychia and dystrophic nail in borderline tuberculoid leprosy.

Mycobacterium tuberculosis

Tuberculosis verrucosa cutis or warty tuberculosis is a paucibacillary form of cutaneous tuberculosis that occurs in previously sensitized individuals having a moderate or high degree of immunity. It usually occurs by traumatic exogenous inoculation into the skin through open wounds. People walking barefoot are particularly at risk. It is also known as "prosector's warts." Rarely, it can also occur by autoinoculation with sputum in a patient with pulmonary tuberculosis. Common sites of lesions are knees, ankles, buttocks, and hands. Tuberculous paronychia associated with warty tuberculosis has been reported as well.[15] The lesion starts as an indurated, warty papule with an inflammatory margin. Gradually, the papule enlarges irregularly forming a firm verrucous plaque with a serpiginous outline. The center may heal with atrophic scarring. At times, exudate and crusting may occur. On histopathological examination, pseudo epitheliomatous hyperplasia with superficial abscess formation is almost always seen. Bacilli are seen only occasionally. Lesions must be distinguished from warts, and

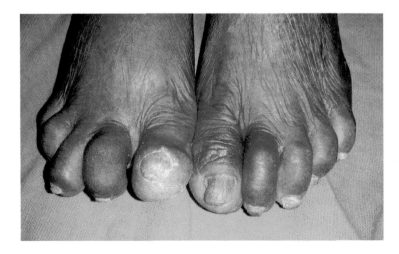

Figure 18.8 Thickened and pigmented nail plate of anesthetic feet in leprosy.

from leishmaniasis when crusted lesions are present. The condition is indolent and lesions may remain dormant for months or years. Spontaneous remission may occur, leaving behind atrophic scars. Response to antitubercular treatment is usually good, except when the disease is caused by non-tuberculous mycobacteria, when culture may be required to confirm the etiological agent. PCR may be helpful if positive but is often negative as this is a paucibacillary form.

Scrofuloderma is a multibacillary form of cutaneous tuberculosis that occurs by contagious spread from an underlying focus of infection, usually lymph nodes, bones, and joints. Scrofuloderma presenting clinically as dactylitis and chronic paronychia has been reported.[16] The exuberant granulation tissue extending from the proximal nail fold to the nail plate resembles a pterygium and therefore has been known to form a "pseudo pterygium." Like any chronic paronychia, tubercular paronychia can lead further to nail matrix abnormalities and subsequently nail dystrophy.[16] Most of the cases presenting as tuberculous dactylitis are of pediatric age group.[17]

Diphtheria

With the advent of immunization, cutaneous diphtheria is rarely encountered these days. However, cases have been reported in travelers to endemic areas.[18] Typically, the disease begins as a pustule and then evolves into an ulcer varying in size from 0.5 cm to a few centimeters in diameter that is covered with a pseudo-membrane that bleeds on removal and has erythematous edges. Within 1–3 weeks, the false membrane turns into a blackish scab and rapidly falls off, leaving behind a residual ulcer that gradually heals with an atrophic scar. Cutaneous diphtheria most often appears on areas afflicted by preexisting dermatological conditions such as traumatic wounds, burns, insect bites, and infection. The commonly involved sites are lower and upper limbs. Differential diagnosis includes impetigo and ecthyma.

VIRAL INFECTIONS

Herpes simplex virus

Herpes simplex virus (HSV) infection may affect the pulp of terminal phalanx as herpetic whitlow or present as an acute paronychia.

Etiopathogenesis: Herpes simplex infection of the digits has a bimodal age of distribution.[19] It occurs more frequently in infants and young children. In this age group, the disease results from autoinoculation from herpetic gingiva-stomatitis during thumb sucking or nail biting. In young adults, the auto-inoculation may occur from lesions of oro-labial or genital herpes. Many cases of herpetic digital infection have been reported among dentists or anesthetists who are prone to trauma while performing various oro-dental procedures or

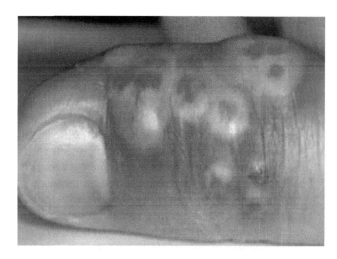

Figure 18.9 Herpetic infection presenting as grouped vesicles and pustules.

intubation in patients with oro-labial herpes, especially if protective hand gear is not worn.[19]

Clinical features: After an incubation period of 3–7 days following inoculation, vesicles appear in crops at the portal of entry, typically around the paronychium or on the volar digital skin (Figure 18.9). Thumb and index finger are more commonly affected compared to other digits.[20] During initial phase, severe throbbing pain, tenderness, erythema, and edema may accompany the vesicles. Vesicles increase in size and number for an initial 1–14 days, often coalescing to form large, honeycomb-like bullae. With time, the fluid inside vesicles may become turbid, sero-purulent, or even hemorrhagic or the vesicles may rupture leading to the formation of erosions with characteristic polycyclic margins. In a subset of patients, the disease may be recurrent, in which case the signs are subtle and acute inflammatory changes accompanying the vesicles may not manifest. Primary herpetic infection of the mouth, fingernails, or genitalia may coexist. Radiating pain along the C7 distribution is sometimes noted and may predict the onset of recurrent herpetic whitlows. Lymphangitis is almost always present and may even precede the vesicles by 1 or 2 days. It usually starts from the wrist and extends to the axilla where axillary lymphadenitis may be appreciated. Persistent lymph-edema may occur. Numbness and hypoesthesia following the acute episode have been reported.[21] Herpetic meningitis has also been reported.[22]

Diagnosis: The diagnosis of herpetic paronychia and herpetic whitlow is mainly clinical. Tzanck smear may help in confirmation of the diagnosis. Multinucleated giant epidermal cells formed by cytopathic effect of the virus are characteristic, but the sensitivity of Tzanck smear is low. Viral culture is confirmatory and is usually positive within 24–48 hours. Negative staining of blister fluid followed by electron microscopy may be performed to visualize viral particles. Monoclonal antibodies or PCR allow confirmation of the diagnosis by immunofluorescence and also differentiation of type 1 from type 2 HSV.

In AIDS patients, herpetic nail infection may have an atypical presentation and lesions tend to be persistent. Ulceration and necrosis are more common, whereas recurrent herpes tends to be severe.

Differential diagnosis: It is important to exclude primary or recurrent herpes simplex infection in the differential diagnosis of every finger infection. Felon presents with increased tension in the finger pulp as there is a frank collection of pus. The typical appearance of the lesions with a disproportionate intensity of pain, presence of vesicles, and lack of increased tension in the finger pulp aid in distinguishing herpetic whitlow from a felon. *Mycobacterium marinum* infection needs to be ruled out.

Treatment: Treatment is primarily supportive and aimed at relief of pain and prevention of secondary bacterial infection. Acyclovir started early in the course of disease at a dose of 400 mg thrice a day for 5–7 days may reduce the duration of lesions and neuropathic pain. Prolonged continuous oral acyclovir (400 mg twice daily) may be required in patients with recurrent herpes simplex infections.

Herpes zoster

Herpes zoster may rarely involve the nail unit and present as grouped vesicles on the proximal nail fold associated with pain. Nail bed involvement may leave behind small grouped subungual hemorrhagic vesicles or crusting.[23] Herpes zoster may produce transverse leukonychia caused by a temporary disturbance in keratinization of nail matrix.[24]

Hand, foot, and mouth disease

Hand-foot-mouth disease is a viral infection of childhood that is caused by viruses of the genus Enterovirus and is commoner in summers and autumn. Coxsackievirus A6 is the most common causative agent followed by Enterovirus A71.[25] It usually occurs in small epidemics and is characterized by erosive stomatitis along with palmoplantar vesicular eruptions. Beau's lines, yellow orange discoloration of the nail plate, and onychomadesis (Figure 18.10) are common long-term sequelae.[26] After 36–39 days of an outbreak in a Spanish nursery, onychomadesis occurred in two-thirds of the patients and Beau's lines in one-third. Enterovirus was detected in stool samples in 47% of the patients.[27] No treatment is required as the pathology is self-limiting and growth of normal nail ensues gradually over a span of a few months.

Orf virus

Orf is a parapox virus that is usually transmitted to humans from sheep or goats. Orf virus infection is known as ecthyma contagiosum and is commonly seen in butchers and herd handlers. In Muslim-predominated communities, orf infection of the hands is seen as a yearly outbreak as goats and sheep are sacrificed as part of festivities.[28] Animals infected with orf virus typically develop scabby sores around their mouth. A break in the skin caused by trivial trauma is required for inoculation in humans. After 3–5 days, a

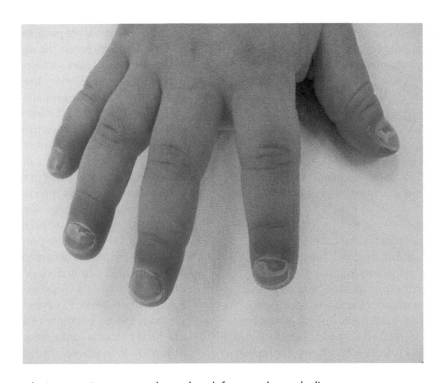

Figure 18.10 Onychomadesis occurring as sequelae to hand, foot, and mouth disease.

pruritic firm papule or nodule surrounded by a halo appears at the site of trauma that ulcerates over a span of days to weeks, revealing a granulomatous lesion. Hands are the most common sites to be involved. Paronychium is often the primary site of inoculation. The disease is self-limiting and the lesion undergoes spontaneous resolution over 6–8 weeks. Failure of spontaneous resolution may be seen in immune-compromised patients, when excision may be required. In a case series, topical imiquimod applied for a week was found to be effective in shortening the time required to healing.[29]

Human papillomavirus

Human papillomavirus is a small epitheliotropic DNA virus that usually causes warts. HPV is transmitted by inoculation following trauma. The virus first infects the basal stem cells of skin. As the cells differentiate and undergo maturation, the viral particles move up along the layers of skin. It's only in the cells of upper layers of the epidermis, i.e., stratum spinosum and stratum granulosum, that the virus replicates. Therefore, in the lower layers of the skin, only viral genome is usually detectable, whereas completely formed viral particles can be found in the upper layers. Besides trauma, those neonates and children who are habitual thumb-suckers or nail-biters are also prone to periungual warts. Occupational meat handlers and wet workers are likely to have impaired barrier function of the nail unit and thus are at risk of developing warts. HPV-1, 2, 4, 5, 7, 27, and 57 cause periungual and subungual warts. They present as firm, verrucous, hyperkeratotic, yellowish-brown, or flesh-colored papules that may coalesce into plaques in the periungual and often extending beneath the nail plate into the nail bed (Figures 18.11 and 18.12). The

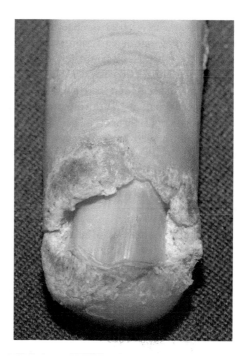

Figure 18.11 Periungual warts.

plaques are typically characterized by the loss of dermatoglyphics. Tiny black dots that represent thrombosed dilated capillaries may be visible at the surface of the lesions and appear when an immune response has been mounted against the viral antigens in an individual lesion. These are pathognomonic of warts. The lesions are generally asymptomatic but can be painful when compressed. Warts, in general, tend to regress and often disappear on their own, although the time

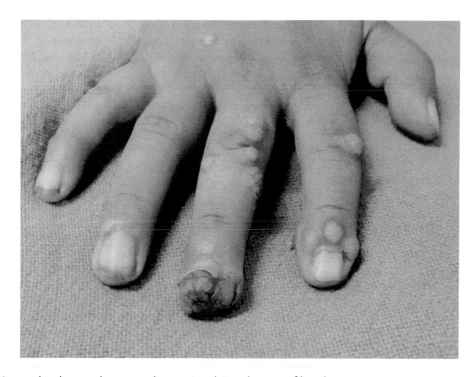

Figure 18.12 Periungual, subungual wart, and warts involving dorsum of hands.

required for the same may vary from a few months to years. The painstakingly slow rate of regression, risk of autoinoculation, and spread to other sites warrant active treatment of all warts. However, periungual warts pose a huge challenge, as the area is difficult to access and there is a possibility of damage to the underlying nail matrix during the treatment, leading to permanent disfigurement of the nail. In addition, these warts have high rate of recurrence. Various treatment modalities have been tried with varying outcomes (Tables 18.4 and 18.5) (Figure 18.13).[30,31,32]

Chikungunya

Nail changes that have been associated with chikungunya include diffuse melanonychia, longitudinal melanonychia, red lunula, black lunula, subungual hemorrhage, periungual ulceration, periungual exfoliation, etc.[33,34]

HIV

Proximal subungual onychomycosis (PSO) is rarely encountered in healthy immune-competent individuals. In contrast, individuals living with AIDS are more likely to develop PSO. Another important association of HIV is with candidal OM, which is more frequent in immunosuppressed states. Particularly, individuals with chronic mucocutaneous candidiasis are at a higher risk of developing candidal OM. Progressive, dose-dependent pigmentation of the nail plate is common secondary to Zidovudine. It has been reported to occur as early as 2 weeks after the initiation of the drug,

Table 18.4 Treatment modalities used for periungual and subungual warts[30,31,32]

Mode	Treatment	Mechanism	Remarks
Topical	Salicylic Acid	• Keratolytic action • May also induce inflammation leading to an immune response	• SA 12%–27% may be applied daily or as a 40% patch • Filing before application or application under occlusion may be required for hyperkeratotic lesions
	Trichloroacetic Acid	• Caustic action • May induce inflammation leading to an immune response	• Used in various concentrations ranging from 70% to 100% • Applied and allowed to dry • Frosting develops as solution dries up
	Dinitrochlorobenzene	• Contact sensitization leading to Type-IV hypersensitivity	• Mutagenic • Not used these days
	Diphenylcyclopropenone	• Contact sensitization leading to Type-IV hypersensitivity	• Most easily available • Affordable
	Squaric acid dibutylester	• Contact sensitization leading to Type-IV hypersensitivity	• Availability an issue • Expensive
	Podophyllin	• Inhibits polymerization of mitotic spindles leading to mitotic arrest (anti-mitotic) • Antiviral properties	• Available as 20% podophyllum resin • Air dried after application • Poor efficacy in hyperkeratotic lesions • Has to be washed after 2–4 hours to prevent systemic absorption
	Imiquimod	• Immunomodulatory activity • Induces IFN-α, TNF-α, IL-1, IL-6, and T_H1 response and aids in killing viral particles and virus-infected cells	• 5% cream used • Inconsistent results
	Cidofovir	• Nucleoside analogue • Competitively inhibits DNA polymerase and thus prevents replication of viral cells	• Applied 5 days a week under occlusion • Not widely available
	Glutaraldehyde	• Virucidal action	• 10% GA applied twice a day • 70% cure rate • Stains the skin brown
	Cantharidin	• Irritant action leads to inflammation	• Kept under occlusion for 24 hours or applied after paring

(Continued)

Table 18.4 (*Continued*) Treatment modalities used for periungual and subungual warts

Mode	Treatment	Mechanism	Remarks

Intralesional	Bleomycin	• Transfers electrons from its Fe^{2+} core to the DNA causing strand scission (anti-mitotic)	• Reconstituted 1 unit/mL solution used
			• Two methods:
			  a. Intralesional injection: Dose as per Table 5
			  b. Prick method[43]: Multiple pricks made on wart followed by spraying bleomycin
			• Maximum 2 mL dose per sitting accepted as safe in terms of systemic adverse effects
			• Response in 1 or 2 sittings
			• Cure rates >90%
			• Very painful. May need mixing with lidocaine
			• Risk of nail matrix and soft tissue necrosis

	5-Fluorouracil	• Incorporates in DNA during its synthesis, leading to inhibition of DNA synthesis and cell death • Predilection for rapidly dividing cells	• Available as 50mg/mL solution for injection • Variable results • Produces intense inflammation and pain. May need mixing with triamcinolone • Risk of ulceration
	MMR vaccine	• Antigenic nature induces immunological reaction	• May be injected into the mother wart or over non-lesional skin (Figure 18.13a and b) • Inconsistent results
	Mw vaccine Tuberculin Candida antigen		
	BCG vaccine	• Antigenic nature induces immunological reaction	• Inconsistent results • Response only in immunocompetent individuals • Risk of inoculation of live bacilli and spread of bacilli
	Auto-implantation of wart tissue	• Intradermal or subcutaneous inoculation leads to an immune response	• Injected directly into the wart or in an intradermal or subcutaneous pocket • Results poor to excellent
Systemic	Zinc	• Immunomodulatory activity	• Variable results
	Cimetidine	• Immunomodulatory activity at high doses	• Dose: 20–40 mg/kg/day • Variable results
Others	Electrosurgery Cryosurgery CO_2 LASER Pulsed Dye LASER KTP LASER Photodynamic therapy		• Risk of nail matrix damage

Table 18.5 Recommended amount of intralesional bleomycin for treatment of periungual and subungual warts[31,32]

Size of wart	Amount of 1 unit/mL of bleomycin injected[a]
Up to 5 mm	0.2 mL
5–10 mm	0.5 mL
>10 mm	1 mL

[a] Injected every 2–4 weeks.

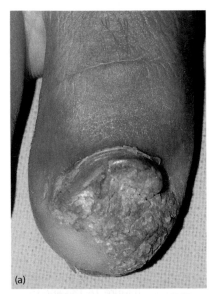

(a)

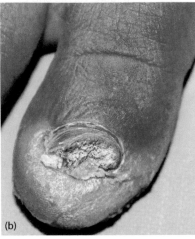

(b)

Figure 18.13 (a) Periungual wart with subungual extension; (b) Result after 1 session of MMR injection. (Courtesy of Dr. Divya Sachdev, AIIMS, Raipur, India.)

but usually occurs after 4–6 month of therapy.[35,36] It is more common in dark-skinned individuals and is reversible. Less often, longitudinal melanonychia in HIV patients, who are not on antiretroviral therapy, has also been reported.[37] Indinavir has been known to cause paronychia and pyogenic granuloma at the nail sulcus, via a mechanism possibly affecting endogenous retinoid metabolism.[38]

PARASITIC INFESTATIONS

Scabies

Scabitic nails have been described in the literature in the past on several occasions. Subungual hyperkeratosis, nail plate deformity/hypertrophy, distal onycholysis, longitudinal nail splitting and periungual scale and crust, and yellowish discoloration of nail plate have been reported in association with scabies. These findings are common in patients with crusted scabies. However, nail lesions have been reported even in the absence of skin lesions and pruritus.[39] Differentiation from onychomycosis and nail psoriasis is important. Microscopic examination of subungual debris reveals mites, eggs, or their fecal matter. Combination of systemic agents with topical scabicidal agents and keratolytic is the most preferred approach. Multiple applications of topical scabicidal agents may be required until the infection is eradicated. When incompletely treated, nails are frequent reservoirs of infection leading to relapse and disease dissemination in the community.

Tungiasis

Tungiasis is caused by the sand flea *Tungapenetrans* that is usually found in the soil near cattle sheds and pigsties. The infestation is common in tropics and subtropical areas including South America, Africa, India, and Pakistan. The causative flea is a female, which penetrates the skin and burrows into the dermis. Later a nodule with a central punctum covered with hemorrhagic crust develops at the site of infestation. Although the presentation is usually limited to a single lesion, multiple such lesions in a cluster are common when treatment is delayed. Common sites include web spaces and periungual skin of toes, soles, and heels. The lesions are associated with intense pruritus and frank inflammation painful enough to hinder walking. Long-term sequelae include deformity of digits, secondary infection, paronychia, and nail dystrophy.[40,41] Diagnosis is usually evident, based on the clinical picture and natural history of the disease. Currently there are no drugs with proven efficacy in the treatment of tungiasis. Oral ivermectin has been tried and reported to be useful, but an RCT found it comparable to placebo.[42] Surgical removal of the fleas and their eggs is the preferred standard of care. However, care should be taken not to leave behind any fragments of the flea inside the lesions, otherwise severe inflammatory reaction ensues.

Pediculosis

Pediculosis of the foot, limited to the hallux, has been reported in a patient with onychomycosis of all toenails with thickened nail plate and subungual hyperkeratosis. Debridement of a toenail exposed multiple cavities, housing body lice.[43]

Subungual myiasis

Subungual myiasis although rare, has been reported in the literature. Various reports have described larvae belonging to flies of various species including *Musca domestica*,

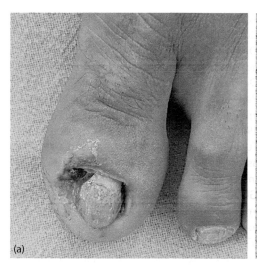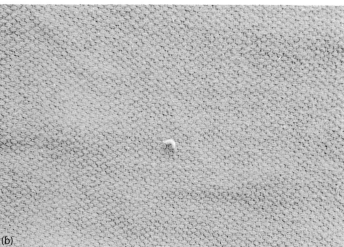

Figure 18.14 **(a)** and **(b)** Myiasis of nail unit. (Courtesy of Dr Shekhar Neema, Command Hospital, Kolkata, India.)

Sarcophaga, and *Calliphora*.[44,45] Myiasis usually occurs in individuals with psychiatric disorders affecting the ability to maintain personal hygiene (Figure 18.14a and b).

REFERENCES

1. Lee HE, Wong WR, Lee MC, Hong HS. Acute paronychia heralding the exacerbation of pemphigus vulgaris. *Int J Clin Pract* 2004; 58(12): 1174–1176.
2. Rockwell PG. Acute and chronic paronychia. *Am Fam Physician* 2001; 63(6): 1113–1116.
3. Brook I. Paronychia: A mixed infection. Microbiology and management. *J Hand Surg Br* 1993; 18(3): 358–359.
4. Wollina U. Acute paronychia: Comparative treatment with topical antibiotic alone or in combination with corticosteroid. *J Eur Acad Dermatol Venereol* 2001; 15(1): 82–84.
5. Sezer E, Bridges AG, Koseoglu D, Yuksek J. Acquired periungual fibrokeratoma developing after acute staphylococcal paronychia. *Eur J Dermatol* 2009; 19(6): 636–637.
6. Pabari A, Iyer S, Khoo CT. Swiss roll technique for treatment of paronychia. *Tech Hand Up Extrem Surg* 2011; 15(2): 75–77.
7. Fitzpatrick JE, Gramstad ND, Tyler H, Jr. Primary extragenital cutaneous gonorrhea. *Cutis* 1981; 27(5): 479–480.
8. Starzycki Z. Primary syphilis of the fingers. *Br J Vener Dis* 1983; 59(3): 169–171.
9. Kingsbury DH, Chester EC, Jr., Jansen GT. Syphilitic paronychia: An unusual complaint. *Arch Dermatol* 1972; 105(3): 458.
10. Noriega L, Gioia Di Chiacchio N, Cury Rezende F, Di Chiacchio N. Periungual lesion due to secondary syphilis. *Skin Appendage Disord* 2017; 2(3–4):116–119.
11. Patki AH, Baran R. Significance of nail changes in leprosy: A clinical review of 357 cases. *Semin Dermatol* 1991; 10(1): 77–81.
12. Patki AH. Pterygium inversum unguis in a patient with leprosy. *Arch dermatol* 1990; 126(8): 1110.
13. Jernigan JA, Farr BM. Incubation period and sources of exposure for cutaneous Mycobacterium marinum infection: Case report and review of the literature. *Clin Infect Dis* 2000; 31(2): 439–443.
14. Hay JR, Baran R. Fungal (onychomycosis) and other infections involving the nail apparatus. In Baran R, de Berker DAR, Holzberg M, Thomas L, editors. *Baran and Dawber's Diseases of the Nails and Their Management*, 4th ed. Oxford, UK: Wiley and Blackwell; 2012. pp. 246–247.
15. Goh SH, Ravintharan T, Sim CS, Chng HC. Nodular skin tuberculosis with lymphatic spread—A case report. *Singapore Med J* 1995; 36(1): 99–101.
16. Khanna D, Chakravarty P, Agarwal A, Gupta R. Tuberculous dactylitis presenting as paronychia with pseudo pterygium and nail dystrophy. *Pediatr Dermatol* 2013; 30(6): e172–e176.
17. Jain AK. Tuberculosis of the skeletal system (bones, joints, spine and bursal sheaths). *Indian J Orthop* 2010; 44(3): 356.
18. Antos H, Mollison LC, Richards MJ, Boquest AL, Tosolini FA. Diphtheria: Another risk of travel. *J Infect* 1992; 25(3): 307–310.
19. Gill MJ, Arlette J, Buchan K. Herpes simplex virus infection of the hand. A profile of 79 cases. *Am J Med* 1988; 84(1): 89–93.
20. LaRossa D, Hamilton R. Herpes simplex infections of the digits. *Arch Surg* 1971; 102(6): 600–601.
21. Muller SA, Herrmann EC, Jr. Association of stomatitis and paronychias due to herpes simplex. *Arch Dermatol* 1970; 101(4): 396–402.

22. Karpathios T, Moustaki M, Yiallouros P, Sarifi F, Tzanakaki G, Fretzayas A. HSV-2 meningitis disseminated from a herpetic whitlow. *Paediatr Int Child Health* 2012; 32(2): 121–122.

23. Hay JR, Baran R. Fungal (onychomycosis) and other infections involving the nail apparatus. In: Baran R, de Berker DAR, Holzberg M, Thomas L, editors. *Baran and Dawber's Diseases of the Nails and Their Management*, 4th ed. Oxford, UK: Wiley and Blackwell; 2012. p.242.

24. Zizmor J, Deluty S. Acquired leukonychia striata. *Int J Dermatol* 1980; 19(1): 49–50.

25. Yan X, Zhang ZZ, Yang ZH, Zhu CM, Hu YG, Liu QB. Clinical and etiological characteristics of atypical hand-foot-and-mouth disease in children from Chongqing, China: A retrospective study. *Biomed Res Int* 2015; 2015: 802046.

26. Shin JY, Cho BK, Park HJ. A clinical study of nail changes occurring secondary to hand-foot-mouth disease: Onychomadesis and Beau's lines. *Ann Dermatol* 2014; 26(2): 280–283.

27. Akpolat ND, Karaca N. Nail changes secondary to hand-foot-mouth disease. *Turk J Pediatr* 2016; 58(3): 287–290.

28. Hawary MB, Hassanain JM, Al-Rasheed SK, Al-Qattan MM. The yearly outbreak of orf infection of the hand in Saudi Arabia. *J Hand Surg Br* 1997; 22(4): 550–551.

29. Erbagci Z, Erbagci I, Almila Tuncel A. Rapid improvement of human orf (ecthyma contagiosum) with topical imiquimod cream: Report of four complicated cases. *J Dermatolog Treat* 2005; 16(5–6): 353–356.

30. Tosti A, Piraccini BM. Warts of the nail unit: surgical and nonsurgical approaches. *Dermatol Surg* 2001; 27(3): 235–239.

31. Herschthal J, McLeod MP, Zaiac M. Management of ungual warts. *Dermatol Ther* 2012; 25(6): 545–550.

32. Sardana K, Garg V, Relhan V. Complete resolution of recalcitrant periungual/subungual wart with recovery of normal nail following "prick" method of administration of bleomycin 1%. *Dermatol Ther* 2010; 23(4): 407–410.

33. Singal A, Pandhi D. Isolated nail pigmentation associated with chikungunya: A hitherto unreported manifestation. *Skin Appendage Disord* 2018; 4: 312–314.

34. Kumar R, Sharma MK, Jain SK, Yadav SK, Singhal AK. Cutaneous manifestations of chikungunya fever: Observations from an outbreak at a tertiary care hospital in Southeast Rajasthan, India. *Indian Dermatol Online J* 2017; 8(5): 336–342.

35. Panwalker AP. Nail pigmentation in the acquired immunodeficiency syndrome (AIDS). *Ann Intern Med* 1987; 107(6): 943–944.

36. Furth PA, Kazakis AM. Nail pigmentation changes associated with azidothymidine (zidovudine). *Ann Intern Med* 1987; 107(3): 350.

37. Glaser DA, Remlinger K. Blue nails and acquired immunodeficiency syndrome: Not always associated with azidothymidine use. *Cutis* 1996; 57(4): 243–244.

38. Sass JO, Jakob-Solder B, Heitger A, Tzimas G, Sarcletti M. Paronychia with pyogenic granuloma in a child treated with indinavir: The retinoid-mediated side effect theory revisited. *Dermatology* 2000; 200(1): 40–42.

39. Oh S, Vandergriff T. Scabies of the nail unit. *Dermatol Online J* 2014; 20(10).

40. Heukelbach J, de Oliveira FA, Hesse G, Feldmeier H. Tungiasis: A neglected health problem of poor communities. *Trop Med Int Health* 2001; 6(4): 267–272.

41. Feldmeier H, Eisele M, Van Marck E, Mehlhorn H, Ribeiro R, Heukelbach J. Investigations on the biology, epidemiology, pathology and control of Tunga penetrans in Brazil: IV. Clinical and histopathology. *Parasitol Res* 2004; 94(4): 275–282.

42. Heukelbach J, Franck S, Feldmeier H. Therapy of tungiasis: A double-blinded randomized controlled trial with oral ivermectin. *Mem Inst Oswaldo Cruz* 2004; 99(8): 873–876.

43. Diemer JT. Isolated pediculosis. *J Am Podiatr Med Assoc* 1985; 75(2): 99–101.

44. Dagci H, Zeyrek F, Gerzile YK, Sahin SB, Yagci S, Uner A. A case of myiasis in a patient with psoriasis from Turkey. *Parasitol Int* 2008; 57(2): 239–241.

45. Balcioglu IC, Ecemis T, Ayer A, Ozbel Y. Subungual myiasis in a woman with psychiatric disturbance. *Parasitol Int* 2008; 57(4): 509–511.

PART 6

Nail in Dermatological and Systemic Diseases; Occupation and Drug Induced Nail Changes

19

Nail in dermatological diseases

PIYUSH KUMAR AND NIHARIKA RANJAN LAL

INTRODUCTION

The nail unit may be involved in several inflammatory as well as non-inflammatory skin disorders. The nail abnormalities may occur in association with skin changes or in isolation. Sometimes, nail findings are disease specific and may be helpful in the diagnosis of dermatologic diseases such as in psoriasis, lichen planus, Darier's disease, scleroderma, lupus erythematosus, and dermatomyositis. There are dermatologic diseases in which nail involvement is common but the nail findings are relatively nonspecific. They are, thus, not diagnostic and include eczema, alopecia areata (AA), lichen striatus, etc. However, nail involvement in these diseases does contribute to morbidity and thus requires treatment.[1]

At times, some dermatologic diseases present with isolated nail involvement like lichen striatus, lichen planus, and AA, posing a diagnostic and therapeutic challenge. A careful clinical history, together with appropriate investigations like dermoscopy and mycology, is mandatory for confirming the diagnosis. Nail biopsy is required in doubtful cases from the representative site.[2]

In this chapter, we have summarized nail findings in various dermatological conditions excluding psoriasis, lichen planus, and infective conditions as they are covered in separate chapters.

ECZEMA

The inflammatory process in eczema may involve the nail fold, matrix, or nail bed in varying combinations, resulting in various nail changes.[3] Nail involvement is common in hand eczema and has been reported in 32.3% cases.[4] Severe nail involvement (nail dystrophy) was noted in up to 16% cases of active atopic patients.[5]

Eczema of proximal and lateral nail folds results in erythema, edema, and loss of cuticle. Secondary bacterial infection can result in acute paronychia. Eczematous changes in nail matrix result in rough, thick, discolored nail plate with surface pitting. Recurrent and intermittent inflammation may result in Beau's line (Figures 19.1 and 19.2) and in severe cases, onychomadesis. Nail changes in various eczema have been listed in Table 19.1.

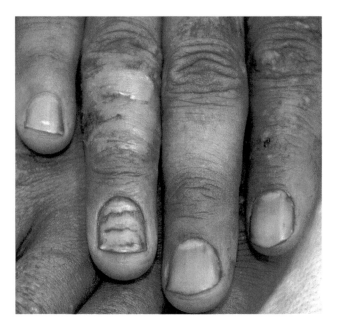

Figure 19.1 Multiple Beau's lines in patient with allergic contact dermatitis to cement.

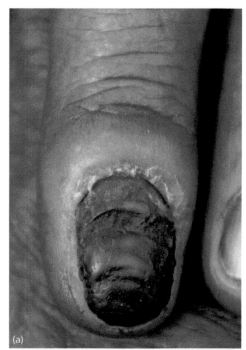

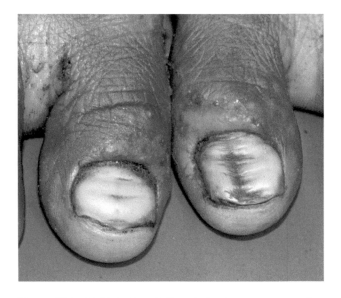

Figure 19.2 Multiple Beau's lines in both great toes and linear groove on the left great toe.

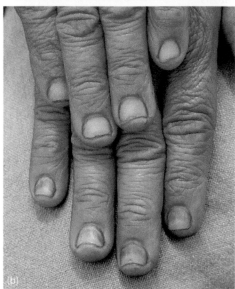

Figure 19.3 (a) Chronic paronychia with Beau's lines and nail dystrophy in irritant contact dermatitis to chronic detergent use; (b) Semilunar thinning and loss of the nail plate due to repeated microtrauma during itching.

Table 19.1 Nail changes in various eczemas

Allergic contact dermatitis	• Splinter hemorrhages, subungual hyperkeratosis, paronychia, onycholysis[1]
	• Less common changes: erythema, scaling, painful fissuring of nail folds
Irritant contact dermatitis	• Paronychia (Figure 19.3a), onycholysis, subungual hyperkeratosis,[4] onychorrhexis[1,4]
	• Features more marked in dominant hand, and in first three fingers[4]
	• Koilonychia: may be seen with use of organic solvents and motor oils[4]
Atopic dermatitis and atopic palmar eczema	• Polished shiny nails[4]
	• Nail pits, transverse grooves, trachyonychia,[4] nail dystrophy[3]
	• Increased prevalence of *Staphylococcus* beneath nails[1,4]
Exfoliative dermatitis	• Polished shiny nails (Figure 19.3b)[4]

The diagnosis will come from a good history and physical examination of the configuration and distribution of the rash on the skin. Patch testing should be performed to identify the offending allergen.[6]

Treatment consists of avoidance of contact with the causative allergen, moisturizers, topical/systemic steroids, and tacrolimus. Hand-care measures like use of gloves and hydration in atopics is equally important.[6]

ALOPECIA AREATA (AA)

Considering the similar structure and growth of nails and hair follicles, it is understandable the nails are targeted by similar inflammatory cells that target hair follicles in AA.[7] The incidence of nail changes in AA reportedly ranges from 7% to 66%.[8,9] Nail involvement in AA may either precede or follow development of alopecia patches.

Pitting (Figures 19.4 and 19.5) is the most common nail abnormality reported in 79.6% of cases in one study, followed by trachyonychia (14.3%) and onychorrhexis (6.1%). Pits presents as fine, grid-like stippling with regular vertical and horizontal rows. Trachyonychia presents as dull, rough, fragile, and friable nails and in severe cases, twenty-nail dystrophy. The severity of nail changes appears to be proportional to the degree of hair loss.[9]

Nail changes in AA are not specific for the disease and can also be seen psoriasis, eczema, lichen planus, and atopic dermatitis.[8] Nail changes in AA have been summarized in Table 19.2.

Histologically spongiotic dermatitis of the matrix (and nail bed) with exudation of serum is seen which becomes incorporated into the nail plate. The inflammation and incorporation of serum and inflammatory cells cause a wavy arrangement of the onychocytes and their keratin fibers resulting in roughened appearance of nails.[7]

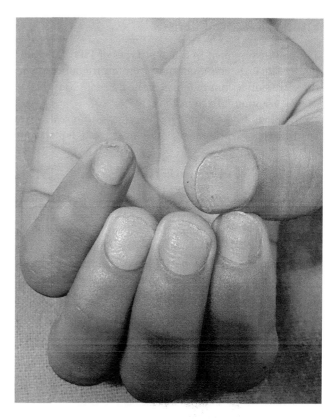

Figure 19.5 Multiple regularly arranged, shallow pits in alopecia totalis. (Courtesy of Prof. Archana Singal.)

Table 19.2 Nail changes in alopecia areata

Common nail changes	• Pits, trachyonychia, onychorrhexis, twenty-nail dystrophy
Less common/ rare	• Beau's lines, nail plate thickening/ thinning, transverse and longitudinal fissuring of nail plate, leukonychia (may be punctate, transverse, or diffuse),[3] spotting of lunula, onycholysis, onychomadesis[9]

As mentioned earlier, the degree of nail involvement directly correlates with the severity of hair loss. Thus, nail involvement is seen much more frequently in alopecia universalis than in circumscribed AA and nail involvement is considered poor prognostic marker for hair regrowth.[8]

Intralesional corticosteroid injections hasten the resolution of the nail changes. Short courses of systemic corticosteroids may also be effective.[9]

DISORDERS OF KERATINIZATION

Nail thickening, subungual hyperkeratosis, and dystrophy are common features of keratinization disorders. These changes along with hyperkeratotic hands and feet (as in PRP and keratodermas) mimic psoriasis and must be differentiated from the same.

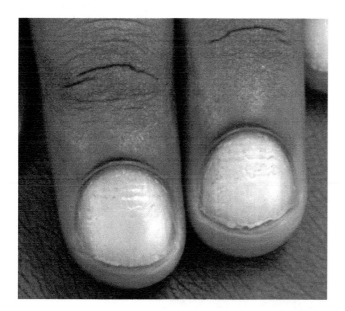

Figure 19.4 Multiple shallow pits arranged regularly in a case of alopecia totalis.

Pityriasis Rubra Pilaris

The nail involvement in different types of Pityriasis Rubra Pilaris (PRP) is common and is more pronounced when there are skin lesions on dorsa of the fingers.[10] Nail changes in PRP are summarized in Table 19.3.

Histologically, the nail bed epithelium reveals parakeratotic areas, acanthosis, and focal basal liquefaction.

Table 19.3 Nail changes in PRP

Common nail changes	• Thick nails, subungual hyperkeratosis (Figure 19.6), splinter hemorrhages, longitudinal ridging, and a distal yellow-brown discoloration[3]
Uncommon findings	• Irregular pitting, Beau's lines, loss of cuticles, and erythema around proximal nail folds[11]

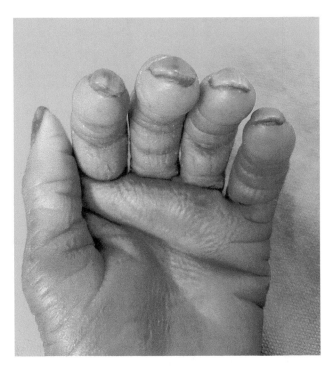

Figure 19.6 Thickened nail plate and subungual hyperkeratosis in a case of pityriasis rubra pilaris. (Courtesy of Dr. Shekhar Neema.)

Keratohyalin granules may be seen. In the dermis, there is a mononuclear inflammatory infiltrate.[3]

Nail changes in PRP must be differentiated from psoriasis. Distal yellow-brown discoloration, subungual hyperkeratosis, nail plate thickening, and splinter hemorrhages indicate a diagnosis of adult (type 1) PRP rather than psoriasis which is rather characterized by onycholysis (particularly marginal), salmon patches, small pits, and larger indentations of the nail plate.[12]

Patients have been treated successfully using etretinate and combined oral retinoid-PUVA treatment. Biological agents are reported to be useful.

Porokeratosis

Though nail involvement has been reported in all clinical types of porokeratosis (Table 19.4), it appears to be particularly common in linear porokeratosis involving the distal portions of the extremities.[13,14]

Histology findings are similar to those of porokeratosis of skin and include hyperkeratotic stratum corneum with a column of poorly staining parakeratotic stratum corneum cells (i.e., cornoid lamella). The granular layer is absent beneath the parakeratotic column.[15]

There is no clear consensus on treatment for nail dystrophy associated with porokeratosis. Topical therapies such as keratolytics, retinoids, vitamin D derivatives, 5-flurouracil ointment, imiquimod cream, and diclofenac gel; systemic retinoids; locally destructive modalities like dermabrasion, cryotherapy, photodynamic therapy, and carbon dioxide laser; and surgical excision and skin grafting have been tried with variable success.[15]

Table 19.4 Nail findings in porokeratosis

Linear porokeratosis	Pterygium, depressed nail plates, onychodystrophy (Figure 19.7), bony narrowing of digits[14]
Porokeratosis of Mibelli	Thickened, opaque, ridged, fissured, or partially destroyed nails,[3] warty debris nail
Porokeratosis plantaris palmaris et disseminata	Pterygium, onychodystrophy[15]

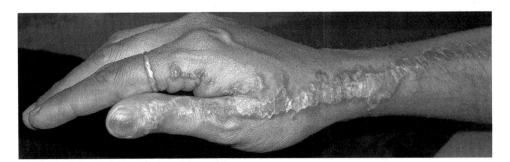

Figure 19.7 Linear porokeratosis with longitudinal nail groove with multiple parallel transverse furrows.

LICHEN NITIDUS AND LICHEN STRIATUS (LS)

Nail changes in lichen nitidus (LN) are uncommon and result from involvement of nail matrix.[16] Nail involvement may precede cutaneous eruptions, or may occur concurrently.[17] LN with palmar involvement is observed more frequently in patients with nail involvement.[18]

LN nail changes are not specific, and maybe similar to those in lichen planus.[16] However, in contrast to lichen planus, nail changes in LN are uncommon and less severe, with no pterygium formation or scarring leading to anonychia.[18] Isolated nail LN presenting with longitudinal nail splitting may resemble median canaliform dystrophy. Biopsy is helpful in confirming diagnosis.[18]

As with LN, nail involvement in lichen striatus is uncommon and Hauber et al. reported nail involvement in 16.67% cases.[19,20] As with LN, nail changes in LS may occur before, simultaneously, or after the cutaneous eruption.[21] Two cases of LS have been reported limited to the nail.[19] Histopathology of nail LS, although similar to skin LS, has a few differences. Compact orthokeratosis and hypergranulosis owing to interference with nail matrix keratinization is a feature of nail LS.[21]

The nail findings of LN and lichen striatus have been summarized in Table 19.5.

Table 19.5 Nail findings in lichen nitidus and lichen striatus

Nail changes	Lichen nitidus	Lichen striatus
Common	• Longitudinal ridges with a rippled or beaded surface (most characteristic)[17] • Pitting,[16,17] thickening,[16] terminal splitting,[16] onychodystrophy (mostly in adults),[16,18] and trachyonychia[18]	• Longitudinal ridging, longitudinal splitting (Figure 19.8), onycholysis, nail plate over-curvature, nail plate thinning, punctate or striate leukonychia, nail bed hyperkeratosis, and total nail loss[20,21] • Onychodystrophy
Uncommon	• Violaceous erythema, swelling and pigmentation of proximal nail fold,[16,18] lichenoid papules on nail folds • Severe linear nail dystrophy resembling lichen planus has been described but presence of numerous giant cells as well as a lichenoid infiltrate might indicate lichen nitidus confined to the nails.[17]	• Longitudinal dystrophy with hyperpigmentation on the lateral portion of the nail • Bilateral nail dystrophy has been reported with unilateral LS.

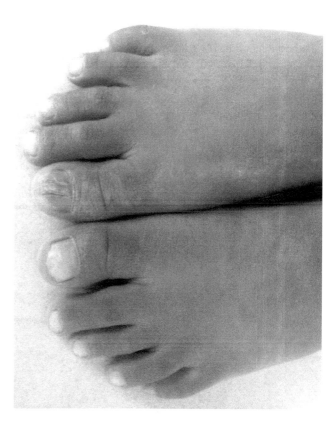

Figure 19.8 Longitudinal splitting of nail in lichen striatus.

Both LN and lichen striatus are asymptomatic and self-healing with less potential for scarring or other permanent sequalae. Usually, no treatment is necessary. However, nail LS may have a protracted course of 6 months to 5 years, leading to patients seeking treatment. Treatment with topical tacrolimus ointment is reported to be successful in resolving nail changes.[21]

GENETIC DISORDERS

Darier's disease

The nail changes in Darier's disease are not only common (reported in 92% to 95% of patients), but also diagnostic. The "candy-cane" appearance of the nails, especially when it ends in a V-shaped notch at the distal nail edge, is considered pathognomonic.[22,23] However, not all nail changes are of diagnostic value. The nail findings of Darier's disease have been tabulated in Table 19.6.

It is noteworthy that nail involvement may occur without other manifestations of Darier's disease. Also, nail involvement may range from 2–3 nails to all 20 nails.[22] In children carrying the gene for Darier's disease, nail changes may be first to appear and precede skin lesions.[24] The differentials for nail changes in Darier's disease include lichen planus and onychomycosis. Longitudinal red or white streaks may occur in tumors of nail matrix or nail bed. Longitudinal white bands are common in Hailey–Hailey disease (HHD).

Table 19.6 Nail findings in Darier's disease

Pathognomonic nail matrix findings	• Longitudinal subungual red and/or white streaks (Figure 19.9) (resembling "candy-cane") associated with a tendency towards longitudinal tears and v-shaped splits of distal ends of nail plate (Figure 19.10)
Other nail matrix findings	• Thinned nail plate, longitudinal ridges, onychorrhexis, increased fragility of nail plate, true leukonychia
Nail bed findings	• Subungual hyperkeratosis, distal cuneiform keratosis, and sometimes splinter hemorrhages (Figure 19.9)
Nail fold	• Keratotic papules on proximal nail fold may present as paronychia
Others	• Secondary infection with dermatophytes, *Candida* and *Pseudomonas* spp.

Source: Baran, R., and Holzberg, M., The nail in dermatological disease, in Baran, R. et al., editors, *Baran & Dawber's Diseases of the Nails and Their Management*, 4th ed., Wiley and Blackwell, Oxford, UK, pp. 280–303, 2012; Baran, R., and Haneke, E., Pits, rough nails, and other surface alterations, in *Nail in Differential Dermatology*, 1st ed., CRC Press, Boca Raton, FL, pp. 1–24, 2006; Baran, R., and Haneke, E., Subungual hyperkeratosis, in *Nail in Differential Dermatology*, 1st ed., CRC Press, Boca Raton, FL, pp. 51–59, 2006.

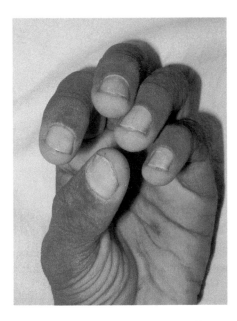

Figure 19.9 Longitudinal erythronychia (4th finger), distal nail plate fragility (1st finger), and distal cuneiform subungual hyperkeratosis (4th and 5th fingers). (Courtesy of Prof. Archana Singal.)

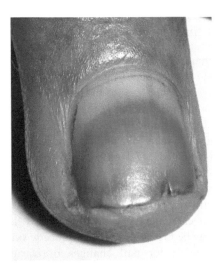

Figure 19.10 Distal nail plate showing V-shaped notch. (Courtesy of Prof. Archana Singal.)

All parts of the nail unit may be affected histologically. The nail bed findings, however, are an exception, revealing the absence of suprabasilar clefts, the presence of multinucleated epithelial giant cells, and the absence of an inflammatory infiltrate. These characteristic changes lead to the diagnosis in rare cases where Darier's disease is limited to the nails. Nail bed epithelium may be hyperplastic and exhibit subungual parakeratosis. Oral retinoids may improve keratotic papules of the proximal nail fold but other nail changes are not improved by treatment.[3]

Hailey–Hailey disease

Both HHD and Darier's disease are rare autosomal dominant acantholytic skin disorders. Nail findings in HHD, unlike Darier's disease, appear to be minimal and have little diagnostic value. The most important finding is multiple longitudinal leukonychia. Other signs like splinter hemorrhages, erythronychia, irregular lunular border, and irregularly spotted lunula are rarely found. In a study by Bel et al., these changes were not found to be more frequent in HHD than controls.[25,26]

Palmoplantar keratoderma

Palmoplantar keratodermas (PPKs) are a group of disorders in which there is gross thickening or hyperkeratosis of palmoplantar skin. Keratodermas can be both hereditary or acquired. The keratodermas can be diffuse, punctate, or focal type.[27]

In a study of pediatric PPKs, nail changes were observed in 60% of children. Nail changes most commonly seen were subungual hyperkeratosis, pitting, and nail plate thickening. Rough and brittle nails were seen in 25% patients each. Nail changes in various types of PPK are listed in Table 19.7.

Conservative treatment includes topical keratolytics, retinoids, and corticosteroids. In recalcitrant cases, oral acitretin or etretinate can be given.[27]

Table 19.7 Nail changes in palmoplantar keratoderma

Diffuse PPK	Nail plate thickening, subungual hyperkeratosis, longitudinal fissures, and nail shedding[3]
Unna Thost syndrome	Parrot beaking of the fingernails and widening of the onychocorneal band, stubby nails[28,29]
Huriez syndrome	Marked scleroatrophy of the hands, diffuse palmoplantar keratoderma and hypoplastic nails, prominent lunula, elongated cuticles, and "V"-shaped notch[30]
Mal de Meleda syndrome	Koilonychia[5] and longitudinal grooving[28]
Olmsted syndrome	Onychodystrophy and thin brittle fingernails[31]
Punctate PPK	
Hereditary punctate palmoplantar keratoderma of Brauer–Buschke–Fischer	Longitudinal ridging, onychorrhexis, onychoschizia, trachyonychia, notching, pitting, onycholysis, and subungual hyperkeratosis[11] Half-moon distal nail plate dystrophy, medial canaliformis, and koilonychia are additional findings reported by Mittal et al.[32]
Keratosis punctata of palmar creases	Pterygium inversum unguis[33]
Focal PPK	
Striate PPK	Ridging and cuticular hyperkeratosis
Vohwinkel-type of PPK	Onychodystrophy[28]

STEVENS–JOHNSON SYNDROME AND TOXIC EPIDERMAL NECROLYSIS

As in skin, inflammation and bulla formation can occur in any portion of the nail unit. The inflammatory reaction can cause damage to the nail fold, matrix, and/or nail bed (Figure 19.11).[34] Nail changes in SJS-TEN have been tabulated in Table 19.8.

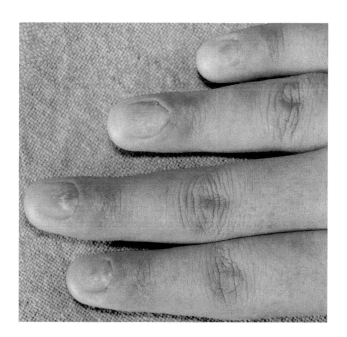

Figure 19.11 Acquired anonychia and nail dystrophy in a case of resolved Stevens–Johnson syndrome.

Table 19.8 Nail changes in SJS-TEN

Common	• Paronychia, onychomadesis
Uncommon	• Nail degloving syndrome
Long-term sequelae	• Nail dystrophy and permanent anonychia • Scarring and pterygium • Onychodystrophy (reported in 10%–37.5% of cases)

Source: Baran, R., and Holzberg, M., The nail in dermatological disease, in Baran, R. et al., editors, *Baran & Dawber's Diseases of the Nails and Their Management*, 4th ed., Wiley and Blackwell, Oxford, UK, pp. 280–303, 2012; Mi, Y.U. et al., *JDA.*, 40, 406–407, 2013.

Nail changes may be treated with intralesional corticosteroids. However, long-standing pterygium of more than one-year duration and nails with severe dystrophy do not respond to treatment.[35,36]

AUTOIMMUNE BLISTERING DISEASES

Many autoimmune blistering disorders can affect nail unit as antigens expressed in nail units are shared with epidermis. The nail findings depend on site of blister formation as summarized in Table 19.9. If nail matrix is affected, paronychia and onychomadesis are seen. Nail bed affection results in onycholysis. The clinical importance of nail involvement in autoimmune blistering disorders is variable; nail involvement signifies poorer prognosis in pemphigus vulgaris (PV), but not in bullous pemphigoid.

Table 19.9 Site of bulla formation and nail findings

Site	Nail findings
Dorsal nail fold	Acute periungual inflammation and bullous lesions
Ventral nail fold	Chronic paronychia
Nail matrix	Beau's lines, onychomadesis, onychoschizia, cross-ridging, pitting, and trachyonychia
Nail bed	Onycholysis (poor prognosis in pemphigus vulgaris)

Source: Seetharam, K.A., *Indian J. Dermatol. Venereol. Leprol.*, 79, 563–575, 2013; Baran, R., and Haneke, E., Severe nail dystrophy, hyponychia and anonychia, and alterations of nail shape, in *Nail in Differential Dermatology*, 1st ed., CRC Press, Boca Raton, FL, pp. 28–48, 2006.

Pemphigus vulgaris

Nail changes in PV have been reported to range from 31.6% to 50% of patients.[3,7] Also, nail changes have been found more frequently in patients with larger number of bullae and longer disease duration, thus correlating with disease severity.[38]

Nail involvement is due to bullous lesions developing in the nail bed, nail matrix, or nail fold (Figure 19.12) as part of the disease process. Nail disease can be part of the initial presentation along with mucosal and cutaneous lesions (47% cases), can precede a flare of the pre-existing disease (33%), or can be the only sign of the disease (20%).[39] The various nail changes in PV have been tabulated in Table 19.10.

Other pemphigus variants exhibit nail affection. Nail shedding, in addition to yellowish nail discoloration, onychorrhexis, and onycholysis, onychomadesis, pterygium, subungual hyperkeratosis, and onychogryphosis may occur in Brazilian pemphigus (fogo selvagem).[40] Vegetating pemphigus of Hallopeau show pustules with onychoatrophy.[3]

Differential diagnosis includes herpetic whitlow.[38] The diagnosis of pemphigus can be made by histological identification and/or by direct immunofluorescence testing. The prognosis of nail changes in PV is generally good, with successful resolution of the nail changes with treatment.[38]

Table 19.10 Nail changes in pemphigus vulgaris

Common	• Acute paronychia (60%, may be the initial presentation of PV, even before cutaneous disease) (Figure 19.13) • Onychomadesis (33%) (Figure 19.13) • Onycholysis and subungual hyperkeratosis
Others	• Onychodystrophy (Figure 19.14) • Subungual, intraungual, and splinter hemorrhages • Beau's lines, pitting, onychoschizia, and longitudinal ridging, trachyonychia • Onycholysis • Nail plate discoloration • Vegetating and verrucous lesions on the nail folds • Pseudopyogenic granuloma of the nail folds (reported to be the first symptom of a relapse of the disease)[40]

Source: Baran, R., and Haneke, E., Severe nail dystrophy, hyponychia and anonychia, and alterations of nail shape, in *Nail in Differential Dermatology*, 1st ed., CRC Press, Boca Raton, FL, pp. 28–48, 2006; Habibi, M. et al., *Int. J. Dermatol.*, 47, 1141–1144, 2008; Cahali, J.B. et al., *Rev. Hosp. Clin.*, 57, 229–234, 2002; Zawar, V. et al., *Skin Appendage Disord.*, 3, 28–31, 2017.

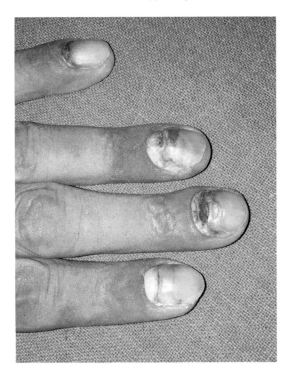

Figure 19.13 Paronychia and onychomadesis in a case with pemphigus vulgaris. (Courtesy of Savant, S.S. et al., *Indian J. Dermatol. Venereol. Leprol.*, 83, 212, 2017. IADVL, Medknow Publications [Wolters Kluwer Health].)

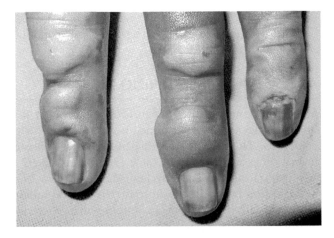

Figure 19.12 Bullous lesions affecting proximal nail fold in a case with pemphigus vulgaris. (Courtesy of Prof. Archana Singal.)

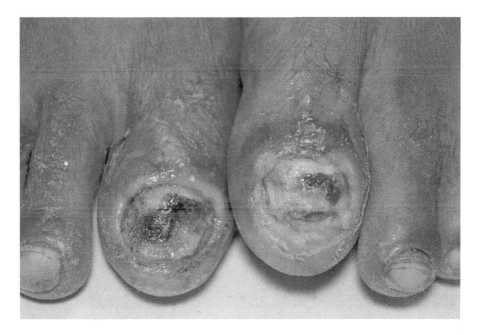

Figure 19.14 Acquired anonychia and nail dystrophy in a case of pemphigus vulgaris.

Bullous pemphigoid

All four regions of the nail, namely the proximal nail fold, nail matrix, nail bed, and hyponychium, express the antigens found in the non-appendageal basement membrane, including BP1Ag and BP2Ag. It is therefore not surprising that the inflammatory process of BP can also involve the nail resulting in nail changes[41] (Table 19.11). Nail involvement has been reported in childhood BP too, and include sloughing, subungual hyperkeratosis, hemorrhage, yellow discoloration, and onychorrhexis.[3]

Differential diagnoses of bullous pemphigoid of the nail include epidermolysis bullosa acquisita (EBA), cicatricial pemphigoid, and erosive lichen planus. Diagnosis can be confirmed by biopsy and immunofluoroscence studies.[42]

Nail changes respond well to systemic treatment for bullous pemphigoid. The prognostic importance of nail involvement is uncertain and further studies are needed to ascertain this.[43]

Table 19.11 Nail changes in bullous pemphigoid

Nail folds	• Paronychia
Matrix	• Longitudinal splitting of the nail, Beau's lines, and onychomadesis
Severe inflammation of nail fold and matrix	• Nail unit scarring with atrophy or even permanent loss of the nails, anonychia, and pterygium
Nail bed	• Onycholysis[43]

Source: Tosti, A. et al., Dermatol. Clin., 29, 511–513, 2011; Henriquez, M.A. et al., J. Am. Acad. Dermatol., 76, AB59, 2017.

Cicatricial pemphigoid

Severe nail dystrophy with ridging and splits has been seen in cicatricial pemphigoid. Pterygium of the fingernails has also been reported.[37,44]

Epidermolysis bullosa acquisita

Nail involvement occurs as a result of periungual/subungual blistering. Nail findings reported in EBA are onycholysis, onychodystrophy, and onychomadesis. Rarely subungual hyperkeratosis may also be seen. Total nail loss, which is rarely described, is the result of nail bed scarring post bullous lesions.[44]

MECHANO-BULLOUS DISORDERS

Nail changes in epidermolysis bullosa (EB) are common, and though they are highly suggestive of the disease, they are not pathognomonic. They are the result of abnormalities of the nail matrix and nail bed, associated with the pathogenetic alterations of the dermo-epidermal junction of EB. In addition, secondary trauma in the areas of epidermal-dermal separation, and chronic inflammation of the nail matrix, are probable contributory factors, even in non-scarring forms of EB.[45]

Nail changes are milder in EB simplex, like onychomadesis. Severe nail changes like onychodystrophy and anonychia (Figures 19.15 and 19.16) are seen in junctional EB (JEB) and dystrophic EB (DEB). Anonychia during neonatal period may be the presenting symptom in JEB. Drumstick appearance of the distal digits covered with granulation tissue is typical of the Herlitz type of JEB. Toenails are dystrophic

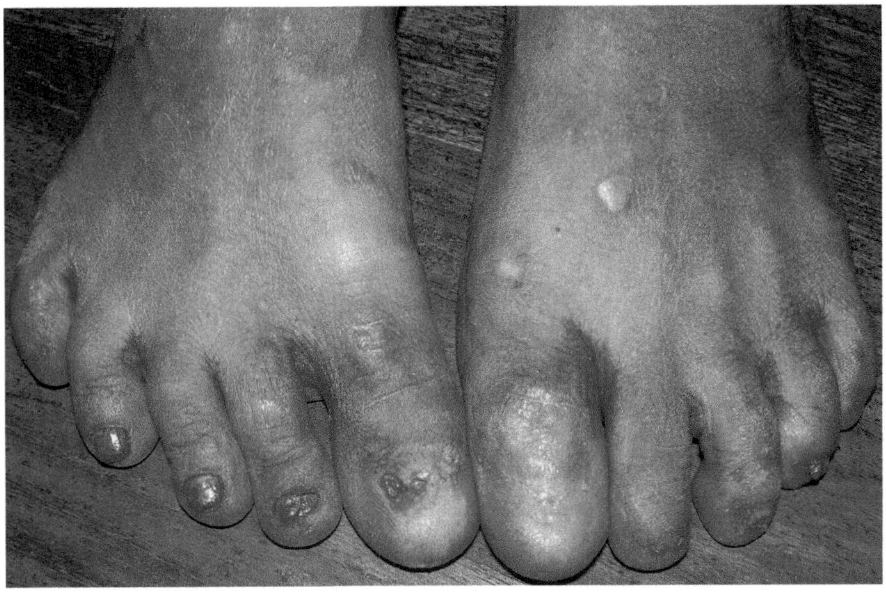

Figure 19.15 Acquired anonychia of both great toes in a case with autosomal dominant dystrophic epidermolysis bullosa.

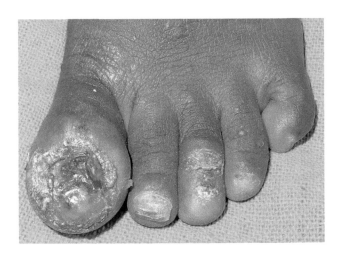

Figure 19.16 Bullous lesions causing loss of nail plate and eroded nail bed in a case of autosomal dominant dystrophic epidermolysis bullosa.

and frequently absent in DEB. Anonychia involving all digits is seen in recessive DEB.[30]

AUTOIMMUNE CONNECTIVE TISSUE DISEASES

The proximal nail fold is the predominantly affected site in various autoimmune connective tissue diseases (AI-CTDs). Nail fold erythema and hemorrhages are common findings in these conditions. Nail fold capillary changes are another major finding and have diagnostic as well as prognostic importance. Two major patterns are seen: lupus type and scleroderma type. Proximal nail fold offers an easily accessible site for biopsy and direct immunofluorescence to diagnose these conditions.

Discoid lupus erythematosus

Discoid lupus erythematosus (DLE) affecting the nail folds and nail unit is very uncommon. Isolated nail involvement has never been reported. Nail changes occur when DLE affects digits (Table 19.12).

Histopathologically, LE of the perionychium shows hyperkeratosis, liquefaction degeneration of the basal cell layer, and a predominantly lymphocytic infiltrate in the superficial dermis with edema and ectatic capillaries in the papillary dermis, while LE of the nail bed causes hyper-orthokeratosis with a corresponding granular cell layer, thinning of the spinous cell layer, and edema of the basal cells, which exhibit ill-defined borders. Hyaline bodies are observed in the superficial dermis.[12]

Table 19.12 Nail findings of discoid lupus erythematosus

Site of involvement	Nail findings
Nail matrix	Scarring, pterygium
Nail bed	Diffuse or punctuate reddish-blue discoloration (Figure 19.17)
Nail fold	• Focal lesions of DLE occurring over the nail fold produce nail plate dystrophy (Figure 19.18) with onychorrhexis • Distally, the nail plates crumble and become fragile, irregular, and split.

Source: Baran, R., and Holzberg, M., The nail in dermatological disease, in Baran, R. et al., editors, *Baran & Dawber's Diseases of the Nails and Their Management*, 4th ed., Wiley and Blackwell, Oxford, UK, pp. 280–303, 2012; Baran, R., and Haneke, E., Subungual hyperkeratosis, in *Nail in Differential Dermatology*, 1st ed., CRC Press, Boca Raton, FL, pp. 51–59, 2006.

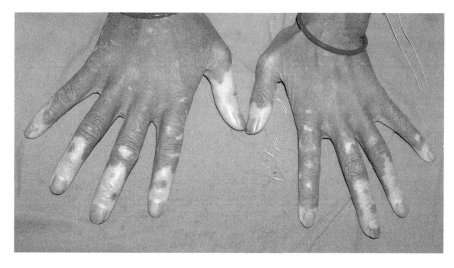

Figure 19.17 Pigmented nail plates in a treated case of discoid lupus erythematosus. (Courtesy of Prof. Archana Singal.)

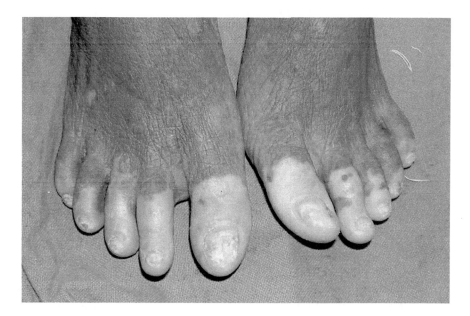

Figure 19.18 Dystrophic nails in a treated case of discoid lupus erythematosus. (Courtesy of Prof. Archana Singal.)

DLE and lichen planus have much in common in the nails, both clinically and histologically. However, nail involvement in discoid lupus is less common than in lichen planus and the focus of scarring is more on the nail fold than on the matrix.[3]

Usually, DLE involving the nail can be diagnosed on the basis of coexisting typical DLE lesions elsewhere, so that nail biopsies are usually not indicated. Potent topical steroids have been used in discoid lupus and may lead to some improvement.[12]

Systemic lupus erythematosus

Although a wide spectrum of nail abnormalities has been described in systemic lupus erythematosus (SLE), none is sufficiently distinctive in the diagnosis of disease. Nail changes may be observed in up to 25%–31% of patients with SLE.[46,47] Nail findings are indicative of active disease and are associated with significantly higher incidence of Raynaud's phenomenon and oral ulceration.[46] Nail changes of SLE have been tabulated in Table 19.13.

The differential diagnosis of LE non-specific nail involvement in LE focuses primarily on other connective tissue diseases with vascular involvement of the proximal nail fold (scleroderma, dermatomyositis, mixed connective tissue disease, rheumatoid arthritis) and are differentiated on the basis of different nail fold capillary patterns.[46]

Systemic sclerosis

Digital ischemia associated with Raynaud's phenomenon and inflammation of the nail matrix may be observed in scleroderma and are responsible for variety of nail changes

Table 19.13 Nail changes in systemic lupus erythematosus

Site affected	Nail changes
Proximal nail fold	• Most important site to get affected in SLE • Nail fold erythema, chronic paronychia, nail fold hyperkeratosis, and ragged cuticles (Figure 19.19)[3]
Nail bed	• Onycholysis (most frequent nail abnormality, almost 25% of cases) • Oil spots and subungual nail bed hyperkeratosis[46]
Nail matrix	• Punctate or transverse leukonychia, nail pitting or ridging, Beau's lines, and onychomadesis[46] • In transverse leukonychia, the width of the leukonychia correlates with the duration and clinical activity of the SLE.[3]
Vasculopathy of nail unit	• Periungual ischemic lesions may present as focal nail fold infarcts, necrosis, and cuticular hemorrhages. • Infarcts in the matrix can lead to permanent nail plate dystrophy. • Subungual splinter hemorrhages (antiphospholipid syndrome secondary to SLE) • Proximal nail fold telangiectasia is common. • Capillary microscopy in SLE reveals a tortuous, meandering loop pattern.[46]
Other findings:	• Clubbing, pincer nail deformity[3] • Dark blue-black hyperpigmentation intermixed with longitudinal pigmented bands noted in up to 52% of black SLE patients (without relationship to disease activity, or to antimalarial therapy).[46] • Red lunula (in up to 19.6% of LE patients)[46,48] • Pterygium inversum unguis (SLE associated with Raynaud's phenomenon)[46]

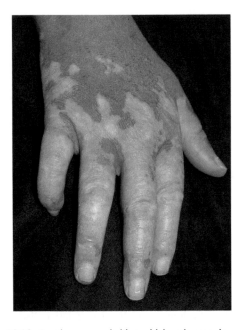

Figure 19.19 Erythema and dilated blood vessels (4th finger) of proximal nail folds.

Table 19.14 Nail findings in systemic sclerosis

Site affected	Nail findings
Blood vessels (Ischemic/ vascular changes)	• Reversible pallor and cyanosis, hyperemic distal nail bed • Prolonged ischemia and subsequent fibrosis results in pseudo-clubbing or "beaking" of the nails (Figures 19.20 and 19.21), fingertip scars, and pterygium inversus unguium[51,52] • Painful, keratotic ulcers (Figure 19.22) that may progress to digital necrosis and gangrene[51,52] • Splinter hemorrhages (proximal ones are more specific) • Ragged cuticle, cuticular hemorrhage • Red lunula
Nail matrix involvement	• Nail plate pitting and beading • Trachyonychia and brachyonychia • Thickened nails • Macrolunula[49]
Others	• Scleronychia, hyponychium hyperkeratosis

observed in scleroderma. In a recent study on 129 patients with systemic sclerosis, nail changes were observed in 80.6% cases. In addition, nail changes in systemic sclerosis were associated with severe esophageal dysmotility, digital ulcers/pitting scars, and calcinosis cutis.[49] Nail findings in SS have been tabulated in Table 19.14.

Nail fold capillaries show characteristic findings under nail fold capillaroscopy. Findings in early disease include enlarged capillaries and some hemorrhages with relatively well-preserved capillary distribution and no evident loss of capillaries. Active cases show frequent giant capillaries and hemorrhage, with moderate loss of capillaries, and mild disorganization of the capillary architecture. Late cases are characterized by severe loss of capillaries with extensive avascular areas, disorganization of the normal capillary array, and ramified/bushy capillaries. Giant capillaries and hemorrhages are minimal. However, this systemic sclerosis pattern (megacapillaries along with decreased capillary density) is not specific to systemic sclerosis and may be seen in other rheumatic conditions like dermatomyositis

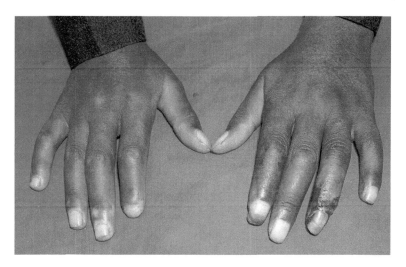

Figure 19.20 Shortening of terminal phalanx with acquired brachyonychia (right 2nd finger), beaking of the nail (left 2nd finger), and crusted ulcer on proximal nail fold (left 4th finger) in systemic sclerosis. (Courtesy of Prof. Archana Singal.)

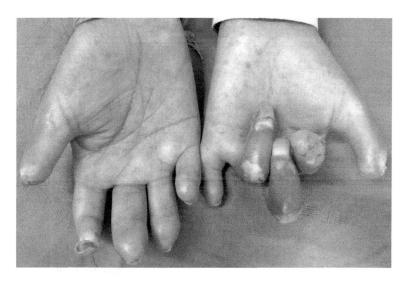

Figure 19.21 Shortening of terminal phalanx with acquired brachyonychia (right 1st finger; left 1st and 2nd finger), beaking of the nails (right 2nd finger; left 3rd and 4th fingers), and pterygium inversum unguis (right 3rd finger) in systemic sclerosis. (Courtesy of Prof. Archana Singal.)

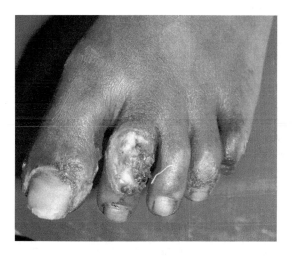

Figure 19.22 Ulceration of proximal nail fold in systemic sclerosis. (Courtesy of Prof. Archana Singal.)

and polymyositis, undifferentiated connective tissue disease (UCTD), and sometimes in SLE too.[50]

Dermatomyositis

Like other connective tissue disorders, proximal nail fold is an important site of affection in dermatomyositis. Nail fold capillary changes are similar to those in scleroderma and include tortuous enlarged and giant capillaries, microhemorrhages, capillary loss, and ramified capillaries. Nail fold capillary changes are considered expression of diffuse microangiopathy, but surprisingly, severe capillary changes were associated with shorter disease duration.[53,54]

Other prominent nail changes include hyperkeratotic cuticle, ragged cuticle, and red lunula (Figure 19.23).[52] Nail matrix might be involved and manifests as nail pitting,

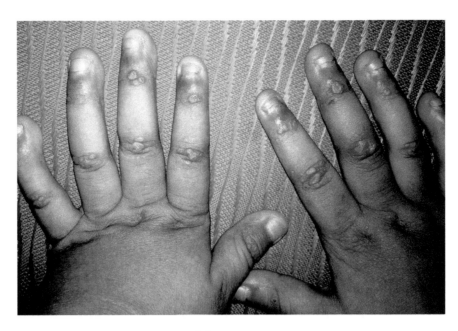

Figure 19.23 Hyperkeratotic ragged cuticle in a case of dermatomyositis.

trachyonychia, onychogryphosis and, in severe cases, onychomadesis. Nail bed too might be affected, resulting in splinter hemorrhages. Rarely, pterygium inversum unguis may develop.[53,54]

Miscellaneous dermatological diseases

Nail involvement in some other dermatological conditions have been summarized in Table 19.15.

CONCLUSION

Nail changes are common in dermatological diseases. It is important to be aware of common nail changes associated with dermatological diseases as it helps supplement the clinical diagnosis. In addition, nail involvement contributes to morbidity and often requires specific treatment. Last but not least, it is important to document and understand the entire spectrum of involvement of integumentary system by a disease process.

Table 19.15 Nail involvement in various dermatoses

Diseases	Nail findings
Acroosteolysis	Pseudoclubbing, racket-nails, koilonychia, pincer nails, and total nail destruction
Acrokeratoelastoidosis	Longitudinal ridging (onychorrhexis), distal onycholysis, and pterygium formation
Granuloma annulare[a] (involving acral area)	Painful nail (subungual pain), blackish discoloration of nails, nail dystrophy, Beaus lines, swelling of digit
Erythema elevatum diutinum	Subungual hemorrhage, onycholysis, and paronychia
Langerhans cell histiocytosis—Nail involvement indicates poor prognosis.	Hemorrhagic and pustular lesions in the nail bed, onycholysis, subungual hyperkeratosis, longitudinal grooving of nail plate, striate nail dystrophy, paronychia, and loss of nail plate
Juvenile xanthogranuloma	Affecting proximal nail fold—hyperkeratotic cuticle, juvenile xanthogranuloma of the proximal nail fold
	Affecting nail bed—subungual nodule lifting nail plate, onychogryphosis
Pityriasis rosea	Multiple transverse grooves, pitting, rectangular areas of dystrophy in the middle third of nail were reported in one case.
Pityriasis lichenoides et varioliformis acuta	Permanent nail dystrophy in one case
Buerger's disease (Figure 19.24a and b)	Subungual splinter hemorrhage, ulceration of nail folds, thickened nails, brittle nails, Beau's lines

Source: El-Komy, M.H., and Baran, R.J., Eur. Acad. Dermatol. Venereol., 29, 2252–2254, 2015; Van Steensel, M.A. et al., Arch. Dermatol., 142, 939–941, 2006; Gutte, R. et al., Indian J. Dermatol. Venereol. Leprol., 78, 468–474, 2012; Futei, Y., and Konohana, I., Br. J. Dermatol., 142, 116–119, 2000; Figueras-Nart, I. et al., JAAD. Case Rep., 2, 485–487, 2016; Piraccini, B.M. et al., Pediatr. Dermatol., 20, 307–308, 2003; Silvers, S.H., and Glickman, F.S., Arch. Dermatol., 90, 31, 1964.
[a] Nail disease was not biopsy confirmed.

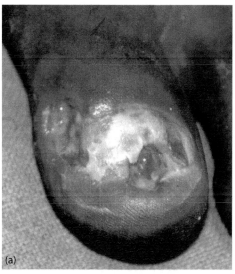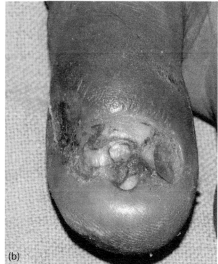

Figure 19.24 **(a)** Ulcer of nail bed and lateral nail fold resulting in partial loss of nail plate in a case of Buerger's disease; **(b)** Three weeks after treatment with nifedipine and ecospirin.

REFERENCES

1. Mortimer PS, Dawber RP. Dermatologic diseases of the nail unit other than psoriasis and lichen planus. *Dermatol Clin* 1985; 3(3): 401–407.
2. Piraccini BM. Nail diseases due to dermatological diseases. In: *Nail Disorders, A Practical Guide to Diagnosis and Management*, 1st ed. Verlag Italia, MI: Springer; 2014. p. 75.
3. Baran R, Holzberg M. The nail in dermatological disease. In: Baran R, de Berker DAR, Holzberg M, Thomas L, editors. *Baran & Dawber's Diseases of the Nails and Their Management*, 4th ed. Oxford, UK: Wiley and Blackwell; 2012. pp. 280–303.
4. Mi YU, Kim SW, Kim MS, Han TY, Lee JH, Son S. Clinical study of patients with hand eczema accompanied by nail dystrophy. *JDA* 2013; 40(5): 406–407.
5. Simpson EL, Thompson MM, Hanifin JM. Prevalence and morphology of hand eczema in patients with atopic dermatitis. *Dermatitis* 2006 17(3): 123–127.
6. Baran R. Nail alteration in hand eczema. In: Alikhan A, Lachapelle JM, Maibach HI, editors. *Textbook of Hand Eczema*. Berlin, Germany: Springer; 2014. pp. 39–46.
7. Seetharam KA. Alopecia areata: An update. *Indian J Dermatol Venereol Leprol* 2013; 79: 563–575.
8. Gandhi V, Baruah MC, Bhattacharaya SN. Nail changes in alopecia areata: Incidence and pattern. *Indian J Dermatol Venereol Leprol* 2003; 69: 114–115.
9. Kasumagic-Halilovic E, Prohic A. Nail changes in alopecia areata: Frequency and clinical presentation. *J Eur Acad Dermatol Venereol* 2009; 23(2): 240–241.
10. Baran R, Haneke E. Pits, rough nails, and other surface alterations. In: *Nail in Differential Dermatology*, 1st ed. Boca Raton, FL: CRC Press; 2006. pp. 1–24.
11. Santoro F, Nallamothu P. A patient presenting with nail changes and type I pityriasis rubra pilaris. *J Am Acad Dermatol* 2012; 66: AB96.
12. Baran R, Haneke E. Subungual hyperkeratosis. In: *Nail in Differential Dermatology*, 1st ed. Boca Raton, FL: CRC Press; 2006. pp. 51–59.
13. Robati RM, Roodsari MR, Ayatollahi A, Hejazi S. Facial and bilateral acral porokeratosis with nail dystrophy: A case report. *Dermatol Online J* 17(1): 5.
14. Kono M, Yokoyama N, Ogawa Y, Takama H, Sugiura K, Akiyama M. Unilateral generalized linear porokeratosis with nail dystrophy. *J Dermatol* 2016; 43: 286–287.
15. Pawar M. Onychodystrophy due to porokeratosis of Mibelli: A rare association. *Acta Dermato Venerologica* 2017; 26: 51–52.
16. Bettoli V, De Padova MP, Corazza M, Virgili A. Generalized lichen nitidus with oral and nail involvement in a child. *Dermatology* 1997; 194(4): 367–369.
17. Munro CS, Cox NH, Marks JM, Natarajan S. Lichen nitidus presenting as palmoplantar hyperkeratosis and nail dystrophy. *Clin Exp Dermatol* 1993; 18: 381–383.
18. Tay EY, Ho MSL, Chandran NS, Lee JS, Heng YK. Lichen nitidus presenting with nail changes—Case report and review of the literature. *Pediatr Dermatol* 2015; 32(3): 386–388.
19. Inamadar AC. Lichen striatus with nail involvement. *Indian J Dermatol Venereol Leprol* 2001; 67: 197.
20. Das S, Adhicari P. Lichen striatus in children: A clinical study of ten cases with review of literature. *Indian J Paediatr Dermatol* 2017; 18: 89–93.

21. Krishnegowda SY, Reddy SK, Vasudevan P. Lichen striatus with onychodystrophy in an infant. *Indian Dermatol Online J* 2015; 6: 333–335.

22. Burge SM, Wilkinson JD. Darier–White disease: A review of the clinical features of 163 patients. *J Am Acad Dermatol* 1992; 27: 40–50.

23. Sehgal VN, Chatterjee K, Chaudhuri A, Verma P, Sharma S. Twenty-nail dystrophy and Darier's (Darier-white) disease. *Skinmed* 2015; 13: 313–315.

24. Munro CS. The phenotype of Darier's disease: Penetrance and expressivity in adults and children. *Br J Dermatol* 1992; 127: 126–130.

25. Kumar R, Zawar V. Longitudinal leukonychia in Hailey-Hailey disease: A sign not to be missed. *Dermatol Online J* 2008; 14(3): 17.

26. Bel B, Soudry-Faure A, Vabres P. Diagnostic value of nail examination in Hailey-Hailey disease. *Eur J Dermatol* 2014; 24(5): 628–629.

27. Puri N. A study on palm plantar keratodermas in childhood in a district hospital. *Indian J Paediatr Dermatol* 2017; 18: 183–186.

28. Kelsell DP, Leigh IM. Inherited keratodermas of palms and soles. In: Wolff K, Goldsmith LA, Katz SI, Gilchrist BA, Paller AS, Lefell DJ, editors. *Fitzpatrick's Dermatology in General Medicine*, 7th ed. New York: McGraw-Hill; 2008. pp. 425–430.

29. Schiller S, Seebode C, Hennies HC, Giehl K, Emmert S. Palmoplantar keratoderma (PPK): Acquired and genetic causes of a not so rare disease. *J Dtsch Dermatol Ges* 2014; 12(9): 781–788.

30. Inamadar AC, Palit A. Nails: Diagnostic cue to geno-dermatoses. *Indian J Dermatol Venereol Leprol* 2012; 78: 271–278.

31. Guerra L, Castori M, Didona B, Castiglia D, Zambruno G. Hereditary palmoplantar keratoder-mas. Part II: Syndromic palmoplantar keratodermas – Diagnostic algorithm and principles of therapy. *J Eur Acad Dermatol Venereol* 2018; 32(6): 899–925. doi:10.1111/jdv.14834.

32. Mittal RR, Jha A. Hereditary punctate palmoplantar keratoderma—A clinical study. *Indian J Dermatol Venereol Leprol* 2003; 69: 90–91.

33. James WD, Berger TG, Elston MD. Pityriasis rosea, pityriasis rubra pilaris, and other papulosquamous and hyperkeratotic diseases. In: *Andrews' Diseases of the Skin: Clinical Dermatology*, 11th ed. London, UK: Elsevier, 2011. p. 208.

34. Gupta LK, Martin AM, Agarwal N, D'Souza P, Kumar P, Pande S et al. Guidelines for the management of Stevens-Johnson syndrome/toxic epidermal necrolysis: An Indian perspective. *Indian J Dermatol Venereol Leprol* 2016; 82: 603–625.

35. Wanscher B, Thormann J. Permanent anonychia after Stevens-Johnson syndrome. *Arch dermatol* 1997; 113: 970.

36. Lerch M, Mainetti C, Terziroli Beretta-Piccoli B, Harr T. Current perspectives on Stevens-Johnson syndrome and toxic epidermal necrolysis. *Clin Rev Allergy Immunol* 2018; 54(1): 147–176.

37. Baran R, Haneke E. Severe nail dystrophy, hypo-nychia and anonychia, and alterations of nail shape. In: *Nail in Differential Dermatology*, 1st ed. Boca Raton, FL: CRC Press; 2006. pp. 28–48.

38. Habibi M, Mortazavi H, Shadianloo S, Balighi K, Ghodsi SZ, Daneshpazhooh M et al. Nail changes in pemphigus vulgaris. *Int J Dermatol* 2008; 47: 1141–1144.

39. Cahali JB, Kakuda EYS, Santi CG, Maruta CW. Nail manifestations in pemphigus vulgaris. *Rev Hosp Clin* 2002; 57(5): 229–234.

40. Zawar V, Pawar M, Kumavat S. Recurrent paronychia as a presenting manifestation of pemphigus vulgaris: A case report. *Skin Appendage Disord* 2017; 3(1): 28–31.

41. Gualco F, Cozzani E, Parodi A. Bullous pemphigoid with nail loss. *Int J Dermatol* 2005; 44: 967–968.

42. Tosti A, André M, Murrell DF. Nail involvement in autoimmune bullous disorders. *Dermatol Clin* 2011; 29: 511–513.

43. Henriquez MA, Alvarez IL, Rodriguez CV, Araya VL, Markthaler M, Peris EG et al. Bullous pemphigoid and nail lesions: Ultrasound correlation. *J Am Acad Dermatol* 2017; 76(6): AB59.

44. Mohor GS, Solovan C. Onychodystrophy and scarring alopecia in epidermolysis bullosa acquisita: A case based review of the literature. *J Clin Case Rep* 2016; 6: 2.

45. Bruckner-Tuderman L, Schnyder UW, Baran R. Nail changes in epidermolysis bullosa: Clinical and patho-genetic considerations. *Br J Dermatol* 1995; 132(3): 339–344.

46. Trueb RM. Involvement of scalp and nails in lupus erythematosus. *Lupus* 2010; 19: 1078–1086.

47. Richert B, André J, Bourguignon R, de la Brassinne M. Hyperkeratotic nail discoid lupus erythemato-sus evolving towards systemic lupus erythemato-sus: Therapeutic difficulties. *J Eur Acad Dermatol Venereol* 2004; 18: 728–730.

48. Garcia-Patos V, Bartralot R, Ordi J, Baselga E, de Moragas J, MD, Castell A. Systemic lupus erythe-matosus presenting with red lunulae. *J Am Acad Dermatol* 1997; 36: 834–836.

49. Marie I, Gremain V, Nassermadji K, Richard L, Joly P, Menard JF, Levesque H. Nail involvement in systemic sclerosis. *J Am Acad Dermatol* 2017; 76(6): 1115–1123.

50. Cutolo M, Sulli A, Secchi ME, Paolino S, Pizzorni C. Nail fold capillaroscopy is useful for the diagnosis and follow-up of autoimmune rheumatic diseases. A future tool for the analysis of microvascular heart involvement? *Rheumatology (Oxford)* 2006; 45 Suppl 4: iv43–iv46.

51. Sherber NS, Wigley FM, Scher RK. Autoimmune disorders: Nail signs and therapeutic approaches. *Dermatol Ther* 2007; 20(1): 17–30.

52. Elmansour I, Chiheb S, Benchikhi H. Nail changes in connective tissue diseases: A study of 39 cases. *Pan Afr Med J* 2014; 18: 150.

53. Manfredi A, Sebastiani M, Cassone G, Pipitone N, Giuggioli D, Colaci M et al. Nail fold capillaroscopic changes in dermatomyositis and polymyositis. *Clin Rheumatol* 2015; 34(2): 279–284.

54. Tunc SE, Ertam I, Pirildar T, Turk T, Ozturk M, Doganavsargil E. Nail changes in connective tissue diseases: Do nail changes provide clues for the diagnosis? *J Eur Acad Dermatol Venereol* 2007; 21(4): 497–503.

55. El-Komy MH, Baran R. Acroosteolysis presenting with brachyonychia following exposure to cold. *J Eur Acad Dermatol Venereol* 2015; 29(11): 2252–2254.

56. van Steensel MA, Verstraeten VL, Frank J. Acrokeratoelastoidosis with nail dystrophy: A coincidence or a new entity? *Arch Dermatol* 2006; 142(7): 939–941.

57. Gutte R, Kothari D, Khopkar U. Granuloma annulare on the palms: A clinicopathological study of seven cases. *Indian J Dermatol Venereol Leprol* 2012; 78: 468–474.

58. Futei Y, Konohana I. A case of erythema elevatum diutinum associated with B-cell lymphoma: A rare distribution involving palms, soles and nails. *Br J Dermatol* 2000; 142(1): 116–119.

59. Figueras-Nart I, Vicente A, Sánchez-Schmidt J, Jou-Muñoz C, Bordas-Orpinell X, Celis-Passini VP et al. Langerhans cell histiocytosis presenting as fingernail changes. *JAAD Case Rep* 2016; 2(6): 485–487.

60. Piraccini BM, Fanti PA, Iorizzo M, Tosti A. Juvenile xanthogranuloma of the proximal nail fold. *Pediatr Dermatol* 2003; 20(4): 307–308.

61. Silvers SH, Glickman FS. Pityriasis rosea followed by nail dystrophy. *Arch Dermatol* 1964; 90: 31.

62. Savant SS, Das A, Kumar P. Paronychia and onychomadesis due to pemphigus vulgaris. *Indian J Dermatol Venereol Leprol* 2017; 83: 212.

20

Nails in systemic disease

BELA J. SHAH

INTRODUCTION

Examination of the nails should be an integral part of physical examination. A few nail changes can be presenting feature of systemic disease before other signs and symptoms become clinically evident. Fingernails usually provide more accurate information than toenails, because clinical signs on toenails are often modified by trauma. Nails should be examined in good light, and in addition to clinical examination, dermatoscopy/onychoscopy may be used as an ancillary tool.

Nail abnormalities in systemic disease can be broadly classified and discussed as summarized in Table 20.1.[1-3]

Before going into details of each change, it is worthwhile to know that certain nail changes are more specific for a particular disease (Table 20.2) and, hence, have diagnostic value. On the other hand, various nail changes are not specific enough for a particular disease (Box 20.1) and their

Table 20.1 Various nail changes in systemic diseases

Abnormalities of nail shape	Abnormalities of nail attachment	Abnormalities of nail surface	Abnormalities of nail color
• Koilonychia	• Onycholysis	• Onychorrhexis	• Leukonychia
• Clubbing	• Pterygium	• Beau's lines	• Melanonychia
• Pincer nails		• Trachyonychia	• Cyanosis
• Dolichonychia		• Onychoschizia	• Icterus
• Brachyonychia			• Nicotine staining of nails
• Parrot beak nail			• Splinter hemorrhages
• Macronychia			• Yellow nail syndrome
• Micronychia			• Red lunula

Source: Singal, A., and Arora, R., *Indian Dermatol. Online J.*, 6, 67–74, 2015; Tosti, A. et al., *Dermatol. Clin.*, 24, 341–347, 2006; Fawcett, R.S. et al., *Am. Fam. Physician*, 69, 1417–1424, 2004.

Table 20.2 Nail changes more specifically associated with systemic disease

Nail changes	Example	Associated systemic condition
True leukonychia	Mees' lines	Arsenic poisoning
Apparent leukonychia	Muehrcke's lines	Hypoalbuminemia
	Half-and-half nails	Renal diseases
	Terry's nails	Hepatic cirrhosis
Clubbing		Cardiopulmonary diseases

Source: Singal, A., and Arora, R., *Indian Dermatol. Online J.*, 6, 67–74, 2015; Tosti, A. et al., *Dermatol. Clin.*, 24, 341–347, 2006.

BOX 20.1: **Nail changes less specific for systemic diseases**[2,3]

- Splinter hemorrhages
- Beau's lines
- Pigmented bands
- Onycholysis
- Pitting
- Koilonychia
- Anonychia
- Micronychia

---

clinical relevance is uncertain. However, they do indicate presence of a systemic condition and efforts should be made to look for an underlying condition. Table 20.3 summarizes common nail changes noted in various systemic conditions.

Details of common nail changes encountered in different systemic diseases are discussed below.

ABNORMALITIES OF NAIL SHAPE

Koilonychia (Greek: *Koilos* = hollow, *Onyx* = nail)[1,5]

It is the presence of reverse curvature in the transverse and longitudinal axes that gives a concave dorsal aspect to the nail[8] (Figure 20.1). These changes result in spooning of the nails capable of retaining a drop of water. It is appreciably more on fingernails than toenails. Occupational softening and iron deficiency are the most common causes. However, the majority of adults with koilonychia demonstrate a familial pattern that may be an autosomal-dominant trait. The petaloid nail is an early stage of koilonychia and is characterized by flattening of the nail.[1] It is believed to result from anoxia and subsequent atrophy

Table 20.3 Nail abnormalities associated with disease of a specific organ system

Organ system	Nail changes
Renal disease	• Half-and-half nail • Muehrcke's nail • Terry's nail • Splinter hemorrhages • Mees' lines
Pulmonary disease	• Clubbing • Yellow nail syndrome
Cardiovascular disease	• Splinter hemorrhages • Koilonychia
Gastrointestinal disease	• Terry's nail • Azure lunula • Muehrcke's line • Brittle nail • Longitudinal striations • True leukonychia
Infectious disease	• Elkynosis • Paronychia • Onychomadesis • Fragility • Racket nails • Subungual abscess • Lilac line of Milan
Endocrine disease	• Longitudinal pigmented bands • Short and brittle nails • Periungual erythema • Telangiectasia • Plummer's nails
Autoimmune disease	• Nail fold capillary abnormality • Beau's line • Periungual telangiectasia • Splinter hemorrhages • Ragged cuticle • Pitted scar • Ventral pterygium • Cuticular hemorrhage • Nail beaking
Central and peripheral nervous system	• Destruction of nails (Lesch–Nyhan syndrome) • Beau's line
Psychological disease	• Onychotillomania • Striated leukonychia

Source: Singal, A., and Arora, R., *Indian Dermatol. Online J.*, 6, 67–74, 2015; Tosti, A. et al., *Dermatol. Clin.*, 24, 341–347, 2006; Fawcett, R.S. et al., *Am. Fam. Physician*, 69, 1417–1424, 2004; Singh, G., *Indian J. Dermatol. Venereol. Leprol.*, 77, 646–651, 2011.

responsible for lowering of the distal matrix as compared to the proximal matrix. Conditions associated with koilonychias include (Box 20.2).

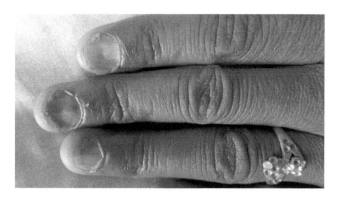

Figure 20.1 Koilonychia in patient of iron deficiency anemia.

BOX 20.2: Causes of koilonychia

- Idiopathic
- Iron deficiency anemia
- Hemochromatosis
- Coronary disease
- Thyroid disorders
- Upper gastrointestinal malignancy
- Traumatic injury
- Nail exposure to chemicals and acitretin
- Occupational
- Raynaud's disease
- Systemic lupus erythematosus
- Nail–patella syndrome
- Old age
- Digital ischemia
- Psoriasis

Clubbing

Clubbing is characterized by increased nail plate curvature longitudinally and transversely with soft tissue hypertrophy of the digital pulp (Figure 20.2), usually involving all 20 digits. It may be associated with hypertrophic osteoarthropathy, in which subperiosteal new bone formation in the distal diaphysis of the long bones of the extremities causes pain and symmetric arthritis-like changes in the shoulders, knees, ankles, wrists, and elbows.[1,2] Clubbing may be an early sign of AIDS in pediatric HIV-positive patients.[2] The common causes of bilateral clubbing is listed in Box 20.3.

The condition may result from megakaryocytes and platelet clumps that have entered the systemic circulation from the pulmonary bed. Platelets then may release platelet-derived growth factor at the nail bed, causing periosteal changes.[6]

BOX 20.3: Causes of clubbing[2,6]

- Cyanotic congenital heart diseases
- Bronchiectasis
- Cystic fibrosis
- Hepatic cirrhosis
- Primary and metastatic lung cancer
- Lung abscess
- Mesothelioma
- Inflammatory bowel disease
- Arteriovenous malformation
- Idiopathic

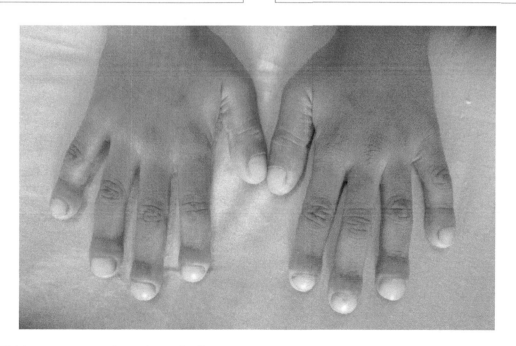

Figure 20.2 Clubbing in patient of Tetralogy of Fallot.

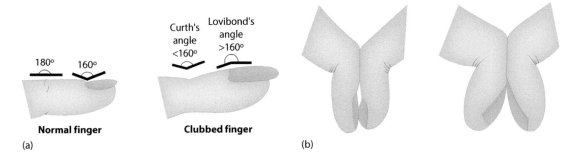

Figure 20.3 **(a)** Clubbed finger showing Curth angle and Lovibond angle. See the corresponding angles in normal nail to appreciate the difference. **(b)** Schamroth sign.

There are three types of geometric assessment (Figure 20.3a and b) used for clubbing[1,6]:

1. Lovibond's angle: This is the angle formed at the junction between nail plate and proximal nail fold and it is normally less than 160°. In clubbing, this is increased to over 180°.
2. Curth's angle: At distal interphalangeal (DIP) joint is normally approximately 180° and this diminishes to less than 160° in clubbing.

3. Schamroth sign refers to the obliteration of normally diamond-shaped space formed when dorsal sides of the distal phalanges of corresponding right and left digits are opposed.

Pincer nail

Pincer nail (also known as omega nails) is a toenail disorder that is characterized by transverse over-curvature along the longitudinal axis, in which the lateral edges of the nail slowly approach each other reaching to its greatest proportion toward the tip (Figure 20.4a and b). This condition

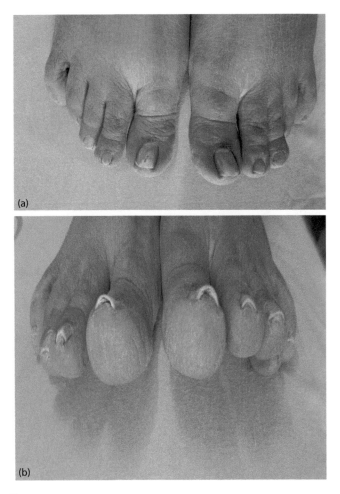

Figure 20.4 **(a and b)** Pincer nails.

is a painful one where it compresses the nail bed and the underlying dermis. Among acquired systemic diseases, pincer nail has been reported in systemic lupus erythematosus and amyotrophic lateral sclerosis.[7,8]

Parrot beaking of the nail

It refers to the excessive forward curvature of the free edge of nail, resembling a parrot's beak. Most commonly, parrot beaking results as an idiopathic finding caused by delayed nail plate trimming, but it may be associated with various systemic conditions. The most common causes include atrophy of digital pulp and absorption of terminal phalanx as noted in vascular insufficiency in scleroderma and repeated microtrauma due to distal neuropathy resulting from diabetes, spinal canal stenosis, leprosy, etc. The condition is usually asymptomatic until the nail grows into soft tissue of the digit.[9]

ABNORMALITIES OF NAIL ATTACHMENT

Onycholysis

Onycholysis refers to the distal separation of the nail plate from the nail bed. Nails with onycholysis are usually smooth, firm, and without nail bed inflammation.

BOX 20.4: Systemic causes of onycholysis[1-3]

- Anemia
- Bronchiectasis
- Lung cancer
- Cutaneous T-cell lymphoma
- Diabetes mellitus
- Thyroid disorders
- Porphyria
- Lupus erythematosus
- Psoriatic arthritis
- Sezary syndrome
- Drugs (psoralens and tetracyclines)
- Vitamin C deficiency

It is not a disease of the nail matrix, though nail discoloration may appear underneath the nail as a result of secondary infection. Areas of separation appear white or yellow due to air beneath the nail and sequestered debris (Figure 20.5). Systemic causes of Onycholysis have been mentioned in Box 20.4.

Pterygium

Pterygium unguis results from scarring involving the nail fold, which extends into the nail matrix (dorsal pterygium). It occurs when a central fibrotic band divides a nail proximally into two, obstructing normal nail growth (ventral pterygium). A large pterygium may destroy the whole nail.[3] The causes of pterygium have been listed in Box 20.5.[2-4]

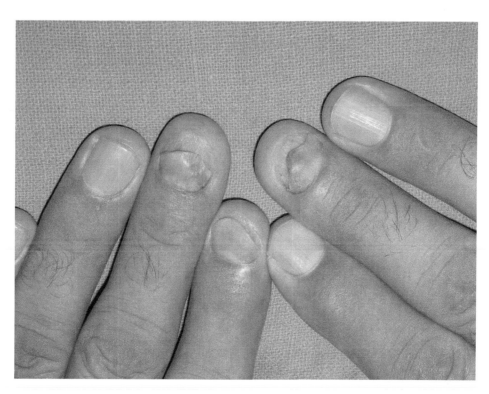

Figure 20.5 Onycholysis in a patient of onychomycosis. (Courtesy of Prof Archana Singal.)

BOX 20.5: **Causes of pterygium**

Dorsal pterygium
- Lichen planus (Figure 20.6)
- Cicatricial pemphigoid
- Dyskeratosis congenita
- Chronic graft versus host disease

Ventral pterygium
- Leprosy
- Neurofibromatosis
- Subungual exostosis
- Lupus erythematosus
- Systemic sclerosis (Figure 20.7)

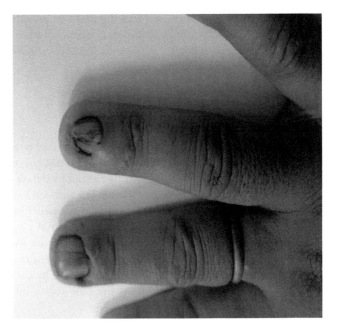

Figure 20.6 Dorsal pterygium in a patient of lichen planus.

ABNORMALITIES OF NAIL SURFACE

Longitudinal ridging

Longitudinal lines, or striations, appear as projecting ridges and may represent long-lasting abnormalities. These ridges that run along the longitudinal axis of all or part of the length of the nail (Figure 20.8). Causes of logitudinal ridging have been mentioned in Box 20.6.

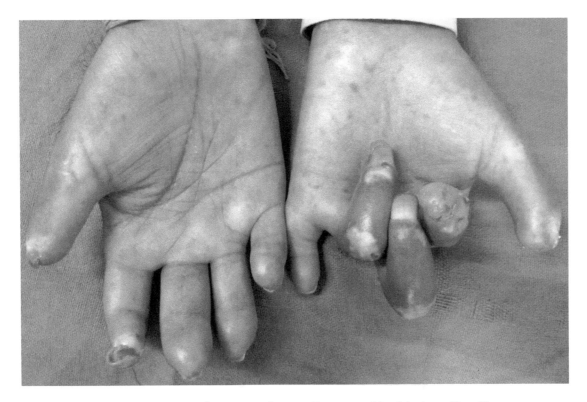

Figure 20.7 Ventral pterygium in a patient of systemic sclerosis. (Courtesy of Prof Archana Singal.)

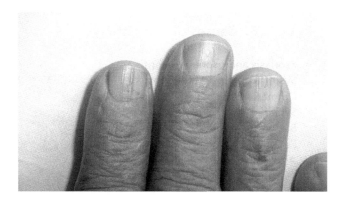

Figure 20.8 Longitudinal ridging.

Beau's lines

These run along the transverse axis of the nail and may be of full or partial thickness. Beau's lines occur at the same spot of the nail plate in most or all the nails and may be caused by any disease severe enough to disrupt normal nail growth. It is the most common and least specific nail change in a systemic disease. They appear first at the cuticle and move distally with nail growth. Beau's lines are more apparent on thumb and great toenails. They have a margin parallel to the lunula, when caused by a systemic disease (Figure 20.9). The time of stress can be calculated after measuring the distance from the cuticle to the Beau's lines. Its exact cause is not known but there is temporary cessation of nail growth in the matrix by various factors. If there is complete inhibition of nail growth for around 2 weeks, Beau's line will reach maximum depth resulting in onychomadesis. Recurrent bouts of illness may lead to the formation of series of transverse furrows/grooves. The width of the transverse groove relates to the duration of the disease that has affected the matrix. The distal limit of the furrow, if abrupt, indicates a sudden attack of disease; if sloping, a more protracted onset.[1,2] Conditions associated with Beau's lines are listed in Box 20.7.

Factors responsible for Beau's lines are (Box 20.7):

Nail pitting

Pits result from a defective keratinization of the proximal matrix with persistence of parakeratotic cells in the nail plate

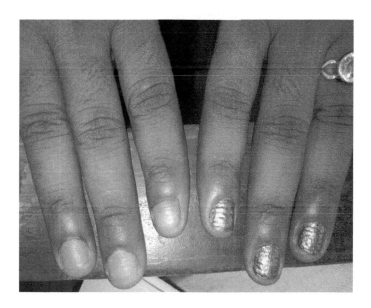

Figure 20.9 Beau's lines.

BOX 20.7: Beau's lines in systemic diseases

- Severe acute illness such as
  - Fever
  - Heart attack
  - Exposure to extreme cold
  - Psychological stress
  - Poor nutritional status
- The presence of Beau's lines on all 20 nails is seen in
  - Mumps
  - Pneumonia
  - Coronary thrombosis
  - Kawasaki disease
  - Syphilis
  - Hypoparathyroidism
- Trauma involving proximal nail fold
- Idiopathic and inherited forms

BOX 20.8: Causes of nail pitting

- Psoriasis and psoriatic arthritis
- Systemic lupus erythematosus
- Dermatomyositis
- Syphilis
- Sarcoidosis
- Pemphigus vulgaris
- Alopecia areata
- Incontinentia pigmenti

surface. These are punctuated by erosions on the nail surface (Figure 20.10). They may be shallow or deep with a regular or irregular outline. An isolated large pit may produce a localized full-thickness defect in the nail plate termed elkonyxis,

which is a feature of Reiter's disease.[1,3,4] Causes of nail pitting have been mentioned in Box 20.8.

Onychoschizia

Horizontal splitting of nail toward its distal portion is also called lamellar splitting of nail (Figure 20.11a and b). It is also called lamellar dystrophy. This can result in discoloration of the nail due to sequestration of debris between the layers.[2,3] The common conditions associated with onychoscizia is listed in Box 20.9.

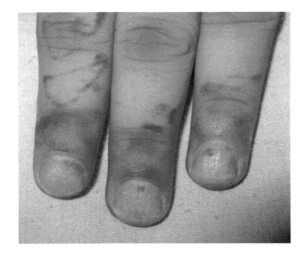

Figure 20.10 Nail pitting.

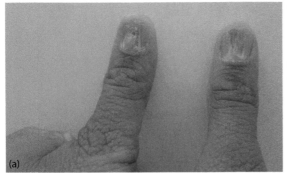
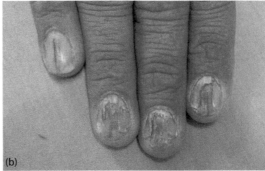

(a) (b)

Figure 20.11 (**a** and **b**) Onychoschizia.

ABNORMALITIES OF NAIL COLOR

Leukonychia

Leukonychia refers to the white discoloration of the nail plate. It is traditionally classified into three subtypes.[1,2]

- **True leukonychia** – Pathology originates in matrix and emerges in the nail plate. Here nails are porcelain white; this may be due to chronic liver disease, but there are rare inherited forms (Figure 20.12).
- **Apparent leukonychia** – Here, the pathology is in the nail bed. On pressure, the leukonychia becomes less apparent and this maneuver differentiates apparent leukonychia from true leukonychia.
- **Pseudo leukonychia** – Nail plate pathology is exogenous, for example, onychomycosis.

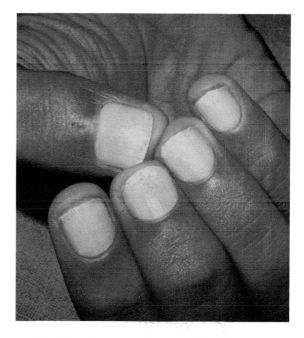

Figure 20.12 Leukonychia (courtesy of Prof. Archana Singal).

Most commonly, leukonychia associated with systemic disease is usually true or apparent leukonychia, as summarized in Table 20.4.

Table 20.4 Leukonychia in systemic diseases

True leukonychia	
Mees' line (Figure 20.13)[1,10]	<ul><li>A single or multiple, transverse, narrow whitish line running along the width of the nail and parallel to the lunula</li><li>Affect multiple nails, although they may also occur singly</li><li>As the defect is in the nail plate itself, the line moves distally as the nail grows. Thus, the timing of the insult can be determined by measuring the distance of the lines from the cuticle.</li><li>Seen in arsenic, thallium, and other heavy metal poisoning</li><li>Can also be seen in renal failures and in patients on chemotherapy. Other rare causes are mentioned in Box 20.10.</li></ul>
Apparent leukonychia	
Muehrcke's lines[1,2] (Figure 20.14)	<ul><li>Seen as double white transverse lines</li><li>Results possibly from a localized edematous state in the nail bed exerting pressure on the vascular bed</li><li>Because the lesion is in the nail bed, it does not move distally with nail growth.</li><li>Specific for hypoalbuminic state (occur in patients with albumin level <2 g/dL)</li><li>These lines disappear when the protein level normalizes. Seen in nephrotic syndrome, glomerulonephritis, liver disease, chemotherapeutic drugs, malnutrition.</li></ul>
Half-and-half nail or Lindsay nail[1,2,11] (Figure 20.15)	<ul><li>Apparent leukonychia with a normal proximal half and abnormal brownish discolored distal half</li><li>It is seen in patients of chronic kidney disease with uremic renal failure.</li></ul>
Terry's nails[1,2,11] (Figure 20.16)	<ul><li>It is an apparent leukonychia characterized by ground glass opacification of nearly the entire nail, obliteration of the lunula, and a narrow band of normal, pink nail bed at the distal border.</li><li>Common causes include congestive cardiac failure, adult-onset diabetes mellitus, peripheral vascular disease, hemodialysis, and HIV.</li></ul>

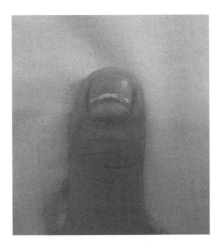

Figure 20.13 Mees' lines.

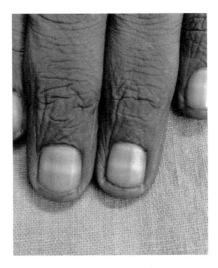

Figure 20.14 Muehrcke's lines (courtesy of Prof. Archana Singal).

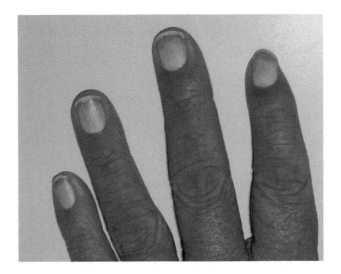

Figure 20.15 Half-and-half nail or Lindsay nail (courtesy of Prof. Archana Singal).

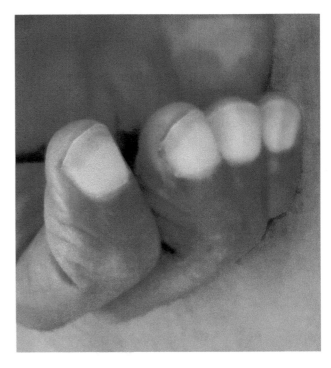

Figure 20.16 Terry's nails (courtesy of Prof. Archana Singal).

BOX 20.10: Uncommon and rare associations of Mees' lines[2,10]

- Hodgkin's disease
- Leprosy
- Tuberculosis
- Malaria
- Herpes zoster
- Chemotherapeutic drugs
- Carbon monoxide (CO) and antimony poisoning
- Renal and cardiac failure
- Pneumonia
- Childbirth

Melanonychia

A longitudinal or transverse brownish-black pigmentation of nail is known as melanonychia. It has been typically attributed to lichen planus.

Melanonychia (Figure 20.17) may be part of racial pigmentation (constitutional) or due to underlying melanocytic nevus or malignant melanoma. Common systemic causes are listed in Box 20.11.[1-3]

Cyanosis

Cyanosis manifests as blue or purple discoloration of the nail bed and digits as a result of lower oxygen saturation causing accumulation of deoxyhemoglobin in the small blood vessels of the extremities.

Central cyanosis is caused by congenital heart diseases and may manifest on mucosa and extremities, whereas

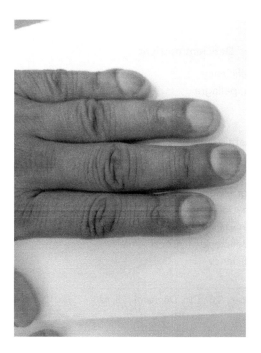

Figure 20.17 Melanonychia.

Splinter hemorrhages

Splinter hemorrhages in nails are tiny bleeding points in the nail bed and hyponychium of the nail unit. They are formed by the extravasation of blood from the longitudinally oriented vessels of the nail bed. A simultaneous occurrence in multiple nails is indicative of a systemic cause, mentioned in Box 20.12.[1–3]

> **BOX 20.12: Systemic causes of splinter hemorrhage**
>
> - Infective endocarditis
> - Rheumatic heart disease
> - Valvular replacement
> - Connective tissue diseases like systemic lupus erythematosus and scleroderma
> - Antiphospholipid syndrome
> - Intravenous drug abusers
> - Congenital heart diseases
> - Drugs – aspirin

Yellow nail syndrome

It is characterized by thickening and yellow to yellow-green discoloration of the nails often associated with systemic disease. Most common causes are lymphedema and compromised respiration due to pleural effusion. The lunula is obscured and there is increased transverse and longitudinal curvature with loss of cuticle.[1,2]

Red lunula

Red lunula result from increased arteriolar blood flow, a vasodilatory capacitance phenomenon, or changes in the optical properties of the overlying nail so that normal blood vessels become more apparent.

It may merge with the nail bed in the distal part of the lunula or be demarcated by a pale line and can be obliterated by pressure on the nail plate. Common systemic causes are mentioned in Box 20.13.[2,12]

> **BOX 20.13: Systemic conditions associated with red lunula**
>
> - Chronic obstructive pulmonary disease
> - Rheumatoid arthritis
> - Systemic lupus erythematosus
> - Cardiac failure
> - Cirrhosis of liver
> - Carbon monoxide poisoning
> - Twenty-nail dystrophy
> - Reticulosarcoma

> **BOX 20.11: Systemic causes of melanonychia**
>
> - Hemochromatosis
> - Malnutrition
> - Thyroid disease
> - Smoking
> - HIV infection
> - Addison's disease
> - Drugs – Antimalarials, Minocycline, Phenytoin, Psoralens, sulfonamides, zidovudine, doxorubicin, methotrexate, azathioprine, etc.[12]

peripheral cyanosis is usually diagnosed by examination of the nail and digits and is caused by vasoconstriction and diminished peripheral blood flow as occurs in cold exposure, shock, congestive cardiac failure, and peripheral vascular disease.[1,2,12]

Icterus

Yellowish discoloration of the mucosae as a result of deposition of bilirubin and may extend to involve the nails in severe cases of liver disease or in patients on hemolysis.[2,12]

Nicotine staining of nails

It is seen in heavy smokers and manifests as yellow discoloration of nail due to nicotine deposition. The discoloration may be a telltale sign of long-term chances of development of cigarette-associated diseases such as carcinoma lung, chronic obstructive airway disease, and coronary artery disease.[12]

Table 20.5 Nail changes in various nutritional deficiencies

Nail findings	Deficient nutrient
Longitudinal melanonychia	Vitamin B12 and vitamin D deficiency
Transverse leukonychia	Acrodermatitis enteropathica, pellagra
Terry's nails	Malnutrition
Half-and-half nail	Pellagra
Muehrcke's line	Hypoalbuminemia, acrodermatitis enteropathica
Splinter hemorrhages	Scurvy
Koilonychia	Iron deficiency anemia, Plummer–Vinson syndrome, riboflavin deficiency, pellagra
Onycholysis	Iron deficiency anemia, pellagra, Cronkhite–Canada syndrome
Beau's line	Protein deficiency, pellagra, hypocalcemia
Onychomadesis	Hypocalcemia, Cronkhite–Canada syndrome
Onychorrhexis	Iron deficiency anemia, zinc deficiency, hypocalcemia
Central ridges	Iron, folic acid, or protein deficiency
Clubbing	Iodine deficiency

Source: Tosti, A. et al., *Dermatol. Clin.,* 24, 341–347, 2006; Cashman, M.W., and Sloan, S.B., *Clin. Dermatol.,* 28, 420–425, 2010; Scheinfeld, N. et al., *J. Drugs Dermatol.,* 6, 782–787, 2007.

NAIL CHANGES IN MALNUTRITION

Varying degrees of nutritional deficiency are common in developing countries like India and awareness of nail changes noted in malnutrition is essential to avoid unnecessary investigations. Nail changes in malnutrition are minor and nonspecific. The most common finding is Beau's lines and Brittle Nail syndrome, characterized by soft, dry, weak, easily breakable nails that show onychorrhexis and onychoschizia. Other nail changes have been summarized in Table 20.5. In general, Kwashiorkor is associated with soft and thin nails; marasmic children have fissured nails and impaired nail growth.[2,13,14]

CONCLUSION

Nail findings may not only be a window to a plethora of possible systemic associations, but also a window of opportunity for an astute dermatologist to identify the uncommon or even rare diseases. Profound knowledge of the associations may be useful in a complete and targeted workup of the patient to clinch a systemic disease, which may be more sinister.

KEY POINTS

- Nail is an important appendage of skin though it may remain an entity that attracts very few dermatologists.
- At times, nails act as a mirror to internal or systemic diseases.
- Nail changes are common in systemic disorders affecting liver, heart, kidney, and lungs.
- A few nail changes are nonspecific and many are specific for systemic disorders.

REFERENCES

1. Singal A, Arora R. Nail as a window of systemic diseases. *Indian Dermatol Online J* 2015;6:67–74.
2. Tosti A, Iorizzo M, Piraccini BM, Starace M. The nail in systemic diseases. *Dermatol Clin* 2006;24(3):341–347.

3. Fawcett RS, Linford S, Stulberg DL. Nail abnormalities: Clues to systemic disease. *Am Fam Physician* 2004;69(6):1417–1424.

4. Singh G. Nails in systemic disease. *Indian J Dermatol Venereol Leprol* 2011;77:646–651.

5. Walker J, Baran R, Vélez N, Jellinek N. Koilonychia: An update on pathophysiology, differential diagnosis and clinical relevance. *J Eur Acad Dermatol Venereol* 2016;30(11):1985–1991.

6. Spicknall KE, Zirwas MJ, English JC 3rd. Clubbing: An update on diagnosis, differential diagnosis, pathophysiology and clinical relevance. *J Am Acad Dermatol* 2005;52(6):1020–1027.

7. Azevedo THV, Neiva CLS, Consoli RV, Couto ACD, Dias AFMP, Souza EJR. Pincer nail in a lupus patient. *Lupus* 2017;26(14):1562–1563.

8. Fujita Y, Fujita T. Pincer nail deformity in a patient with amyotrophic lateral sclerosis. *Neurol Int* 2014;6(4):5716.

9. Chen SX, Cohen PR. Parrot beak nails revisited: Case series and comprehensive review. *Dermatol Ther (Heidelb)* 2018;8(1):147–155.

10. Huang TC, Chao TY. Mees lines and Beau lines after chemotherapy. *CMAJ* 2010;182(3):E149.

11. Pitukweerakul S, Pilla S. Terry's nails and Lindsay's nails: Two nail abnormalities in chronic systemic diseases. *J Gen Intern Med* 2016;31(8):970.

12. Daniel CR, Osment LS. Nail pigmentation abnormalities. Their importance and proper examination. *Cutis* 1982;30(3):348–360.

13. Cashman MW, Sloan SB. Nutrition and nail disease. *Clin Dermatol* 2010;28(4):420–425.

14. Scheinfeld N, Dahdah MJ, Scher R. Vitamins and minerals: Their role in nail health and disease. *J Drugs Dermatol* 2007;6(8):782–787.

21

Occupational nail diseases

DEEPIKA PANDHI AND VANDANA KATARIA

INTRODUCTION

Occupational nail diseases are abnormalities of one or more structures of the nail apparatus, produced and/or aggravated by occupational factors. The occupation must be a major factor in its causation. For example, nail disease would not have occurred if the patient had not been involved in the work pertaining to that occupation.[1] Criteria for diagnosing occupational nail diseases have been summarized in Box 21.1.[1,2]

BOX 21.1: Diagnosis of occupational nail diseases

- Known or highly suspected workplace exposure to potentially noxious substances
- Temporal relationship between exposure and onset of nail symptoms
- Nail changes consistent with work-related exposure to noxious substances
- Exclusion of non-occupational exposure and nail involvement by various dermatoses

---

ETIOLOGY

Very often, multiple etiological factors play a role in pathogenesis of characteristic nail changes. The risk factors for developing occupational nail diseases are similar to occupational disorders elsewhere and are listed as follows:

- Inexperienced workers: Lack of awareness of safety measures to be taken at workplace (gloves, soaps) and indulging in improper handling of tools and chemicals are responsible for various occupational nail diseases. A cycle of occlusion, perspiration, maceration, and subsequent irritation is created by wearing protective gloves; therefore, its overuse or improper use paradoxically increases the risk of development of contact dermatitis.[3]
- Inadequate personal hygiene: Unavailability or inadequacy of basic hygiene methods at workplace.
- Excess use of irritants: Dealing with hazardous cleansing and sanitizing products with a high irritant potential that damages nail fold.
- Temperature and humidity: Low humidity and strong winds also cause the skin to become dry and predispose to skin irritation.

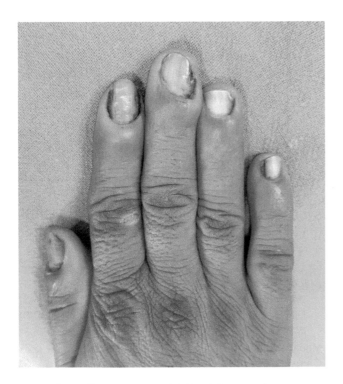

Figure 21.1 Chronic paronychia in a juice merchant. (Courtesy of Archana Singal.)

- Wet work: May impair the epidermal barrier, predisposing to skin irritation and sensitivity and paronychia (Figure 21.1).
- Personal atopy: Increased risk for job change, sick leave, and medical consultations, mainly due to the increased risk of hand eczema.[4]

Occupational factors

Various workplace factors unique to a particular occupation are the immediate cause of occupational nail diseases. Awareness of these factors is critical to prevention and management of these occupational nail diseases. Important workplace factors contributing to occupational nail diseases are summarized in Box 21.2 and are discussed below.

BOX 21.2: Factors responsible for occupational nail diseases[1,2]

1. Trauma
2. Physical
3. Sensitizers
4. Hand eczema
5. Wet work
6. Infections
7. Systemic absorption

TRAUMA

Acute injury in the nail unit of occupational onset may present as partial or total hematoma (25% of the surface of the visible nail plate), lacerating wounds, fractures of the terminal phalanx, denudation of the distal phalanx (nail degloving), and foreign bodies. Onycholysis, dorsal pterygium, and split nail deformity are labelled as delayed post-acute traumatic deformities. Eight digital myxoid cysts affecting the fingers of both hands have been described after 12 months of work, in a patient engaged in a job involving pushing a garment in an embroidery mold, thus exerting a downward force on the fingertips.[5] Similarly, subungual hemorrhages have been described among inexperienced male dishwashers using heavy rubber gloves and are also frequently seen in sportsmen's toes and in the toes of dancers.[6] Also, occupations involving vibrating power tools can lead to nail thickening, brittleness, and splitting of the free edges. Sports-related trauma occurs frequently in the form of golfer's nails, with distal splinter hemorrhages in the fingers used most strongly in the golf grip hand.[7] Exposure to certain plants and woods (e.g., thorns, thistle, sand, sharp-edged leaves of cacti, hyacinth, and narcissus bulbs) may cause foreign body injury.

PHYSICAL FACTORS

Burns, depending on severity, can lead to onycholysis, disfiguring scars, pterygium, and fissured nails. On the other hand, prolonged exposure to cold may result in injury to the nail matrix, leading to derangement of the nail plate ranging from Beau's lines to complete shedding. Interestingly, in Ladakh, India, seasonal koilonychia has been observed due to immersion of hands in cold water at work, for example while washing clothes[8] and subsequent to repairing walls and irrigation canals with wet mud.

SENSITIZERS

A heightened suspicion of allergic contact dermatitis (ACD) should be maintained for nail patients whose condition is not responding to appropriate treatment. Allergens and/or irritants may find their way through nail plate or periungual skin leading to contact dermatitis. For example, Alstroemeria dermatitis can result in onycholysis, in addition to dermatitis of the thumbs and index fingers.[9] Similar changes can also be seen with *Hydrangea*, *Tabernaemontana coronaria*, and "Tulip fingers." "Tulip fingers" is a painful, dry, fissured, hyperkeratotic eczema caused by contact with tulip bulbs and is seen in gardeners and bulb growers[10] with a history of contact with *Narcissus* sap. This irritant sap, as well as many other irritants such as hyacinth dust and pesticides, seemed to be responsible for many nail complaints.[10] It starts beneath the free margin of the nails and extends to the fingertips and periungual regions. Suppurative granulating erosions may be seen on the fingertips in long-standing cases. The highest concentration of the allergen, α-methylene-γ-butyrolactone, is to be found in the outermost cell layers of the inner bulbscales.[6] Common sensitizers of plant origin have been summarized in Box 21.3.

BOX 21.3: Contact dermatitis of plant origin

1. *Alstroemeria* dermatitis: onycholysis of thumb and index fingers
2. *Hydrangea* dermatitis: clinical picture of paronychia and nail dystrophy
3. *Nasturtium* (common plant used in salads): fingertip dermatitis
4. *Rhus* dermatitis: onycholysis and xanthonychia
5. Wooden orange stick (cuticle remover): responsible for persistent eczema of the right hand of manicurist
6. *Tabernaemontana coronaria*: fingertip dermatitis of first three fingers of both hands
7. Tulip fingers: painful, dry, fissured, hyperkeratotic eczema, under free margin of nail and extending up to tips
8. Turpentine (craft workers) eczema of fingers and periungual tissues with subungual hyperkeratosis

Among beauticians, occupational allergic dermatitis has been observed mostly in young trainees who are not using gloves for work such as shampooing, applying dye on hair, etc. A study evaluating contact dermatitis in beauticians by patch testing revealed the following as the most common allergens on patch testing: dyes (as is, open test), cold permanent wave primary solutions (as is, open test), and a shampoo (1% aq., closed test). Positive reactions to allergens were seen with para-phenylenediamine (1% pet), ammonium thioglycolate (5% aq., open test), para-toluenediamine (1% pet), para-aminophenol (1% pet), ortho-aminophenol (1% pet), Quinoline yellow SS (0.5% pet), nickel sulfate (2.5% pet), cobalt sulfate (2.3% pet), thimerosal (0.05% pet), and procaine hydrochloride (1% pet) in decreasing order.[11]

Acrylic monomers used in sculpting artificial nails are important contact and occupational sensitizers that can produce cross-reactions with other acrylic compounds and trigger allergic reactions when re-exposure occurs in a different setting.[12] Artificial nails are an increasingly popular cosmetic enhancement to the natural nail. Nail cosmetics include coatings that harden upon evaporation (nail enamel, base coat, top coat) and coatings that polymerize (sculptured nails, light-curing gels, preformed artificial nails, and nail-mending and nail-wrapping products). Distant ACD is more common with nail enamel than with coatings that polymerize, whereas coatings that polymerize are greater offenders in the nail area. Acrylic monomers used when sculpting artificial nails are important contact and occupational sensitizers that can produce cross reactions with other acrylic compounds.[13]

Amongst acrylics, the methacrylate and acrylate compounds are found in plastic glass for aircraft, paints, coatings, and printing inks, as well as in dentistry. Also, acrylates have a broad area of application in various products, such as the manufacture of dental prostheses and tooth fillings; printing colors; lacquers; paints; orthopedic prostheses and splints; soft contact lenses; histological preparations; floor waxes; floor coatings; surface treatments of leather, textiles, and paper products; nail cosmetics; and as glues, sealants, and adhesives.[14] Nail cosmetics are obviously important allergens of the nail region. Usually, the dorsal aspects of some of the fingers and paronychial tissue, face, and the eyelids may begin to show an ACD.[15] Thumb and index or middle finger of left hand of manicurists, who are constantly exposed to acrylates may also show ACD.[16] Recently, in a study of 66 patients allergic to some acrylic monomer, the most commonly positive allergens were the methacrylates: ethylene glycol dimethacrylate (EGDMA), 2-hydroxyethyl methacrylate 2-HEMA and 2-hydroxypropyl methacrylate (2-HPMA), and the acrylates diethylene glycol diacrylate (DEGDA), and triethylene glycol diacrylate (TREGDA). The three methacrylates were positive in most patients exposed to dental products, glues, or artificial nails, and DEGDA was an important allergen in patients exposed to acrylates in printing work and in the manufacture of UV-cured paints. The patterns of concomitant reactions imply that methacrylates might induce cross-reactivity to acrylates, whereas acrylates do not usually induce sensitization to methacrylates.[17]

Cement dermatitis may be allergic (Figures 21.2 and 21.3), due to the dichromate content, or may result from alkaline irritation and burns. Dermatitis of the dorsum of the proximal nail fold and koilonychia are frequent. Epoxy resin dermatitis[18] especially involves the right first two fingertips, producing erosion and crusting or necrotic-appearing lesions.[6] Formaldehyde is one of the common sensitizers responsible for dermatitis affecting hands including periungual area and thus nail unit, in many occupational groups, including hospital staff.[6]

CHEMICAL IRRITANTS

Prolonged immersion of hands in water containing concentrations of alkalis, alkaline chlorine-containing compounds, or powerful detergents can lead to softening and gradual destruction of nail unit.[19] Thiourea contained in silver polish may produce contact and photo-contact allergy with vesicular eruption of the fingertips and invasion under the fingernails.[6]

WET WORK

As per German regulation of hazardous substances in the workplace, "wet work" is defined as individuals having their skin exposed to liquids longer than 2 hours per day, or using occlusive gloves longer than 2 hours per day, or cleaning the hands very often (e.g., 20 times/day or less if cleaning procedure is more aggressive) or taking care of a less than 4-year-old child at home. Sixteen occupations like laborers, food service workers, machine operators, agricultural workers, health professionals, house cleaners, mechanics, construction workers, and cosmetologists have extensive exposure to water[20] and therefore are more prone to development of contact dermatitis of the hand and the nail unit.

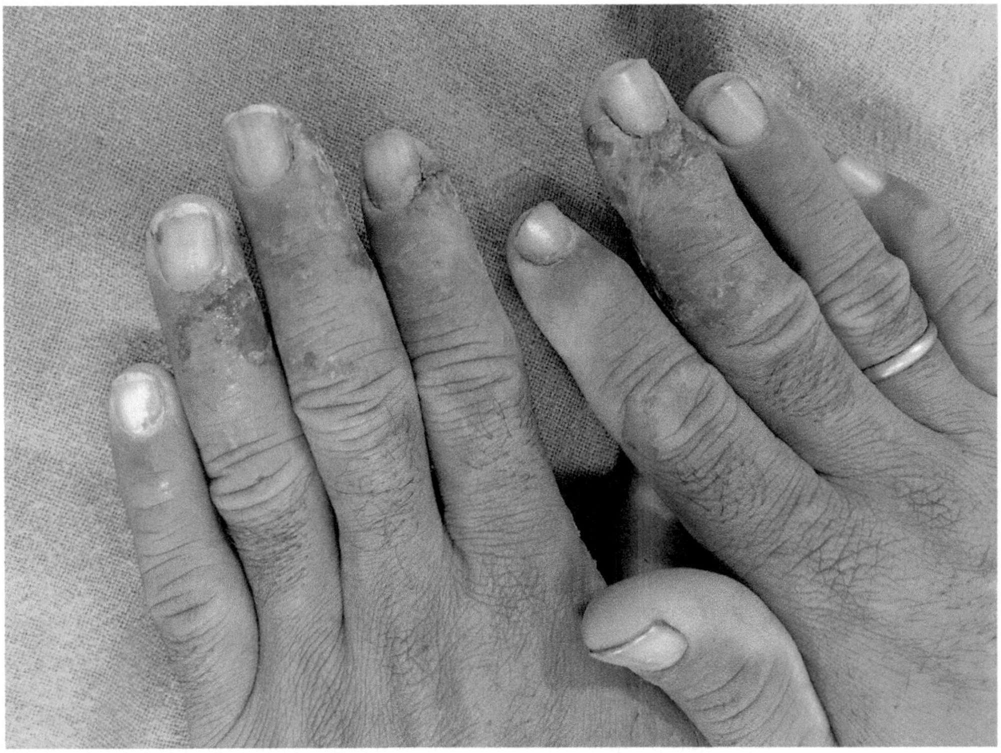

Figure 21.2 Cement worker showing mixed type of hand eczema with marked periungual involvement.

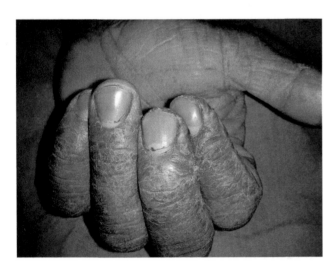

Figure 21.3 Patient with cement dermatitis showing chronic dry fissured eczema of hand with lost cuticle, and shiny nails.

INFECTIONS

Bacterial infections

Even trivial trauma to the periungual skin may act as a portal of infection leading to more severe conditions like cellulitis, erysipelas, and septicemia. Among these, coagulase-positive staphylococci and various streptococci are the usual microorganisms. Healthcare personnel with pseudomonas colonization in their nails may act as a source of nosocomial infections.[6] Paronychia is a common condition affecting nail unit due to occupational onset and is usually caused by a mixture of pathogenic organisms. Persons engaged with household work, kitchen staff, agricultural workers, and pianists are particularly likely to develop this condition. Also, acute paronychia is frequently seen in meat handlers and streptococcal paronychia has been reported in workers in a chicken factory.[21]

There are various uncommon presentations of bacterial infections affecting nail unit. For example, Erysipeloid, also known as fish handler's disease, is a bacterial infection caused by *Erysipelothrix rhusiopathiae*. Occupations at risk are fishers, butchers, and poultry dressers. Other diseases like Leishmaniasis mimic Erysipeloid, usually seen in meat or fish handlers. TB infection: Other diseases involving nail unit like Prosector's wart (*Mycobacterium tuberculosis*), swimming pool granuloma (*Mycobacterium marinum*), Tularemia inoculation by coccobacillus Pasturella tularensis.[6]

Fungal infections

Fungal infections of the nails and periungual region, especially candidiasis, are a common occupational problem. Occupations requiring the hands to be wet or exposed to detergents for prolonged periods, such as dishwashers in restaurants, are more prone to candida paronychia and onycholysis.[6] Also, hot, humid environmental conditions prevailing in occupations like coal mining increase vulnerability to developing dermatophytic toenail infections, with Trichophyton rubrum. Toenails are 25 times more likely to be infected than fingernails as the causative molds are ubiquitous fungi seen in soil, water, and decaying vegetations.[22]

> ## BOX 21.4: Individuals at risk of fungal nail infections[6]
>
> - Armed forces, police
> - Athletes
> - Dustmen
> - Carpet weaving
> - Employees of indoor swimming pools
> - Excavation workers
> - Mine workers
> - Nuclear fuel workers
> - Rubber industry workers
> - Sewer workers
> - Steel and furnace workers
> - Wood cutters
> - Wood pulp workers

Dermatophyte fungi live on the nail plate, and repeated minor trauma permits the fungal organism to invade the nail plate and become established.

The risk factors include occupations requiring tight occlusive footwear that cause crowding of the toes. This promotes fungal infection. Use of communal showers and occupations requiring constant hand washing are also risk factors.

Box 21.4[6] describes the occupations at risk of developing fungal nail infections due to their work-related factors.

Viral infections

Nail unit can be inoculated by viral warts, which are more common in butchers, meat packers, poultry handlers, poultry processing workers, and fish handlers, in whom many of the lesions are periungual or subungual.[6]

SYSTEMIC ABSORPTION

On exposure to cobalt and tungsten, asbestos, talc, beryllium, and silica, pneumoconiotic lung diseases can produce clubbing. In a dental technician exposed to silica, Erasmus syndrome—association of systemic sclerosis following exposure to silica with or without silicosis—was associated with necrosis of the digits.[6] Excessive levels of vinyl chloride, epoxy resin vapor, trichlorethylene, trichlorethane, and silica have been noted as etiological factors in systemic sclerosis. Also, sclerodactyly with nail fold capillary changes, Raynaud phenomenon and acro-osteolysis have also been reported in patients with chronic exposure to vibrations at their workplace.[23]

CLINICAL PRESENTATION

The clinical overview of occupational nail diseases has been summarized in (Table 21.1).

1. The presentation of nail dystrophy[6] is variable and the clinical nail dystrophic patterns of occupational origin includes changes in:

   a. Texture and contour of the nail plate: Onychauxis, worn-down nail plate, brittle nails, koilonychia, clubbing, and pseudoclubbing
   b. Proximal matrix: Pitting/Beau's lines/transverse grooving/trachyonychia/onychomadesis/nail shedding/longitudinal ridging
   c. Distal matrix: leukonychia
   d. Surface of the nail plate and its attachments: Paronychia with occasional onychomadesis leading to nail shedding
   e. Surrounding tissue involvement (pulpitis)
   f. Nail plate staining or subungual alteration
   g. Distal bony phalanx anomalies
   h. Digital ischemia and Raynaud's phenomenon
2. Irritants producing onychia and nail discoloration[1,2,24] may present as follows:

   a. Occupational koilonychia: Spoon-shaped deformity of the nails may be produced by organic solvents in cabinetmakers, motor oils, and in barefoot rickshaw pullers. Occupational koilonychia mostly affects first three fingers of the dominant hand and is usually associated with some subungual hyperkeratosis. Moreover, the changes are more prominent on the distal part of nail plate. Frequently, there are additional associated nail findings that provide a clue to the occupation of the person, as summarized in Table 21.2.
   b. Acute onycholysis from chemicals: Hydroflouric burns, detergent enzymes, hair cosmetics such as dicyanamide (especially useful to restore split and thin hair), depilatories, and thioglycolates used by hairdressers for permanent waving may lead to onycholysis.
   c. "Athletic Nails": Athletic trauma may result in leukonychia of the fingernail in people who practice karate or black discoloration of fingernails in shooters and of toenails in tennis players, jogjoggers etc.
   d. Reaction to "sculptured" acrylate nails: Allergic sensitization to "sculptured" acrylate nails may cause severe onychia and paronychia, with permanent destruction of the nails.
   e. Contact chromonychia: Weed killers and other insecticides may produce nail discoloration that precedes onychia and nail deformity. Other relevant causes include discoloration from nail enamels, nail hardeners, and staining due to hydroquinone.

Nail in hand and foot eczema

Some forms of eczema are altered by regional variation in structure and function of the skin, and these may modify its appearance in regions such as hands and lower legs. Legs and feet are affected by various eczemas. Classically stasis dermatitis affects lower legs. Other eczemas more likely to occur are nummular eczema, juvenile plantar dermatosis, pompholyx, lichen simplex chronicus, and ACD.[25] Hand eczema is a multifactorial, common dermatological

Table 21.1 Overview of occupational nail diseases

Nail findings	Mechanism	Occupations at risk
Alterations in shape of the nail plate		
Koilonychia of fingernails	Repeated micro trauma and/or contact with chemicals that soften the nail plate	Dentists, glass workers, construction workers, mushroom growers, cabinet makers, butchers, oil burner repairers, automotive workers, slaughterhouse workers
Koilonychia of toenails	Repetitive pressure and friction while working barefoot	Rickshaw pullers, farmers working barefoot in mud
Finger clubbing	Exposure to silica, asbestos, and vinyl chloride	Miners
	Trauma	Karate practitioners
Alterations in the color of the nail plate		
Leukonychia	Trauma to distal nail matrix	Manual workers
Yellow discoloration	Exposure to pesticides, chromium salts, textile dyes, 4,4′-methylenedianiline	Farmers, agriculture workers, textile industry, epoxy industry
Orange/red discoloration	Exposure to hair dyes, henna, glutaraldehyde, picric acid, and hydroquinone	Hair dressers, recreational use of henna, petroleum industry
Purple discoloration	Exposure to gold, potassium cyanide	Gold miners, jewelers
Black discoloration	Exposure to tannin and dark woods (ebony and mahogany)	Leather industry, carpenters
Alterations in physical properties of the nail plate		
Onychorrhexis	Exposure to gasoline	Rubber, plastic, and paint manufactures; mechanical repair
Onychoschizia	Exposure to water, detergents, and solvents	Housecleaners, professional swimmers
Nail plate erosions	Mechanical trauma	Manual workers
Nail plate abrasion	Repetitive friction	Guitar players, pottery workers, tailors
Increased nail fragility	Frequent wet works, and exposure to solvents and chemicals	Medical personnel, nurses, chemical personnel, photographers, painters, hairdressers, bartenders, dishwashers food handlers
Nail bed changes		
Subungual hyperkeratosis	Allergic contact dermatitis	Nail salon workers (manicurists), construction workers, painters
Onycholysis of fingernails	Trauma, exposure to wet environment and organic solvents	Butchers, slaughterhouse workers, chicken-processing workers, bartenders, food handlers, dishwashers, hairdressers, gardeners, floriculturists, fishers, nail salon workers (manicurists)
Onycholysis of toenails	Repetitive trauma	Athletes, dancers
Distal splinter hemorrhages of fingers	Mechanical trauma	Golfers, cricket players, gardening and playing percussion instruments
Proximal splinter hemorrhages of fingers	Hypoxia due to high altitude	Mountain climbing
Splinter hemorrhages of toenails	Mechanical trauma	Dancers and athletes, especially in tennis, soccer, or squash players and joggers
Chronic paronychia	Exposure to wet environment and/or irritative compounds (soaps, detergents, and oils), friction	Homemakers, dishwashers, farmers, and other workers involved in wet occupations; food handlers dealing with raw vegetables and fish; pianists and violin players

(Continued)

Table 21.1 (*Continued*) Overview of occupational nail diseases

Nail findings	Mechanism	Occupations at risk
Infective conditions		
Onychomycosis	Exposure to wet environment and fungus	Swimmers
Warts (butchers wart)	Exposure to papilloma viruses (mainly 2 and 7)	Handlers of meat, fish, and poultry
Herpes simplex infection	Exposure to herpes simplex virus	Doctors and nurses, dentists, pathologists, and laboratory technicians
Others		
Digital ischemia	Use of vibrating or drilling tools and chainsaws for years	Forestry workers, miners
Carpal tunnel syndrome	Prolonged use of vibrating tools	Miners

Table 21.2 Occupational koilonychia

Associated finding	Mechanism	Occupation at risk
Longitudinal grooves	Mechanical trauma due to surgical instruments	Dentists
Contact dermatitis of the proximal nail fold and subungual hyperkeratosis	Exposure to cement	Construction workers
Longitudinal splitting and splinter hemorrhages	Rubbing of the nails against heavy plastic bags	Mushroom growers
Onycholysis	Handling of raw meat	Butchers
Nail pigmentation	Exposure to thioglycolates	Hair dressers

Source: Tosti, A., and Pazzaglia, M., Occupational nail disorders, in Scher, R.K., and Daniel III, C.R., editors, *Nails Diagnosis Therapy Surgery*, 3rd edn, Elsevier, Philadelphia, PA, pp. 205–214, 2005.

disorder with a chronic and relapsing course. Predisposing endogenous factors and external factors both play important roles in hand eczema causation. Contact eczema over the hands occurs as a result of exposure to external factors such as allergens or irritants and it contributes to 9%–35% of all occupational disease and up to 80% or more of all occupational contact dermatitis. Almost all types of eczema can affect the nails, although changes are not very specific to any particular subtype and should be considered in relation to the skin changes that usually affect the fingers, hands, or other regions of the body. The most common features are irregular transverse furrows on the nails, thickening, subungual hyperkeratosis, onycholysis, roughness, and furrowing.[26] The proximal nail fold is usually thickened with chronic paronychia. The cuticle then disappears by itself, and the proximal nail wall begins to separate from the underlying nail creating a window for bacterial and fungal infections. Chronic paronychia, which previously was believed to be caused by *Candida albicans* or other candidal organisms, is now largely assumed to be a protein contact dermatitis that is caused by contact with raw vegetables or fruit.[27] In atopic eczema, shiny nails are sometimes seen, which are produced by rubbing of the nail surface on itchy skin and resulting sheen effect. In a personal unpublished observational study in an observational study of hundreds of patients of hand eczema, nail changes were found in 78% of the patients, predominantly more in those engaged in manual work like farming, laborer, homemakers, construction

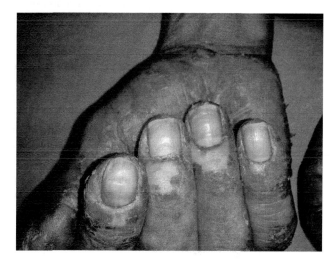

Figure 21.4 Periungual depigmentation, lost cuticle, chronic paronychia, shiny nail plate, Beau's lines, and onycholysis on background of chronic dry fissured eczema of occupational irritant dermatitis in a factory worker dealing with machine oils.

workers, and factory workers (Figure 21.4). Most common patterns of nail changes observed in the same study were cuticle loss (37%), pitting (30%), longitudinal ridging (28%), Beau's lines (26%), paronychia (20%), pulpitis (11%), melanonychia (10%), onycholysis (9%), brittle nails (4%), leukonychia (4%), and onychomadesis (2%). Also, chronic

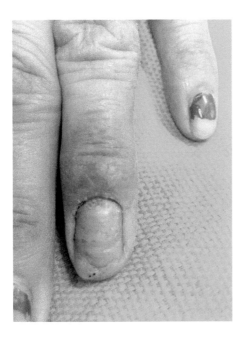

Figure 21.5 Chronic paronychia with loss of cuticle and Beau's lines in a homemaker.

paronychia was significantly higher in manual laborers. Dermatitis in homemakers is common in clinical practice because of their frequent exposure to physical and chemical injury through water and various antigenic substances like vegetables, soaps, and detergents (Figure 21.5). Among various patch-tested antigens, vegetables (garlic and onion) were the most common suspected contactants (50%), followed by soap and detergents (40%) and condiments (10%), in a clinico-etiological study of contact dermatitis in homemakers.[12] Recently, Brans et al.[28] evaluated the prevalence of foot eczema in patients in a retrospective cohort study with occupational hand eczema and found concomitant foot eczema in 27.8%. Interestingly, the majority of patients had similar morphological features over the hands and feet (71.1%). The presence of foot eczema was significantly associated with male sex (odds ratio, atopic hand eczema, hyperhidrosis, and the wearing of safety shoes). Tobacco smoking was associated with foot eczema, in particular with the vesicular subtype. However, as in most series on hand or foot eczema, no data on nail involvement was mentioned.

Diagnosis

WHEN TO SUSPECT

Nail dystrophy should be suspected of occupational origin, if there is history suggestive of factors producing or aggravating the present condition at the workplace or there is temporal correlation of exposure or aggravating factors with present clinical manifestation in the nail unit. Sometimes, a visit to the workplace helps in understanding the etiological role of a particular occupational factor. A heightened suspicion of ACD should be maintained for nail patients who do not respond to appropriate treatment.

Patients with a possibility of ACD should be patch tested to a battery of relevant allergens, and, if possible, their own products. Along with a proper clinical history focusing on nail practices, a thorough understanding of the common allergen and patch testing are necessary to diagnose contact dermatitis. The following indicators may help in diagnosing nail dystrophy of occupational onset:

Work relatedness: Occupational contact dermatitis initially shows greater and more consistent improvement away from work than non-occupational dermatitis, though with chronicity such work relatedness may become less clear.

Prevention: The effects of gloves, other personal protective equipment, or skin care products may help to confirm occupational causation or point to a secondary contact factor.

Other cases: Involvement of fellow workers (and in what proportion) increases the probability of occupational contact dermatitis (with larger proportions favoring irritant rather than allergic).

DIFFERENTIAL DIAGNOSES

Nail changes in dermatoses such as psoriasis, tinea ungium, and lichen planus may be misinterpreted as being induced by work. Dermatoses such as psoriasis or lichen planus of the nails, however, may be exacerbated by occupational trauma due to koebnerization.[6]

Diagnosis

The diagnosis is mainly clinical. Awareness of occupational nail diseases, a detailed clinical history with emphasis on past and present occupation history, and a through nail examination are essential prerequisites for making a clinical diagnosis. Understanding and visualizing the role of occupational factor(s) in the development of nail changes are helpful not only in diagnosis but in formulating a management plan as well. Occupational eczema is a frequent etiological factor that needs patch testing to identify the culprit allergen.

PATCH TESTING

Contact dermatitis may be irritant or allergic in nature. No immune mechanism is involved in contact irritant dermatitis, while ACD reactions results from hypersensitivity reaction of type IV Gell and Coombs, more specifically, type IV a. The time required for a patient to become sensitized is around 14–21 days. But, once sensitized, the reaction time decreases to 24–48 hours. An irritant patch test reaction appears as sharply demarcated erythema with minimal infiltration and small pustules.[29] The only discriminative test between irritant and ACD would be revealing specific T lymphocytes to incriminated allergen in ACD. However, in general, there is no single characteristic in the clinical picture of cumulative irritant contact dermatitis that makes the diagnosis certain, particularly for the hands. Hands are in continuous contact with the external environment with a large range of occupational products; therefore, it is believed that the majority of

BOX 21.5: Important screening allergens in nail products[29]

Name of allergen (vehicle)
Toluene sulfonamide formaldehyde resin (10% pet)
Ethyl acrylate (0.1% pet)
Ethyl methacrylate (2% pet)
2-Hydroxy methacrylate (2% pet)
Ethylene glycol dimethacrylate (2% pet)
Ethyl cyanoacrylate (ECA) (10% pet)

cases are irritant and allergic cases account for approximately 20% of reactions.[29] The distribution of lesions may vary depending on the location of the reaction and occupational circumstances. Epicutaneous patch testing is considered as the gold standard for diagnosis of ACD. A relevant patch test to reach a diagnosis of ACD requires an understanding of the relevant allergens in individual cases, as several thousand allergens may cause an allergic reaction. Also, testing with patients' own products of personal use as well as products at their workplace in appropriate dilutions forms an essential part of evaluation of contact dermatitis in every individualized patient. A rising trend of contact dermatitis to cosmetically relevant antigens further supports the patch testing with patients' own products. A suggested adjunctive panel of screening nail allergens is presented in Box 21.5.[29]

MANAGEMENT

General measures

BARRIER PROTECTION

Gloves and protective footwear are considered to be the best form of protection of nails from existing irritants and/or allergens in the workplace. However, these can only be considered safe to wear if they are made of material appropriate to the agent against which protection is required. Neither natural rubber nor polyvinyl chloride (PVC) gloves, for example, provide good protection against organic solvents.[4] Interestingly, protein contact dermatitis, a chronic recurrent dermatitis caused by contact with a proteinaceous material presenting as paronychia from natural rubber latex has also been reported.[30]

Nearly all forms of hand eczema begin with disruption of the stratum corneum barrier.[31] Thus, initial management usually aims at maintenance and restoration of the barrier and controlling the inflammation. In the prevention of occupational hand dermatitis, the "3-step occupational skin protection concept" includes skin cleansers and skin care products, in addition to barrier creams.[32] The latter are meant as post-exposure products that help to restore the physiological epidermal skin barrier. Barrier creams share some common characteristics with emollients and moisturizers that are used to maintain healthy skin and nail unit. Barrier creams are designed to diminish the irritant impact of the known key factors of skin irritation that are related to wet work, namely, hand washing and exposure to hot water or detergents and other mild irritants. Thus, barrier creams are intended to be applied prior to procedures and exposures that have irritant potential. This would prevent subsequent eczema and associated nail dystrophy. The variation in incidence of cement eczema between Europe and developing countries like India may be attributed to the development of legislation in a European country like Denmark, that down-regulated the content of hexavalent chromate in cement causing contact dermatitis.[33] This highlights the need of such legislative acts to regulate exposure of chromate or any other potential allergens in the causation of occupational ACD.

PRECAUTIONS

The expanding application of methacrylates in cosmetics such as artificial nails is likely to lead to an increase in ACD and stomatitis related to their use. Therefore, patients with suspected allergy to artificial nails should be examined thoroughly, using the methacrylate artificial nail (MAAN) series as well as additional allergens such as ECA and the nail lacquer used by the patient.[12]

Most of the patients with allergic reactions to 2-HEMA will not be able to continue using sculptured acrylic nails. These patients can safely use silk nails if they are not allergic to ECA, which is present in all nail glues. Also, some acrylic nails do not contain 2-HEMA on their list of ingredients, so certain acrylic nails can still be recommended (although these lists of ingredients cannot always be relied on). Patients allergic to ECA and not to acrylates can use acrylic nails, in the event that no repair of broken nails is performed with glues.[12]

TREATMENT

Goal: The goal of treatment should be primarily preventive, with three objectives to achieve:

1. Workers' health promotion through guidance, training, nutrition, hygiene
2. Availability of out-patient care at company itself, periodic inspection of workplace to ensure a safe environment for the workers
3. Active interventions with therapeutic measures for the patients with active lesions along with removal of potential allergens or irritants and further rehabilitation for another activity[34]

Therapeutic measures: The cornerstone of the treatment is identifying and eliminating responsible occupational factors. Sometimes, temporary discontinuation of work or change of occupation in severe cases is needed. Other measures are discussed below:

1. Topical
   - Topical corticosteroids or tacrolimus over nail folds seem to be promising, but always in association with preventive measures.

- Additional topical antimicrobial or systemic antifungal might be required depending on type of secondary infections: bacterial or fungal.
- Also, care should be taken that long-term application of topical steroids might pose risk of secondary infection in itself.
- Structural changes in the nail plate may improve aesthetically with gel nail or nail peeling as discussed in the chapters on nail cosmetics.

2. Surgical
   - Surgical management is only indicated in recalcitrant cases of chronic paronychia, which does not respond to medical management and proper use of general measures. It involves removal of the chronically inflamed tissue, which aids in effective penetration of topical as well as oral medications and regeneration of the cuticle.
   - Various surgical techniques with modifications have been described in the literature. The simplest technique is eponychial marsupialization, in which after anesthesia and tourniquet control, a 3-mm-wide crescent-shaped incision parallel and proximal to the distal edge of the eponychium and extending from the radial to ulnar borders is made. All affected tissue within the boundaries of the crescent and extending down to, but not including, the germinal matrix is excised and packed with gauze pieces. Thus, this procedure exteriorizes the infected and obstructed nail matrix and allows its drainage. Epithelialization of the excised defect occurs over the next 2–3 weeks.
   - Another technique includes marsupialization plus nail removal and en bloc excision of PNF. Eponychial marsupialization has an advantage over en bloc excision in that the former preserves the ventral surface of the PNF, which forms the dorsal roof or surface of the nail plate, thus cosmetically more acceptable result as compared to en bloc excision of PNF (complete removal of the dorsal roof including the eponychium).[35]

CONCLUSION

Occupational nail diseases are frequent diseases with great impact for patients and society. Their treatment is often complex and challenging, thereby leading to a long-term course of disease with the relapsing course placing a heavy burden on patients, often affecting their ability to work. Consequences like sick leave, lost productivity, dermatological treatment, vocational retraining, and workers' compensation have severe economic implications over social security systems.[36] Also, diseases comprise a continuum of symptoms and severities, from very mild disease to severe illness demanding sick leave, change of occupation, or permanent disability, thus in turn affecting the quality of life.[34] Therefore adequate and timely treatment is recommended to prevent longstanding nail sequelae.

REFERENCES

1. Baran R. Occupational nail disorders. In: Rustemeyer T, Elsner P, John SM, Maibach HI, editors. *Kanerva's Occupational Dermatology*. 2nd ed. New York: Springer; 2012. pp. 255–264.
2. Tosti A, Pazzaglia M. Occupational nail disorders. In: Scher RK, Daniel III CR, editors. *Nails Diagnosis Therapy Surgery*. 3rd ed. Philadelphia, PA: Elsevier; 2005. pp. 205–214.
3. Cashman MW, Reutemann PA, Ehrlich A. Contact dermatitis in the United States: Epidemiology, economic impact, and workplace prevention. *Dermatol Clin* 2012; 30(1): 87–98, viii.
4. Nyrén M, Lindberg M, Stenberg B, Svensson M, Svensson Å, Meding B. Influence of childhood atopic dermatitis on future worklife. *Scand J Work Environ Health* 2005; 31(6): 474–478.
5. Connolly M, de Berker DAR. Multiple myxoid cysts secondary to occupation. *Clin Exp Dermatol* 2006; 31(3): 404–406.
6. Baran R, Rycroft RJG. Occupational abnormalities and contact dermatitis. In: Baran R, de Berker DAR, Holzberg M, Thomas L, editors. *Baran & Dawber's Diseases of the Nails and Their Management*. 4th ed. Chichester, UK: John Wiley & Sons; 2012. pp. 443–469.
7. Ryan AM, Goldsmith LA. Golfer's nails. *Arch Dermatol* 1995; 131(7): 857–858.
8. Dolma T, Norboo T, Yayha M, Hubson R, Ball K. Seasonal koilonychia in Ladakh. *Contact Dermatitis* 1990; 22(2): 78–80.
9. Rycroft RJG, Calnan CD. Alstroemeria dermatitis. *Contact Dermatitis* 1981; 7(5): 284–284.
10. Bruynzeel DP, de Boer EM, Brouwer EJ, de Wolff FA, de Haan P. Dermatitis in bulb growers. *Contact Dermatitis* 1993; 29(1): 11–15.
11. Matsunaga K, Hosokawa K, Suzuki M, Arima Y, Hayakawa R. Occupational allergic contact dermatitis in beauticians. *Contact Dermatitis* 1988; 18(2): 94–96.
12. Lazarov A. Sensitization to acrylates is a common adverse reaction to artificial fingernails. *J Eur Acad Dermatol Venereol* 2007; 21(2): 169–174.
13. Cousen PJ, Ramsay HM, Gawkrodger DJ. An unusual cause of fingernail dystrophy. *Clin Exp Dermatol* 2012; 37(5): 589–590.

14. Kanerva L, Jolanki R, Estlander T. 10 years of patch testing with the (meth)acrylate series. *Contact Dermatitis* 1997; 37(6): 255–258.

15. Hemmer W, Focke M, Wantke F, Götz M, Jarisch R. Allergic contact dermatitis to artificial fingernails prepared from UV light-cured acrylates. *J Am Acad Dermatol* 1996; 35(3 Pt 1): 377–380.

16. Baran R. Nail alterations in hand eczema. In: Alikhan A, Lachapelle J-M, Maibach HI, editors. *Textbook of Hand Eczema*. 1st ed. Berlin, Germany: Springer-Verlag; 2014. pp. 37–47.

17. Aalto-Korte K, Henriks-Eckerman ML, Kuuliala O, Jolanki R. Occupational methacrylate and acrylate allergy—Cross-reactions and possible screening allergens. *Contact Dermatitis* 2010; 63(6): 301–312.

18. Brooke RC, Beck MH. Occupational allergic contact dermatitis from epoxy resin used to restore window frames. *Contact Dermatitis* 1999; 41(4): 227–228.

19. Coskey RJ. Onycholysis from sodium hypochlorite. *Arch Dermatol* 1974; 109(1): 96.

20. Belsito DV. Occupational contact dermatitis: Etiology, prevalence, and resultant impairment/disability. *J Am Acad Dermatol* 2005; 53(2): 303–313.

21. Barnham M, Kerby J. A profile of skin sepsis in meat handlers. *J Infect* 1984; 9(1): 43–50.

22. Banu A, Anand M, Eswari L. A rare case of onychomycosis in all 10 fingers of an immunocompetent patient. *Indian Dermatol Online J* 2013; 4(4): 302–304.

23. Nagata C, Yoshida H, Mirbod SM, Komura Y, Fujita S, Inaba R et al. Cutaneous signs (Raynaud's phenomenon, sclerodactylia, and edema of the hands) and hand-arm vibration exposure. *Int Arch Occup Environ Health* 1993; 64(8): 587–591.

24. Rietschel RL, Fowler JF. Preservatives and vehicles in cosmetics and toiletries. In *Fisher's Contact Dermatitis*. 2008. p.892.

25. Chougule A, Thappa DM. Patterns of lower leg and foot eczema in South India. *Indian J Dermatol Venereol Leprol* 2008; 74(5): 458–461.

26. Haneke E. Non-infectious inflammatory disorders of the nail apparatus. *J Dtsch Dermatol Ges* 2009; 7(9): 787–797.

27. Tosti A, Piraccini BM, Ghetti E, Colombo MD. Topical steroids versus systemic antifungals in the treatment of chronic paronychia: An open, randomized double-blind and double dummy study. *J Am Acad Dermatol* 2002; 47(1): 73–76.

28. Brans R, Hübner A, Gediga G, John SM. Prevalence of foot eczema and associated occupational and non-occupational factors in patients with hand eczema. *Contact Dermatitis* 2015; 73(2): 100–107.

29. Militello G. Contact and primary irritant dermatitis of the nail unit diagnosis and treatment. *Dermatol Ther* 2007; 20(1): 47–53.

30. Kanerva L. Occupational protein contact dermatitis and paronychia from natural rubber latex. *J Eur Acad Dermatol Venereol* 2000; 14(6): 504–506.

31. Harding CR. The stratum corneum: Structure and function in health and disease. *Dermatol Ther* 2004; 17 Suppl 1: 6–15.

32. Coenraads P-J. Hand eczema. *N Engl J Med* 2012; 367(19): 1829–1837.

33. Hald M, Agner T, Blands J, Ravn H, Johansen JD. Allergens associated with severe symptoms of hand eczema and a poor prognosis. *Contact Dermatitis* 2009; 61(2): 101–108.

34. Charan UP, Peter CVD, Pulimood SA. Impact of hand eczema severity on quality of life. *Indian Dermatol Online J* 2013; 4(2): 102–105.

35. Relhan V, Goel K, Bansal S, Garg VK. Management of chronic paronychia. *Indian J Dermatol* 2014; 59(1): 15–20.

36. Boehm D, Schmid-Ott G, Finkeldey F, John SM, Dwinger C, Werfel T et al. Anxiety, depression and impaired health-related quality of life in patients with occupational hand eczema. *Contact Dermatitis* 2012; 67(4): 184–192.

22

Chronic paronychia

SANTOSHDEV P. RATHOD AND POOJA AGARWAL

INTRODUCTION

Paronychia (synonym perionychia) is an inflammatory condition involving the folds of tissue surrounding fingernails or toenails; one or more of the three nail folds (one proximal and two lateral) may be involved. The condition may be classified as acute or chronic depending upon the duration of the inflammation. It is termed chronic when inflammation lasts for more than 6 weeks. Acute paronychia is usually of infective origin but chronic paronychia has multifactorial etiology and commonly affects women.

ETIOPATHOGENESIS

Etiopathogenesis is complex and multifactorial. Primary defect lies in the damaged cuticle. In chronic paronychia, the cuticle separates from the nail plate, leaving the region between the proximal nail fold and the nail plate vulnerable to infection, allergens, and irritants, triggering an inflammatory process.[1,2] Various predisposing factors have been summarized in Box 22.1.

> **BOX 22.1: Predisposing factors for chronic paronychia**
>
> - Wet work and retention of moisture as seen in laundry workers, house and office cleaners, cooks, dishwashers, nurses, and swimmers
> - Contact allergy and irritant reactions
> - Immunosuppression
> - Dermatoses like atopic dermatitis, pemphigus, and psoriasis involving digits
> - Finger sucking

The various causes of paronychia are given in Box 22.2.

The retinoid-induced paronychia can be explained by increased nail fragility and minor trauma by small nail fragments. It has also been reported in patients taking Cetuximab, which is an anti-EGFR antibody used in the treatment of solid tumors.[3,4]

It can also occur as a complication of acute paronychia in patients who do not receive appropriate treatment.

Role of *candida albicans*

The role of *Candida albicans* in causing chronic paronychia is debatable. Though *Candida* sp. has been the most frequently cultured organism, it is seen that eradication of the yeast does not cure the condition. The current evidence suggests that *Candida* colonizes the area once there is a physical breach. It plays a key role in perpetuating the inflammation rather than being the primary pathogenic cause.[2] Also, in many cases, *Candida* disappears when the physiologic barrier is restored, thereby suggesting that *Candida* infection is not the primary cause of chronic paronychia.

CLINICAL FEATURES

Any finger may be involved, but index and middle fingers of the right hand and the middle finger of the left hand are most commonly affected as these fingers are more frequently subjected to minor trauma than the remainder. The condition begins as a slight tender swelling at the base of the finger; tenderness is less as compared to acute paronychia. The cuticle is soon lost and pus may form below the nail fold. Clinical manifestations are almost similar to those of acute paronychia: erythema, tenderness, and swelling, with retraction of the proximal nail fold and absence of the cuticle. These changes result in continued exposure of the periungual tissues and the matrix to irritants.

Chronic paronychia may be further sub classified in two categories

1. Simple chronic paronychia: Here, the chronic paronychia is the primary pathology and treatment is aimed at controlling inflammation and getting a favorable environment for cuticle to re-grow. This chapter focuses on simple chronic paronychia only.

2. Complicated chronic paronychia: Here, chronic paronychia is caused by various dermatoses (both local and generalized conditions as described earlier) and drugs, and treatment is directed at underlying dermatosis. Chronic paronychia resolves once underlying dermatosis is controlled and when culprit drug is discontinued.

The severity of chronic paronychia can be graded clinically as described in Box 22.3.[5]

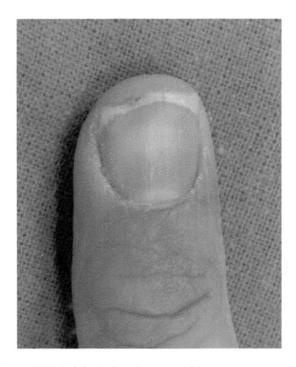

Figure 22.1 Grade 1 chronic paronychia.

Inflammation adjacent to the nail matrix results in nail plate changes, which include thickening or thinning, discoloration, Beau's lines and, sometimes, onychomadesis. In long-standing cases, the size of the nail is reduced.

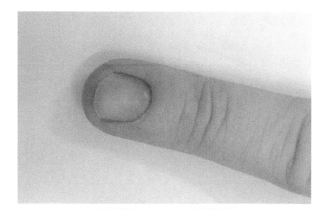

Figure 22.2 Grade 2 chronic paronychia.

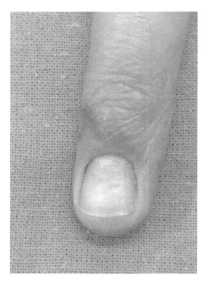

Figure 22.3 Grade 3 chronic paronychia; note slight surface changes in the nail plate in form of partial horizontal grooves.

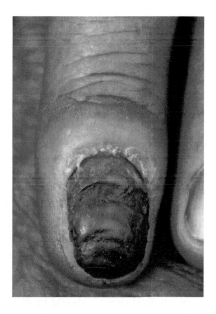

Figure 22.4 Grade 4 chronic paronychia with multiple Beau's lines. (Courtesy of Dr. Piyush Kumar.)

DIFFERENTIAL DIAGNOSIS

- Attempts should be made to identify drugs, infections, irritants, allergens, and various dermatoses that can cause chronic paronychia.
- Pemphigus Vulgaris involving nail unit can be differentiated by the presence of fluid-filled lesions and its distribution elsewhere over the body (Figure 22.5). Similarly, patients on retinoids for psoriasis may develop granuloma pyogenicum like lesions, mimicking chronic paronychia (Figure 22.6).
- Squamous cell carcinoma usually involves a single digit. Biopsy is needed in periungual conditions involving single digits where diagnosis is not clear or paronychia is not responding to the therapy.

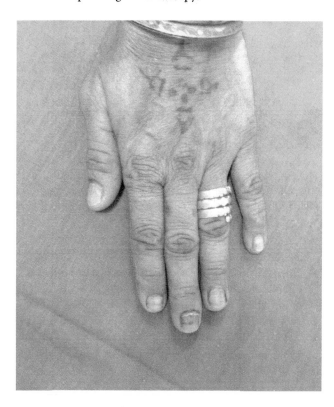

Figure 22.5 Paronychia in a pemphigus patient; note red, indurated proximal and lateral nail folds.

INVESTIGATIONS

The diagnosis is often made clinically. Further investigations are needed to identify underlying dermatoses and culprit allergens.

Onychoscopy: On onychoscopy, loss of cuticle can be confirmed.

Histopathology: In patients presenting with atypical clinical features (e.g., ulceration, excessive inflammation, or desquamation) and in patients with recalcitrant disease, a skin biopsy for histopathologic examination should be performed to rule out malignancy or other conditions mimicking chronic paronychia.

Patch test: Patch test with Indian Standard series can also be done. Nickel, paraphenyldiamine, and formaldehyde

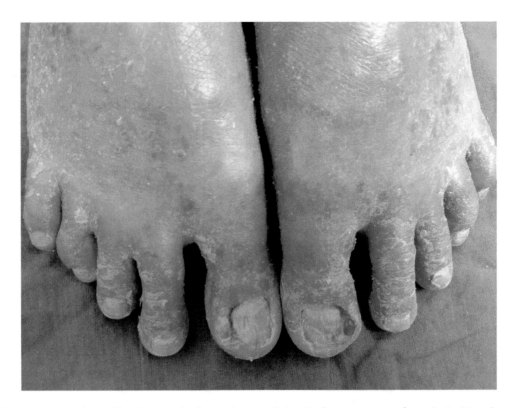

Figure 22.6 Pyogenic granuloma-like changes in the patient on Acitretin for treatment of psoriasis. Note loss of cuticle in the other nails resembling paronychia in 19-year-old female with psoriasis vulgaris. (Courtesy of Dr. Raju Chaudhary, Smt. NHL Municipal Medical College, V.S. Hospital, Ahmedabad.)

are the common allergens found positive in patch test.[5] Open patch test with specific triggers like raw milk can also be done to establish the etiology of chronic paronychia.

Intradermal tests for candida: Positive intradermal skin test for *Candida* may imply hypersensitivity to *Candida*, which may serve as a cause for persistent inflammation of the nail folds.

MANAGEMENT

The recent view holds that chronic paronychia is primarily not a mycotic disease but an eczematous condition with a multifactorial etiology. For this reason, topical and systemic steroids may be used successfully, whereas systemic antifungals are of little value. The treatment plan includes general preventive measures, medical management and, in, recalcitrant cases, surgical management.

General measures

1. Keeping hands and feet dry is the primary requisite in the treatment of paronychia.
2. Avoidance of exposure to contact irritants is an important component in the treatment ladder.
3. Liberal and frequent application of emollients to lubricate the nascent cuticle and the hands is usually beneficial. It also provides a barrier to entry of the pathogens and allergens (and irritants).
4. Avoid any manipulation of the nail, such as manicure, finger sucking, or self-attempts to incise and drain the area.
5. Routine use of barrier creams and protective gloves is advocated.
6. One should keep the nails short and avoid further injuries.

Medical management

As mentioned earlier, medical treatment is aimed at controlling inflammation and controlling *Candida* overgrowth. The medical treatment in different grades of simple chronic paronychia is essentially the same as the nail plate changes revert to normal once inflammation is controlled and do not require separate treatment. However, it may take weeks to months for nail plate surface changes to resolve. Various procedures like chemical peeling and gel nail technique (discussed in different chapters) may be done for a faster improvement in cosmetic appearance of nail plate surface. The management plan has been summarized in flowchart 1.

1. High-potency topical steroids should be the first-line treatment for patients with chronic paronychia for control of inflammation.[6] Clobetasol propionate,

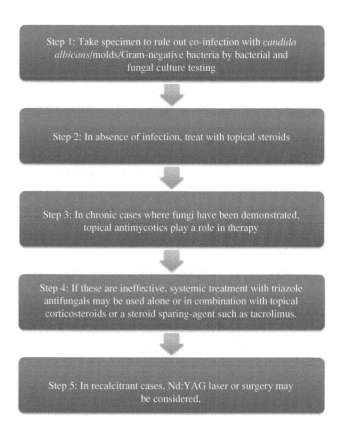

Step 1: Take specimen to rule out co-infection with *candida albicans*/molds/Gram-negative bacteria by bacterial and fungal culture testing

Step 2: In absence of infection, treat with topical steroids

Step 3: In chronic cases where fungi have been demonstrated, topical antimycotics play a role in therapy

Step 4: If these are ineffective, systemic treatment with triazole antifungals may be used alone or in combination with topical corticosteroids or a steroid sparing-agent such as tacrolimus.

Step 5: In recalcitrant cases, Nd:YAG laser or surgery may be considered.

fluocinolone, betamethasone dipropionate and fluticasone propionate are commonly used and therapy should be given for 2–4 weeks. A randomized control trial comparing systemic antifungals with topical steroids for treatment of chronic paronychia found topical steroids to be much more effective.

2. Topical antifungals are used to control overgrowth of *Candida* sp. Amorolfine cream, econazole cream, clotrimazole cream, and ciclopirox suspension are often used twice or thrice daily for 2–4 weeks. Lotion preparations are also used as they can be applied easily.
3. As the accompanying inflammation is pronounced, some authors prefer topical treatment with a combination of steroid and antifungal agents.
4. Topical calcineurin inhibitors (tacrolimus 0.1%) may be used in patients where topical steroids cannot be used.[7] They are important as a steroid sparing agent, too.
5. If the patients do not respond to topical therapy and avoidance of contact irritants, a trial of systemic antifungals may be given for short duration.
6. Acute exacerbations seen in Grade 5 chronic paronychia are often associated with secondary bacterial infection and may require topical and/or systemic antibioics.

Surgical management

Various surgical modalities used in treatment of recalcitrant chronic paronychia include[8]:

1. En bloc excision of the proximal nail fold with or without simultaneous avulsion of the nail plate.[9]

2. Eponychial marsupialization, with or without nail removal.[10] This technique involves excision of a semicircular skin section proximal to the nail fold and parallel to the eponychium, expanding to the edge of the nail fold on both sides.
3. Square flap technique: It removes only the fibrotic tissue of the nail folds, preserving the epidermis and the underlying matrix.[11] In this technique, an incision is made on both sides of the proximal nail fold and a flap is created by making an incision parallel to the epidermis at the distal-thickened proximal nail fold. This incision runs underneath the fibrotic tissue but above the nail, which is used as a guide to avoid matrix damage. The flap is tilted backward and the fibrotic tissue is removed with the scalpel blade. The primary closure is made with a simple interrupted suture.
4. Swiss roll technique: It has been proposed for both chronic paronychia and acute paronychia with runaround abscess.[12] In this technique, the nail fold is elevated by making an incision on either side and reflected proximally over a nonadherent dressing that is rolled up like a Swiss roll and fixed to the skin with two anchoring non-absorbable sutures. The fold is kept open for 48 hours and, if the wound is clean, the sutures are removed and the proximal nail fold falls back to its original position and heals by secondary intention.

Light-based therapy

Recently, Nd-YAG laser has been used to produce varying degrees of improvement in nail fold erythema and swelling in chronic paronychia.[13]

> ### KEY POINTS
>
> - Chronic paronychia has a multifactorial etiology with primary defect being loss of cuticle, which exposes proximal nail area to various irritants, allergens, and infections.
> - Clinically, erythema, tenderness, and swelling of nail folds with loss of cuticle are seen.
> - Keeping hands and feet dry and avoidance of exposure to contact irritants are the primary requisites in the treatment of paronychia.
> - Topical steroid-antifungal combinations form the first ladder of treatment.
> - Surgery and Nd YAG laser are useful in recalcitrant cases.

REFERENCES

1. Habif TP. Nail diseases. In: *Clinical Dermatology: A Color Guide to Diagnosis and Therapy*. 4th ed. Edinburgh, UK: Mosby; 2004: pp. 871–872.
2. Rigopoulos D, Larios G, Gregoriou S, Alevizos A. Acute and chronic paronychia. *Am Fam Physician* 2008; 77: 339–346.

3. Garcia-Silva J, Almagro M, Peña-Penabad C, Fonseca E. Indinavir-induced retinoid-like effects: Incidence, clinical features and management. *Drug Saf* 2002; 25(14): 993–1003.

4. Boucher KW, Davidson K, Mirakhur B, Goldberg J, Heymann WR. Paronychia induced by cetuximab, an antiepidermal growth factor receptor antibody. *J Am Acad Dermatol* 2002; 47(4): 632–633.

5. Daniel CR III, Iorizzo M, Piraccini BM, Tosti A. Grading simple chronic paronychia and onycholysis. *Int J Dermatol* 2006; 45: 1447–1448.

6. Tosti A, Piraccini BM, Ghetti E, Colombo MD. Topical steroids versus systemic antifungals in the treatment of chronic paronychia: An open, randomized double-blind and double dummy study. *J Am Acad Dermatol* 2002; 47(1): 73–76.

7. Rigopoulos D, Gregoriou S, Belyayeva E et al. Efficacy and safety of tacrolimus ointment 0.1% vs. betamethasone 17-valerate 0.1% in the treatment of chronic paronychia: An unblinded randomized study. *Br J Dermatol* 2009; 160: 858.

8. Relhan V, Goel K, Bansal S, Garg VK. Management of chronic paronychia. *Indian J Dermatol* 2014; 59: 15.

9. Grover C, Bansal S, Nanda S, Reddy BS, Kumar V. En bloc excision of proximal nail fold for treatment of chronic paronychia. *Dermatol Surg* 2006; 32(3): 393–398.

10. Bednar MS, Lane LB. Eponychial marsupialization and nail removal for surgical treatment of chronic paronychia. *J Hand Surg [Am]* 1991; 16(2): 314–317.

11. Ferreira Vieira d'Almeida L, Papaiordanou F, Araújo Machado E et al. Chronic paronychia treatment: Square flap technique. *J Am Acad Dermatol* 2016; 75: 398.

12. Pabari A, Iyer S, Khoo CT. Swiss roll technique for treatment of paronychia. *Tech Hand Up Extrem Surg* 2011; 15: 75.

13. El-Komy MH, Samir N. 1064 Nd: YAG laser for the treatment of chronic paronychia: A pilot study. *Lasers Med Sci* 2015; 30(5): 1623–1626.

23

Nail changes due to systemic drugs

VIJAY ZAWAR AND MANOJ PAWAR

NAIL CHANGES DUE TO SYSTEMIC DRUGS

Changes in the nail unit are common during the course of systemic drug therapy. It may be associated with pain and functional impairment. Most nail changes due to drugs are caused by the acute toxicity of the drug or their metabolites to the nail epithelia and thus they may involve many or all nails. Asymptomatic growth rate changes and pigmentation abnormalities are the most common changes. It is often difficult to pinpoint the diagnosis because of nail formation kinetics and its slow growth rate. Fingernails grow at an average rate of 0.1 mm per day (3 mm per month), whereas toenails grow at 0.03 mm per day (1 mm per month). Thus, complete regrowth of fingernail takes 4–6 months while 12–18 months are required for a toenail. Also, the nail changes may appear many weeks after the drug intake, which makes it difficult to establish the temporal association between the abnormalities and the drug. Many times, the nail symptoms resolve on their own even without stopping the drug, and rechallenge of the same drug may not produce similar nail changes. Sometimes only a few nails are involved, complicating the diagnosis. Knowledge of the nail growth rate is useful to help understand why nail plate changes show past events and to establish onset and duration of these events. [1–3]

Nail changes vary according to the nail structure involved. It is imperative to have knowledge about these changes as nail changes may herald serious drug reaction or they can be the initial manifestation of a hidden systemic problem. By knowing drug-induced nail changes, it may prevent us from overt and improper treatment and, last but not least, nails are of cosmetic importance to the patient. [1,4]

We are going to classify the systemic drugs related nail changes according to nail structure involved.

NAIL MATRIX DAMAGE

Beau's lines and onychomadesis

Beau's lines and onychomadesis result from acute and severe toxicity to the nail matrix, leading to transitory decrease in mitotic activity of the nail matrix keratinocytes. It results in arrest of the nail plate production, which ultimately causes transverse depressions of the nail surface, i.e., Beau's lines and whole thickness sulcus, that separate the nail plate from the proximal side with subsequent shedding, i.e., onychomadesis. These changes are dose related and the depth of the depression correlates with the extent of damage whereas the width corresponds to the duration of the insult. When Beau's lines and onychomadesis are present over all nails at the same distance from the proximal nail fold, drugs should always be suspected as a culprit. A drug intake of 2–3 weeks before the appearance of the Beau's lines and onychomadesis should be considered, as nails take several days to emerge from the proximal nail fold. [5]

The most frequently implicated drugs include cancer chemotherapeutic agents (especially taxanes), retinoids, and radiation therapy. It has also been described with the intake of cefaloridine and cloxacillin, sulfonamides, and tetracycline, dapsone, fluorine, itraconazole, carbamazepine, lithium, metoprolol, phenolphthalein, and psoralens. Several Beau's lines can be seen on nails of patients who had repeated courses of chemotherapy (Figures 23.1 through 23.3). [1-3]

These nail changes do not require any treatment as they migrate distally as the nail grows.

Nail fragility

Proximal nail matrix damage-induced nail plate thinning always involves the whole nail length and is often associated with superficial nail plate abnormalities, whereas distal nail matrix damage alters the shape of the free edge

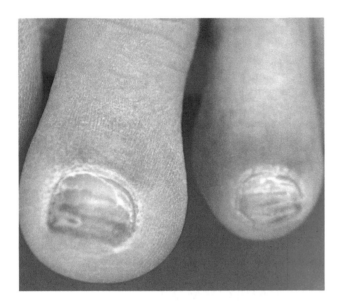

Figures 23.1 Multiple Beau's lines due to taxanes.

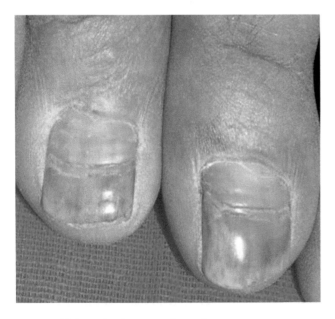

Figures 23.2 Multiple Beau's lines due to taxanes.

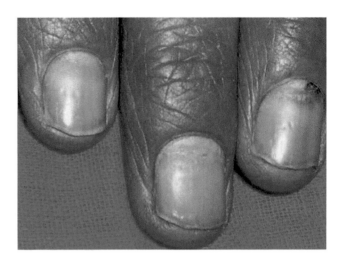

Figure 23.3 Onychomadesis.

of the nail plate. The nails become thin and fragile, which can lead to koilonychias (spoon nails), onychorrhexis (scratched nails), or splitting of the distal plate (onychoschizia). Nail brittleness is common with cancer chemotherapeutic agents, retinoids, and antiretroviral agents. Recently, ibrutinib-treated patients developed the brittle nails, which may result from the drug's ability to disrupt the disulfide bonds between the cysteine residues in the nail. [1,3,6]

Nail growth rate alteration

Both increase and decrease growth rate of nail plate have been observed with the medications. Reduced mitotic activity of the nail matrix cells result in reduced growth rate whereas the cause of increased growth rate is obscure.

Drugs causing slowed growth rate of nail plate are cyclosporine, methotrexate, zidovudine, heparin, and lithium.

Drugs causing increased growth rate of nail plate are azoles, oral contraceptive pills, and levodopa.

Retinoid causes both, i.e., increase and decrease in growth rate of nail plate. [2,7]

True transverse leukonychia

True leukonychia appears as one or several transverse parallel white and opaque bands of 1–2 mm involving all nails at the same level and it moves distally with nail growth. It results from transient impairment of the distal nail matrix keratinization, leading to persistence of cell nuclei in the nail plate. This sign has been commonly reported during treatment with chemotherapeutic agents, especially cyclophosphamide, doxorubicin, and vincristine. Other culprits are cyclosporine, retinoids, corticosteroids, sulfonamides, penicillamine, and fluorine.

Mees' lines are a type of transverse leukonychia, solitary in nature and distributed along the entire width of the nail plate. They are commonly observed after acute arsenic and thallium poisoning (Figure 23.4). [1,3,7]

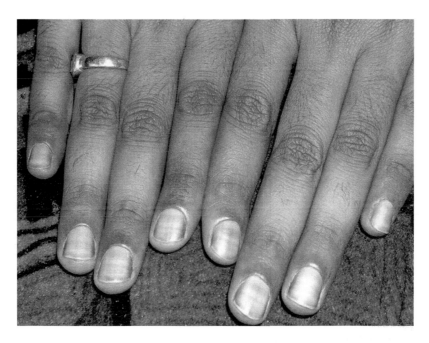

Figure 23.4 Multiple Mees' lines following cyclophosphamide containing CHOP regime for non-Hodgkin's lymphoma.

NAIL BED DAMAGE

Onycholysis

Onycholysis is a result of acute toxicity to the nail bed epithelium with loss of the attachment between the nail bed and the nail plate. As the nail plate detaches from the nail bed it appears white.

Onycholysis with subungual abscess and hemorrhagic onycholysis is characteristic of nail toxic effects induced by taxanes such as docetaxel and paclitaxel. Periarticular thenar erythema with onycholysis (PATEO syndrome) is a distinct taxane-related onycholysis, associated with inflammatory erythema of dorsal hands or perimalleolar and Achilles areas. The proposed pathogenesis for taxen-induced nail changes include activation of nociceptive C-fibers, which enhance neurogenic inflammation by release of neuropeptides or prostaglandins from sympathetic postganglionic terminals. Methotrexate, retinoids, and infliximab are also reported to be associated with this ungual change (Figure 23.5).

Onycholysis often resolves spontaneously or may persist. Soaking the affected digits in topical antiseptic solutions helps prevent secondary bacterial colonization.[1,2,7]

Photo-onycholysis

The mechanism of nail plate detachment is the same as discussed above in onycholysis but it is caused by a photo-mediated toxic or allergic effect of the drug. The possible mechanism of photo-onycholysis is that the lack of melanin and absence of sebum and granular layer in the nail favor the penetration of UV-radiation. Thumbs and lateral nail folds are typically spared.

Four distinct types of photo-onycholysis have been described depending on their appearance. In type-I

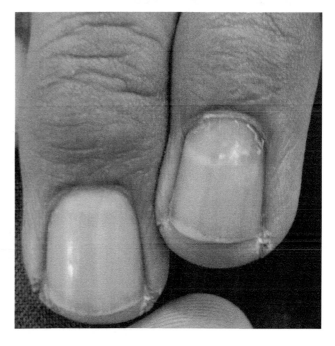

Figure 23.5 Acitretin-induced nail changes in a patient with psoriasis.

photo-onycholysis all fingers are involved with half-moon-shaped separations of the distal nail plate. Type II affects a single finger and is a well-defined, circular notch opening distally that has proximal brownish hue. Type III, which involves the central part of nail bed of several fingers, is defined as round yellow stains of the nail that turn red after 5–10 days. Type IV has been associated with bullae under the nails, mostly caused by the tetracycline hydrochloride.

Photo-onycholysis is commonly seen in patients undergoing psoralen–UVA therapy. Doxycycline, fluoroquinolones,

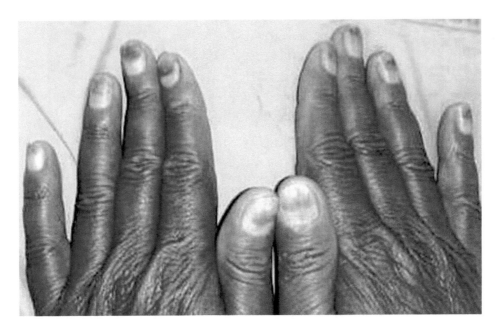

Figure 23.6 Sparfloxacin-induced photo-onycholysis.

captopril, chlorpromazine, thiazide diuretics, and oral contraceptives are also implicated in photo-onycholysis (Figure 23.6).

Avoidance of direct sunlight and topical colored nail varnishes are basic treatment measures. Topical steroids together with soothing lotions reduce the local inflammatory response and pruritus, whereas systemic antihistamines and steroids may be needed in severe cases.[1-4]

Apparent leukonychia

Apparent leukonychia results from abnormalities of the blood flow in the nail bed. It is a white pigmentation of the nail plate that fades with digital compression. It does not migrate with nail growth and is commonly seen after cancer chemotherapy and resolves after drug withdrawal.

It can present in three forms: half-and-half nail (two parts of nail transversely separated by a well-defined border), Muehrcke's (paired narrow white bands that are separated from each other and from the lunula by pink bands of nail), and Terry's nails (nails are an opaque white color that stops 1–2 mm from the distal edge of the nail leaving a pink to brown area 0.5–3.0 mm wide, parallel to the distal part of the nail bed) (Figure 23.7).[1-3]

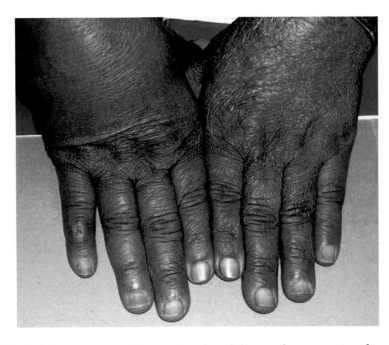

Figure 23.7 Half-and-half nails following carboplatin, paclitaxel, and dexamethasone regime for ovarian cancer.

PROXIMAL NAIL FOLD DAMAGE

Acute paronychia

In drug-induced acute paronychia, usually several nails are involved. The proximal nail fold becomes inflamed, erythematous, and painful, which may result in loss of the nail plate, i.e., onychomadesis ultimately. Toxic effect of the drug on nail epithelia or secondary bacterial infection may play a role.

Paronychia due to retinoids and antiretrovirals is common. Methotrexate causes exudative severe paronychia. Paronychia with pyogenic granulomas has been reported with anti-epidermal growth factor receptor antibodies, i.e., cetuximab, and epidermal growth factor receptor inhibitors used as chemotherapeutic agents such as gefatinib, imatinib, sorafenib, and sunitinib. These nail changes appear 1–3 months after the starting treatment and fade with discontinuation of treatment (Figure 23.8a and b).

Paronychia resolves with the stoppage of the drug. Topical alitretinoin and potent topical corticosteroids are useful in alleviating the local inflammation, while mupirocin is helpful in treating microbial colonization. Re-challenge is often positive.[1,7,8]

NAIL BLOOD FLOW ALTERATIONS

Ischemic changes

Impairment of digital blood supply due to drugs may damage the nail unit and results in digital ischemia, which initially results in Raynaud's phenomenon and is followed by chronic course necrosis. These side effects are commonly seen with β-blockers and bleomycin. β-blockers cause vasoconstriction, which is commonly seen with propranolol, whereas bleomycin results in collagen and glycosaminoglycan deposition with scleroderma-like manifestations and ischemia. Dapsone-induced methemoglobinemia results in both central and peripheral cyanosis and affects nail unit, too (Figure 23.9a).

Splinter hemorrhages

Splinter hemorrhages appear as the reddish-brown lines of blood that run in a vertical direction under the nails and are caused by tiny blood clots that damage the small capillaries under the nails. It is most often evident in the distal nail bed. The subungual hematoma appears after trauma, as a blue-black discoloration due to trapping of

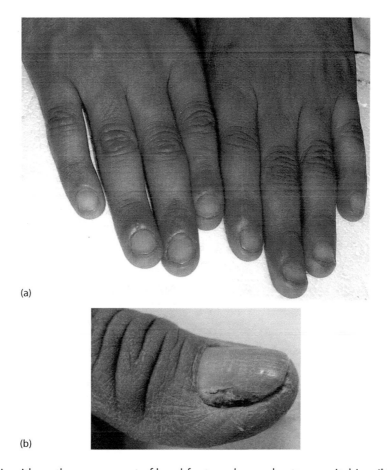

(a)

(b)

Figure 23.8 (a) Paronychia with erythema as a part of hand-foot syndrome due to gemcitabine; (b) Onychomycosis due to mold with paronychia in a patient receiving DCP.

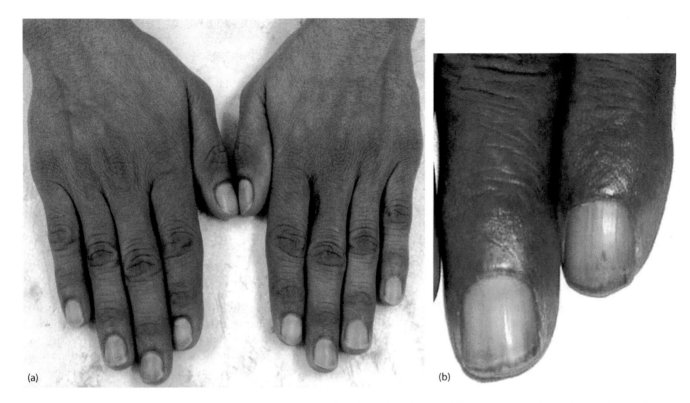

(a)
(b)

Figure 23.9 **(a)** Nail cyanosis in a patient on dapsone who developed methemoglobinemia; **(b)** Splinter hemorrhage due to doxorubicin, cyclophoshamide, vincristine, and prednisolone regime.

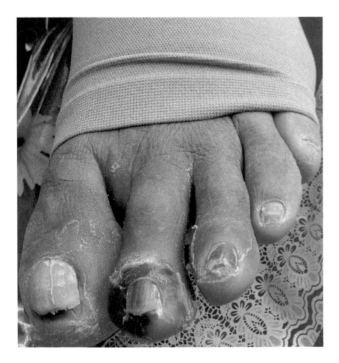

Figure 23.10 Subungual hemorrhage in a patient of DVT receiving heparin.

blood at the junction of the nail plate and nail bed. With time it slowly migrates distally with the growth of the nail plate. These changes are seen in the fingernails almost exclusively. The impairment in blood supply of the nail bed may damage the nail unit resulting in splinter hemorrhages and subungual hematoma (Figure 23.9b). These nail changes are dose-related and disappear after drug withdrawal. Antithrombotics, anticoagulants such as aspirin and warfarin, cancer chemotherapeutic agents, especially the taxanes, and tetracyclines are common causes of both splinter hemorrhage and subungual hematoma (Figure 23.10).[4,7]

NAIL PIGMENTATION

Melanonychia

Drug-induced melanonychia appears 3–8 weeks after the drug intake and presents as single or multiple light brown- or black-colored longitudinal or transverse bands (melanonychia striata), which mostly affect several nails. A diffuse nail matrix melanocyte activation causes pigmentation of the whole nail plate (total melanonychia),

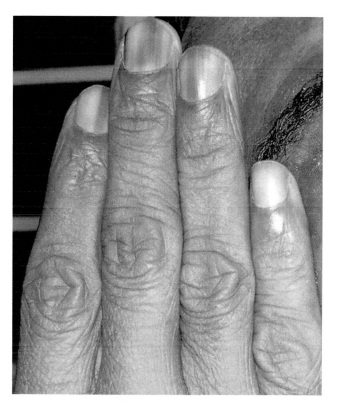

Figure 23.11 Longitudinal melanonychia following antiretroviral (zidovudine) therapy.

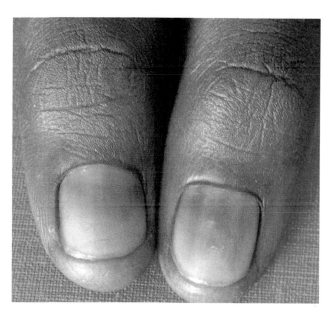

Figure 23.12 Jet-black discoloration following cisplatin/carboplatin, and 5-FU therapy.

whereas activation of clusters of nail matrix melanocytes produce bands of melanonychia. This pigmentation usually fades within 6–8 weeks, but may persist for longer duration even after withdrawal of the drug. Rechallenge is usually negative. Zidovudine, cancer chemotherapeutic agents, hydroxyurea, and psoralens are common causes of melanonychia (Figure 23.11).[7,8]

Non-melanic pigmentation

Non-melanic nail pigmentation due to drugs occurs as a consequence of storage of drugs within the nail plate as some of the drugs get excreted via the nail unit. This pigmentation moves distally with nail growth. Clofazimine causes dark-brown pigmentation, minocycline causes blue-gray pigmentation of the nail bed, and antimalarials produce a blue-brown pigmentation. Tetracyclines and gold salts cause a yellow discoloration of the nail plate. Xanthochromia, i.e., yellow nail discoloration, has been reported in patients treated with mTOR inhibitors such as everolimus and temsirolimus (Figures 23.12 and 23.13).

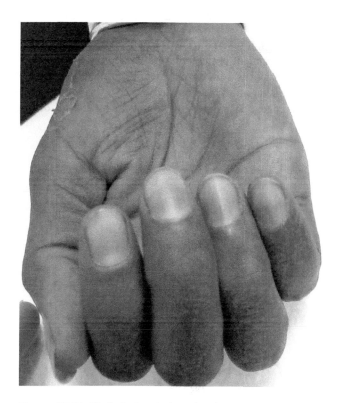

Figure 23.13 Clofazimine-induced nail pigmentation sparing lunula in patients of leprosy.

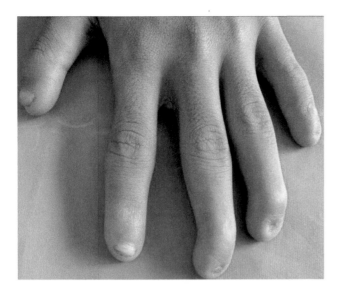

Figure 23.14 Anonychia of the middle, index, and little finger of the left hand with flexion deformity of the middle and ring finger due to phenytoin exposure in a mother of patient during pregnancy.

Topical tar and anthralin, produce an exogenous brown-black pigmentation that moves distally with nail growth.[3–6]

ANONYCHIA OR NAIL HYPOPLASIA

Some drugs, if taken during pregnancy, may interfere with nail development of the fetus and result in nail abnormalities of newborns. Nail development begins at 8–10 weeks of gestational age and is completed by the fifth month of gestational age; hence, intake of teratogens by mother during the 1st and 2nd trimester of pregnancy adversely affects nail development. The nail abnormalities range from mild hypoplasia to complete absence of the nails, i.e., anonychia. Anonychia secondary to teratogenic drugs commonly occurs with phenytoin and warfarin and has also been reported with valproate, carbamazepine, morphine, and trimethadione (Figure 23.14).[4,5]

REFERENCES

1. Piraccini BM, Tosti A. Drug-induced nail disorders: Incidence, management and prognosis. *Drug Saf* 1999;21(3):187–201.
2. Piraccini BM, Iorizzo M, Antonucci A, Tosti A. Drug-induced nail abnormalities. *Expert Opin Drug Saf* 2004;3(1):57–65.
3. Piraccini BM, Iorizzo M, Tosti A. Drug-induced nail abnormalities. *Am J Clin Dermatol* 2003;4(1):31–37.
4. Drug-induced nail disorders. *Prescrire Int* 2014;23(151):180–182.
5. Valeyrie-Allanore L, Sassolas B, Roujeau JC. Drug-induced skin, nail and hair disorders. *Drug Saf* 2007;30(11):1011–1030.
6. Piraccini BM, Iorizzo M, Starace M, Tosti A. Drug-induced nail diseases. *Dermatol Clin* 2006;24(3):387–391.
7. Piraccini BM, Iorizzo M. Drug reactions affecting the nail unit: Diagnosis and management. *Dermatol Clin* 2007;25(2):215–221.
8. Robert C, Sibaud V, Mateus C, Verschoore M, Charles C, Lanoy E, Baran R. Nail toxicities induced by systemic anticancer treatments. *Lancet Oncol* 2015;16(4):e181–e189.

PART 7

Nail in Special Populations

24

Nail in children: Congenital and hereditary diseases

TARU GARG AND SARITA SANKE

INTRODUCTION

Nail development begins by the ninth week of gestation. The nail plate development is evident by 14 weeks and is complete by the 20th week. The nail defects that occur before the 20th week are known as "embryopathies," while the defects occurring after the 20th week are known as "fetopathies." The congenital and hereditary nail dystrophies can be classified based on the embryology of the nails as shown in Figure 24.1.[1] Congenital nail abnormalities can occur in up to 1% of newborns. These nail abnormalities can be present as the only manifestation of a disease, but more commonly they occur as a part of various syndromes in association with other anomalies.[2] The defects in the nails are usually associated with developmental changes of other organs like skin, teeth, brain, and bones. A few of the congenital and hereditary syndromes associated with nail abnormalities are listed in Table 24.1, while the important syndromes are described below in detail.

NAIL–PATELLA SYNDROME

(Syn: hereditary onycho-osteodysplasia (HOOD), Fong disease, or Turner-Kieser syndrome)

Nail–patella syndrome (NPS) is a disorder of nail and bone dysplasia.

Epidemiology: It is a rare autosomal dominant (AD) syndrome with an incidence of 1 in 50,000.[3] Males and females are affected equally.

Etiopathogenesis: Mutation in LMX1B gene at chromosome 9q33.3 is usually responsible for the syndrome.[4] LMX1B is required for the development of kidneys, eyes, and bones.

Clinical features: It is characterized by a tetrad involving the nails, knees, elbows, and iliac horns. Involvement of finger- and toenails is described in 95%–100% of the affected patients. Changes are bilateral and symmetrical and can be present since birth. The thumb and index finger are most commonly involved. There may be anonychia/hyponychia/micronychia of the nails, discoloration, longitudinal nail cleft, and pitting. The triangular lunulae with the apex at the midline is a pathognomonic feature of NPS. These changes are usually present at birth.[5] The other associated findings include hypoplastic/aplastic patella, hypoplasia of proximal radius and ulna, posterior iliac horns, and webbing of digits. Renal changes can occur in 30%–50% of patients manifesting as proteinuria, hematuria, hypertension, or end-stage renal disease.

Investigations: Clinical features along with radiological evaluation to detect iliac horns suffice for making the diagnosis.

Treatment: Nail changes usually do not need any treatment. Physiotherapy for orthopedic problems and monitoring of hypertension are usually recommended.

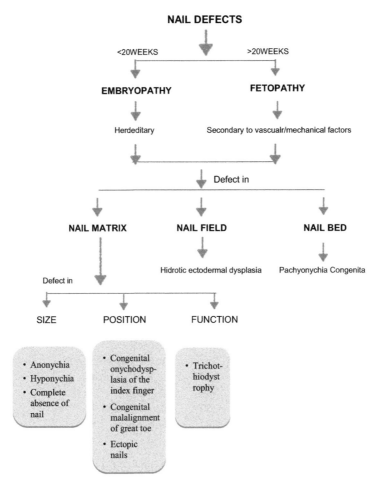

Figure 24.1 Classification of congenital and hereditary nail disorders based on embryology.

Table 24.1 Congenital and hereditary syndromes associated with nail anomalies

	Nail changes	Associated features
Nail involvement only		
Kikuchi congenital onychodysplasia of the index finger syndrome	Anonychia/micronychia of only the index finger	
Nail and skin involvement (including hair)		
Adams Oliver syndrome	Aplastic nails	Aplasia cutis, syndactyly, brachydactyly, abnormalities of fingers and toes
Acro-dermato-ungual-lacrimal-tooth syndrome (ADULT)	Dysplastic nails	Ectrodactyly, syndactyly, mammary hypoplasia, excessive freckling, hypodontia, lacrimal duct anomalies, hypotrichosis
Ankyloblepharon-ectodermal defects-cleft lip and palate syndrome	Dystrophic nails	Ankyloblepharon, cleft lip, palmo-plantar keratoderma, xerosis
Epidermolysis bullosa dystrophica	Anonychia, dystrophy, atrophy	Bullae with scarring, hand and feet contractures, dental anomalies, milia
Epidermolysis bullosa junctional	Dystrophic nails	Blisters, keratoderma, and dental defects
Focal dermal hypoplasia	V nicking, longitudinal ridging, micronychia, anonychia	Dermal hypoplasia, aplasia cutis, telangiectasias, oligodactyly, syndactyly
Erythrokeratoderma Variabilis	Porcelain white nails	Transient figurate erythema, palmoplantar keratoderma

(*Continued*)

Table 24.1 (*Continued*) Congenital and hereditary syndromes associated with nail anomalies

	Nail changes	Associated features
Hypohidrotic ectodermal dysplasia	Dystrophic or fragile/brittle nails	Smooth dry skin with absence of dermal appendages, lack of sweating, dental defects
Witkop syndrome	Longitudinal ridging, nail pitting, koilonychia, fragile nails (Toenails>fingernails)	Hypodontia, large teeth, absent teeth
Darier's disease	Longitudinal erythronychia, leukonychia, V-shaped nick	Greasy hyperkeratotic papules in seborrheic distribution
Clouston syndrome	Hypoplastic nails, paronychia	Hypotrichosis, palmoplantar hyperkeratosis

Nail and systemic involvement

CHILD syndrome	Dystrophic nails (unilateral)	Icthyosiform erythroderma with hemidysplasia
Acrogeria	Atrophic nails	Premature aging predominantly over extremities
Incontinentia pigmenti	Dystrophic nails and occasionally koilonychia	Vesicular, hyperkeratotic, and atrophic skin lesions in blaschkoid pattern in stages. Ocular and CNS anomalies
Nail–patella syndrome	Triangular lunula, anonychia, ulnar nail dystrophy	Hypoplastic patella, iliac horns
Rothmund–Thomson syndrome	Aplastic nails	Poikilodermatous skin, premature canities, baldness, short stature, hypogonadism, cataracts
Progeria	Yellow and atrophic nails	Premature aging syndrome with bird facies, hydrocephalus, short stature, and bony anomalies
Autoimmune polyendocrinopathy-candidiasis-ectodermal dystrophy syndrome (APECED)	Subungual hyperkeratosis, thickened and dystrophic nails	Chronic mucocutaneous candidiasis (CMC), hypoparathyroidism, and adrenal gland insufficiency
Deafness, osteodystrophy, onychodystrophy (DOOR) syndrome	Anonychia, hyponychia, discoloration	Dysplastic distal phalanges, absent dermatoglyphics, deafness
Dyskeratosis congenita	Dystrophic nails with atrophy, thinning, ridging	Poikilodermatous skin changes, oral leukokeratosis, bone marrow failure
Ellis–van Creveld Syndrome (Chondroectodermal dysplasia)	Hypoplastic/dysplastic nails	Dwarfism, polydactyly, narrow chest, dental abnormalities
Epidermolysis bullosa simplex with muscular dystrophy	Occasional nail dystrophy	Blisters, alopecia, muscular dystrophy
Keratitis icthyosis syndrome (KID)	Anonychia, leukonychia, nail plate thickening, dystrophy	Icthyosiform erythroderma, deafness, keratitis
Odonto-onychodermal dysplasia	Dystrophic nails	Palmoplantar skin thickening, mental retardation, hypotrichosis
Mucocutaneous candidiasis syndrome	Onychomycosis	Candidal infections of skin and mucous membranes
Kindler syndrome (Figure 24.2.)	Thick cuticles, dystrophic nails	Poikiloderma, photosensitivity, congenital blistering
Tuberous sclerosis	Periungual fibromas (Koenen's tumor) (Figure 24.3)	Angiofibromas, hypomelanotic macules, shagreen patch, focal seizures, and spasms
Osler–Weber–Rendu Syndrome (hereditary hemorrhagic telangiectasia)	Subungual splinter hemorrhages, cyanosis, clubbing	Mucocutaneous telangiectasias, anemia, intestinal bleeding

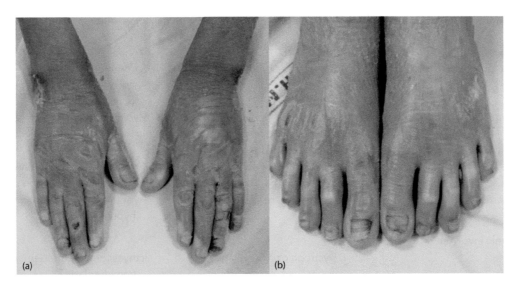

Figure 24.2 Dystrophic nails in Kindler syndrome. **(a)** Fingernails; **(b)** Toenails.

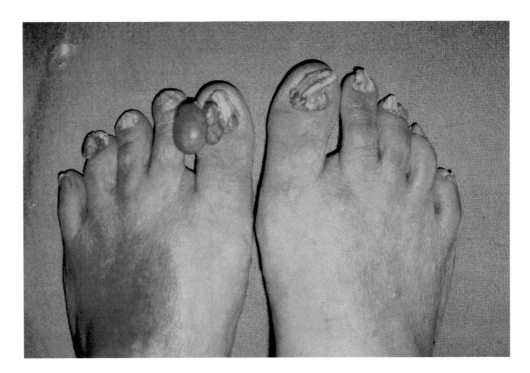

Figure 24.3 Koenen's tumor in tuberous sclerosis.

YELLOW NAIL SYNDROME

Yellow nail syndrome (YNS) is a triad of thickened yellow nails, primary lymphedema, and recurrent respiratory infections.

Epidemiology: An estimated prevalence of YNS is <1/1,000,000.[6] It usually occurs in adults over 50 years of age, with no sex predilection.

Etiopathogenesis: It is an acquired condition of unknown etiology. The pathogenesis has been ascribed to impaired lymphatic drainage leading to thickened nails with slow growth causing subungual nail bed sclerosis leading to further lymphatic obstruction. The yellowish discoloration is ascribed to secondary accumulation of lipofuscin pigment.

Clinical features: YNS is a triad of thickened yellow nails, primary lymphedema, and recurrent respiratory infections. Any two of these are sufficient to make the diagnosis, but yellow nails are a characteristic feature (Figure 24.4). However, the possible interval between the first clinical sign (lymphedema, lung manifestations) and nail discoloration hinders affirmation of the YNS diagnosis. The discoloration of nails can vary

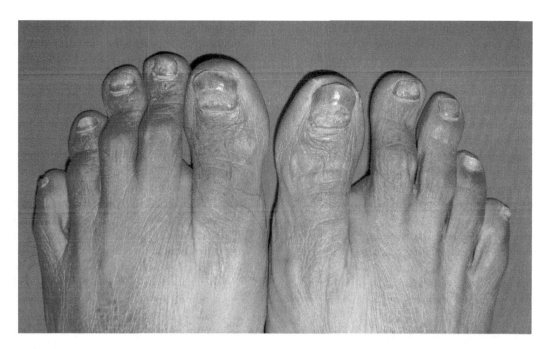

Figure 24.4 Thick yellow nails in yellow nail syndrome.

from pale yellow (xanthonychia) to green. The nail plate is thickened with increased curvature, cross-ridging, scleronychia, and loss of cuticles. The lunula is usually absent (disappears due to nail hyperkeratosis). Onycholysis, partial or complete, is also sometimes noted.

Differential diagnosis: Yellowish discoloration of nails can be secondary to certain drugs (d-penicillamine, bucillamine, gold), infections (candida), psoriasis, and alopecia areata.

Treatment: Spontaneous resolution of nail changes can be seen in around 30% of patients. Oral vitamin E (1000–1200 IU/day) is found to be successful in patients not responding.[6] Oral zinc sulfate supplementation (300 mg) has found to decrease the yellowing of nails and the lymphedema.

Complications: Recurrent respiratory infections, sinusitis, and pleural effusion can result from the pulmonary involvement. Lymphedema can cause difficulty in walking and social embarrassment.

DYSKERATOSIS CONGENITA

Dyskeratosis congenita (DKC) is an inherited bone marrow failure syndrome characterized by the classic triad of abnormal skin pigmentation, nail dystrophy, and oral leukoplakia.

Epidemiology: The prevalence is estimated to be 1 in 1,000,000 individuals. Approximately half of the cases are males.

Etiopathogenesis: DKC is inherited either as X-linked pattern, AD, or autosomal recessive patterns. Mutations in at least 10 telomere and telomerase-associated genes have been described in DKC and hence it is considered to be "telomeropathy."[7]

Clinical features: Minimum criteria for the diagnosis of DKC includes at least two major and two minor features (Table 24.2).[8] The nail dystrophy in DKC is seen in approximately 90% of patients and fingernail involvement precedes the toenail involvement.[9] The onset of nail changes tend to begin in the first decade with a median of 6 years. The dystrophic nails can show longitudinal ridging, splitting, nail plate atrophy, pterygium, and

Table 24.2 Clinical features of dyskeratosis congenita (at least two major and two minor criteria should be present for the diagnosis)

Major features (>75% patients)	Minor features
Bone marrow failure	Short stature
Nail dystrophy	Hyperhidrosis
Oral leukokeratosis	Developmental delay
Reticulate/poikilodermatous skin changes	Pulmonary disease
	Esophageal stricture
	Epiphora
	Gastrointestinal disease
	Ataxia
	Hypogonadism
	Microcephaly

thinning. Anonychia, hyponychia, distortion in shape, and pterygium can also be usually noted. Reticular or poikilodermatous skin changes are noted over the face, neck, back, and thighs usually during late childhood or teenage years. Leukokeratosis with blisters and erosions are noted in the oral mucosa. Severe aplastic anemia with neutropenia, splenomegaly, myelodysplastic syndrome, and squamous cell carcinoma has also been described.

Differential diagnosis: Rothmund–Thomson syndrome, epidermolysis bullosa simplex with mottled pigmentation, and Naegeli–Franceschetti–Jadassohn (NFJ) syndrome can be confused with DKC due to their poikilodermatous presentation.

Investigations: Screening can usually be done with the help of flow cytometry and fluorescence in situ hybridization to detect telomere shortening.

Treatment: Allogenic stem cell transplantation is recommended for bone marrow failure.

PACHYONYCHIA CONGENITA

Pachyonychia congenita (PC) is a rare type of ectodermal dysplasia caused by mutations in genes encoding the nail keratin.

Epidemiology: Although the exact frequency of PC is unknown, it appears to be rare. An estimated 5,000–10,000 cases have been reported worldwide.[10]

Etiopathogenesis: The inheritance of PC is AD with incomplete penetrance but autosomal recessive and sporadic cases have also been reported. PC is caused due to mutations in keratin genes (K6a, K6b, K16, K17) that are expressed in the suprabasal layer of nail bed epithelium. These genes are responsible for the strength and resilience of skin, hair, and nail. Thus, defect in these genes result in abnormal thickening of nails.

Clinical features: PC is divided into three types based on the specific keratin gene involved: PC-K6a, PC-K6b, PC-K6c, PC-K16, and PC-K17. Table 24.3 enumerates the differences in three types of PC.

- Type I (Jadassohn and Lewandowsky type): It is due to mutations in keratin 6a and 16. The nails in this syndrome are normal at birth but become progressively discolored and thickened with age, usually in the first year. Wedge-shaped or V-shaped subungual hyperkeratosis is the characteristic finding (Figure 24.5). This may develop in one of two ways: nails that grow to full length but have an upward inclination due to prominent subungual distal hyperkeratosis or "early ending of the

Table 24.3 Major types of pachyonychia congenita and associated features

	Mutation	Nail features	Cutaneous features
PC Type I	Keratin 6a and 16	Wedge-shaped or V-shaped subungual hyperkeratosis	Palmoplantar hyperhidrosis, keratoderma, oral leukokeratosis
PC Type II	Keratin 6b and 17	Mild subungual hyperkeratoses	Natal teeth, steatocystoma multiplex, and pili torti, no oral leukokeratosis
PC Tarda	1A domain of K17	Nail dystrophy	Palmoplantar hyperkeratosis, oral leukokeratosis, hyperhidrosis

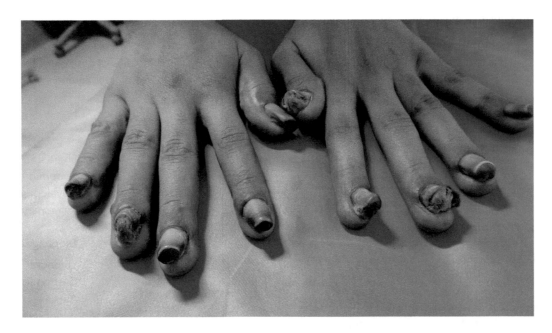

Figure 24.5 Wedge-shaped subungual hyperkeratosis in pachyonychia congenita.

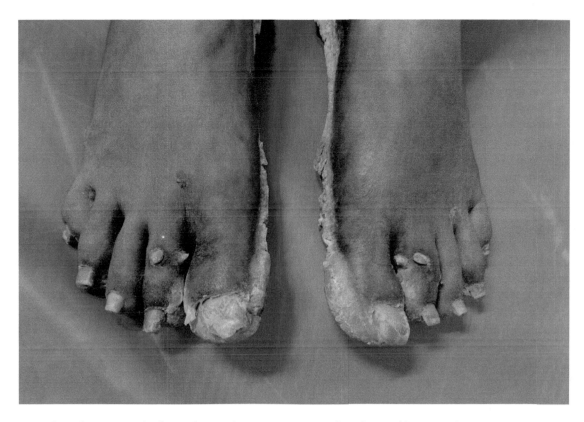

Figure 24.6 Nail involvement with plantar keratoderma in a patient of pachyonychia congenita.

nail" and the curving of distal hyperkeratosis. The other associated features include palmoplantar hyperhidrosis, acral bulla, and oral leukokeratosis. Plantar keratoderma poses another limitation in these patients and can be present in 10.4% of affected patients (Figures 24.5 and 24.6). The keratoderma is more prominent at pressure points on the heel and ball of great toe.

- Type II (Jackson–Lawler syndrome): It is due to mutations in keratin 6b and 17. Type 2 additionally present with natal teeth, steatocystoma multiplex, and woolly hair with other manifestations being less severe.[11]
- PC Tarda: It is late onset variant of PC. It is characterized by nail dystrophy, palmoplantar hyperkeratosis, leukokeratosis of mucous membranes, follicular hyperkeratosis, and hyperhydrosis of palms and soles.

Investigations: Genotyping can be performed for definite diagnosis.

Differential diagnosis: Clouston syndrome can present with nail changes and keratoderma at birth and cause confusion with PC. However, hearing loss and sparse hair are additional features that can help in differentiating it from PC.

Treatment: Mechanical options like filing and grinding of the nails can be done. Oral Vitamin A analogues (retinoids) and Vitamin E have shown some benefit in reducing the nail thickness and the keratoderma. Topical keratolytics, moisturizers, and retinoids can be used for keratoderma.

Complications: Nail changes cause social embarrassment while painful erosions, bullae, and fissures can occur over areas of keratoderma. It can impede walking and playing.

HEREDITARY ECTODERMAL DYSPLASIA

Hereditary ectodermal dysplasia (HED) is a term used to denote a group of disorders (at least 90) that have at least one of the following features: hypotrichosis, hypodontia, hidrotic changes, and onychodysplasia, plus at least one sign affecting other ectodermal tissues.[8] A few of the important disorders under HED having nail defects have been listed in Table 24.4.

EPIDERMOLYSIS BULLOSA (EB)

Epidermolysis bullosa includes a group of inherited mechano-blistering skin diseases. It is distinguished into three different types: epidermal, junctional, and dystrophic.

Etiopathogenesis: Mutations have been described in genes encoding for keratin filaments, adhesion contact, desmosomes, hemidesmosomes, and anchoring fibrils.

Table 24.4 Hereditary ectodermal dysplasias with nail changes

Cutaneous disorder	Associated nail changes
Cardio-faciocutaneous syndrome	Dysplastic nails with koilonychia
Ectrodactyly clefting syndrome	Brittle, dystrophic nails, pitting
Dermatopathia pigmentosa reticularis	Lamellar splitting and ridging
Naegeli–Franceschetti–Jadassohn syndrome	Subungual hyperkeratoses, onycholysis
Palmoplantar keratoderma (Unna-thost)	Thickened nail plate
Maleda-type palmoplantar keratoderma	Subungual hyperkeratosis, onychogryphosis, koilonychia
Papillon–Lefévre syndrome	Punctate depressions, koilonychia
Keratoderma with leuconychiatotalis	Leukonychia of all nails
Lamellar icthyosis	Thick and striated subungual hyperkeratoses
Olmsted's syndrome	Thick and striated subungual hyperkeratoses
Oculo-dento-digital syndrome	Fusion of nails of fourth and fifth fingers
Aplasia cutis	Thin and short grey nails, occasional onychogryphosis
Chondrodysplasia punctate	Flat nails with splitting
Trichodystrophy, BIDS syndrome	Brittle short nails
Trichothiodystrophy, IBDS, or Tay syndrome	Brittle dystrophic nails, convex curvature
Trichothiodystrophy with PIBIDS syndrome	Hypoplasia/dystrophy with leukonychia and lamellar splitting

BIDS: Brittle hair, intellectual impairment, decreased fertility, and short stature; IBIDS: Icthyosis, brittle hair, intellectual impairment, decreased fertility, and short stature; PIBIDS: Photosensitivity, icthyosis, brittle hair, intellectual impairment, decreased fertility, and short stature.

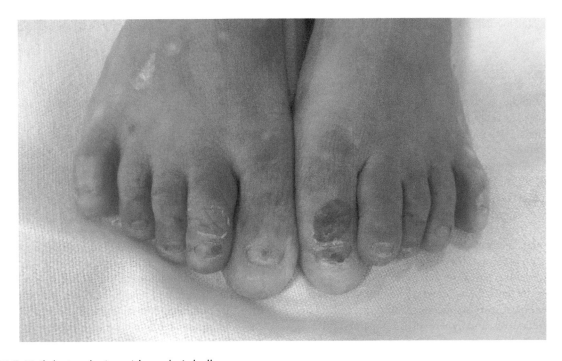

Figure 24.7 Nail dystrophy in epidermolysis bullosa.

Clinical features: These disorders are characterized by increased skin fragility, and blisters can be induced mechanically. The nail changes are usually seen in the dystrophic and sometimes in junctional variant of EB. The associated nail findings may include anonychia, subungual or periungual hemorrhagic blisters producing onycholysis, erosions, nail atrophy, nail hyperkeratosis, onychomadesis, etc. (Figure 24.7). Onychogryphosis can be seen in the Ogna variant of EB simplex. Pseudo syndactyly is a feature of non-Herlitz junctional EB. Mitten deformity of hands and feet points to the

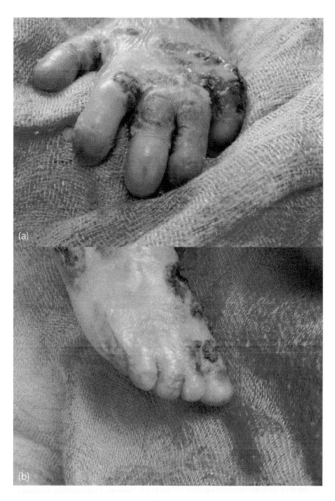

Figure 24.8 Anonychia with distal resorption of fingers/toes in epidermolysis bullosa dystrophic. **(a)** Fingernails; **(b)** Toenails.

Table 24.5 Nail findings in various types of epidermolysis bullosa

	Disease type	Nail findings
Epidermal variants (simplex)	Dowling Meara type	Dystrophic nails
	EB simplex with mottled pigmentation	Curved and dystrophic
	Ogna variant	Onychogryphosis
	EB superficialis	Dystrophic
	EBS with neuromuscular disease	Dystrophic
Junctional variants (localized)	Junctional localized Inversa	Dystrophic, anonychia
	Acral	Anonychia
	Progressive	Dystrophic and fragile nails
Junctional (generalized)	Gravis	Anonychia, hypoplastic fragile nails
	Cicatricial	Anonychia
EB dystrophic variants	Inversa	Thick, dystrophic
	Acral	Dystrophic
	Pretibial	Thick, dystrophic
	Hyperplastic	Thick, dystrophic
	Bart type	Anonychia, dystrophic
	Gravis	Split nail, anonychia
	Mitis	Dystrophic

diagnosis of the generalized recessive form of DEB (Hallopeau-Siemens variant) (Figure 24.8a and b).[12] Table 24.5 summarizes the various types of EB with the associated nail defects.

CHRONIC MUCOCUTANEOUS CANDIDIASIS

Chronic mucocutaneous candidiasis (CMC) is characterized by candida infection of the mucous membrane, scalp, skin, and nails with *candida* species, especially *C. Albicans*.

Epidemiology: It can be AD or recessive in nature.
Etiopathogenesis: Abnormality in cell mediated immunity secondary to abnormal complement function and neutrophil phagocytosis can cause the disease. Recently, it has been proposed that STAT1 mutations are responsible for CMC.[13]

Clinical features: Candidal infection of the mucosae, scalp, and nails are the characteristic features. However, endocrine dysfunctions, alopecia, vitiligo, malabsorption syndromes, neoplasms, and other infections may also occur in patients with CMC. Nail involvement presents as onychomycosis with or without paronychia. The nails become thickened, fragmented, hyperkeratotic, and brittle.
Investigations: Potassium hydroxide (KOH) mount and fungal culture of skin swabs and nail plate scrapings can be done to confirm the organism.
Treatment: Oral antifungal agents like itraconazole work well, but recurrence is common.

ISO–KIKUCHI SYNDROME

Also known as congenital onychodysplasia of the index finger (COIF), Iso–Kikuchi syndrome is a syndrome characterized by dysplasia/absence of fingernails with underlying bone abnormalities.

Etiopathogenesis: Several pathogenetic mechanisms have been postulated, such as in-utero ischemic injury secondary to abnormal fetal vascular supply from the palmar digital artery affecting the radial side of finger, impairment of "WNT signaling pathway" due to genetic mutation that plays a role in embryonic growth and development and, lastly, intra-uterine fetal exposure to teratogens. It can be sporadic in onset or hereditary. When inherited, transmission pattern of this condition seems to be AD.[14]

Clinical features: The clinical criteria for diagnosing COIF are unilateral or bilateral hypoplasia/aplasia of the index fingernails and/or other fingernails and toenails, radiographic abnormalities of the distal bony phalanx of the affected fingers, and congenital occurrence.

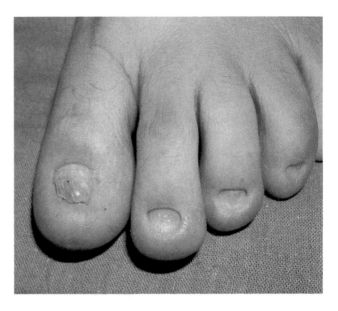

Figure 24.9 Anonychia of nails in hereditary anonychia.

COOKS SYNDROME

The syndrome was first described by Cooks et al.[15] in 1985 in a family with "onychonychia" and absence or hypoplasia of distal phalanges.

Etiopathogenesis: It is an AD condition with initial spontaneous mutation.[15] Recently, microduplications on chromosome 17q involving non-coding element of SOX9 gene resulting in an abnormal digit and nail development have been associated with Cooks syndrome.[16]

Clinical features: The nail changes described in this syndrome include hypoplasia or complete absence of fingernails; total absence of all toenails; congenital onychodystrophy; hypoplasia of distal phalanges in hands, especially fifth finger; brachydactyly; digitalization of the thumb; or absence of all distal phalanges of feet with normal hair, teeth, and sweat glands. Anonychia involving all the 20 digits is a rare occurrence.

HEREDITARY ANONYCHIA

It is characterized by isolated congenital absence of the fingernails/toenails.

Etiopathogenesis: Mutation in the R-spondin-4 (RSPO4) gene on chromosome 20p13, which is expressed in the mesenchymal tissue at tip of the digits, is responsible for the disease. It can be inherited as AD, AR, or sporadic in onset.

Clinical features: The hypoplasia or anonychia is usually congenital and involves all the nails. Rudimentary nails can be found occasionally (Figure 24.9); underlying bone abnormality of the digits is usually associated.

Anonychia is usually associated with other features like polydactyly, syndactyly, broad and small hands, and brachydactyly.

KEIPERT SYNDROME

It is an autosomal recessive syndrome comprising sensorineural deafness with facial and digital abnormalities. It is characterized by broad thumbs and halluces, brachydactyly, short stature, macrocephaly, and facial dysmorphic features. The thumbs and great toenails are more involved than the other nails.[17]

DOOR SYNDROME

It is an autosomal recessive disorder and refers to deafness, onychodystrophy, osteodystrophy, and mental retardation. It (OMIM220500) is an extremely rare genetic condition with just over 40 cases reported to date since its first description in 1961. The abnormalities in the nails can present as anonychia, hypoplasia, hyponychia, and discoloration or variation in texture or shape of one or more nails. Osteodystrophies can be in the form of absent or dysplastic distal phalanges, triphalangeal thumb, or great toe.[18]

CONCLUSION

In addition to all the above-described syndromes, various morphological abnormalities of the nails in the form of discoloration (Figure 24.10), short/broad nails, clubbing, koilonychia, etc. can be present in certain disorders that have been listed in Table 24.6.

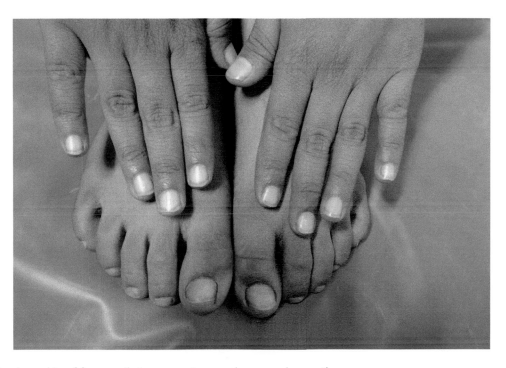

Figure 24.10 Leukonychia of fingernails in comparison to the normal toenails.

Table 24.6 Hereditary syndromes associated with specific morphological abnormality

Morphological abnormality	Associated syndromes
Clubbing	Cartilage hair hypoplasia
	Hereditary clubbing of digits
	Palmoplantar keratoderma with clubbing
	Pachydermoperiostosis
	Cleidocranial dysostosis
	Peutz–Jeghers–Touraine syndrome
Broad Nails	Acrodysostosis
	Acrocephalosyndactyly
	Dwarfism-brachydactyly syndrome
	Megalodactyly
	Rubinstein–Taybi syndrome
	Keipert syndrome
	Larsen's syndrome
	Familial mandibuloacral dysplasia
Koilonychia	Keratoderma palmoplantare progressiva
	Familial koilonychia
	Monilethrix
	Nail–patella syndrome
	Incontinentia pigmenti
	Trichoepithelioma multiplex
Anonychia-Micronychia	DOOR syndrome
	Dermolytic epidermolysis bullosa
	Amniotic bands
	Ectodermal dysplasias
	Iso–Kikuchi syndrome
	Nail–patella syndrome

(Continued)

Table 24.6 (*Continued*) Hereditary syndromes associated with specific morphological abnormality

Morphological abnormality	Associated syndromes
Dolichonychia	Ehlers–Danlos syndrome
	Marfan's syndrome
	Eunuchoidism
	Hypopituitarism
	Hypohidrotic ectodermal dysplasia
Leukonychia (Figure 24.10)	Ectodermal dysplasia
	Hailey–Hailey disease
	White nail syndrome
	Congenital lamellar icthyosis
	Alagille syndrome
Discolored Nails	Leopard syndrome—white
	Keratitis, icthyosis, and deafness—white
	Leuconychiatotalis—milky
	Leuconychiastriatus—milky
	Incontinentia pigmenti—yellow
	Pachyonychia congenita—yellow/brown
	Progeria—yellow
	Yellow nail syndrome—yellow
	Darier's disease—brown/red/white
	Gunther's disease—brown
	Klippel–Trenaunay syndrome—bluish

To summarize, nail abnormalities can manifest in various genetic and hereditary syndromes. Detailed evaluation of the nails at birth can provide a clue in diagnosing various syndromes. One should always look for various cutaneous and extra cutaneous features in a child with nail abnormalities.

KEY POINTS

- Congenital nail abnormalities can occur in up to 1% of newborns.
- The congenital and hereditary nail defects can be classified into "embryopathies" (occurring before 20th week) or "fetopathies" (occurring after 20th week).
- These nail abnormalities can be present as the only manifestation of a disease or can occur as a part of various syndromes.
- The defects in the nails can also be associated with developmental changes of other organs like skin, teeth, brain, and bones.
- Detailed evaluation of the nails at birth can provide a clue in diagnosing various syndromes.
- One should always look for various cutaneous and extra cutaneous features in a child with nail abnormalities.

REFERENCES

1. Telfer NR, Barth JH, Dawber RPR. Congenital and hereditary nail dystrophies: An embryological approach to classification. *Clin Exp Dermatol* 1988;13(3):160–163.
2. Juhlin L, Baran R. Hereditary and congenital nail disorders. In: *Baran and Dawber's Diseases of the Nails and Their Management*, 3rd ed. (Baran R, Dawber RPR, de Berker DAR, Haneke E, Tosti A, Eds.), Blackwell Science Ltd, Oxford, UK. 2001: pp. 370–424.
3. Padmanabhan LD, Yesodharan D, Nampoothiri S. Prenatal diagnosis of nail patella syndrome: A case report. *Indian J Radiol Imaging* 2017;27(3):329–331.
4. Witzgal R. Nail-patella syndrome. *Pflugers Arch* 2017;469(7–8):927–936.
5. Inamadar AC, Palit A. Nails: Diagnostic clue to genodermatoses. *Indian J Dermatol Venereol Leprol* 2012;78:271–278.
6. Vignes S, Baran R. Yellow nail syndrome: A review. *Orphanet J Rare Dis* 2017;12(1):42.
7. Dokal I. Dyskeratosis congenita. *Hematol Am Soc Hematol Educ Prog* 2011;2011:480–486.
8. Rubin A, Paller AS. Genetic defects of nails and nail growth. In: *Rooks Textbook of Dermatology*, 9th ed. (Griffiths C, Barker J, Bleiker T, Chalmers R, Creamer D, Eds.), Wiley-Blackwel, Chichester, UK. 2016: p. 69.4.

9. Dokal I. Dyskeratosis congenita in all its forms. *Br J Haematol* 2000;110:768–779.

10. Kaspar RL. Challenges in developing therapies for rare diseases including pachyonychia congenita. *J Investig Dermatol Symp Proc* 2005;10(1):62–66.

11. Sravanthi A, Srivalli P, Gopal K, Rao TN. Pachyonychia congenita with late onset (PC Tarda). *Indian Dermatol Online J* 2016;7:278–280.

12. Inamadar AC, Palit A. Nails: Diagnostic clue to genodermatoses. *Indian J Dermatol Venereol Leprol* 2012;78:271–278.

13. Van de Veerdonk FL, Netea MG. Treatment options for chronic mucocutaneous candidiasis. *J Infect* 2016;72 Suppl:S56–S60.

14. Valerio E, Favot F, Mattei I, Cutrone M. Congenital isolated Iso–Kikuchi syndrome in a newborn. *Clin Case Rep* 2015;3(10):866–869.

15. Cooks RG, Hertz M, Katznelson MBM, Goodman RM. A new nail dysplasia syndrome with onychonychia and absence and/or hypoplasia of distal phalanges. *Clin Genet* 1985;27:85–91.

16. Kurth I, Klopocki E, Stricker S, van Oosterwijk J, Vanek S, Altmann J et al. Duplications of noncoding elements 5¢ of SOX9 are associated with brachydactyly-anonychia. *Nat Genet* 2009;41:862–863.

17. Amor DJ, Dahl H-HM, Bahlo M, Bankier A. Keipert syndrome (nasodigitoacoustic syndrome) is X-linked and maps to Xq22.2–Xq28. *Am J Med Genet A* 2007;143A:2236–2241.

18. Nair LD, Sagayaraj B, Kumar R. Absence of nails, deaf-mutism, seizures, and intellectual disability: A case report. *J Clin Diagn Res* 2015;9(4):SD01–SD03.

25

Nail in elderly population

SAVITHA AS AND SHASHIKUMAR BM

INTRODUCTION

There is no universally accepted chronological age to consider an individual as elderly. Most countries have accepted the age of 65 years as the definition of an elderly or older person. With the improvement in medical care over the last few decades, there has been a constant rise in the geriatric population throughout the world. In an Egyptian study, nail changes were present in 88% of subjects of elderly population in contrast with only 39% of younger subjects in the control group.[1] Onychodystrophies due to chronic faulty biomechanics, recurrent trauma, and infections are common in elderly. Nail abnormalities that were present at an earlier age might get modified further with advancing age. Routine nail care can be hampered in the elderly due to difficulty in reaching feet, nails that become too thick to cut, or poor vision. Nail changes can either cause severe symptoms hampering the daily activities or they may be asymptomatic causing cosmetic concern.

Nail changes in the elderly may be described under the following headings.

NAIL CHANGES DUE TO AGING

Age-associated characteristic changes in nail occur as the person becomes older, and these changes pertain to the composition, growth rate, color, vasculature, contour, thickness, surface, and histology, as summarized in Table 25.1.

Changes in chemical composition

Average water content of nail is approximately 18% (10%–30%). Nails become brittle when the water content is less than 16% and become soft when it is above 25%. Brittle nails are common in elderly due to reduced water content and reduced lipid (cholesterol sulfate). There is a reduction in iron concentrations also. The concentration of magnesium and calcium increases in nail with age.[2]

Change in growth rate

Nail growth decreases by approximately 0.5% per year between the ages of 20 and 100 years. It has been observed that thumbnail growth decreases on an average by 38%

Table 25.1 Common nail changes in the elderly

Characteristics	Changes
Color	Yellow to gray with dull, opaque appearance
	"Neapolitan" nails: nails with loss of lunulae and a white proximal portion, a normal pink central band, and an opaque distal free edge
Contour	Increased transverse convexity
	Decreased longitudinal curvature
Histology	Nail plate keratinocytes—increased size, increased number of pertinax bodies (keratinocyte nuclei remnants)
	Nail bed dermis—thickening of the blood vessels, degeneration of elastic tissue
Linear growth	Decreases
Surface	Increased friability with splitting and fissuring
	Longitudinal furrows that are superficial (onychorrhexis) and deep (ridges)
Thickness	Variable: normal, increased, or decreased

Source: Ohgitani, S. et al., J. Bone Miner. Metab., 23, 318–322, 2005.

between the third and the ninth decade. Females have a more pronounced decrease in the rate of nail growth as compared to men up to the sixth decade, which makes females more prone for fungal infections. Some co-existent systemic diseases and certain drugs also may affect linear nail growth rate.[3]

Changes in color

Nail color changes vary from shades of yellow to grey with aging. Pale, dull, opaque, and lusterless nails were the most common nail changes in elderly group in a study.[1] The lunular size decreases with age and this has been previously noted as an aging-related nail change[4] (Figure 25.1). The white nails of old age, similar to those reported in cirrhosis, azotemia, and hypoalbuminemia, have been termed "Neapolitan nails" because of the three bands as in Neapolitan ice cream. These are characterized by an absent lunula in addition to three horizontal bands of white (proximal), pink (middle), and opaque (distal) discolorations. These changes occur without detectable protein, liver, or kidney abnormalities.[5]

Transverse leukonychia (Figure 25.2) and multiple transverse white bands paralleling the distal shape of the lunula result from repeated microtrauma on the untrimmed distal nail edge. Frictional longitudinal melanonychia occurs due to recurrent trauma (Figure 25.3).

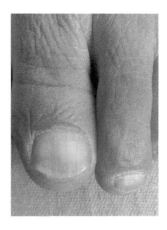

Figure 25.1 Absence of lunulae.

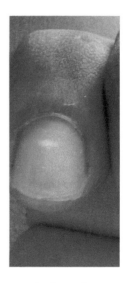

Figure 25.2 Transverse leukonychia.

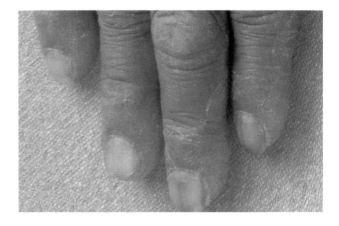

Figure 25.3 Longitudinal melanonychia.

Changes in blood vessels

Senile nail changes can be attributed to arteriosclerosis. Short tortuous capillary loops and ill-defined subpapillary venous plexus are the frequent distortions of nail bed capillaries in the elderly. These changes, favored by frequent

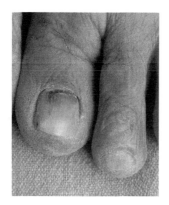

Figure 25.4 Subungual hematoma.

trauma to nails and intake of multiple drugs like anticoagulants, explain the increased frequency of distal splinter hemorrhages in the elderly. Splinter hemorrhages, which are most commonly traumatic in the elderly, are black and located in the middle or distal third of the fingernail. In contrast, splinter hemorrhages induced by systemic disorders are red in color and proximal in location.

Anticoagulants are often responsible for subungual hematomas. Hematomas also result from acute trauma and can be very painful (Figure 25.4).

Acral arteriolar ectasia is a distinct vascular malformation consisting of purple serpiginous vessels on the dorsum of digits, which first arrive in the fifth decade of life. The vessels are ectatic arterioles and believed to represent a rare vascular malformation.[6]

Contour changes

Loss of the normal double curvature of nails resulting in platynychia or koilonychia is common in the elderly (Figure 25.5).

Changes in nail plate thickness

Fingernails often become thinner, soft, and fragile and thus prone to longitudinal fissuring and splitting into layers.

Toenails usually become thicker compared to fingernails and the thickness increases with age, probably due to repeated trauma from footwear.

1. **Onychauxis** is thickening of the nail plate with discoloration that occurs in the elderly (Figures 25.6a, b and 25.7). It is often associated with subungual hyperkeratosis of the nail bed. Presenting features may include pain, onycholysis, underlying fungal infection, hemorrhage, or ulceration of the nail bed.[7]

   Treatment: Periodic partial or total debridement of the thickened nail should be done with the help of electric drills or burrs. Moistening the nail helps to prevent dispersion of infective material, if any, during drilling. Chemical (40% urea paste) or surgical avulsion gives temporary relief. Permanent ablation with chemical (phenol) or surgical matricectomy may be required for recurrent and troublesome onychauxis. As subungual hyperkeratosis is a common manifestation of onychomycosis, onychauxis can be misdiagnosed as fungal infection and patients inappropriately treated with antifungals. Therefore, microscopic confirmation of onychomycosis in elderly patients should be obtained before antifungal therapy is begun.

2. **Onychogryphosis** is characterized by thickened, uneven, discolored, severely elongated, curved nails with claw-like deformity (oyster-like or ram's horn deformity). It is often associated with multiple striations and hypertrophy

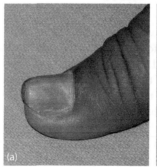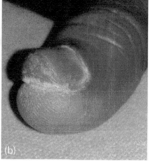

Figure 25.6 **(a)** Onychauxis—dorsal view and **(b)** onychauxis—ventral view.

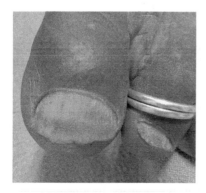

Figure 25.5 Platynychia- flat dull lusterless nail.

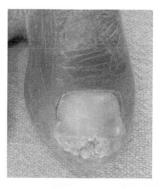

Figure 25.7 Onychauxis, nail plate is dystrophic.

of nail bed. Toenail is most commonly involved. Onychogryphosis occurs mainly due to infrequent cutting of the nails due to physical factors. The nail plate initially grows upwards and thereafter deviates laterally towards the other toes, the direction of growth being influenced by pressure from footwear and matrix activity. Other etiologies include trauma, hypertrophy of the nail bed, and bony deformities like hallux valgus. It can be sometimes painful, be associated with fungal infection, and interfere with shoe wearing. A few patients who have underlying peripheral vascular disease and diabetes develop subungual gangrene due to pressure effects.[8]

Treatment: Treatment is required to avoid complications like subungual gangrene and for cosmetic reasons. Management is similar to that of onychauxis, which includes trimming the nails with an electric burr, filing subungual hyperkeratosis, avulsion of the nail plate, and surgical or chemical destruction of the nail matrix with phenol. The choice of treatment should take into account peripheral vascular circulation, treatment compliance, and potential complications. Any coexisting fungal infection should be treated appropriately.[9]

In hemi-onychogryphosis, a condition mimicking onychogryphosis, the nail plate grows laterally from the beginning. This may be a complication of persistent congenital malalignment of the great toenails. This condition can be prevented by regular nail plate trimming and foot care.

Changes in nail plate surface

The senile nail may have more pronounced and numerous longitudinal striations due to altered turnover rate of the matrix cells or may be related to whorls of generative cells in the most proximal region of the nail matrix.[3] The striations are termed "onychorrhexis" if they are superficial and "ridges" or "sausage-link ridges" or "beading" if deep[10] (Figures 25.8 through 25.10a, b). Aging is the most common cause of onychorrhexis. Beau's lines (transverse ridges), pitting, and trachyonychia are also found frequently (Figure 25.11).

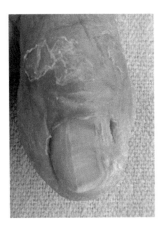

Figure 25.8 Prominent longitudinal striations.

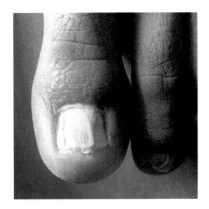

Figure 25.9 Lustreless nail with prominent striations.

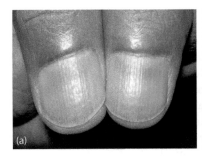
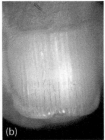

Figure 25.10 **(a)** Beaded appearance of striations and **(b)** dermoscopy of beaded appearance.

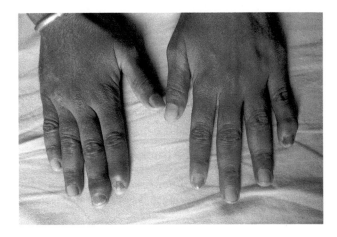

Figure 25.11 Trachyonychia.

Brittle nails are more common in the elderly. Due to increased fragility there will be lamellar splitting—onychoschizia—and irregularity of distal nail plate (castle battlement appearance) (Figure 25.12a and b). Several endogenous factors and recurrent exogenous factors acting on the nail plate and nail matrix result in brittle nails. Repeated cycles of hydration and dehydration—as occurs during excessive domestic wet work or with overuse of dehydrating agents, nail enamel, nail enamel removers, or cuticle removers—may precipitate brittle nails.[8]

Treatment: The primary treatment in the management of brittle nails is elimination of any habits or agents that are

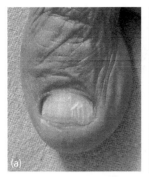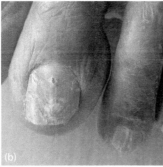

Figure 25.12 **(a and b)** Onychoschizia.

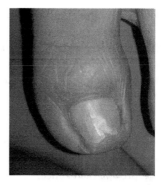

Figure 25.13 Lateral deviation of nail plate.

precipitating brittle nails. Hydration of the nails by applying a moisturizer (containing lactic acid, paraffin, or urea) to nail unit including nail beds should be initiated. Soaking the nails for 10–15 minutes in lukewarm water before applying moisturizers and occlusion enhances the effect. Application of nail enamel slows evaporation of water from nail plate. Frequent changing of nail enamels (more than once a week) should be discouraged. There is a risk of allergic contact dermatitis with nail enamels and enamel removers. Oral biotin, iron, thiamine, cysteine, pantothenic acid, and para-aminobenzoic acid (PABA) have been found to be effective in brittle nails.[7]

Histopathology of senile changes

The nail plate contains an increased number of "pertinax bodies" compared with the normal adult nail. They could be interpreted as remnants of nuclei of keratinocytes. Retarded nail plate growth results in larger corneocytes.[11]

AGE-RELATED TOENAIL DISORDERS LINKED TO REPEATED TRAUMA AND FOOT BIOMECHANICS

Footwear

Footwear plays a major role in contour and surface nail changes. The higher the heel, the more damage will occur on the anterior part of the foot, especially around the nail apparatus and the apices. Poor toe box design with inadequate width and depth can result in unusual external pigmentation acquired from rubbing on the leather of new shoes. More commonly, a single toenail with a very "polished" sheen to it, or a redness of the distal portion, may be the result of continuous rubbing on the soft lining of a shoe.[3]

Hallux abducto valgus

The progressive lateral deviation of the big toe is accompanied by valgus rotation of the nail. This places great stress on the nail apparatus of the big toe and adjacent nails, which frequently become distorted, thickened, onychogryphotic, or ingrown (Figure 25.13). This is predominantly seen in women. There is medial deviation of the first

metatarsal with lateral deviation of hallux. Where excessive pronation coexists, the use of orthoses may give relief from symptoms. Surgery is indicated where severe deformity develops or when pain relief is not achieved with conservative methods.

Hammer toe

Hammer toe is a deformity arising through increased extension at the metacarpophalangeal joint and corresponding flexion at the proximal interphalangeal joint. In the extreme form, the tip of the digit is directed downwards and develops an "end corn" beneath the pulp of the toe just below the nail plate edge associated with thickening of the nail plate and the distal nail bed. This is called claw deformity.

Onychophosis[8]

This refers to localized or diffuse hyperkeratosis on the lateral or proximal nail folds, in the space between the nail folds and nail plate, and also subungually. It results from repeated minor trauma and nail fold and adjacent soft tissue deformities such as nail fold hypertrophy, onychomycosis, onychocryptosis, and xerosis. The first and the fifth toes are commonly affected.

Treatment: Onychophosis can be prevented by the use of appropriate footwear to minimize pressure effects. It is treated by debridement of the hyperkeratotic tissue by means of keratolytics (urea 20%, lactic acid 12%, or salicylic acid 6%–20%), followed by application of emollients, thinning of the nail plate, packing of the nail and, if necessary, surgery to remove the hyperkeratotic tissue.

Onychoclavus (subungual heloma/corn)

Repeated minor trauma may produce a subungual corn (heloma or onychoclavus) of the distal nail bed. It is a hyperkeratotic process in the nail area, mostly under the distal nail margins, due to a bony deformity or abnormal foot function. The corn typically affects the great toe and appears as a painful dark spot under the nail, resembling a foreign body. A circumscribed area of intense pain corresponding to the location of the corn can be elicited by applying pressure with a probe. In addition, the onychoclavus may cause the overlying nail plate to be elevated or split.

It should also be differentiated from subungual melanoma, subungual exostosis, and an epidermoid cyst. Subungual exostosis will not yield to pressure and an X-ray helps to confirm diagnosis.

Treatment: It can be enucleated by removing the corresponding section of the nail plate with excision of the hyperkeratotic tissue. Any bony abnormality should be corrected and modified footwear, protective pads, or tube foam should be used to prevent recurrence.

Subungual exostosis[12]

A subungual exostosis is a benign, tender, bony proliferation that most commonly occurs on the great toe and is associated with onychodystrophy of the corresponding nail plate. In older persons, it may be associated with an overlying onychoclavus. Subungual exostosis is of two types: genetic (type 1) or acquired (type II). The acquired lesions typically present during the fourth through sixth decades of life. In older patients, the pathogenesis of acquired subungual exostosis is probably related to faulty pedal biomechanics. The exostosis usually produces hypertrophy of the entire nail bed such that the appearance of the nail is an "inverted U" with incurvation of the medial and lateral aspects of the nail plate. Another feature seen during cutaneous examination of the digit with an acquired subungual exostosis is accentuation of the dorsal interphalangeal joint skin crease. Although inflammation of the nail folds is typically absent in acquired subungual exostosis, the patients often have chronic onychocryptosis and pincer nail. Radiographic findings reveal a blunted or sharp protuberance on the distal dorsal and central ungual tuberosity.

Treatment: The treatment involves removal of the excess bone aseptically. Initially the nail plate is avulsed and the exostosis is exposed via a longitudinal incision of the overlying nail bed. The lesion is then separated from the underlying bone with a bone rongeur, chisel, or mastoid curette, the rough edges are curetted flush with the surrounding bone, and the nail bed is sutured.

INGROWN TOENAILS (ONYCHOCRYPTOSIS)

Ingrowing toenails cause pressure on the periungual area and can be debilitating in elderly patients. This condition results when part of the nail plate presses the lateral nail fold. Thick nails and difficulty in bending result in improper cutting of nails, which along with improper fitting footwear are major predisposing factors for ingrown nails in elderly. Other etiologic factors include abnormally long toes, hereditary conditions (congenital excessive convexity of the nail plate and congenital malalignment of the great toenail), hyperhidrosis, imbalance between the width of the nail plate and that of the nail bed, pointed-toed or high-heeled shoes, poor foot hygiene, and prominence of the nail folds. Typically, onychocryptosis is characterized by inflammation with or

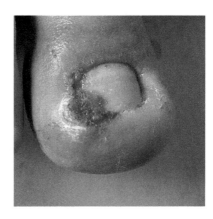

Figure 25.14 Onychocryptosis with granulation tissue.

without accompanying granulation tissue, tenderness at rest, and pain on ambulation or with pressure to the digit (Figure 25.14). In the elderly patient with decreased sensation of their feet or toes secondary to an underlying systemic disease such as diabetes mellitus, peripheral vascular disease, or arteriosclerosis, onychocryptosis can be a devastating problem with significant morbidity. These persons are often unaware that a problem exists because their neuropathy results in minimal pain. Consequently, they often do not come for treatment until more serious complications such as deep infection, osteomyelitis, or gangrene have occurred.[7]

Treatment: Treatment has to be individualized taking into consideration the age, associated systemic diseases, and degree of morbidity. Prophylactic care includes correcting predisposing factors and proper nail trimming so that the corners of the nail plate are beyond the distal edge of the lateral nail folds; this is performed by cutting the distal nail plate straight across. Conservative measures include placing a small wisp of cotton beneath the edge of the nail plate. Elevation of the lateral border of the nail results; subsequently, as the nail grows out, the lateral edge does not penetrate into the soft tissue of the lateral nail fold. Secondary bacterial and fungal infections should be treated appropriately. If onychocryptosis is more severe then surgical approach may be required. Surgical measures include partial or complete nail avulsion with matrix ablation.

PINCER NAIL

Pincer nail refers to the over-curvature of the nail resulting in pinching the nail bed. It may affect only the great toe or all toes and cause distress to the patient due to pain. The nail thickens and turns inwards, pinching the nail bed and causing difficulty to cut it. There may be associated bone pathology like exostosis and hyperostosis (Figure 25.15a and b).

Treatment: Various nail braces with series of adjustments are available to maintain constant tension on the nail plate and correct the inward distortion. If the underlying bone pathology remains untreated, relapse is usual. Therefore, the permanent phenol removal of the lateral matrix horn is considered to be the simplest, least painful, but effective treatment modality. In recalcitrant cases, total nail avulsion may be required.

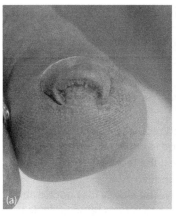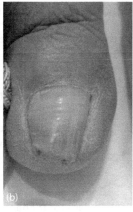

Figure 25.15 (a) Pincer nail—nail incurves pinching the soft tissue and (b) dorsal view of pincer nail.

TUMORS OF NAIL UNIT

Benign: Myxoid pseudocysts (mucous cysts or periungual ganglion) are probably the most common benign tumors. They are more common in females and usually involve the proximal nail fold of fingers. These are asymptomatic, soft to firm, cystic/fluctuant, sometimes causing transverse nail depressions. They can be treated with intralesional injections of triamcinolone or surgical removal.

Malignant: As many chronic diseases occur in the periungual region, a high degree of suspicion is required to detect malignancies early.

- Carcinoma of the nail apparatus is not rare; more than 150 cases have been reported, with a peak incidence in the seventh decade.
- Subungual melanoma, mostly affecting the great toe, is common in the elderly white population.
- Bowen's disease and squamous cell carcinoma, are also more frequent in this age group.[3]

INFECTIONS AND INFESTATIONS

The nail apparatus may get primarily infected or involved in infections of the adjacent structures.

Onychomycosis

The various nail dystrophies in the elderly predispose the nail to fungal infections. The prevalence of onychomycosis increases with age, reaching nearly 20% in patients over 60 years. In the study of Rao et al., onychomycosis was seen in 16%, followed by chronic paronychia in 9%. The most common change in onychomycosis was loss of lustre, subungual hyperkeratosis, onycholysis, brittleness, and color change with blackish-brownish or yellowish discoloration. The great toenail is the most common one involved. Distal subungual onychomycosis (DSO) (Figure 25.16) is the most common presentation.

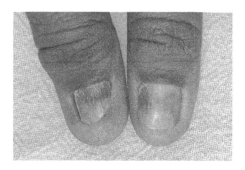

Figure 25.16 Distal and lateral onychomycosis.

Non-dermatophyte molds, such as *Scopulariopsis brevicaulis*, *Hendersonula toruloidea*, and *Scytalidium hyalinum*, are found more frequently in the elderly.[7]

Treatment: In view of the prolonged duration of therapy and multiple drug interactions in the elderly, antifungal therapy has to be carefully chosen. Nail avulsion can be employed for severe disease.

Paronychia

Paronychia is infection of the nail fold; it may be acute or chronic. Acute paronychia is usually bacterial and caused by *Staphylococcus aureus* or *Pseudomonas* species (Figure 25.17).

Treatment is similar to that of other bacterial infections of the skin and involves draining of the abscess, warm saline soaks, systemic antibiotics, and topical antibiotics such as 2% mupirocin ointment.

Chronic paronychia, caused by *candida* species or Gram-negative bacteria (*Proteus* sp. or *Klebsiella* sp.), appears as red, swollen, boggy, tender nail folds with loss of cuticle and a patent proximal nail groove. Common nail plate changes due to paronychia are transverse furrows, loss of luster, and thickening[13] (Figure 25.18).

Treatment is prolonged and includes keeping the nail olds and the surrounding skin dry, application of a topical antifungal, and excision of the chronic hypertrophic proximal nail fold in resistant cases. In cases with severe inflammation, topical or intra-lesional steroids can be used.[8]

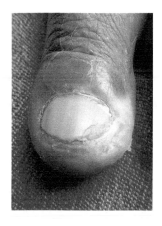

Figure 25.17 Acute paronychia.

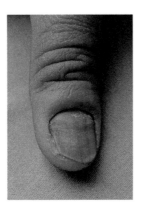

Figure 25.18 Chronic paronychia.

Scabies

Subungual hyperkeratosis is a niche for scabies mites, especially in Norwegian scabies. Failure to treat the subungual hyperkeratosis leads to persistent infestations or epidemics. The nails should be cut short and fingertips should be brushed with a scabicide in affected patients.

Warts

Periungual warts are due to infection with human papillomavirus.

FINGERNAIL VS TOENAIL CHANGES[1]

Domyati et al. documented nail changes to affect the fingernails more than toenails (Table 25.2).

ASSOCIATED SYSTEMIC ABNORMALITIES

In the elderly group, systemic diseases such as anemia, ischemic heart disease, diabetes mellitus, hypertension, renal disorders, chronic liver disease, and cardiopulmonary diseases are more prevalent and may give rise to various nail changes such as koilonychia, brittleness, paronychia, onychomycosis, half-and-half nails, and clubbing.

Table 25.2 Fingernail versus toenail changes in elderly

Fingernail changes	Toenail changes
Nail pitting	Green nails
Onychomadesis	Anonychia
Half-and-half nails	Pyogenic granuloma
Yellow nails	Pincer toe
Splinter hemorrhage	Onychocryptosis
Subungual warts	Onychoclavus
	Onychogryphosis

RECOMMENDED NAIL CARE REGIMEN

Recommended nail care practices have been summarized in Box 25.1

BOX 25.1: Nail care for the elderly

- Nails to be inspected regularly. Check for excessive thickness, change in color, hemorrhages.
- Use mild soap to wash the feet and dry thoroughly.
- Wear proper-fitting shoes.
- Trim toenails regularly. The elderly may not be able to care for toenails due to various reasons like failing eyesight and arthritis causing reduced flexibility; they should be encouraged to take help of a family member (trained by dermatologist) or to contact a podiatrist.
- Soaking feet in warm water helps to soften nails before trimming, or nails can be cut after bath.
- Nails to be trimmed straight to avoid further injury of ingrowing.

CONCLUSION

Prevalence of nail changes is high among the elderly population. Sometimes these may be overlooked due to the other more severe comorbidity. The cosmetic aspect of the nails is significant even in the elderly, as it may affect social as well as intra-family interactions. Dermatologists should be aware of the various nail changes related to aging and those associated with other dermatoses or systemic diseases to avoid inappropriate prescriptions.

KEY POINTS

- Age-associated characteristic changes occur in composition, growth rate, color, vasculature, contour, thickness, surface, and histology.
- Histopathologic and microbiological examination helps to enhance the accuracy of diagnosis and prevent inadvertent prescription of antifungals.
- Associated secondary factors that contribute to nail pathologies, including improper footwear, faulty biomechanics, bony anomalies, or infections, should be dealt with accordingly.

REFERENCES

1. El-Domyati M, Abdel-Wahab H, Abdel-Azim E. Nail changes and disorders in elderly Egyptians. *J Cosmet Dermatol* 2014;13(4):269–276.
2. Ohgitani S, Fujita T, Fujii Y et al. Nail calcium and magnesium content in relation to age and bone mineral density. *J Bone Miner Metab* 2005;23:318–322.

3. Baran R, Dawber RP. The nail in childhood and old age. In: Baran R, Dawber RPR, editors. *Diseases of the Nails and Their Management*, 2nd ed. Oxford, UK: Blackwell Science; 1994. pp. 81–96.

4. Lewis BL, Montgomery H. The senile nail. *J Invest Dermatol* 1955;24:11–18.

5. Horan MA, Puxly JA, Fox RA. The white nails of old age (Neapolitan nails). *J Am Ger Soc* 1982;30:734–737.

6. Paslin DA, Heaton CL. Acral arteriolar ectasia. *Arch Dermatol* 1972;106:906–908.

7. Singh G, Haneef NS, Uday A. Nail changes and disorders among the elderly. *Indian J Dermatol Venereol Leprol* 2005;71(6):386–392.

8. Cohen PR, Scher RK. Geriatric nail disorders: Diagnosis and treatment. *J Am Acad Dermatol* 1992;26:521–531.

9. Mumoli N. Ram's horn nails. *Med J Aust* 2011;195(4):202.

10. Cohen PR, Scher RK. Aging. In: Hordinsky MK, Sawaya ME, Scher RK, editors. *Atlas of Hair and Nails*. Philadelphia, PA: Churchill Livingstone; 2000. pp. 213–225.

11. Lynch MH, O'Guin WM, Hardy C et al. Acidic and basic hair/nail ('hard') keratins: Their colocalization in the upper cortical and cuticle cells of the human hair follicle and their relationship to 'soft' keratins. *J Cell Biol* 1986;103:2593–2606.

12. Salasche SJ, Garland LD. Tumors of the nail. *Dermatol Clin* 1985;3:521–530.

13. Rao S, Banerjee S, Ghosh SK et al. Nail changes and nail disorders in the elderly. *Indian J Dermatol* 2011;56:603–606.

PART 8

Nail Unit Tumors

Benign tumors

ECKART HANEKE

The tip of the digit including its dorsally located nail unit can give rise to many different tumors. Most nail tumors are relatively rare and may also occur on other sites of the body, but some are specific to the nail.[1,2]

Tumors are of epithelial, fibroepithelial, fibrous and other mesenchymal, vascular, neurogenic, lymphatic, and melanocytic origin. Also, a variety of reactive and degenerative conditions (pseudotumors) may present in a similar manner (Figure 26.1). The clinical diagnosis is often challenging as the macroscopic appearance of these tumors is often non-specific and is modified by the specific anatomy of the nail apparatus, rendering histopathology the gold standard of diagnosis. In addition, secondary alterations due to trauma or infection may change the clinical appearance and, hence, a thorough personal history of the patient along with histopathology of the lesion is key to the diagnosis.

A tumor may have a site-dependent effect on nail growth and appearance. Swelling of the nail bed lifts the nail plate and is often associated with subungual hyperkeratosis. Pseudoclubbing may result from a tumor of the matrix. A circumscribed neoplasm in the proximal nail fold causes a longitudinal groove in the nail plate due to pressure on the matrix. Matrix damage may cause surface alterations, a split, or a pterygium. Slow-growing benign tumors usually cause nail deformation whereas malignant neoplasms may result in nail destruction.

An important potential source of error is pigmentation of a tumor that is usually not pigmented. Although the skin type of the patient is obvious when the patient consults the dermatologist it may not be known by the pathologist. A peroxidase reaction can be performed by the clinician and can distinguish blood from melanin pigmentation; however, any bleeding tumor including melanomas are positive with the benzidine reaction.[2–4]

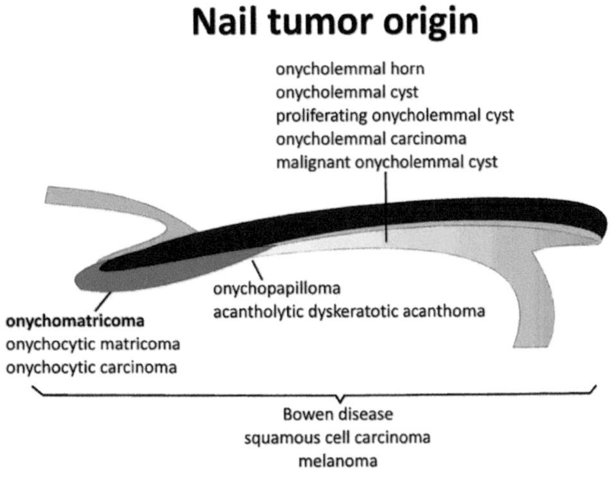

The subungual space can be occupied by benign solid tumors, benign cystic lesions (epidermal and mucoid cysts), swellings, and malignant tumors (squamous cell carcinoma [SCC], malignant melanoma, metastases). Modern imaging techniques are important for the detection, exact localization, and differentiation of subungual tumors. High-resolution ultrasonography (US) and color-coded Doppler give information on tumor size, location, shape, and internal characteristics (cystic, solid, or mixed, vascular flow). Magnetic resonance (MR) imaging allows tumors to be differentiated according to their anatomic location, pathologic origin, and signal characteristics. Although there is some overlap between US and MR, their combination often permits a better diagnosis and management, particularly when correlated with clinical and pathologic findings.[5]

NAIL-SPECIFIC TUMORS

Benign nail-specific tumors are divided into matrix- and nail bed-derived neoplasms. They are mostly epithelial or rarely fibroepithelial.

Matrix-derived tumors

ONYCHOCYTIC MATRICOMA

Onychocytic matricoma is an acanthoma of the matrix epithelium. It was first described under the term of subungual linear keratotic melanonychia,[6] then as subungual seborrheic keratosis.[7] As the latter is associated with hair follicles and this does not exist in the nail unit, the term onychocytic matricoma was coined.[8]

Clinically, a longitudinal pale to yellowish to brownish subungual keratotic lesion is seen emerging from under the proximal nail fold and extending to the free margin of the nail plate. End-on dermatoscopy usually shows a slight thickening of the nail as the lesion is confluent with the plate (Figure 26.2). Histologically, an acanthoma-like thickening of the matrix epithelium is seen mainly made up of basaloid cells. The architecture is regular with some nail keratin inclusions. Mitoses, cellular atypias, or dyskeratoses are lacking. Pigmentation varies from almost absent to very pronounced[9] (Figure 26.3).

The main clinical differential diagnoses are onychopapilloma and Bowen's disease.[10]

Nail tumor origin

Figure 26.1 Origin of nail-specific tumors.

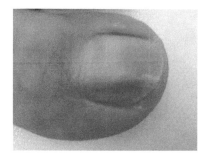

Figure 26.2 Clinical aspect of onychocytic matricoma. There is a light brown longitudinal streak in the nail; end-on dermatoscopy reveals a circumscribed slight thickening of the nail.

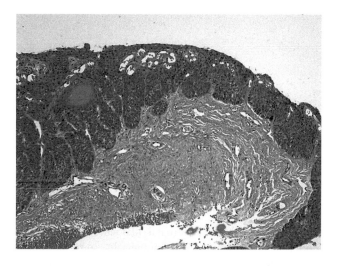

Figure 26.3 Histopathology of onychocytic matricoma shows a pigmented acanthoma made up of mainly basaloid and suprabasaloid cells and a "squamous eddy" formed by a pearl of nail keratin.

ONYCHOPAPILLOMA

Onychopapilloma was described in 2000 as a longitudinal erythronychia with distal subungual keratosis.[11] Although first disputed as an entity,[12] onychopapilloma is now generally accepted.[13,14] It is fairly common and most cases occur on fingers. The most common clinical presentation is a longitudinal whitish, yellowish, reddish, or sometimes light brown streak in the nail originating in the distal matrix as a pink band with a cuneiform distal end.[15,16] It is usually 3 to 4 mm wide not exceeding 5 to 6 mm. Splinter hemorrhages are frequently seen. At the undersurface of the free nail margin, a narrow keratotic rim and a circumscribed thinning of the nail plate are observed that render the nail liable to split. A wedge-shaped distal onycholysis may be associated. The nail fissure and onycholysis may be embarrassing (Figure 26.4a and b). The treatment of choice is horizontal excision after partial nail detachment, which leads to normal nail growth without recurrence. Simple nail avulsion leads to nail regrowth with the same appearance of the onychopapilloma.

Histopathologically, a circumscribed acanthosis of the matrix epithelium with finger-like rete ridges spreading slightly outward like a fan is observed in its most proximal level. Along the nail bed, multinucleated cells are present (Figure 26.5). The overlying nail plate exhibits a slight but well-circumscribed indentation, which remains visible all along the nail plate until its free margin. At the level of the hyponychium, the hyperkeratosis is compact to verruciform but still adheres to the nail plate (Figures 26.6 and 26.7). Splinter hemorrhages appear as small lakes of blood at the border between the epithelium and the keratosis or in the hyperkeratosis. When the lesion was removed tangentially after partial nail avulsion, only the epithelial portion is commonly seen. Pigmentation is usually mild but may mimic longitudinal melanonychia.[17]

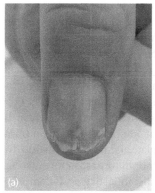
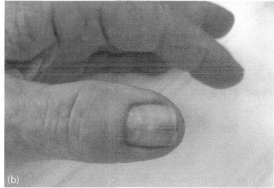

Figure 26.4 (a) Clinical aspect of an onychopapilloma with distal nail plate defect; (b) A case of onychopapilloma with pink longitudinal band and wedge-shaped onycholysis and longitudinal split.

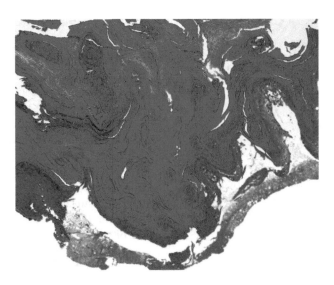

Figure 26.5 Onychopapilloma at the level of the distal nail bed demonstrating a thick thread of whorled keratin.

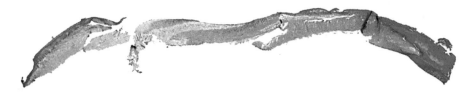

Figure 26.6 Histopathology of an onychopapilloma. This is a longitudinal section of a tangentially excised onychopapilloma (matrix left, hyponychium right).

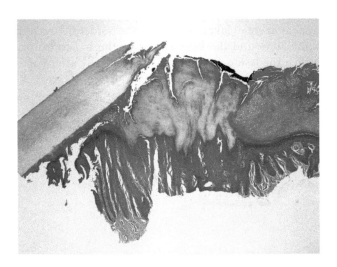

Figure 26.7 Histopathology of an onychopapilloma. This transverse section is made at the level of the distal matrix.

The differential diagnosis comprises onychocytic matricoma, subungual acantholytic dyskeratotic acanthoma (SADA), warty dyskeratoma, subungual filamentous tumor, and Bowen's disease.[13,18]

SUBUNGUAL FILAMENTOUS TUMOR

Described in 1972,[19] subungual filamentous tumor is an underdiagnosed lesion now thought by some authors to be a narrow onychopapilloma. However, these two lesions are sufficiently different both on clinical as well as histological grounds to consider them to be entities of their own. Subungual filamentous tumor is seen as a 1- to 1.5-mm-wide streak in the nail. It runs from the distal matrix to the free end of the nail plate. Its color is whitish to yellowish, rarely light brown or reddish. At the undersurface of the free nail margin, a small keratotic rim is seen that can be easily and painlessly pared off. Growth is apparently slow and the onset and duration of the lesion are usually not remembered. A small V-shaped notch may be seen in the nail margin being the reason to consult the dermatologist. Cautious nail plate avulsion reveals a very narrow rim all along the undersurface of the nail that causes a slight longitudinal depression in the nail bed. Its origin in the matrix is can be visualized with a head magnifier lens. Histology reveals a rim of keratin with a somewhat whorled structure on transverse sections through the nail plate and no pigmentation. In the distal matrix a tiny hood-like or filiform structure is seen (Figures 26.8 and 26.9).

The differential diagnosis comprises onychopapilloma and other longitudinal keratotic structures. Both dyskeratosis follicularis of Darier and benign familial pemphigus of Hailey–Hailey can also cause longitudinal keratotic striations.

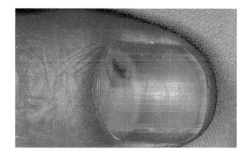

Figure 26.8 Subungual filamentous tumor causing a fine longitudinal white line in the nail. This patient came for consultation after he had hit his thumb with a hammer several weeks prior and the dark pigmentation due to hematoma had not yet disappeared. The fine white line on top of the figure represents the subungual filamentous tumor.

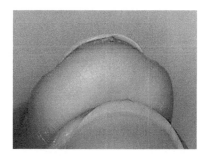

Figure 26.9 Subungual filamentous tumor. End-on view shows a small thread-like subungual keratin bud.

SUBUNGUAL ACANTHOLYTIC DYSKERATOTIC ACANTHOMA

Three cases of SADA were recently described in subungual location. All were clinically diagnosed as onychopapillomas. The time of evolution was about 6 to 9 months. They were 3 to 5 mm in width, yellowish over the nail bed, and reddish over the matrix. One case presented with splinter hemorrhages.[20] The histopathological changes involve the distal matrix, nail bed, hyponychium, and digital pulp. The epithelium is acanthotic with pronounced subungual parakeratotic and dyskeratotic-acantholytic hyperkeratosis that lifted the nail plate up (Figures 26.10 and 26.11).

The main clinical differential diagnosis is onychopapilloma; in fact, they cannot be distinguished clinically. Subungual warty dyskeratoma is extremely rare[21,22]; its origin is in the nail bed as opposed to that of SADA and onychopapilloma, which is in the distal matrix.

ONYCHOMATRICOMA

Onychomatricoma is a fairly common but underdiagnosed benign tumor of the nail matrix.[23] Since its first description, probably more than 200 cases have been described.[24–27] Men and women are equally affected, and most patients are middle-aged Caucasians. Fingers are twice as frequently involved as toes.[28] It is a slowly growing, painless tumor exhibiting a

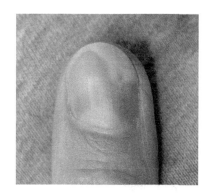

Figure 26.10 Subungual acantholytic dyskeratotic acanthoma. The clinical aspect is indistinguishable from an onychopapilloma.

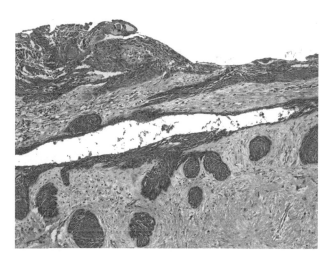

Figure 26.11 Histopathology of acantholytic dyskeratotic acanthoma demonstrating long obliquely running epithelial formations with an acantholytic split formation as well as small round epithelial buds in the nail bed dermis.

funnel-shaped, yellow streaky, thickened nail with transverse overcurvature and splinter hemorrhages in its proximal portion. Usually, only a segment of the nail is involved, but also the entire matrix may be affected (Figure 26.12a–c). End-on view exhibits tiny holes (woodworm like holes) in the nail plate (Figure 26.12d). On cutting such a nail, it may bleed from such a hole[29] as the long filiform projections of the tumor may extend to the free margin of the nail and dilated capillaries may remain patent. The filiform projections of the tumor can be visualized with the naked eye, giving an appearance of a "sea anemone" (Figure 26.12e). Pigmented and mucinous onychomatricomas, a pterygium-like appearance, and nail fold swelling have been described.[30,31] A cutaneous horn is an exceptional presentation.[27] A polypoid variant was also reported.[32] Onychomycosis is not rare in onychomatricoma. MR imaging shows the characteristic channels in the nail plate.[26] The bone is not involved. Ultrasound may help to make the correct diagnosis.[33]

Histopathology of onychomatricoma has distinctive features allowing the diagnosis to be made both from the nail plate as well as the tumor itself. It is a benign fibro-epithelial neoplasm. Its stroma consists of densely packed, but mainly

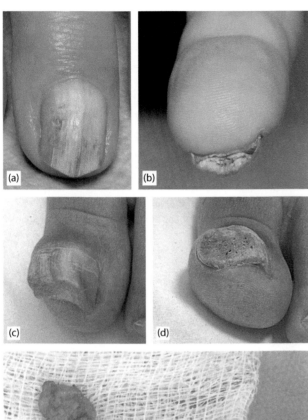

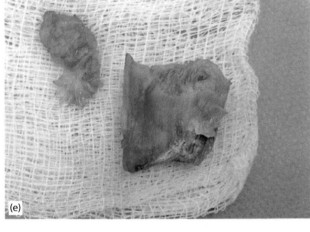

Figure 26.12 Onychomatricoma of the middle finger demonstrating a yellow discoloration and thickening of the nail with longitudinal striation. **(a)** Dorsal View; **(b)** End-on (frontal) view; **(c)** Onychomatricoma of great toes showing yellowish discoloration and thickening of the nail; **(d)** End-on (frontal view) shows tiny holes, resembling woodworm holes; **(e)** Nail avulsion shows a filiform tumor with multiple filamentlike digitations (resembling a sea anemone).

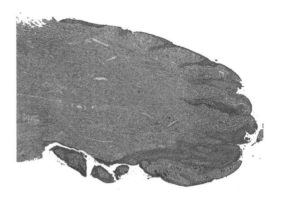

Figure 26.13 Histopathology of the tumor mass of an onychomatricoma showing a protuberant lesion with dense cellular stroma covered by normal matrix epithelium with deep indentations and splits.

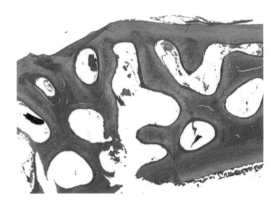

Figure 26.14 Transverse section of the nail of the same onychomatricoma showing the holes lined by the superficial compartment of matrix epithelium.

fine, wavy collagen fibers and many fibroblasts with a relatively well-pronounced cytoplasm in its more superficial portion. The deeper part of the stroma has coarse collagen fibers. The stroma is characteristically positive for both CD10 and CD34.[34] The epithelial component is identical to normal matrix epithelium and apparently produces nail substance at a normal rate.[24] The peculiarity of this tumor is its unique architecture. It forms long slender filiform digitations both outwards as well as into the connective tissue stroma. This leads to a tremendous increase in matrix epithelium surface, which is the reason for the circumscribed nail thickening.[24] In sections containing both the tumor together with its nail, the filiform projections are seen to extend into the nail substance and to form channels in the nail plate. The nail plate reveals characteristic changes.[35] On transverse cuts, round to oval holes are seen in the nail plate, which particularly in the more proximal portion of the nail plate are lined by the superficial compartment of the matrix epithelium (Figures 26.13 and 26.14). This epithelial lining is seen to gradually degenerate toward the distal margin of the nail.

Several variants such as onychoblastoma,[36,37] unguioblastic fibroma and unguioblastoma,[38,39] have been described, the independence of which remain, however, disputed.[40] They are most probably just variants of onychomatricoma with variable amounts of connective tissue stroma or epithelial component.

MATRIX CYSTS

Matrix cysts are usually due to a surgical intervention in the matrix region. Clinically, they appear as an asymptomatic swelling on one side of the proximal nail fold, often after previous surgery for an ingrown nail. They are indistinguishable

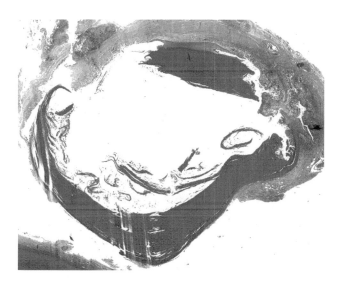

Figure 26.15 Postoperative matrix cyst; the cyst wall consists of matrix epithelium and epidermis.

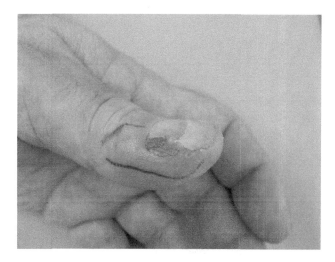

Figure 26.16 Onycholemmal horn in the lateral side of the nail bed of the thumb. The clinical diagnosis was squamous cell carcinoma and the lesion was excised with an adequate safety margin (excision margins marked preoperatively).

from epidermal inclusion cysts. Histopathology shows a cyst lining that at least in part consists of matrix and may show true nail formation within its lumen. In addition, there may also be a structure similar to nail bed, to which the intracystic nail is attached (Figure 26.15). All other cysts, particularly epidermal cysts, have to be considered in the clinical and histopathologic differential diagnosis.

Specific tumors of the nail bed

In analogy to the nomenclature of follicular tumors, nail bed-specific tumors are commonly referred to as onycholemmal.

ONYCHOLEMMAL HORN

This is the first nail-specific tumor described.[1] It is a rare slow-growing asymptomatic lesion originating from the nail bed, mostly its lateral part. It clinically resembles a wart or another hyperkeratotic tumor including keratoacanthoma (KA) and SCC.[1] The term "onycholemmal horn" was coined as it architecturally and cytologically closely resembles a trichilemmal horn.[41] The nail bed is analogous to the outer root sheath of the hair follicle in its way of keratinization[42] (Figure 26.16).

Histopathology shows a markedly hyperkeratotic and acanthotic lesion. The epithelium resembles that of a trichilemmal horn with large, pale cells becoming larger toward the surface and keratinizing abruptly, usually without forming a granular layer although this may in part be present. The basal layer consists of one or two rows of small cuboid cells. Mitoses and cell atypias are lacking (Figure 26.17).[1] Differential diagnoses include common wart, KA, and SCC.

PROLIFERATING ONYCHOLEMMAL TUMOR

Proliferating onycholemmal tumor is a very rare lesion deriving from the nail bed. It grows slowly without causing

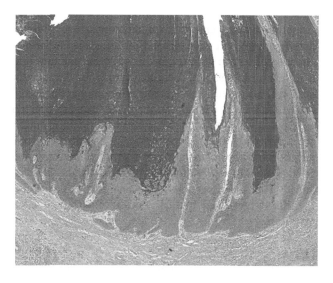

Figure 26.17 Histopathology of the onycholemmal horn showing an endo-exophytic tumor with massive horn production and cells that enlarge from the basal to the superficial layers to keratinize abruptly.

symptoms. Clinically it resembles a wart, onycholemmal horn, Bowen's disease, KA, or SCC.

Histopathologically, proliferating onycholemmal tumor presents as an exophytic lesion with striking resemblance with a proliferating trichilemmal tumor. It is a solid growth with small and regularly arranged basal cells with round basophilic nuclei. The cells gradually enlarge and become paler until they abruptly keratinize. There are no mitoses and cellular atypias. The border to the neighboring epidermal and nail bed keratinocytes is clearly discernable. As the lesion originates from the nail bed the nail plate itself is not involved (Figure 26.18).

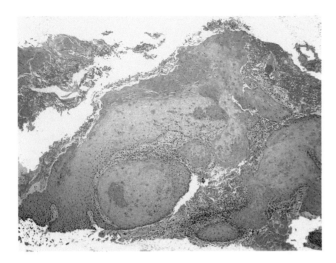

Figure 26.18 Histopathology of a proliferating onycho-lemmal tumor shows a close resemblance to proliferating trichilemmal cyst with small basal cells and large suprabasal cells with marked premature keratinization.

SUBUNGUAL VERRUCOUS PROLIFERATIONS OF INCONTINENTIA PIGMENTI

Incontinentia pigmenti of Bloch–Sulzberger is an X-linked dominant multi-organ syndrome; it is usually lethal for male offspring. The skin lesions show three stages: the first stage is seen at birth or shortly thereafter as multilocular intraepidermal blisters with characteristic eosinophilia, the second stage is verrucous with almost identical changes as seen in young women with subungual lesions, and the third stage is characterized by linear hyperpigmentations that with time may become hypopigmented and are sometimes referred to as stage 4. Skin lesions are distributed along the Blaschko lines.[43] The underlying molecular defect is a mutation of the *NEMO* gene required for nuclear factor κB (NFκB) activation.

The nails are affected between the ages of 15 to 35 years (3 to 45 years[44]) and may be the sole manifestation.[45] Fingers are mostly involved.[46] The tumors are usually painful warty or tumorous lesions elevating the nail from its bed.[47] Matrix involvement leads to nail destruction. Bone erosion may be responsible for the pain. Spontaneous resolution followed by recurrence was observed in a patient during her two pregnancies. Many cases have finally resolved, but retinoids appear to be the treatment of choice.[48] Histopathology is very similar to proliferating onycholemmal tumor although this is painless and grows very slowly.

Differential diagnosis comprises of KA (which is also characterized by pain and often shows many single dyskeratoses), warts, acantholytic dyskeratotic acanthoma, subungual epidermoid inclusions, subungual fibroma, Bowen's disease, and SCC.

ONYCHOLEMMAL CYSTS (SUBUNGUAL EPIDERMOID INCLUSIONS)

Subungual epidermoid inclusions are a frequent incidental finding in nail biopsies commonly without clinical

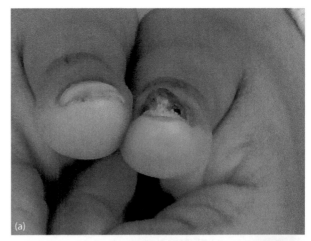

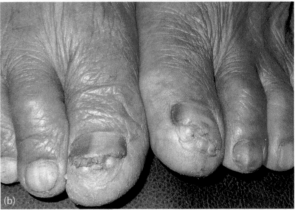

Figure 26.19 (a) Overcurvature of the left thumb nail with underlying multiple onycholemmal cysts; (b) Bilateral subungual inclusion cysts lifting the nail plates up. (From Kumar, P. et al., *Indian J. Dermatol. Venereol. Leprol.*, 83, 472–473, 2017. IADVL, Medknow Publications [Wolters Kluwer Health].)

significance. They do not cause signs or symptoms; in some cases, they led to subungual hyperkeratosis or were observed in association with finger clubbing.[49] They probably derive from epidermal buds of the rete ridges as is often seen in onychopapillomas.[2] Whether trauma is etiologically important is not clear (Figure 26.19a and b).

Histopathologically, multiple onycholemmal cysts are mainly found in the nail bed. They are small round-to-oval epithelial structures resembling minute epidermal cysts. In contrast to these, they do not grow bigger than approximately a millimeter in diameter. There is an elongation of the rete ridges with pinching off of the lower parts thus giving rise to free-lying cysts in the nail bed dermis. Another variant with marked subungual hyperkeratosis, hyperplasia of the nail bed, and short and dystrophic nails was also described, a traumatic origin was assumed[50] (Figure 26.20).

Differential diagnosis comprises all conditions with subungual hyperkeratosis, particularly nail psoriasis, eczema, and onychomycosis. Epidermoid inclusions were assumed to mimic miniature trichilemmal cysts.[57]

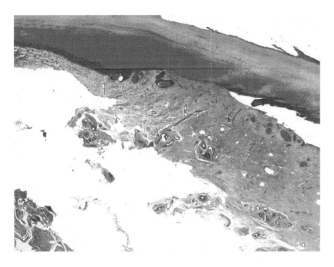

Figure 26.20 Histopathology of multiple onycholemmal cysts.

PROLIFERATING ONYCHOLEMMAL CYST

This is an exceedingly rare tumor of the nail bed with insidious symptomless growth. It resembles a wart, Bowen's disease, or SCC; its very slow progression and absence of pain distinguishes it from KA. Histopathology shows a lesion morphologically very similar to proliferating trichilemmal cyst, hence its designation. It appears solid and mainly exophytic, though many small and medium-sized cyst-like formations are seen. The peripheral cells are relatively small with dense nuclei. Towards the center of the neoplasm, the cells increase in size to finally keratinize abruptly without a granular layer (Figure 26.21).

Onycholemmal horn and proliferating onycholemmal tumor have to be differentiated. Careful evaluation of the different criteria will allow onycholemmal horn to be distinguished.[1] Malignant onycholemmal cyst exhibits cellular atypias and pathological mitoses.

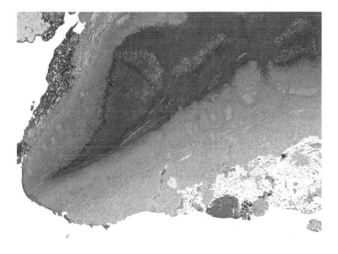

Figure 26.21 Proliferating onycholemmal cyst is similar to proliferating trichilemmal cyst with small regular basal cells and large, non-flattened superficial cells that may focally exhibit a granular layer as a sign of irritation.

CHARACTERISTIC EPITHELIAL TUMORS OF THE NAIL

Epidermal nevi

Although various types of epidermal nevi occur, involvement of the distal dorsal digit and the nail is only described in verrucous epidermal nevi. Most are present since birth, but they may also occur in later life. Depending on their localization in the nail apparatus, they may cause wart-like lesions on the proximal nail fold, ridging of the nail plate when its undersurface is affected, or nail splitting in case of matrix and/or nail bed involvement.[51] A clinically similar condition was observed in a little girl with a porokeratotic eccrine duct and hair follicle naevus.[52] The histology shows marked epidermal papillomatosis with hyperorthokeratosis, but acanthosis is usually not very pronounced.

Epidermal cysts

Epidermal cysts of the nail unit are mainly due to a penetrating trauma, which is not always remembered by the patient. A heavy trauma may cause intraosseous implantation of squamous epithelium.[53] Postoperative epidermal cysts are found in the very vicinity of the scar.[54] Most epidermal cysts are slow-growing, symptomless lesions. Rapidly enlarging cysts may cause discomfort and pain and may lead to nail loss.[55] When localized under the matrix, transverse overcurvature or clubbing may develop. Radiograph may show indentation of the bone. Ultrasound is said to have a high sensitivity. Histopathology shows a cyst lined with a regular thin epidermis with a normal stratum granulosum. Cyst rupture may lead to partial disappearance of the epidermal lining with formation of a keratin granuloma.

All space-occupying lesions may clinically mimic an ungual epidermal cyst.

Subungual trichoadenoma

Trichoadenoma is a rare tumor that mainly develops in the face or on the buttocks, rarely on the neck, arm, or thigh. Only one case was reported describing a subungual trichoadenoma as a very tender, hyperkeratotic nodule under a fingernail without bone destruction or ossification in the distal phalanx.[56] It was mentioned that the origin of this "trichoadenoma" remains unclear as there are no hair follicles in the nail region; whether this can be seen as another hint at the developmental similarity between the hair and nail[1] or was just a case of multiple small subungual epidermoid inclusions in very distal location is not clear.

Histopathologically, numerous small keratin-filled cysts, longitudinal cystic structures, and solid tumor islands were scattered in the nail bed dermis. There was no continuity between the nail bed epithelium and the tumor.

Syringoma

Syringomas are small benign tumors arising from the excretory ducts of eccrine sweat glands. Their stroma is sclerotic. They are almost always multiple. Subungual hyperkeratosis and onycholysis was observed in the nail bed of the big toe of a middle-aged woman after trauma.[57] Histopathology showed the classical round-to-oval islands of mainly cuboid eosinophilic tumor cells that were either solid or showed small (duct) lumina filled with keratin. The differential diagnosis is mainly subungual epidermoid inclusions.

Chondroid syringoma

This tumor was previously also called cutaneous mixed tumor. It is a benign adnexal tumor composed of epithelial and connective tissue elements. There appears to be an analogy to mixed tumors of the salivary glands although they do not tend to recur after local excision. A 25-year-old black woman was described with a deformed big toe and osteolytic changes in the distal phalanx. The diagnosis was made by histopathology after amputation of the big toe.[58]

Eccrine syringofibroadenoma and eccrine syringofibroadenomatosis

This rare benign tumor of eccrine ductal differentiation has a variable clinical appearance, but its histology is characteristic. Most commonly, lesion develops on acral skin of elderly persons and presents as solitary, sometimes verrucous nodule. Eccrine syringofibroadenomatosis is seen as large plaques with an irregular papillomatous or verrucous surface on the foot and may be a reactive lesion to chronic edema, chronic ulcers, burn scars, SCC, and even pincer nail.[59] It may involve the periungual skin, but solitary eccrine syringofibroadenoma of the nail is exceptional.[60] It may cause a whitish longitudinal band similar to onychopapilloma.[61] The histopathology is characteristic with long, slender anastomosing strands of mostly cuboid cells and abundant fibrovascular stroma.[62] Multiple narrow cords and strands of uniformly cuboid cells often forming a small lumen between their two cell rows extend from the epithelium into the dermis.

The clinical differential diagnosis of eccrine syringofibroadenoma comprises any potentially papular hyperkeratotic or verrucous lesion.

Eccrine poroma

This benign tumor derives from the upper eccrine sweat ducts. They are usually solitary neoplasms appearing as small dome-shaped nodules less than 10 mm in diameter. Nail bed involvement elevates the nail plate[55] or may look like a pyogenic granuloma,[63] whereas periungual localization led to an enlarged distal phalanx with destroyed nail.[64] One case each was observed on the nail fold[65] and one at the hyponychium mimicking an angiofibroma.[66] Histopathologically, eccrine poroma is a well-circumscribed basophilic tumor with cuboid basaloid cells and small regular nuclei. Poromas may be connected to the overlying epidermis or lie in the mid-to-deep dermis; the latter are often called dermal duct tumor. Clinically as well as histologically, seborrheic keratosis and basal cell carcinoma may be considered as differentials.

Eccrine angiomatous hamartoma

This lesion is also called angio-eccrine hamartoma. It is composed of mature eccrine sweat glands and a variable amount of mostly capillary vessels among and around the eccrine glands. It may appear as an induration, plaque, or nodule, single or multiple. Tenderness or pain, itching, hypertrichosis, and hyperhidrosis are common.[67] Nail involvement is rare[68] and may cause nail destruction.[69] Misdiagnosis led to unnecessary amputation.[70]

Histopathology demonstrates a deep dermal proliferation of normal sweat glands and small blood vessels, mostly capillaries. The stroma may be myxoid and/or lipomatous. Both the eccrine gland as well as the vascular component show normal immunohistochemical staining. A peculiar painful subungual lesion of the big toe was described consisting of a well-circumscribed proliferation of densely packed eccrine sweat glands, thick-walled arterial vessels, and thick myelinated nerves; it was termed neuro-arteriosyringeal hamartoma.[71]

Any painful ungual lesion has to be considered in the clinical differential diagnosis. Histologically, eccrine nevus on one side and a capillary malformation on the other side have to be ruled out. Sudoriparous angioma exhibits vessels of large-caliber and dilated eccrine sweat glands.[72] In contrast, congenital hemangioma of sweat glands is characterized by abundant wide capillary vessels with prominent endothelial cells located around the secretory portion of the sweat glands; this lesion slowly regresses spontaneously.[73] One case of mucinous eccrine nevus involving four toes including the periungual skin was described.[74]

Ungual keratoacanthoma (distal digital keratoacanthoma)

KA is a tumor of chronically sun-exposed hair-bearing skin of elderly persons. It is considered a variant of SCC by some authors. Its localization in the nail apparatus is rare, but not exceptional.[75,76] It grows rapidly and often aggressively, most commonly under the free edge of the nail, in the distal nail bed, or the lateral nail groove (Figure 26.22).[77] Localization in the proximal nail fold causes a paronychia-like chronic swelling.[78] Multiple subungual KAs are very rare.[79,80] One subungual KA was observed in a patient with Muir–Torre syndrome and a germline mutation in the *MSH* mismatch repair gene.[81]

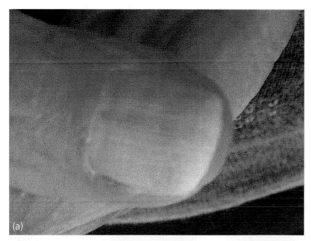

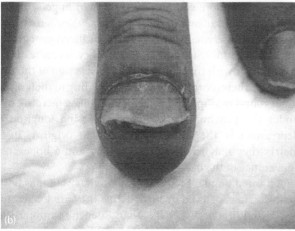

Figure 26.22 **(a)** and **(b)** Subungual keratoacanthoma is painful but otherwise non-specific in most cases.

Ungual KA is characteristically painful probably due to its rapid growth and frequent bone erosion.[119] Clinically, a keratotic nodule is commonly seen that may be tender on palpation. The central keratotic plug may be expressed from the tumor crater by lateral pressure. The treatment of choice is total excision as spontaneous involution of ungual KAs is rare. Mohs micrographic surgery may be indicated in case of recurrence.[82] Histopathology shows an endophytic growth in ungual KA with a growth direction that is more vertical or oblique in proximal-deep direction. A narrow central keratin plug is regularly seen extending deep into the dermis under the nail bed. Lip formation is pronounced though without an overhanging shoulder. The tumor cells are large and pale and some may contain keratohyalin granules. The blunt tumor downgrowths have an irregular lower border. The peripheral cells are basaloid. The rare mitoses are normal, an important differential diagnostic criterion between KA and SCC. A mixed inflammatory infiltrate with neutrophils and eosinophils is observed at the base of the tumor, sometimes even with abscess formation. Perineural invasion is rare in ungual KAs. Immunohistochemically, KAs stain with a cytokeratin cocktail. The proliferation markers p53 and Ki67 are positive with a regular distribution

from the basal cell layers gradually decreasing to the more superficial tumor cells.

Many attempts were made to reliably distinguish subungual KA from SCC.[83–85] KA patients are usually younger, the tumor grows faster, the duration of symptoms is shorter, bone invasion is more rapid and more common, and multiple KAs do occur though rarely. The clinical differential diagnosis comprises virtually all painful nail lesions plus SCC, onycholemmal horn, subungual tumors of incontinentia pigmenti, and hypertrophic lichen planus. Histologically, the classical architecture of KA with its relatively well-circumscribed oval shape, lateral lip formation, and central keratin plug are typical enough to make the correct diagnosis, provided the biopsy/excision specimen allows the entire architecture to be evaluated. Atypical mitoses and infiltration or single cell formations are seen in SCC. The proliferation index in KA is slightly higher than in hypertrophic lichen planus and penetrating elastic fibers are very rare in hypertrophic lichen planus as compared to KA.[86] Verrucous (hyperkeratotic) lupus erythematosus may be clinically similar to KA and SCC.[87] The differential diagnosis is particularly difficult when there is a sequence of wart–KA–verrucous carcinoma at the same site.[88] Immunohistochemistry has often been claimed to be of discriminative value, but the differences are usually only quantitative.

CHARACTERISTIC FIBROEPITHELIAL TUMORS OF THE NAIL

Viral warts

Verrucae vulgaris are the most frequent reactive tumors of the nail apparatus, both in children and adults. Their etiology is the common benign human papillomavirus (HPV) types 1, 2, 4, and 7, with the latter occurring in butchers. They are slowly growing, weakly contagious fibroepithelial lesions with a natural life-span of 2 to 5 years. Their clinical appearance depends on their localization within the nail apparatus. On the proximal nail fold, they are round (Figure 26.23a) and similar to other body sites, on the lateral nail folds they are more oval and fissured, and at the hyponychium they may appear as a slightly hyperkeratotic rim that swells and takes on a white color more rapidly than the surrounding skin after immersion in water. Subungual warts often raise the nail plate (Figure 26.23b and c). The most important differential diagnoses in adults are Bowen's disease and SCC, but verrucous melanoma, many infectious and benign lesions such as tuberculosis cutis verrucosa also called prosector's wart or butcher's nodule, onychopapilloma, onycholemmal horn,[1] subungual corn (heloma subunguale), subungual warty hyperkeratoses in incontinentia pigmenti, subungual vegetations in amyloidosis, inflammatory linear verrucous epidermal nevus, or lichen striatus may rarely present in a similar manner. Multicentric reticulohistiocytosis causes a rim of small verrucous nodules along the free margin of the proximal

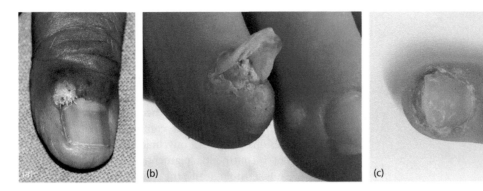

Figure 26.23 (a) Viral wart on proximal nail fold. (Courtesy of Piyush Kumar.) (b) Subungual wart lifting the nail plate. (c) Subungual and periungual viral warts.

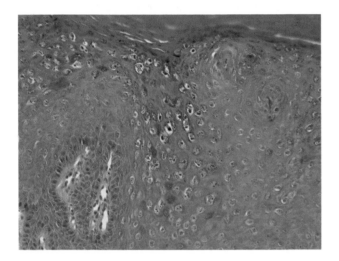

Figure 26.24 Histopathology of a subungual wart with many inclusion bodies.

nail fold. Onychophosis is a painful keratotic lesion in the lateral nail groove of the toenails. Mucinous eccrine metaplasia was seen to clinically appear like a subungual wart.[89] Vacuolization of keratinocytes, called pagetoid dyskeratosis, of the tip of the toe is a frequent chance observation without pathologic relevance and must be differentiated from a flat wart at the hyponychium.

Treatment of subungual and periungual warts is challenging. They frequently persist for longer than 2 to 5 years and may be a source of spread during this period.[3,90]

Histopathology is similar to warts elsewhere (Figure 26.24). Many patients tend to traumatize their ungual warts with resulting bleeding and inflammation. A lichenoid infiltrate is considered to be a sign of wart regression.

Fibrokeratoma

Two types of ungual fibrokeratoma (FK) exist: multiple FKs in tuberous sclerosis complex (TSC; Koenen tumors) and sporadic, mostly solitary FK. They are common tumors of the nail unit originating from the nail folds, matrix, nail bed, or hyponychium. Koenen's tumors occur in 50% of the patients with tuberous sclerosis from the age of 12 years

onwards, are more common on toes than fingers, and are more frequent in females than in males.[91] Koenen's tumors exhibit no difference between TSC1 localized on chromosome 9q34 and TSC2 on 16p13.3.[92] They increase in size and number with time and may be the sole sign of tuberous sclerosis. Their morphology varies according to their origin: small round multiple lesions, 1–5 mm long, emerging from under the proximal nail fold, and causing longitudinal depressions in the nail plate; when their origin is in the matrix they may cause nail thickening and a honeycomb appearance of the nail on plate avulsion.[93]

Acquired ungual FKs are usually solitary but may have a double, triple, or even quadruple tip. They are longer, narrower, and more sausage-like than Koenen's tumors. Their tip is either hyperkeratotic or black. FKs arising from the depth of the nail pocket cause a longitudinal depression (Figure 26.25). Those originating in the mid-matrix run intraungually until the overlying nail lamella breaks off showing the tip of a narrow FK and giving rise to a distal longitudinal depression (Figure 26.26). FKs arising in the nail bed cause a rim in the nail plate. All FKs are easily detachable from the overlying and underlying epithelium or nail plate; this easily distinguishes it from onychopapilloma. The etiology of acquired ungual FKs is not yet understood; trauma may play a role.[94,95] The differential diagnosis comprises viral warts and a supernumerary digit, particularly when located on one side of the distal phalanx. Bowen's diseases and SCC may mimic FK.[96,97] Other clinical differential diagnoses are keloids, other fibromas (Figure 26.27),

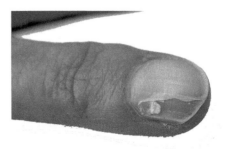

Figure 26.25 Ungual fibrokeratoma emerging from under the proximal nail fold.

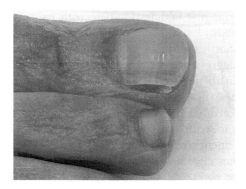

Figure 26.26 Intraungual fibrokeratoma in a young dark-skinned woman.

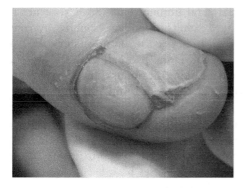

Figure 26.27 Fibroma of the lateral matrix and nail bed.

recurring digital fibromas of childhood, exostosis, pseudomalignant osseous soft tissue tumor, cutaneous horn, pyogenic granuloma, eccrine poroma, fibrosarcoma, and dermatofibrosarcoma protuberans.[98,99] Onychomatricoma has a peculiar cell-rich stroma.[100]

Histopathology shows a fibroma surrounded by thinned epidermis (Figure 26.28a). In some cases, overlying epidermis may be acanthotic (Figure 26.28b). The tip often contains clotted serum and blood explaining why it clinically looks black. Ossification, though rare, may be seen at the base.

BENIGN FIBROUS TUMORS

Although fibrous tumors are common on skin they are relatively rare in the nail apparatus. Clinical examination rarely allows a definite diagnosis to be made. Also, histologically, they may pose considerable diagnostic challenges.

Fibrous histiocytoma

Although common on the extremities, histiocytoma is very rare in the nail unit. Its localization within the nail apparatus determines its clinical appearance.[101] Histiocytoma may cause a circumscribed hard swelling in the nail fold. Histologically, it is an ill-defined dermal lesion of spindle shaped and round cells. Epidermal hyperplasia may be obvious, but hyperpigmentation is uncommon.[101]

Storiform collagenoma

This rare form of dermal fibromas is also called sclerotic fibroma or plywood fibroma. It occurs spontaneously[102] or in association with Cowden's syndrome[103,104] and is mainly observed in young and middle-aged adults. It grows slowly and does not exceed a diameter of 1 cm. It is rare in the nail.[105] It needs to be distinguished from other types of fibromas, particularly old sclerotic histiocytoma.

Keloids

Keloids have been observed in the nail region with sometimes extreme size. They are elevated scars (Figure 26.29) extending beyond the confines of the original trauma or wound, grow insidiously, and show no tendency to spontaneous involution. Most patients are young individuals and keloids are more frequent in dark-skinned persons. There is a genetic predisposition to develop keloids.[2] They are usually due to trauma, particularly to the heat trauma of electrosurgery for viral warts. However, keloids may

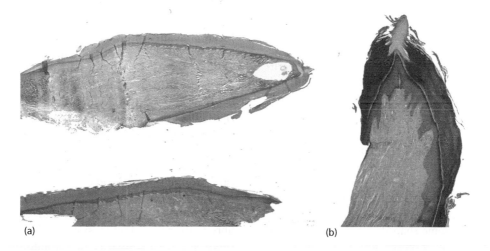

(a) (b)

Figure 26.28 **(a)** Scanning microscopy of a fibrokeratoma; **(b)** Scanning view of an acquired digital fibrokeratoma.

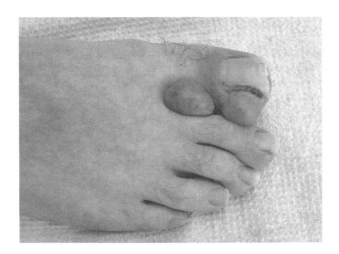

Figure 26.29 Periungual keloid of the big toenail after ingrown nail surgery. (Courtesy of Dr Zografakis, Athens, Greece.)

occur spontaneously. They may completely destroy the nails. Treatment has a recurrence rate between 45%–95%.[106] Keloids have to be distinguished from chronic sclerotic scar tissue as later is often seen in very long-standing ingrown toenails.[107] The histopathology is distinctive with thick eosinophilic hyalinized collagen type I bundles, which are haphazardly arranged but may form nodular or whorled masses. The border is often ill defined.

Knuckle pads

Knuckle pads occur mainly on the dorsal surface of the metacarpophalangeal and interphalangeal joints and may extend to the proximal nail fold. They are persistent, asymptomatic, slightly hyperpigmented, keratotic plaques more often seen in men. They are probably due to chronic rubbing and other chronic repeated traumas.[108] Similar lesions on the finger joints and clubbing of the nails were associated with epidermolytic palmar and plantar keratoderma of Vörner.[109] Pseudo-knuckle pads, called chewing pads[110] or pachydermodactyly,[111] may be a sign of obsessive-destructive behavior.[112]

Knuckle pads are similar to lichen simplex chronicus and friction induced acanthomas. In pseudo-knuckle pads due to biting, the epidermis shows signs of excessive superficial traumatization. The dermal changes are very similar to those of Dupuytren's contracture and the two disorders may occur in association.[113]

Recurrent digital fibrous tumors of childhood of Reye

Reye's tumors or infantile digital fibromatosis occurs mainly in young children,[114,115] rarely in adults.[116] They are round, smooth, shiny, dome-shaped, usually skin-colored or red, firm-to-tense nodules on the dorsal and lateral surfaces of the digits 2 to 5, sparing the thumbs and the big

toes. Periungual nodules interfere with nail growth and joint mobility.[117–120] They may already be present at birth or appear shortly thereafter. Spontaneous regression is the rule and no aggressive surgery is indicated.[121] The digital fibromas seen in terminal osseous dysplasia and pigmentary defects also disappear spontaneously.[122]

Clinical differential diagnosis includes hypertrophic lip of the great toe with overgrowth of the lateral nail fold, keloids, juvenile aponeurotic fibroma, pachydermodactyly, cerebriform connective tissue nevus, proteus syndrome, multiple mucinous periungual tumors in systemic sclerosis, and terminal osseous dysplasia and pigmentary defects.[123,157]

Superficial acral fibromyxoma

Superficial acral fibromyxoma (SAFM) occurs mainly in middle-aged adults. Men are slightly overrepresented. Virtually all tumors occur on fingers or toes, particularly the big toe, and more than half of them in periungual or subungual location. The tumors range from 0.5 to 5 cm and approximately 40% are painful. They are seen as a dome-shaped mass growing insidiously and finally distorting or even destroying the nail. Roughly one third erode the bone.[124] Complete extirpation is the treatment of choice. Recurrences are observed in approximately one quarter of the cases. No metastases have been observed so far[125–127] (Figure 26.30a and b).

Pleomorphic fibroma

Pleomorphic fibroma is very rare in subungual location.[128] It is a solitary, dome-shaped or polypoid, asymptomatic, slow-growing, and flesh-colored lesion. Its size ranges from 4 to 16 mm. One subungual pleomorphic fibromas had been present for 40 years.[129] Clinically, dermal nevus, solitary neurofibroma, or angioma may be considered. Incomplete excision may be followed by a recurrence.[130]

Histopathology shows a well-circumscribed, dome-shaped fibrous tumor. Mitoses are rare.

Juvenile hyaline fibromatosis

Juvenile hyaline fibromatosis (JHF) is a rare autosomal-recessive disease caused by mutations in the gene of the anthrax toxin receptor 2 protein (capillary morphogenesis gene 2) located on chromosome 4p21.[131,132] It starts between 3 months to 5 years, rarely later. Hyaline material is deposited in skin, mucous membranes, and other organs, causing skin lesions, among others. They are multiple cutaneous papules, nodules, large plaques with a transparent appearance and gelatinous consistency on ears, around the nose and on fingers.[133] Periungual lesions and distal onycholysis have repeatedly been observed[134,135] and were clinically similar to recurrent infantile digital fibromatosis.[136] Infantile systemic hyalinosis, an allelic syndrome with similarity to myofibromatosis has to be differentiated.

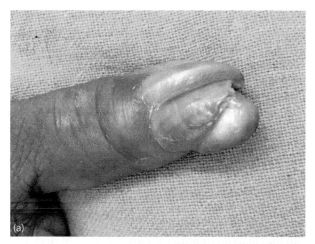

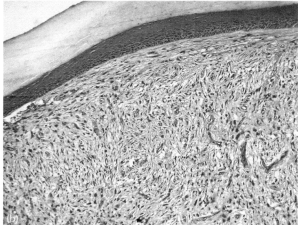

Figure 26.30 (a) Superficial acral fibromyxoma presenting as a flesh-colored soft-to-firm growth arising from the medial half of subungual area of right thumb. (From Kumar, P. et al., *Skin Appendage Disord.*, doi:10.1159/000489899.) (b) Histopathology showing spindle cells arranged in a random, loose storiform pattern in a myxoid stroma with scant collagen. Overlying epidermis is stretched and shows orthohyperkeratosis. (H&E x100) (From Kumar, P. et al., *Skin Appendage Disord.*, doi:10.1159/000489899.)

Pseudomalignant osseous tumor of soft tissue

This lesion also called digital pseudotumor is a benign reactive condition although it is characterized by an aggressive periosteal reaction and benign soft-tissue inflammation.[137] It is probably not so rare as several reports refer to this disease with a variety of different terms such as benign fibro-osseous pseudotumor, digital pseudotumor, florid reactive periostitis, parosteal fasciitis, fasciitis ossificans, myositis ossificans, and bizarre parosteal osteochondromatous proliferation.[138–140] To avoid this confusing nomenclature, some authors have placed it into the heterogeneous group of pseudomalignant osseous tumors of soft tissue, proliferative periosteal processes,[141,142] metaplastic bone formation in chronic fibroblastic inflammation[143] or classify it into the myositis ossificans

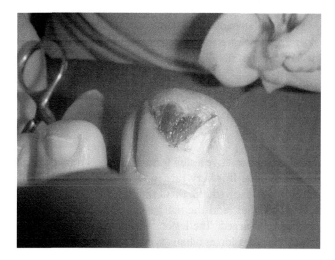

Figure 26.31 Subungual pseudomalignant osseous soft tissue tumor. After removing the overlying part of the distal nail plate, a pyogenic granuloma-like lesion is seen in the distal nail bed.

group.[144] Most digital pseudotumors occur in the phalanges of the fingers although subungual location is rare. The term "pseudomalignant" was coined as the speckled appearance on radiographs may resemble that of an extraskeletal osteosarcoma or chondrosarcoma. It is a tender or painful, fusiform, often erythematous lesion of the volar aspect of the proximal phalanx of fingers and infrequently the toes (Figure 26.31). Ulceration is rare. Most patients are young adults with a slight female preponderance. It is thought that repeated minor trauma is the cause. When occurring in subungual location, its clinical appearance is totally nonspecific with the most common misdiagnosis being pyogenic granuloma.[182] Radiographically and histopathologically, an exostosis may be suspected (Figure 26.32).[145]

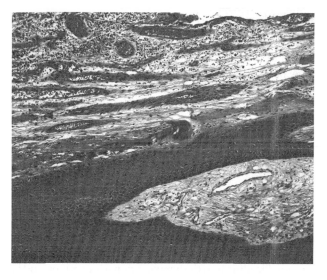

Figure 26.32 Histopathological aspect of a subungual pseudomalignant osseous soft-tissue tumor.

VASCULAR TUMORS

Most vascular neoplasms that are so frequent in glabrous skin are very rare in the nail apparatus, and many have never been described in this particular localization.

Intravascular papillary endothelial hyperplasia (pseudoangiosarcoma of Masson)

This peculiar reactive lesion was originally thought to be an angiosarcoma. It is very rare in the nail apparatus. In the single case observed, the tip of the index finger was slightly tender, bulbous, and the nail bed was bluish red. The nail appeared enlarged. The lesion was embarrassing with the patient's profession as a hair stylist.[146]

Acral arteriovenous shunting

Acral arteriovenous shunting (AAS) develops after a trauma or is due to autonomic nerve damage as the result of luxury blood supply with relatively high pressure or as a chronic stasis dermatitis associated with venous insufficiency.[147,148] It results in a pseudo-Kaposi-like appearance with dark red to almost black papules and plaques sometimes developing keloid-like areas. Acroangiodermatitis of Mali[149] and Stewart-Bluefarb syndrome[150] are variants. The toes and perionychium may be involved. The nails are rarely directly affected, but may show a purple hue or be leukonychotic. One 52-year-old woman with terminal renal insufficiency developed a pincer nail due to a pseudo-Kaposi sarcoma thought to be due to an arteriovenous fistula placed to perform hemodialysis.[151] Doppler ultrasound can diagnose an acral hyperstomy syndrome.[152] The clinical differential diagnoses are Kaposi's sarcoma, stasis dermatitis, lichen purpuricus, purpura pigmentosa, lichen aureus, vasculitis, lichen simplex chronicus, actinic keratosis, basal cell carcinoma, hemangioma, lymphangioma, and lymphangiosarcoma.[153]

Histopathology exhibits regularly built capillary vessels with thick walls, edematous stroma, and loosely structured lobuli in the papillary and reticular dermis. The epidermis may be acanthotic and hyperkeratotic. Extravasated erythrocytes lead to massive hemosiderin deposits, both within macrophages (siderophages) as well as in the interstitium. With time, the dermis becomes more fibrotic and finally sclerotic. Chronic spongiotic dermatitis (stasis eczema) may develop, particularly in acroangiodermatitis.

Lymphangioma circumscriptum

This is a common developmental anomaly of the deep muscular lymph collectors,[154] which leads to dilatation of the superficial lymph capillaries clinically simulating frog spawn. Bleeding into the lymphangioma is common and has led to the erroneous designation hemangiolymphangioma, which should better be termed hematolymphangioma. It is one of the functions of lymph vessels to take up extravasated erythrocytes and to re-introduce them into the circulation. Involvement of the digital tip is rare and may lead to nail deformation or even gross enlargement, finally progressing to elephantiasis nostras. Superficial lacerations may lead to recurrent erysipelas. Therapeutically, "circumscribed" lymphangiomas are difficult to extirpate as their limits in the tissue are usually very ill defined and the underlying malformation of the large lymph collectors may be missed or impossible to remove.

Histopathology demonstrates multiple round to oval cavities lined with a very thin, sometimes incontinuous-appearing endothelium. They are often directly in contact with the epidermis mimicking intraepidermal blisters. Long-standing lesions often develop hyperkeratosis.

Hemangioma

Infantile hemangioma is the most frequent vascular tumor of infancy and childhood, affecting roughly 1% of all newborns and more than 10% of premature babies. It makes up for approximately one third of all vascular neoplasms.[155] They have a characteristic course. Occurrence in the nail organ is extremely rare. They may then present as a reddish to violaceous, soft lesion under the nail and at the tip of the digit.

Histopathologically, infantile hemangioma has a lobular architecture. Endothelial proliferation around small capillary lumina or in solid strands and clusters is seen during the growth phase with large endothelial cells and frequent mitoses. In the maturing phase, the endothelial cells flatten, the lumina become wider, and mitoses decrease in number. In mature hemangiomas, some lumina are grossly dilated mimicking a cavernous hemangioma. Finally, in regressing lesions, there is more and more fibrosis and the blood vessels gradually disappear. At the end, a fibrotic lobular lesion is seen.

Cirsoid angioma

These arteriovenous tumors that are mainly found in the fronto-temporal area as a solitary, dark red nodule, may occur in acral[156] and subungual location.[157] A periungual or subungual mass not sufficiently characteristic to make the diagnosis is seen. They cause a nodular vascular lesion in the lateral nail fold of the little finger, under the nail, or both thumb nails are overcurved with a central wide split. There is neither clinical nor histological resemblance with pyogenic granuloma.

Histopathology is needed to make the diagnosis. Densely packed thick-walled and some thin-walled vessels are observed in the nail bed and matrix connective tissue. Glomus cells are not present. However, we have seen a patient with a subungual angioma, the vessels of which were intermediate between small arteries and early glomus bodies.

Pyogenic granuloma

Pyogenic or telangiectatic granuloma is an eruptive lobular angioma, not a granuloma.[158] It is commonly seen in association with a previous penetrating trauma that may be remembered, particularly in case of transungual growth. The lesion is most common in adolescents and young adults, but they may occur at any age and particularly during pregnancy. It is a rapidly growing, bright-red papule of 10 to 20 mm in diameter that often breaks through the horny layer of the skin giving the typical aspect of a collaret. The surface becomes eroded, crusted, even ulcerated, and tends to bleed (Figure 26.33). Although some lesions may regress with time, removal is advocated if this is not the case. The main differential diagnoses are granulation tissue, coccal nail fold angiomatosis, bacillary angiomatosis, Kaposi's sarcoma and angiosarcoma. Granulation tissue is quite common around the nails, most frequently as part of an ingrown nail. The so-called periungual pyogenic granulomas[159] under treatment with synthetic retinoids,[160,161] antiretrovirals,[162–165] taxanes,[166] other cytostatic drugs,[167] and epidermal growth factor receptor (EGFR) inhibitors[168,169] are in fact granulation tissue. Also, lectitis purulenta et granulomatosa[170] is most probably granulation tissue induced by trauma and nail avulsion. Acral angioosteoma is clinically similar to pyogenic granuloma and histologically demonstrates a capillary proliferation with metaplastic bone formation and was once described in subungual location as a dome-shaped ulcerated lesion on the left fourth toe. It lacks the lobular pattern of vascular proliferation typical for pyogenic granuloma.[171] Histopathology of pyogenic granuloma shows an elevated or polypoid lobular angiomatous tumor of mostly capillary vessels covered by a thinned or eroded epidermis. At the base, a collaret of acanthotic epidermis is frequently seen. When the lesion is erosive or ulcerated there may be an inflammatory infiltrate with plenty of neutrophils similar to granulation tissue. Feeder vessels can often be observed reaching deep into the dermis. In older and regressing lesions, the fibrotic septa become wider and the walls of the capillary vessels thicker (Figure 26.34).

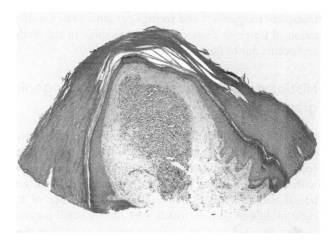

Figure 26.34 Small pyogenic granuloma of the nail. Histopathology shows a lobular angioma covered with a thinned epidermis that tends to erode.

Coccal nail fold angiomatosis

This condition is characterized by pyogenic granuloma-like lesions usually occurring on several fingers after a cast was removed, which had been applied for one to three months to treat a phalanx, metacarpal bone, or wrist fracture. Most patients had mild pain or paresthesia during cast wearing.[172] Between 7 to 30 days after cast removal, oozing peculiar, sometimes painful, small tumors (Figure 26.35) grow out from under the proximal nail fold, which in contrast to classical pyogenic granuloma are never covered with an epidermis. Later, onychomadesis is seen. Etiologically, a mild nerve injury and a reaction similar to reflex sympathetic dystrophy were suggested.[173,174] Histology shows capillary vessels in a myxoid stroma with lymphoid cells, plasma cells, and some neutrophils; cultures grew ß-hemolytic *streptococci* and *Staphylococcus aureus*. It is not a lobular angioma like pyogenic granuloma. Other differential diagnoses are bacillary angiomatosis, now rarely seen as antibiotic prophylaxis has become the rule in severely immunodepressed patients with HIV infection, leukemia,[175] other malignancies, and in organ

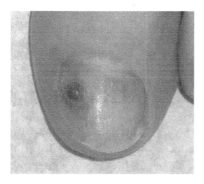

Figure 26.33 Transungually growing pyogenic granuloma after a penetrating trauma.

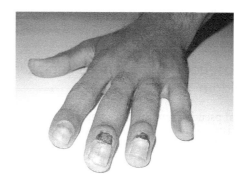

Figure 26.35 Coccal nail fold angiomatosis after removal of a cast for a wrist fracture.

transplant recipients[176] and verruga peruana, a late manifestation of Carrion's disease, which is endemic in the Andes and occurs due to *Bartonella bacilliformis*.[177]

Histiocytoid hemangioma (pseudopyogenic granuloma)

Originally described under the term of pseudopyogenic granuloma, histiocytoid hemangioma is now the accepted term.[178–180] Involvement of the distal phalanx and the nail with angiomatous nodules in the fingertip, nail bed, and lateral nail folds,[181] with multiple painless lesions of the right middle fingernail, which were mostly small measuring between 1–3 mm, and a larger vegetating angiomatous nodule of 5 mm (that was bright red, smooth, and eroded destroying the nail plate),[182] causing distal onycholysis, subungual and periungual reddening, longitudinal splitting of the nail, swelling of the nail folds and purulent secretion were observed.[183] Radiation treatment led to disappearance of the nodules. Histopathology is indispensable to make the diagnosis. It shows nests and cords of endothelial cells and abnormal vessels that are lined by large endothelial cells. A variable number of inflammatory cells is usually present, which was the reason for the first designation of pseudopyogenic granuloma.

Angiolymphoid hyperplasia with eosinophilia

Angiolymphoid hyperplasia with eosinophilia presents with bright-red or violaceous nodules, quite often in the head and neck region. Distal digital localization is rare. Nail bed involvement leads to a reddish or bluish-red discoloration or to nail splitting and nail deformity.[184] One case was described in association with pachydermoperiostosis.[185] A circumscribed proliferation of blood vessels and a chronic inflammatory infiltrate rich in eosinophils characterize this reactive benign lesion. Synonyms were epithelioid angioma, inflammatory angiomatous nodule, pseudo-pyogenic granuloma, atypical pyogenic granuloma, and intravenous atypical vascular proliferation.[186–188] Trauma and inflammation are thought to play an etiological role.

Acral pseudolymphomatous angiokeratoma of children

The acral pseudolymphomatous angiokeratoma of children (APACHE) lesion is mainly observed in children and is characterized by multiple small hyperkeratotic angiomatoid lesions on the tips of several digits with striking clinical similarity with angiokeratoma of Mibelli.[189] Single digit plus nail involvement is very rare.[190] Histopathology exhibits marked hyperkeratosis, thinning of the epidermis over the lesion itself with elongated rete pegs at the margin of the lesion. A well-circumscribed, dense infiltrate of mature

T and B lymphocytes is present around dilated vessels that extend from the papillary dermis down to the subcutaneous tissue. The epidermis is not invaded. The multiple lesions rule out angiokeratoma of Mibelli.

Angiokeratoma circumscriptum

Involvement of the toes, fingers, and perionychium has been observed in angiokeratoma circumscriptum.[191] It is a hyperkeratotic lesion with an angiomatous base mainly occurring on the lower extremity in young adults. Verrucous hemangioma is indistinguishable clinically. An important clinical differential diagnosis is melanoma.

Histopathology demonstrates abundant ectatic, thin-walled capillaries filled with erythrocytes in the papillary dermis bulging the thin epidermis up. There is often acanthosis at the margins and a variable degree of hyperkeratosis. Verrucous hemangioma is characterized by marked hyperkeratosis, parakeratosis, papillomatosis, and elongation of the rete ridges extending from the dermo-epidermal junction into the deeper dermis, where numerous small to large vascular channels are seen.[192]

Aneurysmal bone cyst (arterio-venous fistula)

Aneurysmal bone cyst is a rare benign, locally aggressive bone lesion sometimes occurring in the distal phalanx of young individuals. It grows rapidly, is painful, and markedly enlarges the tip of the digit and the nail.[193] Radiographs show a distension of the bone resembling the secular protrusion of the walls of an aneurysm. The phalanx appears almost completely substituted by an osteolytic process.[194] The etiology is not clear, but trauma may play a role.[195] Treatment is by curettage of the lesion.

Histopathology shows a stroma of proliferating fibroblasts, histiocytes, and multinucleated giant cells and dilated, blood-filled vascular spaces without endothelial cells separated by fibrous septa and small osteoid or bone strands. Giant cell reparative granuloma is a solid aneurysmal bone cyst and thus almost identical except for the lack of blood-filled spaces.

Angioleiomyoma

Angioleiomyoma of the nail was described more than 130 years ago. More cases were reported,[196] of which several were mistaken for glomus tumor because they were painful.[197,198] Depending on their localization within the nail apparatus, angioleiomyomas of the nail may elevate the nail plate, appear as a small nodule at the tip of the digit just under the hyponychium or distort the nail.

Histopathologically, they are well circumscribed lesions made up of a ball of densely packed mature smooth muscle cells with some small blood vessel lumina. Subungual angioleiomyomas are often much less compact and are more similar to cirsoid angiomas.

Glomus tumor

Glomus tumors make up for approximately 2% of all hand tumors. They were first described 200 years ago as a painful subcutaneous tubercle,[199] later as colloid sarcoma or angiosarcoma. Most patients are between 30 and 50 years old. Women are more frequently affected than men. Glomus tumors mostly occur in the nail matrix and nail bed of fingers. Most patients consult the dermatologist or surgeon because of the intense pain that is both spontaneous as well as elicited by minor trauma or cold. The pain can radiate up to the shoulder. A tourniquet at the base of the finger or a blood pressure cuff inflated to 300 mm Hg stops the pain. The glomus tumor is often seen in the distal matrix as a bluish or violaceous round to oval spot of 3 to 8 mm in diameter, from which a reddish band extends distally that is sometimes slightly elevated (Figure 26.36a and b). The nail may even split distally (Figure 26.37). Probing provokes intense pain, but can localize the tumor very exactly. Dermatoscopy, ultrasound, thermography, dynamic thermography, arteriography, MR, and particularly angio-MRI help to visualize the lesion, but are rarely more precise than probing. An impression of the phalangeal bone may be seen in approximately one third of the cases on X-ray. Up to 10% of glomus tumors are multiple, being the cause for presumed recurrence.[200,201] The diagnosis is virtually always obvious as there are no other lesions with this highly specific symptomatology. Surgical removal is not demanding as the glomus tumor is a round, very well-delineated, encapsulated lesion standing out by its grayish color from the surrounding connective tissue or fat. The overlying nail is gently detached from the matrix and proximal nail bed and a slightly arched shallow incision parallel to the lunula border is made over the bluish spot. The glomus tumor is seen popping out. The overlying thin matrix epithelium is cautiously dissected from the glomus tumor, then the tumor is shelled out using blunt curved scissors. The matrix is closed with 6-0 vicryl rapid and the detached nail laid back and stitched to fix it. Healing is usually fast within 10 to 14 days.

The clinical differential diagnosis comprises virtually all painful conditions of the nails such as subungual warts, KA, subungual exostosis, enchondroma, neuroma, Pacinian neuroma, caliber-persistent artery, leiomyoma, paronychia, osteitis terminalis, subungual felon, herpetic whitlow, causalgia, gout, melanoma,[202] and several more. Glomangioma is often multiple, sometimes in linear distribution involving an extremity including the periungual skin, usually are not painful or are only tender on deep palpation, and the main clinical differential diagnosis is venous malformation or blue rubber bleb nevus.[203] Familial glomangioma has been described.[204] Minute synovial sarcomas may have some similarity with glomus tumors.[205]

A genetically different subset of glomus tumors occurs in von Recklinghausen's neurofibromatosis I, which is characterized by a bi-allelic mutation in the tumor suppression gene NF1.[206] These patients have a higher risk of developing multiple glomus tumors.[207] In a cohort of glomus tumor patients, 29% had neurofibromatosis I giving an odds ratio of 168:1.[208]

Histopathology shows a well circumscribed, encapsulated lesion. It has an afferent arteriole, vascular channels that are surrounded by cuboidal basophilic cells with dark round nuclei and lined with a flat endothelium, and efferent veins leading into small veins of the dermis (Figures 26.38 and 26.39). These structures of the glomus tumor are,

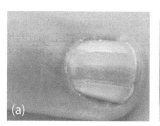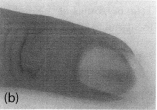

Figure 26.36 **(a)** Glomus tumor of the matrix. There is an exceedingly tender circumscribed spot just under the free margin of the proximal nail fold from where a reddish streak extends distally all along the lunula and nail bed. **(b)** Glomus tumor of the nail bed in a 39-year-old female immigrant from India. Note that the reddish streak has a slight brown tinge and only starts in the nail bed. Here was the point of maximum pain when probing.

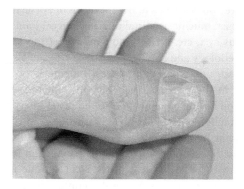

Figure 26.37 Glomus tumor of distal nail bed causing split in the nail plate.

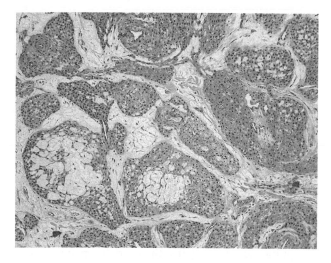

Figure 26.38 Histopathology of a glomus tumor reveals nests of cuboid cells with round dark nuclei and small vessel lumina with a flat endothelium.

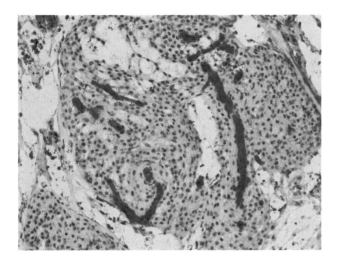

Figure 26.39 Immunohistochemistry with the endothelial marker CD31 demonstrates the narrow vessels in the glomus cell agglomerates.

however, often not seen in routine sections. Special stains show myelinated and unmyelinated nerves; they may be responsible for the pain. Thus, the glomus tumor is held to be a true hamartoma rather than a tumor.

Caliber-persistent artery

Caliber-persistent artery is not a tumor (Dieulafoy's lesion, cirsoid aneurysm, or submucosal arterial malformation), but an acquired or inborn lesion where the terminal artery caliber does not diminish with each branching but remains wide. It is relatively common in the intestinal tract but is rare in skin, mainly seen on the lower lip.[209] A small nodule with chronic superficial ulceration develops. Gentle palpation may reveal pulsation.[210] Ultrasound also helps to make the diagnosis.[211] Two patients presenting with subungual lesions and a split nail were histologically diagnosed as caliber-persistent artery. MR imaging had shown a longitudinal lesion of suspected vascular origin. The diagnosis was completely unexpected; as nail surgery is performed with a tourniquet bleeding was not an intraoperative feature suggesting the correct diagnosis. Treatment of choice is ligation of the artery on both ends. The diagnosis of subungual caliber-persistent artery is an unexpected finding. As a split in the nail can have many different causes, caliber-persistent artery should be included into the list of differential diagnoses.

Histopathology of the specimens from the matrix and nail bed showed a disproportionately large artery in the distal matrix, which was otherwise anatomically normal. The pathogenesis of the split nail is due to pressure from the pulsating artery against the overlying nail plate leading to circumscribed matrix epithelium atrophy, which eventually results in insufficient nail formation and finally in a split nail.

BENIGN TUMORS WITH ADIPOCYTE, MUSCULAR, OSSEOUS, AND CARTILAGINOUS FEATURES

The clinical diagnosis of these tumors in the nail unit is difficult. Simple examinations like probing, dermatoscopy, and transillumination are often helpful as are imaging techniques such as radiography, ultrasound, computed tomography, and MR imaging.[212] However, the diagnostic gold standard is histopathology.

Lipoma

Lipomas, so frequent elsewhere in the skin, are exceptional in the nail apparatus.[213,214] They deform the nail depending on their size and location or resemble nevus lipomatodes superficialis.[215] Subungual lipoma was also observed in association with a SCC of the nail bed of the same digit.[216] MR imaging allows the diagnosis to be made as there is a very intense signal in T1-weighted images.[217]

Histopathology shows a neoplasm made up of mature adipocytes separated by thin fibrous septa. There may or may not be a thin fibrous capsule. One case of subungual spindle cell lipoma was described.[218]

Myxoma

True myxomas of the nail are rare. Their distinction from focal mucinosis is often arbitrary. Most myxoid lesions of the nail apparatus are, however, so-called myxoid pseudocysts (MPCs).[219] Subungual myxomas either elevate or deform the nail or enlarge the nail and fingertip.[220] Treatment is by cautious extirpation with preservation of the matrix.[221] The differential diagnosis comprises SAFM and other myxoid lesions.

Histopathology shows abundant hyaluronic acid-rich ground substance, in which stellate or fusiform cells are loosely distributed. Toluidine blue, Giemsa as well as colloidal iron stains are positive for acid mucopolysaccharides.

Myxoid pseudocyst (dorsal finger cyst)

MPCs are also described under the terms of dorsal finger cyst, digital focal mucinosis, distal interphalangeal joint ganglion, mucinous cyst, etc. These synonyms reflect the opinions as to their etiology and pathogenesis. Two types of lesions were postulated, one type being a focal mucinosis of the distal phalanx in the proximal nail fold (myxomatous type), the other type having a connection to the distal interphalangeal joint (ganglion type). Roughly 85% show a connecting stalk to the joint by intraarticular injection of 0.05 to 0.1 mL of sterile methylene blue solution. This connection is probably secondary to wear-and-tear of the joint capsule in a long-standing lesion. MPC is the most common pseudotumor of the nail apparatus. Women are slightly more often involved than men. Most MPCs are solitary although more than one finger can be affected, and very rarely two lesions are found on one finger. When the toes are involved, there is usually a firm protuberant cystic lesion. Almost always, a degenerative distal interphalangeal osteoarthritis with Heberden nodes is present. Three clinical types are distinguished: Type A is localized in the proximal nail fold and is seen as a round dome-shaped skin-colored lesion pressing on the matrix and causing a regular longitudinal depression in the nail plate (Figure 26.40). Type B is also localized in the proximal nail fold but ruptures at the undersurface of the nail fold releasing part of its content into the nail pocket. This leads to an irregular depression in the nail often with narrow transverse ridges in the canaliform depression reflecting the period of diminished pressure on the matrix (Figure 26.41). Type C is the submatrical MPC clinically seen as a violaceous swelling under a hemi-overcurved nail. Transillumination is positive (Figure 26.42). MR imaging clearly demonstrates the lesion, rarely also the connecting stalk to the joint (Figure 26.43). Treatment depends on their stage and extent. Early and multiple MPCs respond to intralesional triamcinolone acetonide injection (Kenacort 10 mg/mL®) after puncture and

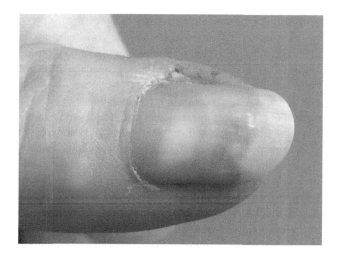

Figure 26.42 Subungual myxoid pseudocyst (type C) leading to overcurvature of the nail and a violaceous tint of the matrix; this area shines up on transillumination (diaphanoscopy).

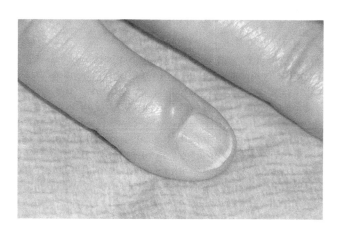

Figure 26.40 Myxoid pseudocyst (type A).

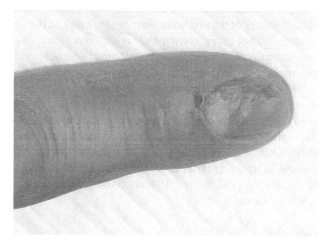

Figure 26.41 Myxoid pseudocyst of the proximal nail fold that had ruptured into the nail pocket (type B). The variable pressure due to emptying and refilling of the lesion leads to irregular depressions in the nail plate.

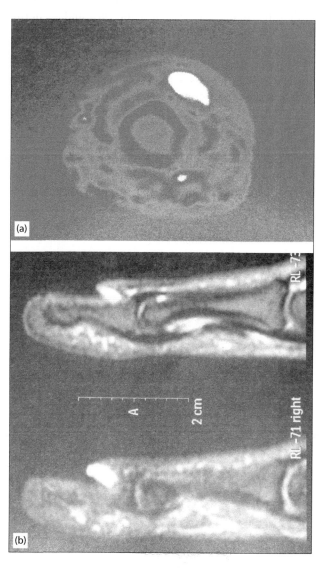

Figure 26.43 Magnetic resonance image of a myxoid pseudocyst. (a) Transverse view and (b) Side view.

expression of the content. Circumscribed pressure for several weeks is useful. Other therapies include repeated puncture and expression, injection of a sclerosant agent, cryosurgery with carbon dioxide ice or liquid nitrogen, coagulation with an infrared coagulator, or different lasers. Surgery by simple excision and suture is commonly followed by recurrence. The treatment of choice is intraarticular injection of sterile methylene blue from the volar distal interphalangeal joint crease to visualize a potential communication with the joint, raising a flap over the lesion, meticulously dissecting any blue stained myxoid tissue and ligating the stalk to the joint, which is visible as a dark-blue spot, and finally close the defect with the flap. A padded dressing is performed that is changed the next day. Postoperative finger stiffness is exceptional in contrast to the method of simply removing the osseous Heberden nodes.

Histopathology of complete excision specimens reveals myxomatous areas in the wall of the pseudocyst in more than 80% of the cases. In many cases, there is a central lake of mucin surrounded by myxomatous tissue containing scattered stellate and spindle-shaped cells. Particularly in toe MPCs, the mucin has expanded the surrounding normal connective tissue giving rise to a pseudocapsule. The overlying epidermis is often considerably thinned (Figure 26.44). The myxoid areas are positive with alcian blue and Hale's colloidal iron stain. In the so-called ganglion type, the myxomatous areas are sparse or not seen. A cyst lining is not seen.[222]

Chondroma

Chondroma is relatively frequent in the hands. Three types of subungual chondroma have been observed: enchondroma, parosteal chondroma, and soft tissue (extraskeletal) chondroma.

ENCHONDROMA

Enchondroma is the most frequent of the subungual chondromas. It is a solitary intraosseous proliferation of

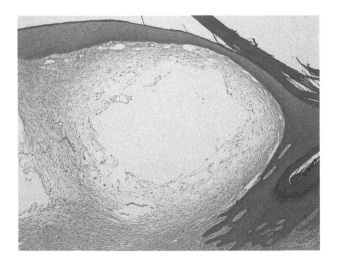

Figure 26.44 Myxoid pseudocyst: histopathology of an early lesion reveals a nodular mucinosis with a central lake of mucin.

cartilage. Multiple enchondromas are observed in enchondromatosis (chondrodysplasia of Ollier, OMIM 166000) and chondrodysplasia with multiple soft tissue and intraosseous hemangiomas (Maffucci–Kast syndrome, OMIM 614569); both syndromes are due to cartilage that fails to undergo normal ossification and both tend to progress to chondrosarcoma—almost 25%—and have a higher malignancy rate in general.[223] Solitary enchondromas of the distal phalanx with enlargement of the tip of the digit is rare.[224] About 20% of the lesions remain asymptomatic, but paronychia, clubbing, and secondary nail changes with longitudinal ridging are seen.[225] Pathologic fractures are the result of progressive thinning of the cortical bone. Radiography demonstrates well-defined to cloudy radiolucent defects with expansion of the terminal phalanx, in most cases close to the articular surface of the distal interphalangeal joint.[5]

PAROSTEAL CHONDROMA

Parosteal chondroma of the distal phalanx is very rare. It slowly and insidiously occupies the subungual or periungual space with resulting nail deformation. X-ray may show an impression of the distal phalangeal bone.

EXTRASKELETAL CHONDROMA

Extraskeletal or soft tissue chondroma is thought to derive from the connective tissue, not preexisting chondrocytes.[226] Clinically, it mimics parosteal chondroma. The clinical differential diagnosis comprises a number of other chondromatoses that rarely affect the digits, such as synovial chondromatosis. Histopathologically, all chondromas are characterized by a proliferation of hyaline cartilage irregularly arranged cells, but without mitoses or cellular atypias. In the differential diagnosis, chondroblastoma and chondrosarcoma are important.

Osteoma cutis

Osteomas of the skin are small round to oval nodules with all characteristics of normal bone. They are very rare in the distal digit.[227] They may present merely as a splinter hemorrhage extending from the site of the osteoma to the hyponychium.[228] Subungual osteomas can only be suspected radiographically.

Histopathology demonstrates a round to oval, well-demarcated lesion of mature bone with a few osteocytes in the bone trabeculae. Osteoblasts are rare. Subungual calcifications constitute the main differential diagnosis that are very common under the toe- and fingernails. They usually present as irregular basophilic von Kossa-positive deposits of clumpy material. Some calcifications may have been mistaken for osteoma.[229]

Subungual calcifications

They are a common phenomenon usually remaining unnoticed. Women are affected considerably more frequently and earlier than men. Most cases represent dystrophic calcinosis, but also subungual onycholemmal cysts undergo calcification. Even a congenital tumorous calcification of the distal lateral nail fold was observed.[230,231]

Histopathology shows dystrophic lesions and, rarely, metastatic calcifications in case of disturbances of calcium metabolism. The calcium deposits are of various size and shape, often scattered in the dermis without an inflammatory reaction. Some are partly surrounded by macrophages and an occasional giant cell, some are calcified onycholemmal cysts.

Subungual exostosis

Subungual exostosis is the most frequent reactive bony lesion of the toes,[232] but is rare in fingers.[233] Adolescents are most commonly affected. Trauma is thought be an etiologic factor[234]; however, recent research demonstrated a chromosomal translocation t(X;6)(q13-14;q22) suggesting that it is a true tumor.[235] The distal dorsal medial aspect of the distal phalanx of the hallux is the most common localization, but in principle all digits may be involved. Usually, the nail plate is lifted and slightly deformed. A small onycholytic area is often present. The overlying epidermis is smooth, shiny, and stretched out. A collaret-like delimitation to the ridged skin of the tip of the toe is highly characteristic. Ulceration of the overlying skin occurs spontaneously or is trauma-induced. Although the clinical diagnosis is obvious in most cases as there is hardly any other lesion as hard on palpation as an exostosis, the list of misdiagnoses reaches from viral wart to other tumors and even onychomycosis[236] (Figure 26.45a and b). A radiograph is recommended to confirm the diagnosis and determine its extension. The removal consists of generous extirpation at the base of the lesion. Radiographically, bone fragments after fracture of the distal subungual tuft, subungual calcifications as seen quite frequently in elderly women,[237] posttraumatic subungual calcifications, primary osteoma cutis, and calcified subungual

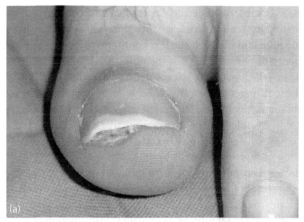

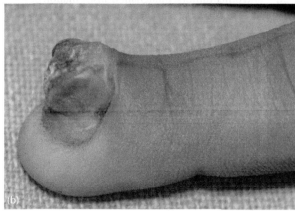

Figure 26.45 (a) Subungual exostosis; (b) Subungual exostosis in a young child. Affection of finger is uncommon. (From Kumar, P. et al., *Indian J. Dermatol. Venereol. Leprol.*, 84, 232–233, 2018.)

epidermoid inclusions have to be ruled out. The differentiation from osteochondroma depends on its localization as summarized in Table 26.1.[238] Subungual exostoses usually appear as

Table 26.1 Differential diagnosis of subungal exostoses

	Subungual exostosis	Subungual osteochondroma	Enchondroma
Onset age (years)	Early 20s	10–25	20–40
Male: female ratio	1:2	2:1	1:1
History of trauma	Frequent	Frequent	Frequent
Clinical appearance	Nodule on distal medial phalanx	Nodule on proximal phalanx	Swelling of the phalanx
Growth	Slow, continues	Slow, stops after epiphyseal fusion[a]	Rapid
Radiology	Sessile or pedunculated well-circumscribed osseous growth that lacks a clear contiguity of both the medullary cavity and cortex. Fibrocartilaginous cap is usually radiolucent, but may rarely be calcified.	Sessile or pedunculated osseous growth seen in the metaphyseal region and shows continuity with medullary cavity of parent bone (better appreciable on computed tomography scan)	Expansile and usually lytic (radiolucent) lesion affecting the phalanx. Expansion of overlying cortex is observed and sometimes, rings and arcs calcification of the lesion is noted.
Pathology	Osseous bone with fibrocartilage cap	Osseous bone with hyaline cartilage	Fibrovascular bundles surrounding hyaline cartilage

[a] Continued growth after skeletal maturity is considered an indicator of malignant transformation and requires histopathological evaluation of the lesion.

well circumscribed, sessile, or pedunculated bony growth originating from metaphysis, but they lack well-formed cortex and medulla and hence, lack clear continuity with the medullary cavity of parent bone. On the other hand, osteochondromas have well-developed cortex and medulla, communicating with those of parent bone, which helps to distinguish them from subungual exostoses. Enchondromas affecting phalanges present in a similar clinical manner, but are radiolucent (lytic) and causes expansion of phalanx itself (Figure 26.46). MR image shows a high signal of the hyaline cartilage, cap in osteochondroma as compared to the low signal of the fibrocartilage cap in a typical exostosis.[239] Clinical differential diagnoses are melanoma, SCC, pyogenic granuloma, warts, digital pseudotumor,[240] and other tumors. Malignant transformation of solitary subungual exostoses has not been observed in contrast to the hereditary multiple exostoses syndrome (diaphyseal aclasis), which rarely affects the distal phalanx.[241]

Histopathology demonstrates mucopolysaccharide deposition and osteoid formation in the early lesion. A gradual continuum of highly cellular chondroid and osteoid follows. The mature subungual exostosis reveals a three-zonal pattern: a fibrocartilaginous cap on its surface, a rim of hyaline cartilage, and below trabeculae of bone with a rim of osteoblasts and some osteoclasts (Figure 26.47). Among the bone lamellae, some lipomatous medulla is present, but blood formation does not occur.

Osteochondroma

Osteochondroma is a benign bone tumor originating from the epiphyseal cartilage. When located subungually the signs and symptoms are virtually indistinguishable from subungual exostosis although the latter originates from the distal portion of the terminal phalanx.[242] MR shows a cap of hyaline cartilage in contrast to subungual exostosis with its fibrocartilaginous cap (see above) (Figures 26.48 and 26.49).

Histopathology exhibits a cap of hyaline cartilage; if this is not visible the differential diagnosis is not possible.

Osteoid osteoma

Osteoid osteoma occurs in virtually all bones, making up 1%–2% of all hand tumors; 8% of them occur in the phalanges, but localization in the distal phalanx is rare.

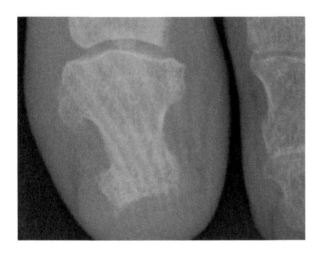

Figure 26.46 Subungual exostosis, X-ray.

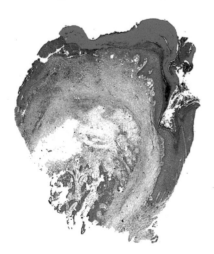

Figure 26.47 Subungual exostosis, histopathology, scanning magnification.

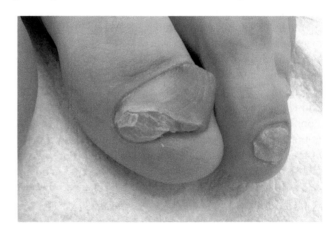

Figure 26.48 Subungual osteochondroma in a 12-year-old boy.

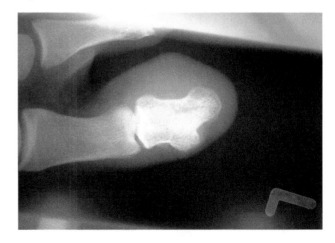

Figure 26.49 X-ray of the subungual osteochondroma demonstrating its relatively proximal origin.

Most develop in young adults, but there was also one probable congenital case.[243] Osteoid osteomas of the nail region cause enlargement of the tip of the digit and nail, clubbing, and nail thickening.[244] This unique bone lesion is characterized by marked pain,[245] which is nagging to pulsating at night and reacts promptly to non-steroidal antiinflammatory agents including acetylsalicylic acid. The pain was attributed to the effect on nerves and vessels by prostaglandin E2 produced by the osteoblasts.[246] Osteoid osteomas of the distal phalanx present diagnostic difficulties because of their atypical radiological appearance, presence of soft tissue enlargement and nail deformity, the small size of the distal phalanx, and consequent close approximation of lesions to the nail plate and distal interphalangeal joint.[247] Subperiosteal localization may mimic an exostosis.[248] Probing elicits pain and helps to localize the tumor. Radiography exhibits a small area of contrast rarefaction surrounded by a narrow sclerotic ring.[249] Arteriography, thermography, scintigraphy, color-coded duplex US,[250] fine-layer computed tomography, and MR imaging help to make the diagnosis and to find the lesion. Preoperative administration of a tetracycline and examination of the lesion under UV light during surgery allows the nidus to be visualized intraoperatively.[251] Complete extirpation is the treatment of choice, either by surgery or radiofrequency ablation.

Histopathology reveals a sharply delineated central growth area, the nidus, consisting of a meshwork of trabeculae of osteoid with a variable degree of calcification and surrounded by plump osteoblasts that are dispersed in a very vascular connective tissue usually without any sign of inflammation.[252] Osteoblastoma is histologically almost identical to osteoid osteoma, but it lacks the characteristic pain, the nidus is larger, and the rim of reactive sclerotic bone formation is lacking. The differential diagnosis of osteoblastoma and well differentiated osteosarcoma can pose extreme difficulties.[253]

Giant cell tumor of the bone

Giant cell tumor of the bone (GCTB), also called osteoclastoma, is uncommon and distal phalanx affection is exceedingly rare.[254] The distal phalanx is massively enlarged and radiographically lytic with a very thin bone lamella without any sclerosis or periosteal reaction. Pain is marked and probing reveals a very tender lesion. Spontaneous fracture is common. The surgical specimen is solid, tan, or light brown, often with small hemorrhagic areas. The clinical differential diagnosis is aneurysmal bone cyst, osteoid osteoma, intraosseous epidermal cyst, other intraosseous cysts, enchondroma, and intraosseous glomus tumor.

Histopathology shows two main tumor cell components: the stromal cells, which are now thought to constitute the "real neoplastic and proliferative component," and the obvious osteoclast-like giant cells that derive from fusioned macrophages. A number of other giant cell lesions of bones and adjacent tissues such as chondromyxoid

fibromas, chondroblastoma, nonossifying fibromas, metaphyseal fibrous defect, Langerhans cell histiocytosis, solitary bone cyst, osteitis fibrosa cystica in hyperparathyroidism, giant cell reparative granuloma, aneurysmal bone cyst, osteoid osteoma, and osteoblastoma, have to be considered.[255]

Solitary bone cyst

Solitary bone cysts are pseudotumors seen in young males. A single case was described in the distal phalanx of the second left toe. The phalanx was tender and enlarged, and the nail clubbed. X-ray showed a cystic loss of bone with only an extremely thin bone lamella left.[256] The cyst contains a clear yellowish fluid. The main differential diagnosis is aneurysmal bone cyst.

Histopathology shows a cyst lined by a smooth membrane-like material. The connective tissue is well vascularized, often with hemosiderin in macrophages and cholesterol clefts.

Synovialoma (giant cell tumor of the tendon)

Synovialoma, also called benign xanthomatous giant cell tumor or villonodular pigmented synovitis, derives from the synovial membrane of the joints or tendon sheath. It is frequent in the hand and more common in women. When located on the dorsal aspect of the distal digit it appears as a solitary or lobulated, firm to hard, skin-colored tumor, to which the skin is firmly attached. When the tumor is located in the digital pulp it is easily movable and when extirpated it appears as a corymbiform yellow-brownish lesion. It is not tender except when pressed too hard and does not usually interfere with nail growth. Localization in the lateral nail fold may cause a paronychia-like lesion.[257] When under the nail, it causes nail deformity.[258] Treatment is by meticulous extirpation. Radiographs do not show calcifications in contrast to its very rare malignant counterpart synovial sarcoma. Clinical differential diagnosis comprises MPC, epidermal cyst, neuroma, rheumatoid nodules, Heberden nodes, FK, epidermal cyst, tendon sheath fibroma, multicentric reticulohistiocytosis, tendinous xanthoma, epithelioid sarcoma, and other sarcomas as well as metastases, but in rare cases also granuloma anulare and erythema elevatum diutinum.[259]

Histopathology reveals a lobulated mass extending into the subcutaneous tissue around the tendon in volar location and more into the lower dermis in dorsal location. In the former site there is usually a dense fibrous capsule that often also divides the tumor into lobules. The microscopic aspect of the lesion varies according to the number of mononuclear cells, giant cells, hemosiderin deposition, xanthomatous cells, and collagen. Xanthoma cell-rich areas are irregularly distributed and may even contain cholesterol clefts. The xanthoma cells also often contain fine hemosiderin granules. Reticulohistiocytoma has an almost identical histopathology.

NEUROGENIC TUMORS

A large number of different peripheral nerve tumors can be observed in the nail region. Their diagnosis may be difficult and is based on morphologic similarity with structures of the peripheral nerves, on the development of their neurocristic precursors and reactions of nerves to injury and regeneration.[260] Neurosustentacular, some mesenchymal cells and melanocytes are of neuroectodermal origin thus sharing a common progenitor and having many cell markers in common. Some neural tumors are tender or painful, others are completely asymptomatic.

Neuroma

Neuromas of the distal phalanx of the digits usually occur after trauma or surgery.[261] They develop at any age. When located under the nail they elevate the nail and cause tenderness and nail dystrophy. Postoperative neuromas of the distal phalanx are palpated as tender areas or firm papules in or next to the scar. Lancinating pain may indicate an amputation neuroma.[262] An encapsulated palisaded neuroma of the proximal nail fold resembled a MPC.[263] Thickening of the proximal nail fold was observed in the multiple mucosal neuroma syndrome.[264] Clinical differential diagnosis is glomus tumor and a variety of other painful nail lesions.

Histopathologically, traumatic neuromas are not true tumors, but a reparative process. They demonstrate an increased and disorganized number of myelinated nerve fascicles of various sizes and shapes running in various directions. Mucin may be found in the nerves. A true capsule does not exist. Neural markers are strongly positive. The neurofilament positivity allows neuromas from neurofibromas and schwannomas to be distinguished.

Rudimentary supernumerary finger

The rudimentary supernumerary finger is localized at the lateral aspect of the fifth metacarpo-phalangeal joint. It is seen as a symmetrical small, slightly hyperkeratotic or verrucous nodule. Pain is not pronounced.[265] As it is usually treated by suture ligation and left for auto-amputation, an amputation neuroma may develop. Early excision and removal of the accessory digital nerve can prevent the development of this peculiar type of amputation neuroma.[266] The main differential diagnosis is neuroma, particularly when the location of the excision specimen was not indicated.

Pacinian neuroma

Pacinian neuroma or hyperplasia is rare. It mostly occurs in areas where Pacini bodies are found normally. It grows asymptomatically or causes tenderness and pain spontaneously or on probing (Figure 26.50).[267] On extirpation, many tiny sand-grain-like ivory-colored structures can be seen

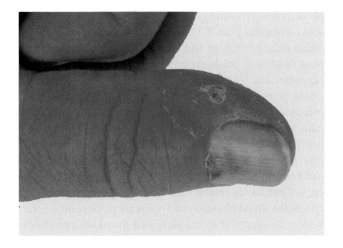

Figure 26.50 Pacinian neuroma in the lateral aspect of the proximal nail fold. This led the patient to continuously manipulate the skin in this area.

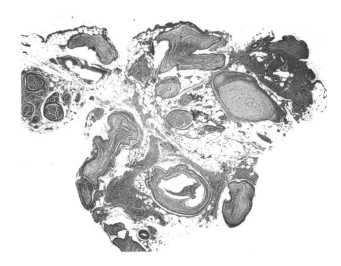

Figure 26.51 Histopathology shows a conglomerate of otherwise normal appearing Pacinian bodies in an atypical anatomic site.

with the naked eye that seem to fall apart when removed from their "host site." About half of the cases were seen to develop after a trauma.

Histologically, four types of Pacinian neuroma were described: A. a single enlarged corpuscle, B. a grape-like structure of normal-sized Pacinian corpuscles, C. slightly enlarged corpuscles arranged in tandem, and D. hyperplastic Pacinian corpuscles arranged along the entire length of a digital nerve[268] (Figure 26.51).

Neurofibroma

Neurofibromas are common tumors of the Schwann cells of cutaneous nerves. They occur as solitary lesions or by the hundreds or thousands in neurofibromatosis. In the nail, however, virtually all the neurofibromas observed were isolated, so-called extraneural sporadic cutaneous neurofibromas, and not in association with any type of neurofibromatosis. Clinically, they may occur as a Koenen tumor-like lesion, grow subungually elevating the nail or causing nail dystrophy. Those of the proximal nail fold cause a longitudinal depression in the nail. Location in the lateral nail fold may imitate paronychia. Ulcerated neurofibromas look like periungual pyogenic granuloma. Enlargement of the distal phalanx is a rare finding.[269] Pain is rare. Neuromas and schwannomas are the main differential diagnosis in ungual neurofibromas.

Histopathology demonstrates faintly eosinophilic, circumscribed, but not encapsulated tumors. They consist of loosely and haphazardly arranged thin spindle cells with elongated wavy nuclei that are regularly spaced in a meshwork of fine wavy collagen fibers. PAS stain shows that the Schwann cells have a fine basal membrane. Mast cells can easily be discerned and are moderately increased in number. Immunohistochemistry is positive for protein S100 and a variety of other neural and Schwann cell markers.

Schwannoma

Subungual schwannoma is a chance observation as the diagnosis cannot be made clinically. Depending on its specific localization within the nail unit, the nail may be deformed, lifted, or a paronychia-like presentation may be seen. Histopathology is characterized by the formation of Verocay bodies, with or without Antoni A and B bodies, of the Schwann cells.

Granular cell tumor

Granular cell tumor has been described twice in the nail. One was a verrucous periungual growth in the deep medial portion of the proximal nail of a big toe causing a longitudinal depression in the nail, the other caused an enlargement of the middle toe with overgrowing of the nail. There may be tenderness of the lesion.[270,271]

Histopathologically, large granular Schwann cells are seen that may look like striated muscle cells. They are arranged in poorly cohesive nests, strands, and sheets of large cells. Rhabdomyoma may have a strikingly similar cytology.

Perineurioma

Perineurioma is a fibroma that expresses the immunocytochemical markers of perineurial cells, i.e., epithelial membrane antigen. Subungual location is very rare.[272] One case caused clubbing of the involved digit.[273]

Histopathology exhibits a well-circumscribed tumor with a thin fibrous capsule. Within it, a delicate fibrous matrix of fine collagen fibers and slender fusiform cells with bipolar cytoplasmic processes and plump angulated basophilic nuclei may be observed. The myxoid component can be important.

HISTIOCYTIC LESIONS

Histiocytes are cells with the potential to variable specialization. The differentiation of histiocytic and non-histiocytic lesions is often arbitrary as many cells, particularly those of bone and synovial tumors often display histiocytic markers that need to be used for accurate classification. CD14 is a marker for monocytes from which all other histiocytes are derived. Macrophages stain with CD14, CD68, and CD163. Dermal and interstitial dendritic cells are positive for CD14, CD163, factor XIIIa, and fascin. Langerhans cells stain with antibodies to CD1a, langerin, and protein S100 and are also demonstrable with peanut agglutinin (PNA).[274]

Histiocytic tumors

JUVENILE XANTHOGRANULOMA

Juvenile xanthogranuloma (JXG) is a benign proliferative disorder mostly seen in young children as a yellow to reddish-tan, painless, dome-shaped nodule in the face and on the trunk. Subungual xanthogranuloma is very rare.[275] It causes elevation and deformation of the nail plate. The clinical diagnosis, among others, concerns Spitz's nevus.

Histopathology reveals a characteristic granuloma-like infiltrate composed of lymphocytes, some eosinophils, foam cells, and giant cells both of foreign and Touton type. The latter exhibit a central homogeneously eosinophilic cytoplasm, a wreath of nuclei and an outer ring of foamy cytoplasm.

VERRUCIFORM XANTHOMA

Verruciform xanthoma (VX) is a reactive lesion seen in conditions with hyperplastic epidermis such as inflammatory linear verrucous nevus, congenital hemidysplasia with ichthyosiform erythroderma and limb defects (CHILD syndrome). One case involving the toenails was observed in a female patient with lymphedema.[276] Another patient had multiple lesions and an almost complete nail dystrophy in the involved digit[277]; this is also a common feature in CHILD syndrome. We have seen a young woman with a subungual VX of a fingernail causing onycholysis (Figure 26.52) and marked bacterial contamination. Most

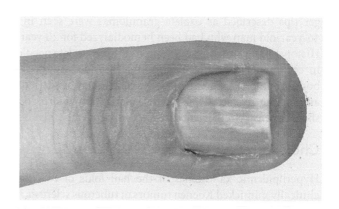

Figure 26.52 Subungual verruciform xanthoma.

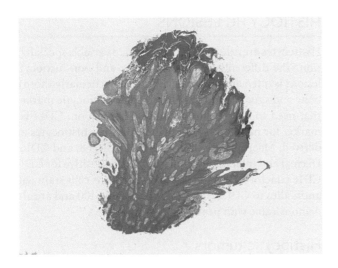

Figure 26.53 Subungual verruciform xanthoma, scanning magnification.

commonly, xanthoma cells are seen in elongated dermal papillae. The suprapapillary epidermis is thinned and may be parakeratotic (Figure 26.53). Hypercholesterolemia or hyperlipidemia are not observed.

TUMOR-LIKE DEPOSITIONS

Mucin

Mucin deposition is a characteristic for pretibial myxedema. It can be so extensive as to involve the toes and overgrow the nails. Histopathology of a biopsy is identical with focal mucinosis and myxoma.

Urate

Urate crystal deposition is a typical feature of gout. Tophi are exceptionally seen in the distal interphalangeal joint and the tip of the digits. A blood test reveals elevated uric acid levels.

Oxalate

Oxalate deposition is a feature of chronic renal failure. Tender, grouped, yellow-to-tan nodules at the finger tips described as oxalate granulomas were seen in a 46-year-old man who had been hemodialyzed for 20 years. Histopathology revealed crystalloid calcium oxalate needles in corymbiform arrangement and surrounded by foreign body granulomas. Foreign body giant cells may be scattered among the oxalate depositions. Polarization microscopy shows intense birefringence.[278]

Cholesterol

Hyperlipidemic xanthomas of the nail folds of two toes clinically mimicked Koenen tumors of tuberous sclerosis.[279] Histopathology is identical with hyperlipidemic xanthomatosis elsewhere.

BENIGN HEMATOGENOUS TUMORS

Benign tumorous hematogenous lesions are generally called pseudolymphoma. They are very rare in the nail region and do not display a characteristic clinical pattern.

BENIGN MELANOCYTIC LESIONS OF THE NAIL

Benign melanocytic lesions are of particular concern as they may be the hallmark of the most serious nail tumor, nail unit melanoma (NUM; see Nail dyschromias and malignant tumors, 8). Melanocytic lesions may be located anywhere in and around the nail unit. Depending on their specific localization the clinical aspect varies considerably. However, it is very important to note that the intensity of the brown to black color is not an indicator of its dignity. Histologically, three different types of lesions may cause a brown spot or a melanonychia: activation of melanocytes without numerical increase, lentigo and nevus, or melanoma. When this occurs in the nail matrix, a longitudinal brown streak develops in the nail as the overproduction of melanin leads to its incorporation in the newly formed nail plate. Localization in the nail bed is seen as a slightly blurred dark spot under the nail and localization around the nail appears as a brown spot or nevus similar to any other acral melanocytic lesion.

Melanocyte activation

Melanocyte activation is an extremely frequent phenomenon, particularly in individuals with dark complexion (Figure 26.54). When it occurs on the proximal nail fold, for instance like in Lifa's sign, it may be mistaken for a Hutchinson sign. In contrast to the latter, Lifa's sign is not well delimited and may be lighter in the cuticle region (Figure 26.55). Melanocyte activation in the matrix leads to functional melanonychia, which is physiologic in

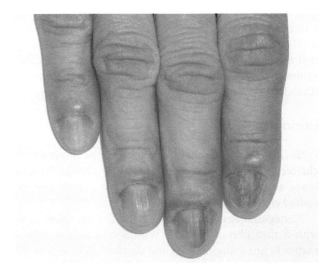

Figure 26.54 Melanocyte activation leading to longitudinal melanonychia in a 53-year-old Thai man.

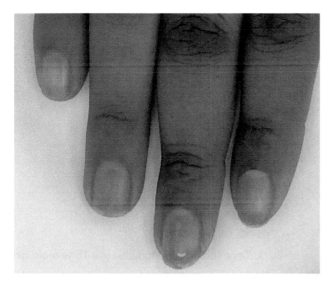

Figure 26.55 Lifa's disease (or sign) in a 21-year-old woman from Ethiopia.

dark-skinned races. It is seen on many nails, usually with many light brown bands on several or even all nails. In these persons, also friction from ill-fitting shoes or professional strain may cause functional melanonychia, which is more limited than the racial melanonychia. Drugs, malnutrition, pregnancy, nail picking, and many other events may also cause melanocyte activation in the matrix. In most cases of Laugier–Hunziker–Baran syndrome, there is only a functional melanonychia (Figure 26.56). Dermatoscopy usually demonstrates a band of greyish-brown lines on a grey background; in dark-skinned persons the background may also be brown (Figure 26.57). The problem of functional melanonychia is the clinical and histopathological differential diagnosis with NUM (see Malignant tumors).

Histopathology is often disappointing at first glance. In hematoxylin and eosin stained sections, the hyperpigmentation of the matrix specimen is barely visible,

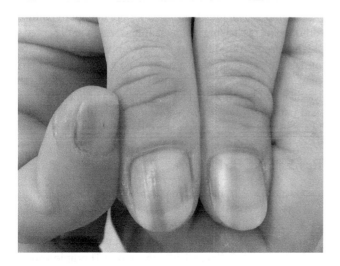

Figure 26.56 The nails in Laugier–Hunziker–Baran syndrome.

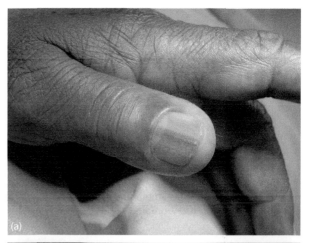

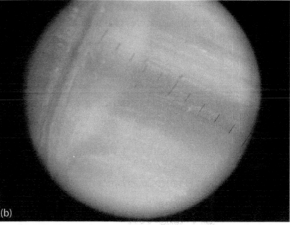

Figure 26.57 Longitudinal melanonychia in a Brazilian man. (a) Macrophotography; (b) Dermatoscopy.

individual melanocytes are not discernable, and the nail plate also reveals no or very little melanin. It is the differential staining with Fontana–Masson argentaffin reaction revealing the pigment and a melanocyte marker such as MelanA or HMB45 showing a normal number of melanocytes that allows the correct diagnosis to be made with certainty.[2]

Lentigo of the nail unit

Lentigines of the nail apparatus are rare. Around and under the nail they appear as a pigmented spot. In the matrix, they cause a circumscribed area of increase in pigment-producing melanocytes giving rise to a well-delimited longitudinal brown streak (Figure 26.58). This is seen as a brown band composed of brown lines on a brown background by dermatoscopy. Most matrix lentigines are seen in children and they have a propensity to fade between the age of 10 to 16 years.

Histopathology reveals an increase in the number of pigmented melanocytes without atypia and mitoses mainly in the basal and suprabasal layers of the matrix. The melanocytes are positive for MelanA and HMB45, but staining with S100 antibodies is less reliable.[2]

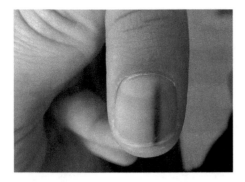

Figure 26.58 Longitudinal melanonychia due to a matrix lentigo in a fair-skinned woman.

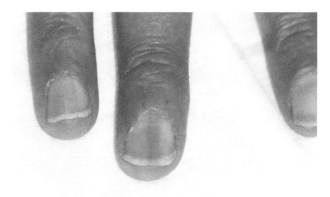

Figure 26.60 Longitudinal melanonychia in a 15-year-old girl.

The main differential diagnosis is early subungual melanoma, in which the melanocytes can look very bland and be equidistally distributed.

Nevi

Nevi are usually differentiated into congenital and acquired and may be further subclassified into various subtypes of melanocytic nevi including blue nevi. They are all relatively rare in the nail region and even the acquired nevi mostly occur in children.

Congenital nevi (Figure 26.59) are often very dark, almost black, may be very large and even distort the nail and distal phalanx. When they occupy the matrix, the nail plate is usually black. However, when they shine through the plate the nail may look like dirt, embarrassing the patient.

Acquired nevi are rare around the nail. When they are localized in the matrix they may cause a longitudinal melanonychia (Figure 26.60). Dermatoscopy shows a brown band made up of regularly distributed brown lines on a brown background; in children, often dark-brown spots are seen in the nail plate as a sign of transungual elimination of nevus cell nests. Some matrix nevi disappeared around puberty. Nevi of the nail bed remain visible as brown areas under the nail.

Histopathology reveals a proliferation of melanocytes in a lentiginous and nest-like pattern. Almost all matrix nevi in children and young adults are junctional nevi. Melanocyte atypia and mitoses are not seen.

A blue nevus is a collection of highly pigmented melanocytes in the dermis without junctional nests. Cases of "blue nevi with associated melanonychia" were most probably combined nevi.

As follows from the previous lines, histopathology is necessary in any suspicious case of melanonychia. This requires an adequate biopsy. It has to be stressed that it has to be taken from the matrix; a nail bed or plate biopsy does not allow a diagnosis to be made. There are different biopsy techniques that depend on the localization within the nail unit and the degree of suspicion. The melanocytic lesion of a very narrow band may be excised with a 3-mm punch as this is said not to leave a major nail dystrophy. If the brown band is in the lateral quarter of the nail, a lateral longitudinal biopsy is optimal. For all other lesions, we recommend the tangential nail matrix biopsy as described in 1999.[280,281] This technique yields a specimen of approximately 0.8 mm thickness that permits the diagnosis of virtually all melanocytic lesions in the matrix.[282]

Brown nail streaks are a particularly delicate problem in children. It is generally held that they are benign in children although metastasizing nail melanomas were also observed in this age group. This difficulty is even compounded in children of dark color in whom melanocyte activation in the matrix may occur. A general rule is that the browner the streaks the less likely they are malignant; however, when one stands out as a particularly dark one—the "ugly duckling sign"—or is black and rapidly growing a biopsy is indicated.[283,284]

REFERENCES

1. Haneke E. 'Onycholemmal' horn. *Dermatologica* 1983;167:155–158.
2. Haneke E. *Histopathology of the Nail–Onychopathology*. Boca Raton, FL: CRC Press;2017.
3. Haneke E. Differentialdiagnose und Therapie von Schwielen, Hühneraugen und Plantarwarzen. *Z Hautkr* 1982;57:263–272.

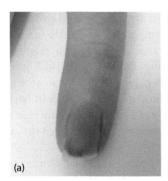
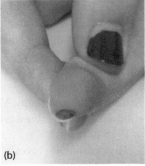

(a)   (b)

Figure 26.59 Congenital nevus of the distal nail bed and hyponychium in a 16-year-old girl. (a) Dorsal view; (b) Frontal view.

4. Poudyal S, Elpern DJ. Simple diagnostic tests for subungual pigmentation. *Dermatol Res Pract* 2009;2009:278040.

5. Baek HJ, Lee SJ, Cho KH et al. Subungual tumors: Clinicopathologic correlation with US and MR imaging findings. *Radiographics* 2010;30:1621–1636.

6. Baran R, Perrin C. Linear melanonychia due to subungual keratosis of the nail bed: A report of two cases. *Br J Dermatol* 1999;140:730–733.

7. Bon Mardion M, Poulalhon N, Balme B, Thomas L. Ungual seborrheic keratosis. *J Eur Acad Dermatol Venereol* 2010;24:1102–1104.

8. Perrin C, Cannata GE, Bossard C, Grill JM, Ambrossetti D, Michiels J-F. Onychocytic matricoma presenting as pachyonychia longitudinal. A new entity. *Am J Dermatopathol* 2012;34:54–59.

9. Spaccarelli N, Wanat KA, Miller CJ, Rubin AI. Hypopigmented onychocytic matricoma as a clinical mimic of onychomatricoma: Clinical, intraoperative and histopathologic correlations. *J Cutan Pathol* 2013;40:591–594.

10. Wanat KA, Reid E, Rubin AI. Onychocytic matricoma: A new, important nail-unit tumor mistaken for a foreign body. *JAMA Dermatol* 2014;150:335–337.

11. Baran R, Perrin C. Longitudinal erythronychia with distal subungual keratosis. Onychopapilloma of the nail bed and Bowen's disease. *Br J Dermatol* 2000;143:132–135.

12. Gee BC, Millard PR, Dawber RP. Onychopapilloma is not a distinct clinicopathological entity. *Br J Dermatol* 2002;146:156–157.

13. Criscione V, Telang G, Jellinek NJ. Onychopapilloma presenting as longitudinal leukonychia. *J Am Acad Dermatol* 2010;63:541–542.

14. Cohen PR. Longitudinal erythronychia: Individual or multiple linear red bands of the nail plate: A review of clinical features and associated conditions. *Am J Clin Dermatol* 2011;12:217–231.

15. Higashi N, Sugai T, Tamamoto T. Leukonychia striata longitudinalis. *Arch Dermatol* 1971;104:192–196.

16. de Berker D, Perrin C, Baran R. Localized longitudinal erythronychia: Diagnostic significance and physical explanation. *Arch Dermatol* 2004;140:1253–1257.

17. Miteva M, Fanti PA, Romanelli P, Zaiac M, Tosti A. Onychopapilloma presenting as longitudinal melanonychia. *J Am Acad Dermatol* 2012;66:e242–e243.

18. Jellinek NJ. Longitudinal erythronychia: Suggestions for evaluation and management. *J Am Acad Dermatol* 2011;64:167.e1–e11.

19. Samman PD. *The Nails in Disease*. 3rd ed. London, UK: Heinemann Publishing; 1978: p. 153.

20. Sass U, Kolivras A, Richert B, Moulonguet I, Goettmann-Bonvallot S, Anseeuw M, Theunis A, André J. Acantholytic tumor of the nail: Acantholytic dyskeratotic acanthoma. *J Cutan Pathol* 2009;36:1308–1311.

21. Higashi N. Focal acantholytic dyskeratosis. *Hifu* 1990;32:507–510.

22. Baran R, Perrin C. Focal subungual warty dyskeratoma. *Dermatology* 1997;195:278–280.

23. Baran R, Kint A. Onychomatrixoma. Filamentous tufted tumour in the matrix of a funnel-shaped nail: A new entity (report of three cases). *Br J Dermatol* 1992;126:510–515.

24. Haneke E, Fränken J. Onychomatricoma. *Dermatol Surg* 1995;21:984–987.

25. Kint A, Baran R, Geerts ML. The onychomatricoma: An electron microscopic study. *J Cutan Pathol* 1997;24:183–188.

26. Goettmann S, Drapé JL, Baran R, Perrin C, Haneke E, Belaïch S. Onychomatricome: Deux nouveaux cas. Intérêt de la résonancemagnétiquenucléaire. *Ann Dermatol Venereol* 1994;121(suppl 1):145.

27. Perrin C, Goettmann S, Baran R. Onychomatricoma: Clinical and histopathologic findings in 12 cases. *J Am Acad Dermatol* 1998;39:560–564.

28. Cloetingh D, Helm KF, Ioffreda MD, Billingsley E, Rubin AI, Haneke E. Onychomatricoma. *J Am Acad Dermatol* 2014;70:395–397.

29. Raison-Peyron N, Alirezai M, Meunier L, Barneon G, Meynadier J. Onychomatricoma: An unusual cause of nail bleeding. *Clin Exp Dermatol* 1998;23:138.

30. Fayol J, Baran R, Perrin C, Labrousse F. Onychomatricoma with misleading features. *Acta Derm Venereol* 2000;80:370.

31. Perrin C, Baran R. Onychomatricoma with matricial pterygium: Pathogenetic mechanism in 3 cases. *J Am Acad Dermatol* 2008;59:990–994.

32. Gaertner EM, Gordon M, Reed T. Onychomatricoma: Case report of an unusual subungual tumor with literature review. *J Cutan Pathol* 2009;36(Suppl. 1):66–69.

33. Soto R, Wortsman X, Corredoira Y. Onychomatricoma: Clinical and sonographic findings. *Arch Dermatol* 2009;145:1461–1462.

34. Perrin C, Baran R, Balaquer T et al. Onychomatricoma: New clinical and histological features. A review of 19 tumors. *Am J Dermatopathol* 2010;32:1–8.

35. Miteva M, Cadore de Farias D, Zaiac M, Romanelli P, Tosti A. Nail clipping diagnosis of onychomatricoma. *Arch Dermatol* 2011;147:1117–1118.

36. Misciali C, Fanti PA, Iorizzo M, Piraccini BM, Tosti A. Onychoblastoma–hamartoma of the nail unit: A new entity? (Abstr). *J Cut Pathol* 2005;32:104.

37. Misciali C, Iorizzo M, Fanti PA, Piraccini BM, Ceccarelli C, Santini D, Tosti A. Onychoblastoma (hamartoma of the nail unit): A new entity? *Br J Dermatol* 2005;152:1077–1078.

38. Ko CJ, Shi L, Barr RJ, Mölne L, Ternesten-Bratel A, Headington JT. Unguioblastoma and unguioblastic fibroma—An expanded spectrum of onychomatricoma. *J Cutan Pathol* 2004;31:307–311.

39. Petersson F, Tang ALY, Jin ACE, Barr RJ, Lee VK. Atypical cellular unguioblastic fibroma—A rare case with more atypical histological features than previously reported. *Am J Dermatopathol* 2010;32:387–391.

40. Baran R. Is onychoblastoma really a new entity? *Br J Dermatol* 2006;154:384–385.

41. Baran R, Dawber RPR, Richert B. Physical signs. In: Baran R, Dawber RPR, de Berker D, Haneke E, Tosti A, Eds. *Diseases of the Nails and Their Management*, 3rd ed. Oxford, UK: Blackwell Science; 2001: pp. 48–103.

42. Achten G, André J, Parent D et al. Le poil et l'ongle. *Dermatologica* 1985;171:494–495.

43. Hadj-Rabia S, Rimella A, Smahi A, Fraitag S, Hamel-Teillac D, Bonnefont JP, de Prost Y, Bodemer C. Clinical and histologic features of incontinentia pigmenti in adults with nuclear factor-κB essential modulator gene mutations. *J Am Acad Dermatol* 2011;64:508–515.

44. Chun SR, Rashid RM. Delayed onychodystrophy of incontinentia pigmenti: An evidence-based review of epidemiology, diagnosis and management. *J Drugs Dermatol* 2010;9:350–354.

45. Nicolaou N, Graham-Brown RA. Nail dystrophy, an unusual presentation of incontinentia pigmenti. *Br J Dermatol* 2003;149:1286–1288.

46. Piñol-Aguadé JP, Mascaró JM, Herrero C, Castel T. Tumeurs sous-unguéales dyskératosiques douloureuses et spontanément résolutives: Ses rapports avec l'incontinentia pigmenti. *Ann Dermatol Syphiligr* 1973;100:159–168

47. Mascaró JM, Palou J, Vives P. Painful subungual keratotic tumors in incontinentia pigmenti. *J Am Acad Dermatol* 1985;13:913–918.

48. Malvehy J, Palou J, Mascaró JM. Painful subungual tumour in incontinentia pigmenti. Response to treatment with etretinate. *Br J Dermatol* 1998;138:554–555.

49. Bukhari IA, Al-Mugharbel R. Subungual epidermoid inclusions. *Saudi Med J* 2004;25:522–523.

50. Fanti PA, Tosti A. Subungual epidermoid inclusions: Report of 8 cases. *Dermatologica* 1989;17:209–212.

51. Ocampo-Garza J, Di Chiacchio Ng, Di Chiacchio N, Haneke E. Verrucous epidermal nevus—A misleading diagnosis for 28 years. *J Eur Acad Dermatol* 2018;32(3):e109–e111.

52. Vicente MA, Baselga E, Garcia-Puig R et al. Porokeratotic eccrine duct and hair follicle naevus. A familial case with systematized involvement. *Ann Dermatol Vénéréol* 1998;125(Suppl 1):S176.

53. Berghs B, Feyen J. Intraosseous epidermal inclusion cyst following surgery for ingrowing toenail. *Foot* 1998;8:138–140.

54. Wadhams PS, McDonald JF, Jenkin WM. Epidermal inclusion cysts as a complication of nail surgery. *J Am Podiatr Med Ass* 1990;80:610–612.

55. Chavallaz O, Borradori L, Haneke E. Subungual epidermoid cyst: Report of a case with rapid growth and nail loss mimicking a malignant tumor. *J Clin Dermatol* 2010;1(2):73–75.

56. Miyazaki-Nakajima K, Hara H, Terui T. Subungual trichoadenoma showing differentiation toward follicular infundibulum. *J Dermatol* 2011;38:1118–1121.

57. Blatière V, Baran R, Barnéon G, Perrin C. A syringoma of the big toenail. *J Eur Acad Dermatol Venereol* 1999;12(Suppl 2):S128.

58. Barreto CA, Lipton MN, Smith HB, Potter GK. Intraosseous chondroid syringoma of the hallux. *J Am Acad Dermatol* 1994;30:374–378.

59. Theunis A, André J, Forton F, Wanet J, Song M. A case of subungual reactive eccrine syringofibroadenoma. *Dermatology* 2001;203:185–187.

60. Chen S, Palay D, Templeton SF. Familial eccrine syringofibroadenomatosis with associated ophthalmologic abnormalities. *J Am Acad Dermatol* 1998;39:356–358.

61. Fouilloux B, Perrin C, Dutoit M, Cambazard F. Clear cell syringofibroadenoma (of Mascaró) of the nail. *Br J Dermatol* 2001;144:625–627.

62. Mascaró JM. Considérations sur les tumeurs fibro-épithéliales: Le syringofibroadénome eccrine. *Ann Dermatol Syphilol* 1963;90:146–153.

63. Goettmann S, Marinho E, Grossin M, Bélaich S. Porome eccrine sous-unguéal. A propos de deux observations. *Ann Dermatol Vénéréol* 1995;122(Suppl1):S147–S148.

64. Arenas R. *Dermatología. Atlas, Diagnostico y Tratamiento*. Mexico: McGraw-Hill; 1987: pp. 539–540.

65. Al-Qattan MM, Al-Turaiki TM, Al-Oudah N, Arab K. Benign eccrine poroma of the dorsum of the hand: Predilection for the nail fold and P53 positivity. *J Hand Surg Eur* 2009;34:402–403.

66. Haim H, Chiheb S, Benchikhi H. An unusual case of eccrine poroma. *21st Cong Eur Acad Dermatol Venereol*, Prague, September 27–30, 2012: p. 371 Histopathology with clear cells.

67. Lin YT, Chen CM, Yang CH, Chuang YH. Eccrine angiomatous hamartoma: A retrospective study of 15 cases. *Chang Gung Med J* 2012;35:167–177.

68. Sanmartin O, Botella R, Alegre V, Martinez A, Aliaga A. Congenital eccrine angiomatous hamartoma. *Am J Dermatopathol* 1992;14:161–164.

69. Sezer E, Koseoglu RD, Filiz N. Eccrine angiomatous hamartoma of the fingers with nail destruction. *Br J Dermatol* 2006;154:1002–1004.

70. Gabrielsen TO, Elgjo K, Sommerschild H. Eccrine angiomatous hamartoma of the finger leading to amputation. *Clin Exp Dermatol* 1991;16:44–45.

71. Haneke E. Neuro-arterio-syringeal hamartoma in subungual location. *14th Int Cong Dermatol Surg*, Book of Abstracts, Sevilla, October 1–4, 1993: p. 85.

72. Domonkos AN, Suarez IN. Sudoriparous angioma. *Arch Dermatol* 1967:92:552–553.

73. Rositto A, Ranelleta M, Drut R. Congenital hemangioma of eccrine sweat glands. *Pediat Dermatol* 1993;10:341–343.

74. Man X-Y, Cai S-Q, Zhang A-H, Min Zheng M. Mucinous eccrine naevus presenting with hyperhidrosis: A Case Report. *Acta Derm-Venereol* 2006;86:554–555.

75. Baran R, Goettmann S. Distal digital keratoacanthoma: A report of 12 cases and review of the literature. *Br J Dermatol* 1998;139:512–515.

76. André J, Richert B. Kératoacanthome sous-unguéal. *Ann Dermatol Venereol* 2012;139:68–72.

77. Haneke E, Mainusch O, Hilker O. Subunguale Tumoren: Keratoakanthom, Neurofibrom, Nagelbett-Melanom. *Z Dermatol* 1998;184:86–102.

78. Gonzales-Ensenat A, Vilalta A, Torras H. Kératoacanthome péri et sous-unguéal. *Ann Dermatol Vénérél* 1988;115:329–331.

79. Hilker O, Winterscheidt M. Familiäre multiple Keratoakanthome. *Z Hautkr* 1987;62:284–289.

80. Haneke E. Multiple subungual keratoacanthomas. XIIth Int Cong Dermatol Surg, Munich 1991. *Zbl Haut- GeschlKr* 1991;159:337–338.

81. Stoebner PE, Fabre C, Delfour C, Joujoux JM, Roger P, Dandurand M, Meunier L. Solitary subungual keratoacanthoma arising in an MSH2 germline mutation carrier: Confirmation of a relationship by immunohistochemical analysis. *Dermatology* 2009;219:174–178.

82. Cecchi R, Troiano M, Buralli L, Innocenti S. Recurrent distal digital keratoacanthoma of the periungual region treated with Mohs micrographic surgery. *Australas J Dermatol* 2012;53:e5–e7.

83. Connolly M, Narayan S, Oxley J, de Berker DA. Immunohistochemical staining for the differentiation of subungual keratoacanthoma from subungual squamous cell carcinoma. *Clin Exp Dermatol* 2008;33:625–628.

84. Underhill T. Subungual keratoacanthoma: The importance of accurate diagnosis. *J Hand Surg Eur Vol* 2010;35:599–600.

85. González-Rodríguez AJ, Gutiérrez-Paredes EM, Montesinos-Villaescusa E, Burgués Gasión O, Jordá-Cuevas E. Subungual keratoacanthoma: The importance of distinguishing it from subungual squamous cell carcinoma. *Actas Dermosifiliogr* 2012;103(6):549–551.

86. Bowen AR, Burt L, Boucher K, Tristani-Firouzi P, Florell SR. Use of proliferation rate, p53 staining and perforating elastic fibers in distinguishing keratoacanthoma from hypertrophic lichen planus: A pilot study. *J Cutan Pathol* 2012;39:243–250.

87. Miteva L, Broshtilova V, Schwartz RA. Verrucous systemic lupus erythematosus. *Acta Dermatovenereol* 2009;17:301–304.

88. Baran R, Tosti A, De Berker D. Periungual keratoacanthoma preceded by a wart and followed by a verrucous carcinoma at the same site. *Acta Derm Venereol* 2003;83:232–233.

89. Scully C, Assad A. Mucinous syringometaplasia. *J Am Acad Dermatol* 1984;11:503–508.

90. Haneke E, Baran R. Subunguale Tumoren. *Z Hautkr* 1982;57:355–362.

91. Aldrich S, Hong CH, Groves L, Olsen C, Moss J, Darling T. Acral lesions in tuberous sclerosis complex: Insights into pathogenesis. *J Am Acad Dermatol* 2010;63:244–251.

92. Sampson JR, Harris PC. The molecular genetics of tuberous sclerosis. *Hum Mol Gen* 1994;3:1477–1480.

93. Haneke E. Intraoperative differential diagnosis of onychomatricoma, Koenen's tumours, and hyperplastic Bowen's disease. *J Eur Acad Dermatol Venereol* 1998;13 Suppl:S119.

94. Baykal C, Büyükbabani N, Yazganoglu KD, Saglik E. Acquired digital fibrokeratoma. *Cutis* 2007;79:129–132.

95. Sezer E, Bridges AG, Koseoglu D, Yuksek J. Acquired periungual fibrokeratoma developing after acute staphylococcal paronychia. *Eur J Dermatol* 2009;19:636–637.

96. Haneke E. Epidermoid carcinoma (Bowen's disease) of the nail simulating acquired ungual fibrokeratoma. *Skin Cancer* 1991;6:217–221.

97. Dominguez-Cherit J, Garcia C, Vega-Memije ME, Arenas R. Pseudo-fibrokeratoma: An unusual presentation of subungual squamous cell carcinoma in a young girl. *Dermatol Surg* 2003;29:788–789.

98. Cahn RL. Acquired periungual fibrokeratoma. *Arch Dermatol* 1977;113:1564–1568.

99. Haneke E. Subungual pseudomalignant osseous soft tissue tumor: Treatment for complete cure. *Eur J Clin Med Oncol* 2011;3(2):77–81.

100. Fraga GR, Patterson JW, McHargue CA. Onychomatricoma: Report of a case and its comparison with fibrokeratoma of the nail bed. *Am J Dermatopathol* 2001;23:36–40.

101. Rupp M, Khalluf E, Toker C. Subungual fibrous histiocytoma mimicking melanoma. *J Am Podiat Med Ass* 1957;3:141–142.

102. Metcalf JS, Maize JC, LeBoit PE. Circumscribed storiform collagenoma (sclerosing fibroma). *Am J Dermatopathol* 1991;13:122–129.

103. Al-Daraji WI, Ramsay HM, Ali RB. Storiform collagenoma as a clue for Cowden disease or PTEN hamartoma tumour syndrome. *J Clin Pathol* 2007;60:840–842.

104. Trufant JW, Greene L, Cook DL, McKinnon W, Greenblatt M, Bosenberg MW. Colonic ganglioneuromatous polyposis and metastatic adenocarcinoma in the setting of Cowden syndrome: A case report and literature review. *Hum Pathol* 2012;43:601–604.

105. Tosti A, Cameli N, Peluso AM. Storiform collagenoma of the nail. *Cutis* 1999;64:203–204.

106. Niessen FB, Spauwen PH, Schalkwijk J, Kon M. On the nature of hypertrophic scars and keloids: A review. *Plast Reconstr Surg* 1999;104:1435–1458.

107. Haneke E. Controversies in the treatment of ingrown nails. *Dermatol Res Pract* 2012:1–12. doi:10.1155/2012/783924.

108. Rushing ME, Sheehan DJ, Davis LS. Video game induced knuckle pad. *Pediatr Dermatol* 2006;23:455–457.

109. Küster W, Zehender D, Mensing H, Hennies HC, Reis A. Keratosis palmoplantaris diffusa Vörner. Klinische, formalgenetische und molekularbiologische Untersuchungen bei 22 Familien. *Hautarzt* 1995;46:705–710.

110. Meigel WN, Plewig G. Kauschwielen, eine Variante der Fingerknöchelpolster. *Hautarzt* 1976;27:391–395.

111. Yanguas I, Goday JJ, Soloeta R. Pachydermodactyly: Report of two cases. *Acta Derm Venereol* 1994;74:217–218.

112. Calikoğlu E. Pseudo-knuckle pads: An unusual cutaneous sign of obsessive-compulsive disorder in an adolescent patient. *Turk J Pediatr* 2003;45:348–349.

113. Hueston JT. Some observations on knuckle pads. *J Hand Surg Br* 1984;9:75–78.

114. Reye RD. Recurring digital fibrous tumors of childhood. *Arch Pathol* 1965;80:228–231.

115. Beckett JH, Jacobs AH. Recurring digital fibrous tumors of childhood: A review. *Pediatrics* 1977;59:401–406.

116. Sarma DP, Hoffmann EO. Infantile digital fibroma-like tumor in an adult. *Arch Dermatol* 1980;116:578–579.

117. Poppen NK, Niebauer JJ. Recurring digital fibrous tumor of childhood. *J Hand Surg Am* 1977;2:253–255.

118. Coskey RJ, Nabai H, Rahbari H. Recurring digital fibrous tumor of childhood. *Cutis* 1979;23:359–362.

119. Mehregan AH. Superficial fibrous tumors in childhood. *J Cutan Pathol* 1981;8:321–334.

120. Burgert S, Jones DH. Recurring digital fibroma of childhood. *J Hand Surg Br* 1996;21:400–402.

121. Niamba P, Léauté-Labrèze C, Boralevi F, Lepreux S, Chamaillard M, Vergnes P, Taieb A. Further documentation of spontaneous regression of infantile digital fibromatosis. *Pediat Dermatol* 2007;24:280–287.

122. Bacino CA, Stockton DW, Sierra RA, Heilstedt HA, Lewandowski R, Van den Veyver IB. Terminal osseous dysplasia and pigmentary defects: Clinical characterization of a novel male lethal X-linked syndrome. *Am J Med Genet* 2000;94:102–112.

123. Marzano AV, Berti E, Gasparini G, Vespasiani A, Scorza R, Caputo R. Unique digital skin lesions associated with systemic sclerosis. *Br J Dermatol* 1997;136:598–600.

124. Oteo-Álvaro A, Meizoso T, Scarpellini A, Ballestín C, Pérez-Espejo G. Superficial acral fibromyxoma of the toe, with erosion of the distal phalanx. A clinical report. *Arch Orthop Trauma Surg* 2008;128:271–274.

125. André J, Theunis A, Richert B, de Saint-Aubain N. Superficial acral fibromyxoma: Clinical and pathological features. *Am J Dermatopathol* 2004;26:472–474.

126. Kroft EBM, Haneke E, Pruszczinski M, Blokx WAM, Pasch MC. Een zeldzame subunguale tumor. *Ned T Dermatol Venereol* 2007;17:169–172.

127. Hollmann TJ, Bovée JV, Fletcher CD. Digital fibromyxoma (superficial acral fibromyxoma): A detailed characterization of 124 cases. *Am J Surg Pathol* 2012;36:789–798.

128. Hassenein A, Telang G, Benedetto E, Spielvogel R. Subungual myxoid pleomorphic fibroma. *Am J Dermatopathol* 1998;20:502–505.

129. Hsieh YJ, Lin YC, Wu YH, Su HY, Billings SD, Hood AF. Subungual pleomorphic fibromas. *J Cutan Pathol* 2003;30:569–571.

130. Kamino H, Lee JY, Berke A. Pleomorphic fibroma of the skin: A benign neoplasm with cytologic atypia. A clinic-pathologic study of eight cases. *Am J Surg Pathol* 1989;13:107–113.

131. Fong K, Rama Devi AR, Lai-Cheong JE, Chirla D, Panda SK, Liu L, Tosi I, McGrath JA. Infantile systemic hyalinosis associated with a putative splice-site mutation in the ANTXR2 gene. *Clin Exp Dermatol* 2012. doi:10.1111/j.1365-2230.201104287x.

132. Denadai R, Raposo-Amaral CE, Bertola D et al. Identification of 2 novel ANTXR2 mutations in patients with hyaline fibromatosis syndrome and proposal of a modified grading system. *Am J Med Genet A* 2012;158A:732–742.

133. Finlay AY, Ferguson SD, Holt PJ. Juvenile hyaline fibromatosis. *Br J Dermatol* 1983;108:609–616.

134. Puretic S, Puretic B, Fišer-Herman M et al. A unique form of mesenchymal dysplasia. *Br J Dermatol* 1962;74:8–19.

135. Rimbaud P, Jean R, Meynadier J, Rieu D, Guilhou JJ, Barnéon G. Fibro-hyalinose juvénile. *Bull Soc Fr Dermatol Syphiligr* 1973;80:435–436.

136. Ribeiro SLE, Guedes EL, Botan V, Barbosa A, Guedes de Freitas EJ. Juvenile hyaline fibromatosis: A case report and review of the literature. *Acta Reumatol Port* 2009;34:128–133.

137. Moosavi CA, Al-Nahar LA, Murphey MD, Fanburg-Smith JC. Fibroosseous pseudotumor of the digit: A clinicopathologic study of 43 new cases. *Ann Diagn Pathol* 2008;12:21–28.

138. Prevel CD, Hanel DP. Fibro-osseous pseudotumor of the distal phalanx. *Ann Plast Surg* 1996;36:321–324.

139. Abramovici L, Steiner GC. Bizarre parosteal osteochondromatous proliferation (Nora's lesion): A retrospective study of 12 cases, 2 arising in long bones. *Human Pathol* 2002;33:1205–1210.

140. Solana J, Bosch M, Español I. Florid reactive periostitis of the thumb: A case report and review of the literature. *Chir Main* 2003;22:99–103.

141. Patel MR, Desai SS. Pseudomalignant osseous tumor of soft tissue: A case report and review of the literature. *J Hand Surg* 1986;11:66–70.

142. Dupree WB, Enzinger FM. Fibro-osseous pseudotumor of the digits. *Cancer* 1986;58:2103–2109.

143. Ernstberger H. Metaplastische Knochengewebsbildung bei chronisch-narbenbildender Entzündung der rechten Großzehe. *Hautarzt* 1985;36:248.

144. Schütte HE, van der Heul RO. Reactive mesenchymal proliferation. *J Belge Radiol* 1992;75:297–302.

145. Shin J, Kim EH, Kim YC. A bonelike protrusion on the toe-Fibro-osseous pseudotumor (FOPT) of the digit. *Arch Dermatol* 2011;147:975–980.

146. Haneke E. Subungual intravascular papillary endothelial hyperplasia. *Z Dermatol* 184:141–157.

147. Landthaler M, Stolz W, Eckert F, Schmoeckel C, Braun-Falco O. Pseudo-Kaposi's sarcoma occurring after placement of arteriovenous shunt. *J Am Acad Dermatol* 1989;21:499–505.

148. Pimentel MIF, Cuzzi T, Azeredo-Coutinho RBG, Vasconcellos ECF, Benzi TSCG, Carvalho LMV. Acroangiodermatitis (Pseudo-Kaposi sarcoma): A rarely-recognized condition. A case on the plantar aspect of the foot associated with chronic venous insufficiency. *An Bras Dermatol* 2011;86(S1):S13–S16.

149. Mali JWH, Kuiper JP, Hamers AA. Acro-angiodermatitis of the foot. *Arch Dermatol* 1965;92:515–518.

150. Bluefarb SM, Adams LA. Arteriovenous malformation with angiodermatitis. Stasis dermatitis simulating Kaposi sarcoma. *Arch Dermatol* 1967;96:176–181.

151. Hwang SM, Lee SH, Ahn SK. Pincer nail deformity and pseudo Kaposi sarcoma: Complication of an artificial arteriovenous fistula for haemodialysis. *Br J Dermatol* 1999;141:1129–1132.

152. Alioua Z, Lamsyah H, Sbai M, Rimani M, Baba N, Ghfir M, Sedrati O. [Pseudo-Kaposi's sarcoma secondary to superficial arteriovenous malformation: Stewart-Bluefarb syndrome]. *Ann Dermatol Vénéréol* 2008;135:44–47.

153. Rao B, Unis M, Poulos E. Acroangiodermatitis: A study of ten cases. *Int J Dermatol* 1994;33:179–183.

154. Whimster IW. The pathology of lymphangioma circumscriptum. *Br J Dermatol* 1976;94:473–486.

155. Coffin CM, Dehner LP. Vascular tumors in children and adolescents: A clinicopathologic study of 228 tumors in 222 patients. *Pathol Annu* 1999;28:97.

156. Gurbuz Y, Muezzinoglu B, Apaydin R, Yumbul AZ. Acral arteriovenous tumor (cirsoid aneurysm): Clinical and histopathological analysis of 6 cases. *Adv Clin Path* 2002;6:25–29.

157. Burge SM, Baran R, Dawber RPR, Verret JL. Periungual and subungual arteriovenous tumours. *Br J Dermatol* 1986;115:361–366.

158. Mills SE, Cooper PH, Fechner RE. Lobular capillary hemangioma: The underlying lesion of pyogenic granuloma. A study of 73 cases from the oral and nasal mucous membranes. *Am J Surg Pathol* 1980;4:470–479.

159. Piraccini BM, Bellavista S, Misciali C, Tosti A, De Berker D, Richert B. Periungual and subungual pyogenic granuloma. *Br J Dermatol* 2010;163:941–953.

160. Baran R. Action thérapeutique et complications du retinoïde aromatique sur l'appareil unguéal. *Ann Dermatol Vénéréol* 1982;109:367–371.

161. Baran R. Pyogenic granuloma-like lesions associated with topical retinoid therapy. *J Am Acad Dermatol* 2002;47:970.

162. Tosti A, Piraccini BM, D'Antuono A, Marzaduri S, Bettoli V. Periungual inflammation and pyogenic granulomas during treatment with the antiretroviral drugs lamivudine and indinavir. *Br J Dermatol* 1999;140:1165–1168.

163. Williams LH, Fleckman P. Painless periungual pyogenic granulomata associated with reverse transcriptase inhibitor therapy in a patient with human immunodeficiency virus infection. *Br J Dermatol* 2007;156:163–164.

164. Bouscarat F, Bouchard C, Bouhour D. Paronychia and pyogenic granuloma of the great toes in patients treated with indinavir. *N Engl J Med* 1998;338:1776–1777.

165. Calista D, Boschini A. Cutaneous side effects induced by indinavir. *Eur J Dermatol* 2000;10:292–296.

166. Paul LJ, Cohen PR. Paclitaxel-associated subungual pyogenic granuloma: Report in a patient with breast cancer receiving paclitaxel and review of drug-induced pyogenic granulomas adjacent to and beneath the nail. *J Drugs Dermatol* 2012;11:262–268.

167. Curr N, Saunders H, Murugasu A, Cooray P, Schwarz M, Gin D. Multiple periungual pyogenic granulomas following systemic 5-fluorouracil. *Australas J Dermatol* 2006;47:130–133.

168. Segaert S, Van Cutsem E. Clinical signs, pathophysiology and management of skin toxicity during therapy with epidermal growth factor receptor inhibitors. *Ann Oncol* 2005;16:1425–1433.

169. High WA. Gefitinib: A cause of pyogenic granulomalike lesions of the nail. *Arch Dermatol* 2006;142:939.

170. Eichmann A, Baran R. Lectitis purulenta et granulomatosa (granulomatous purulent nail bed inflammation). *Dermatology* 1998;196:352–353.

171. Lee EJ, Lee JH, Shin MK, Lee SW, Haw CR. Acral angioosteoma cutis. *Ann Dermatol* 2011;23(Suppl 1):S105–S107.

172. Davies MG. Coccal nail fold angiomatosis. *Br J Dermatol* 1995;132:162–163.

173. Tosti A, Baran R, Peluso AM, Fanti PA, Liguori R. Reflex sympathetic dystrophy with prominent involvement of the nail apparatus. *J Am Acad Dermatol* 1993;29:865–868.

174. Camacho F, Ordoñez E. Reflex sympathetic dystrophy with nail involvement: Its role in atopic dermatitis. *Eur J Dermatol* 1996;6:172–174.

175. LeBoit PE, Berger TG, Egbert BM, Beckstead JH, Yen TSB, Stoler MH. Bacillary angiomatosis. The histopathology and differential diagnosis of a pseudoneoplastic infection in patients with human immunodeficiency virus disease. *Am J Surg Pathol* 1989;13:909–920.

176. Moulin C, Kanitakis J, Ranchin B, Chauvet C, Gillet Y, Morelon E, Euvrard S. Cutaneous bacillary angiomatosis in renal transplant recipients: Report of three new cases and literature review. *Transpl Infect Dis* 2012. doi:10.1111/j.1399-3062.2011.00713.x.

177. Seas C, Villaverde H, Maguiña C. A 60-year-old man from the highlands of Peru with fever and hemolysis. *Am J Trop Med Hyg* 2012;86:381.

178. Wilson-Jones E, Bleehen SS. Pseudo-pyogenic granuloma. *Br J Dermatol* 1969;81:804–816.

179. Rosai J, Gold J, Landy R. Histiocytoid haemangiomas. *Hum Pathol* 1979;10:707–729.

180. Verret JL, Avenel M, François H, Baudoin M, Alain P. Hémangiomes histiocytoïdes des pulpes digitales. *Ann Dermatol Vénéréol* 1983;110:251–257.

181. Avenel M, Verret JL, Fortier P. Finger localisation of Wilson–Jones pseudo-pyogenic granuloma. *XVI Int Congr Dermatol*, Tokyo, 1982. Tokyo, Japan: University of Tokyo Press.

182. Tosti A, Peluso AM, Fanti PA, Torresan F, Solmi L, Bassi F. Histiocytoid hemangioma with prominent fingernail involvement. *Dermatology* 1994;189:87–89.

183. Dannaker C, Piacquadio D, Willoughby CB, Goltz RW. Histiocytoid hemangioma: A disease spectrum. *J Am Acad Dermatol* 1989;21:404–409.

184. Risitano C, Gupta A, Burke F. Angiolymphoid hyperplasia with eosinophilia in the hand. *J Hand Surg* 1990;15B:376–377.

185. Kanekura T, Mizumoto J, Kanzaki T. Pachydermoperiostosis with angiolymphoid hyperplasia with eosinophilia. *J Dermatol* 1994;21:133–134.

186. Wilson Jones E, Bleehen SS. Inflammatory angiomatous nodules with abnormal blood vessels occurring about the ears and scalp (pseudo or atypical pyogenic granuloma). *Br J Dermatol* 1969;81:804–815.

187. Rosai J, Akerman LR. Intravenous atypical vascular proliferation. A cutaneous lesion simulating a malignant blood vessel tumor. *Arch Dermatol* 1974;109:714–717.

188. Bendl BJ, Asano K, Lewis RJ. Nodular angioblastic hyperplasia with eosinophilia and lymphofolliculosis. *Cutis* 1977;19:327–329.

189. Ramsay B, Dahl MG, Malcolm AJ, Soyer HP, Wilson-Jones E. Acral pseudolymphomatous angiokeratoma of children (APACHE). *Br J Dermatol* 1983;119(Suppl 33):13.

190. Hara M, Matsunaga J, Tagami H. Acral pseudolymphomatous angiokeratoma of children (APACHE). A case report and immunohistological study. *Br J Dermatol* 1991;124:387–388.

191. Dolph JL, Demuth RJ, Miller SH. Angiokeratoma circumscriptum of the index finger in a child. *Plast Reconstr Surg* 1981;67:221–223.

192. Pavithra S, Mallya H, Kini H, Pai GS. Verrucous hemangioma or angiokeratoma? A missed diagnosis. *Indian J Dermatol* 2011;56:599–600.

193. Leeson MC, Lowry L, McCue RW. Aneurysmal bone cyst of the distal thumb phalanx. A case report and review of the literature. *Orthopedics* 1988;11:601–604.

194. Schajowicz F, Aiello C, Slullitel I. Cystic and pseudocystic lesions of the terminal phalanx with special reference to epidermoid cysts. *Clin Orthop Rel Res* 1970;68:84–92.

195. Fuhs SE, Herndon JH. Aneurysmal bone cyst involving the hand: A review and report of two cases. *J Hand Surg Am* 1979;4:152–159.

196. Requena L, Baran R. Digital angioleiomyoma: An uncommon neoplasm. *J Am Acad Dermatol* 1993;29:1043–1044.

197. Sawada Y. Angioleiomyoma masquerading as a painful ganglion of the great toe. *Eur J Plast Surg* 1988;11:175–177.

198. Baran R, Requena L, Drapé J.L. Angioleiomyoma mimicking glomus tumour in the nail matrix. *Br J Dermatol* 2000;142:1239–1241.

199. Wood W. On painful subcutaneous tubercle. *Edinb Med J* 1812;8:28.

200. Parsons ME, Russo G, Fucich L, Millikan LE, Kim R. Multiple glomus tumors. *Int J Dermatol* 1997;36:894–900.

201. Di Chiacchio N, Loureiro WR, Di Chiacchio NG, Bet DL. Synchronous subungual glomus tumors in the same finger. *An Bras Dermatol* 2012;87(3):475–476.

202. Smalberger GJ, Suszko JW, Khachemoune A. Painful growth on right index finger. Subungual glomus tumor. *Dermatol Online J* 2011;17(9):12.

203. Miyamoto H, Wada H. Localized multiple glomangiomas on the foot. *J Dermatol* 2009;36:604–607.

204. Namazi MR, Hinckley ML, Jorizzo JL. Multiple collections of soft bluish nodules on the body. *Arch Dermatol* 2008;144:1383–1388.

205. Michal M, Fanburg-Smith JC, Lasota J, Fetsch JF, Lichy J, Miettinen M. Minute synovial sarcomas of the hands and feet: A clinicopathologic study of 21 tumors less than 1 cm. *Am J Surg Pathol* 2006;30:721–726.

206. Brems H, Park C, Maertens O et al. Glomus tumors in neurofibromatosis type 1: Genetic, functional, and clinical evidence of a novel association. *Cancer Res* 2009;69:7393–7401.

207. Harrison B, Sammer D. Glomus tumors and neurofibromatosis: A newly recognized association. *Plast Reconstr Surg Glob Open* 2014;2:e214.

208. Harrison B, Moore AM, Calfee R et al. The association between glomus tumors and neurofibromatosis. *J Hand Surg Am* 2013;38:1571–1574.

209. Lovas JG, Rodu B, Hammond HL, Allen CM, Wysocki GP. Caliber-persistent labial artery. A common vascular anomaly. *Oral Surg Oral Med Oral Pathol Oral Radiol Endod* 1998;86:308–312.

210. Lewis DM. Caliber-persistent labial artery. *J Okla Dent Assoc* 2003;93(3):37–39.

211. Wortsman X, Calderón P, Arellano J, Orellana Y. High-resolution color Doppler ultrasound of a caliber-persistent artery of the lip, a simulator variant of dermatologic disease: Case report and sonographic findings. *Int J Dermatol* 2009;48:830–833.

212. Ragsdale BD. Tumors with fatty, muscular, osseous, and/or cartilaginous differeniation. In: Elder DE, Ed. *Lever's Histopathology of the Skin*, 10th ed. Philadelphia, PA: Wolters Kluwer Lippincott Williams & Wilkins; 2009: pp. 1057–1106.

213. Richert B, André J, Choffray A, Rahier S, de la Brassinne M. Periungual lipoma: About three cases. *J Am Acad Dermatol* 2004;51(2 Suppl):S91–S93.

214. Bardazzi F, Savoia F, Fanti PA. Subungual lipoma. *Br J Dermatol* 2003;149:418.

215. Baran R. Periungual lipoma, an unusual site. *J Dermatol Surg Oncol* 1984;10:32–33.

216. Failla JM. Subungual lipoma, squamous carcinoma of the nail bed, and secondary chronic infection. *J Hand Surg A* 1996;21:512–514.

217. Bancroft LW, Kransdorf MJ, Peterson JJ, O'Connor MI. Benign fatty tumors: Classification, clinical course, imaging appearance, and treatment. *Skeletal Radiol* 2006;35:719–733.

218. Kwon NH, Kim HS, Kang H, Lee JY, Kim HO, Kang SJ, Park YM. Subungual spindle cell lipoma. *Int J Dermatol* 2011. doi:10.1111/j.1365-4632.2011.04963.x.

219. Haneke E. Operative Therapie der myxoiden Pseudozyste. In: Haneke E, Ed. *Gegenwärtiger Stand der operativen Dermatologie. Fortschritte der operativen Dermatologie* 4. Heidelberg, Germany: Springer; 1988: pp. 221–227.

220. Gourdin IW, Lang PG. Cylindrical deformity of the nail plate secondary to subungual myxoma. *J Am Acad Dermatol* 1996;35:846–848.

221. Rozmaryn LM, Schwartz MA. Treatment of subungual myxoma preserving the nail matrix: A case report. *J Hand Surg* 1998;23A:178–180.

222. Haneke, E. Dorsal finger cyst. *13th Ann Meet Soc Cutan Ultrastruct Res & Eur Soc Comp Skin Biol*, Paris, France, May 28–31, 1986, Abstract.

223. Cremer H, Gullotta F, Wolf L. The Mafucci-Kast syndrome. Dychondroplasia with hemangiomas and frontal lobe astrocytoma. *J Cancer Res Oncol* 1981;101:231–237.

224. Koff AB, Goldberg LH, Ambergel D. Nail dystrophy in a 35-year-old man. Subungual enchondroma. *Arch Dermatol* 1996;132:223, 226.

225. Dumontier CA, Abimelec P. Nail unit enchondromas and osteochondromas: A surgical approach. *Dermatol Surg* 2001;27:274–279.

226. Ishii T, Ikeda M, Oka Y. Subungual extraskeletal chondroma with fingernail deformity: Case report. *J Hand Surg* 2010;35A:296–299.

227. Burgdorf W, Nasemann T. Cutaneous osteomas: A clinical and histopathologic review. *Arch Dermatol Res* 1977;260:121–135.

228. Blatière V, Baran R, Barneon G. An osteoma cutis of the nail matrix. *J Eur Acad Dermatol Venereol* 1999;12(Suppl 2):126.

229. Cambiaghi S, Imondi D, Gangi S et al. Fingertip calcinosis cutis. *Cutis* 2000;66:465–467.

230. Fischer E. Subunguale Verkalkungen im normalen Nagelbett der Finger. *Hautarzt* 1983;34:625–627.

231. Fischer E. Weichteilverkalkungen am Rand der Tuberositas phalangis distalis der Finger. *Fortschr Röntgenther* 1983:139:150–157.

232. Di Giovanni C, Laudati A. L'esostosi subungueale dell'alluce. *Arch Putti Chir Organi Mov* 1986;36:137–142.

233. Stieler W, Reinel D, Jänner M, Haneke E: Ungewöhnliche Lokalisation einer subungualen Exostose. *Akt Dermatol* 1989;15:32–34.

234. Sebastian G. Subunguale Exostosen der Großzehe, Berufsstigma bei Tänzern. *Dermatol Mschr* 1977;163:998–1000.

235. Mertens F, Möller E, Mandahl N, Picci P, Perez-Atayde AR, Samson I, Sciot R, Debiec-Rychter M. The t(X;6) in subungual exostosis results in transcriptional deregulation of the gene for insulin receptor substrate 4. *Int J Cancer* 2011;128:487–491.

236. Ippolito E, Falez F, Tudisco C, Balus L, Fazio M, Morrone A. Subungual exostosis. Histological and clinical considerations on 30 cases. *Ital J Orthop Traumatol* 1987;13:81–87.

237. Fischer E. Subunguale Verkalkungen. *Fortschr Röntgenol* 1982;137:580–584.

238. Apfelberg DB, Druker D, Maser M, Lash H. Subungual osteochondroma. *Arch Dermatol* 1979;115:472–473.

239. Richert B, Baghaie M. Medical imaging and MRI in nail disorders: Report of 119 cases and review of the literature. *Dermatol Ther* 2002;15:159–164.

240. Unlu S, Demirkale I, Kalkan T, Tunc B, Bozkurt M. Large subungual exostosis of the great toe: A case report. *J Am Podiatr Med Ass* 2010;100:296–298.

241. Solomon L. Chondrosarcoma in hereditary multiple exostosis. *S Afr Med J* 1974;48:671–676.

242. Schulze KE, Hebert AA. Diagnostic features, differential diagnosis, and treatment of subungual osteochondroma. *Pediatr Dermatol* 1994;11:39–41.

243. Szabó RM, Smith B. Possible congenital osteoid osteoma of a phalanx; case report. *J Bone Joint Surg* 1985;67A:815–816.

244. Becce F, Jovanovic B, Guillou L, Theumann N. Painful finger tip swelling of the middle finger. Osteoid osteroma of the distal phalanx of the middle finger. *Skeletal Radiol* 2011;40:1479–1480.

245. Jaffé HL. Osteoid osteoma. A benign osteoblastic tumor composed of osteoid and atypical bone. *Arch Surg* 1935;31:709–728.

246. Wold LE, Pritchard DI, Bergert I, Wilson DM. Prostaglandin synthesis by osteoid osteoma and osteoblastoma. *Mod Pathol* 1988;1:129–131.

247. Burger IM, McCarthy EF. Phalangeal osteoid osteomas in the hand: A diagnostic problem. *Clin Orthop Relat Res* 2004;427:198–203.

248. Shankman S, Desai P, Beltran J. Subperiosteal osteoid osteoma: Radiographic and pathologic manifestations. *Skeletal Radiol* 1997;26:457–462.

249. Meng Q, Watt I. Phalangeal osteoid osteoma. *Br J Radiol* 1989;62:321–325.

250. Gil S, Marco SF, Arenas J, Irurzun J, Agullo T, Alonso S, Fernandez F. Doppler duplex color localization of osteoid osteomas. *Skelet Radiol* 1999;28:107–110.

251. Ayala AG, Murray JA, Erling MA, Raymond AK. Osteoid osteoma: Intraoperative tetracycline fluorescence demonstration of the nidus. *J Bone Joint Surg* 1986;68A:747–751.

252. Di Gennaro GL, Lampasi M, Bosco A, Donzelli O. Osteoid osteoma of the distal thumb phalanx: A case report. *Chir Organi Mov* 2008;92:179–182.

253. Cheung FMF, Wu WC, Lam CK, Fu YK. Diagnostic criteria for pseudomalignant osteoblastoma. *Histopathology* 1997;31:196–200.

254. Goettmann S, Baran R, Fraitag S et al. Tumeurs à cellules géantes osseuses avec atteinte unguéale. *Ann Dermatol Vénéréol* 1995;122(Suppl 1):S148–S149.

255. Rosai J. Bone and joints. In: Rosai J, Ed. *Rosai and Ackerman's Surgical Pathology*, 10th ed. Chapter 24. Edinburgh, UK: Elsevier Mosby; 2011: pp. 2043–2046.

256. Goldsmith E. Solitary bone cyst of the distal phalanx. A case report. *J Am Podiatr Ass* 1966;5:69–70.

257. Richert B, André J. Laterosubungual giant cell tumor of the tendon sheath: An unusual location. *J Am Acad Dermatol* 1999;41:347–348.

258. Abimelec P, Cambiaghi S, Thioly D, Moulonguet I, Dumontier C. Subungual giant cell tumor of the tendon sheath. *Cutis* 1996;58:273–275.

259. Pulitzer DR, Martin PC, Reed RJ. Fibroma of tendon sheath. A clinicopathologic study of 32 cases. *Am J Surg Pathol* 1989;13:472–479.

260. Reed RJ, Pulitzer DR. Tumors of neural tissue. In: Elder DE, Ed. *Lever's Histopathology of the Skin*, 10th ed. Philadelphia, PA: Wolters Kluwer Lippincott Williams & Wilkins; 2009: pp. 1107–1149.

261. Zook EG. Complications of the perionychium. *Hand Clin* 1988;2:407–427.

262. Sreedharan S, Teoh LC, Chew WY. Neuroma of the radial digital nerve of the middle finger following trigger release. *Hand Surg* 2011;16:95–97.

263. Jokinen CH, Ragsdale BD, Argenyi ZB. Expanding the clinicopathologic spectrum of palisaded encapsulated neuroma. *J Cutan Pathol* 2010;37:43–48.

264. Runne U. Syndrom der multiplen Neurome mit metastasierendem medullärem Schilddrüsenkarzinom ('Multiple mucosal neuroma-syndrome'). *Z Hautkr* 1977;52:299–301.

265. Hartzell TL, Taylor H. Traumatic amputation of a supernumerary digit: A 16-year-old boy's perspective of suture ligation. *Pediatr Dermatol* 2009;26:100–102.

266. Leber GE, Gosain AK. Surgical excision of pedunculated supernumerary digits prevents traumatic amputation neuromas. *Pediatr Dermatol* 2003;20:108–112.

267. Haneke E. Pacinian neuroma of the nail apparatus. *19th Sem Dermatopathol*, Vars, France, 2012.

268. Rhode CM, Jennings WD, Jr. Pacinian corpuscle neuroma of digital nerves. *South Med J* 1975;68:86–89.

269. Baran R, Haneke E. Subungual myxoid neurofibroma on the thumb. *Acta Derm Venereol* 2001;81:210–211.

270. Hasson A, Arias MC, Guttierez A et al. Periungual granular cell tumour. A light microscopic, immunohistochemical and ultrastructural study. *Skin Cancer* 1991;6:41–46.

271. Peters JS, Crowe MA. Granular cell tumor of the toe. *Cutis* 1998;62:147–148.

272. Baran R, Perrin C. Perineurioma: A tendon sheath fibroma-like variant in a distal subungual location. *Acta Derm Venereol* 2003;83:60–61.

273. Baran R, Perrin C. Subungual perineurioma: A peculiar location. *Br J Dermatol* 2002;146:125–128.

274. Burgdorf WHC, Zelger B. The histiocytoses. In: Elder DE, Ed. *Lever's Histopathology of the Skin*, 10th ed. Philadelphia, PA: Lippincott Williams & Wilkins; 2009: pp. 667–688.

275. Chang P, Baran R, Villanueva C, Samayoa M, Perrin C. Juvenile xanthogranuloma beneath a fingernail. *Cutis* 1996;58:173–174.

276. Chyu J, Medenica M, Whitney DH. Verruciform xanthoma of the lower extremity: Report of a case and review of literature. *J Am Acad Dermatol* 1987;17:695–697.

277. Mountcastle EA, Lupton GP. Verruciform xanthomas of the digits. *J Am Acad Dermatol* 1989;20:313–317.

278. Sina B, Lutz LL. Cutaneous oxalate granuloma. *J Am Acad Dermatol* 1990;22:316–317.

279. Keller PH. Hypercholesterinämische Xanthomatose. *Dermatol Wochenschr* 1960:14:336–337.

280. Haneke E. Operative Therapie akraler und subungualer Melanome. In: Rompel R, Petres J, Eds. *Operative und onkologische Dermatologie. Fortschritte der operativen und onkologischen Dermatologie.* Berlin, Germany: Springer; 1999: pp. 210–214.

281. Haneke E, Baran R. Longitudinal melanonychia. *Dermatol Surg* 2001;27:580–584.

282. Di Chiacchio N, Refkalefsky Loureiro W, Schwery Michalany N, Kezam Gabriel FV. Tangential biopsy thickness versus lesion depth in longitudinal melanonychia: A pilot study. *Dermatol Res Pract* 2012;2012, Article ID 353864.

283. Haneke E. Melanonychia. In: Baran R, Hadj-Rabia S, Silverman R, Eds. *Pediatric Nail Disorders.* Boca Raton, FL: CRC Press; 2017: pp. 169–180.

284. Di Chiacchio N, Tosti A, Eds. *Melanonychias.* Cham, Switzerland: Springer; 2017.

Malignant tumors

ECKART HANEKE

Malignant tumors of the nail apparatus are relatively rare.[1,2] The main reason for the scarcity of malignant nail neoplasms is that the nail plate is a very effective ultraviolet protective shield that does not permit harmful doses to penetrate.[3] Also, other potential carcinogens are exceptional. On the other hand, virtually all tissues of the tip of the digit may give rise to malignant tumors and also metastases are occasionally seen.

New or recurrent swellings and lesions not responding to treatment based on an initial clinical impression should be subjected to biopsy.[4]

MALIGNANT NAIL-SPECIFIC TUMORS

The nail-specific malignant neoplasms have only recently been described and their characteristics are not yet fully defined.[1,2]

Onychocytic carcinoma

Onychocytic carcinoma (OCC) is a rare low-grade neoplasm that requires histopathology for its diagnosis.[1,2] The nail plate is thickened, discolored, and rough.[5] End-on dermatoscopy shows minute holes in the nail plate that are much smaller than those of onychomatricoma. The main clinical differential diagnosis is Bowen's disease. Treatment is complete excision, best performed by Mohs surgery. Most cases were in situ, but one showed invasion.[6] Histopathology demonstrates a circumscribed matrix tumor with small extensions into the nail plate. It exhibits a keratogenous zone like its benign counterpart, the onychocytic matricoma.[2]

Onycholemmal carcinoma

Onycholemmal carcinoma (OLC) is an uncommon neoplasm of the nail bed in elderly individuals. It is seen as a warty, crusted, nodular, or ulcerated lesion (Figure 27.1a). Half of the lesions are asymptomatic. Treatment is by surgery, but radiation and curettage were also successfully performed. Amputation is not warranted. Recurrences were not observed after any of these therapeutic approaches.[7] The most important differential diagnoses are squamous cell carcinoma (SCC), Bowen's disease, and onycholemmal horn. It is probably identical with malignant proliferating onycholemmal cyst.[8]

Histologically, invasive cell complexes with abrupt keratinization are seen that may form small cysts or remain solid. Areas of clear cells are often seen. Atypical mitoses are present (Figure 27.1b and c).[2]

MALIGNANT EPITHELIAL NAIL TUMORS

Bowen's disease and SCC are the most common malignancies of the nail. As a whole, they are relatively rare and a high index of clinical suspicion is necessary to make an early correct diagnosis, which in many cases is the prerequisite for a good prognosis.

Actinic keratosis

Actinic keratosis, the most common precancerous lesion, is very rare in the nail region and does not occur under it. It may present as a hyperkeratotic or crusted rough lesion with telangiectasiae on an erythematous base on the proximal nail fold. The clinical differential diagnosis is broad and comprises of warts, chronic radiodermatitis, arsenical keratosis, keratoacanthoma, Bowen's disease, SCC,

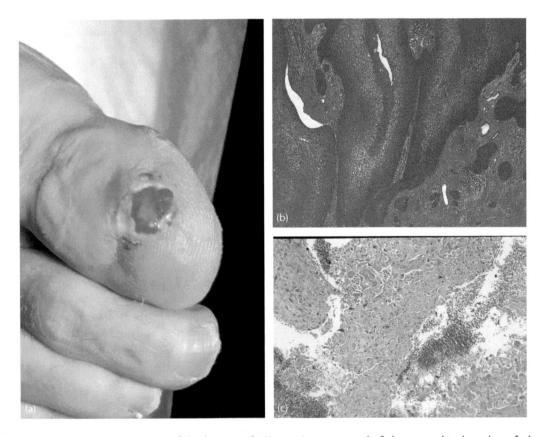

Figure 27.1 (a) Onycholemmal carcinoma of the big toe; (b) Tumor is composed of sheets and trabeculae of pleomorphic, poorly differentiated carcinoma with abrupt eosinophilic keratinization (H&E × 100); (c) The infiltrating carcinoma is composed of atypical squamous cells with eosinophilic onycholemmal keratinization (H&E × 400).

other carcinomas, other cutaneous horns, and a variety of other lesions that may occasionally develop hyperkeratosis. Patients with insufficient DNA repair, e.g., xeroderma pigmentosum, are prone to develop hundreds of actinic keratoses including on the distal phalanx that tend to degenerate to invasive SCC.[2]

Histopathology shows a keratinocytic intraepidermal neoplasia (KIN) or dermal intraepithelial neoplasia (DIN) and is graded from I to III. There are different types of solar keratoses but in the nail region it is either hyperkeratotic or atrophic.[2]

Arsenical keratosis

Arsenical keratoses are mainly seen in regions with a high content of arsenic in the drinking water [India (West bengal), Bangladesh] or after professional exposure.[9,10] This may be associated with arsenical melanosis. The therapeutic administration of arsenical compounds such as Fowler's solution or Asiatic pills was declared obsolete many decades ago, although there are countries in which they are still used to treat psoriasis and lichen planus. With the advent of Ayurvedic medicine, a new source of chronic arsenicism has appeared.[11] Patients with arsenical keratoses have a very high risk to develop various cutaneous as well as internal cancers. The diagnosis must therefore prompt a general check-up of the patient. Arsenical keratoses appear as small, hard keratotic papules that develop anywhere on the skin, but particularly on the palms and soles. They are said to exhibit a higher autofluorescence with ultraviolet light than the surrounding epidermis of the palms and soles.[10] Around and under the nails, keratotic papules and plaques develop that may eventually degenerate to Bowen's disease and/or SCC.[12] Nail dystrophy is an unspecific sign. Actinic keratosis, Bowen's disease, SCC, and basal cell carcinoma (BCC) are the most important differential diagnoses.

The histopathology resembles that of actinic keratosis or even Bowen's disease with loss of polarity of the basal cells, large hyperchromatic nuclei, clumping, atypical mitoses, and dyskeratoses, but there are often larger areas of hyperkeratosis without obvious nuclear atypia.[13] Some lesions may progress to a mixture of Bowen's disease and BCC. Actinic elastosis is usually absent.[2]

Bowen's disease

Bowen's disease is an in situ carcinoma and said to be the most frequent malignancy of the nail. Arsenic, other potential carcinogenic compounds, chronic X-irradiation,[14] and high-risk human papillomaviruses are etiologic agents. It is seen in middle-aged to elderly persons with a peak incidence between 50 and 70 years. Males predominate and fingers are more often affected than toes. The diagnosis

of ungual Bowen's disease is very often delayed for many months or years. Bowen's disease on palms and soles is very obvious as a reddish plaque with irregular hyperkeratosis. Localization in the webspace of the toes exhibits a macerated white keratosis. Ulceration may be a sign of beginning invasion. On the finger pulp and at the hyponychium, it usually looks like a flat, fissured wart. On the proximal nail fold, its clinical appearance is often that of a red, flat, hyperkeratotic, or verrucous plaque, but it may also present as a reddish macule, particularly in association with an erythematous plaque.[15] In the lateral groove, the most frequent nail localization, it may be verrucous, macerated or even fibrokeratoma-like (Figures 27.2 through 27.4).[16] Where it affects the cuticle this appears whitish. Longitudinal leukonychia and nail dystrophy[17] are the result of matrix involvement. Erythronychia, either as a single red line or several lines, may be observed.[18] Subungual localization often presents as onycholysis (Figure 27.5).[19] Marked hyperkeratosis may resemble pachyonychia congenita or a cutaneous horn.[20] Pigmented Bowen's disease of the nail causes regular or irregular longitudinal melanonychia or pigmentation of the skin surrounding the nail.[21] Multiple digits are rarely affected by ungual Bowen's disease.[22] In recent years, many cases of ungual Bowen's disease due to high-risk human papillomaviruses such as HPV 16, 18, 26, 33, 34, 35, 45, 51, 53, 73, and more were identified.[23] They are also found in genital lesions indicating a genital-to-digital infection or auto-inoculation.[24] Co-infection of different HPV types is possible.[25] HPV 56-induced ungual Bowen's disease is often associated with longitudinal melanonychia.[26] Longitudinal melanonychia was also seen in a patient with epidermodysplasia verruciformis of Lewandowsky-Lutz and subungual Bowen's disease.[27] Bowen's disease is very rare in toes. Although Bowen's disease of the nail is more likely to progress to invasive carcinoma,[28] it is less likely to metastasize. The treatment of choice of ungual Bowen's

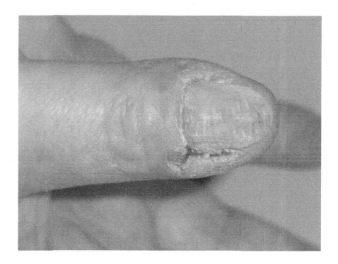

Figure 27.2 Subungual and periungual Bowen's disease mimicking an atypical wart.

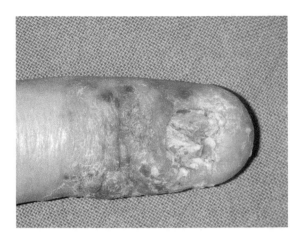

Figure 27.3 Long-standing pigmented Bowen's disease in a 38-year-old Brazilian woman.

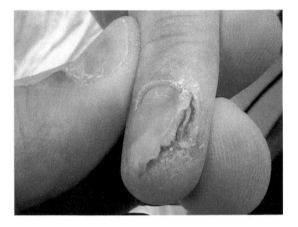

Figure 27.4 Bowen's disease of the nail. (Courtesy of Dr Yiannis Neofytou, Greece.)

disease is Mohs micrographic surgery,[29] but other surgical and non-surgical methods have also been used. Clinical differential diagnoses depend on the localization in the nail apparatus and comprise viral warts, paronychia, psoriasis, onychomycosis and other infections, arsenical keratosis, actinic keratosis, subungual exostosis, onychomatricoma, SCC, and many more.

Bowen's disease is a classical in situ carcinoma or intraepithelial neoplasia grade IV. Around the nail, it shows an acanthotic thickening of the epidermis that lacks an orderly architecture in its entire thickness. Papillomatosis and hyperkeratosis are common. There is crowding and loss of polarity of the basal cells large and pleomorphic, often hyperchromatic nuclei. Some cells have more clumped nuclei, and all stages of mitoses including many pathologic ones are seen in all layers. Dyskeratoses and necrotic keratinocytes in mitosis are a frequent finding; dyskeratosis may be the only sign in some areas. In many cases, perinuclear vacuolization is seen suggesting a viral cause. Subungual Bowen's disease is similar but its hyperkeratosis is much less pronounced. When the nail is clipped with the nail bed keratosis it contains dyskeratoses and some large nuclei allowing the diagnosis of Bowen's diseases to be suspected. Clear-cell Bowen's disease has been described, both with large round Paget-like and trichilemmal sheath-like cells.[17] Bowen's disease of the matrix results in inclusion of dyskeratotic cells into the nail plate clinically appearing as leukonychia. Pigmented Bowen's disease is due to dendritic melanocytes populating the lesion. Immunohistochemistry for HPV and PCR are positive in HPV-related Bowen's disease.[2]

Bowenoid papulosis of the periungual skin was described both with (HPV 42) and without[30] concomitant genital

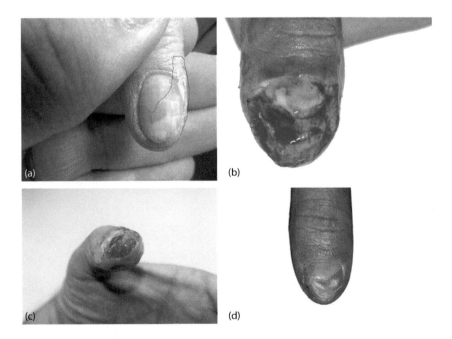

Figure 27.5 Bowen's disease of the nail. (a) The extent of the planned excision is marked; (b) Two days after surgical removal of the lesion; (c) Frontal view; (d) One month after surgery, dorsal view.

lesions as well as in an HIV patient.[31] It is said to exhibit more focal and less intense changes; however, this distinction is apparently often not made.

Squamous cell carcinoma

SCC is very frequent in light-skinned Caucasians. Most SCCs develop in sun-exposed skin as hard keratotic nodules with a tendency to ulcerate. They are very common in organ transplant recipients[32] and other immunodeficiency states such as epidermodysplasia verruciformis. In the nail unit, SCCs occur in subungual location, on the proximal or lateral nail folds, and very rarely in the hyponychium/finger pulp region. The common sign of subungual SCC is onycholysis with oozing—a sign shared with subungual Bowen's and rarely other subungual diseases. Bleeding and formation of a nodule or ulceration indicate invasion (Figures 27.6 through 27.8). Bone invasion is rare.[33] Metastases have been observed in SCC patients with ectodermal dysplasia,[34] but more recently also independently.[35] Removal of the overlying onycholytic nail plate is essential to make the diagnosis (Figure 27.6). The diagnostic delay may be up to

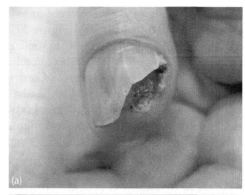

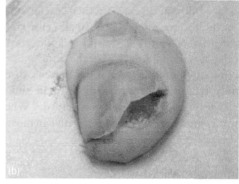

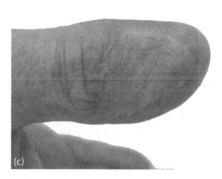

Figure 27.7 Invasive subungual squamous cell carcinoma. (a) Preoperative view; (b) Surgical specimen; (c) Two years after wide local excision and defect repair with a full-thickness skin graft.

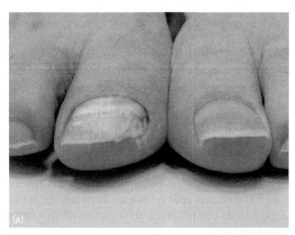

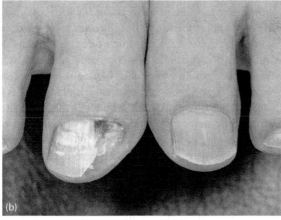

Figure 27.6 Subungual squamous cell carcinoma of the big toe. (a) Clinical aspect; (b) Removal of the overlying nail plate reveals the extent of the carcinoma.

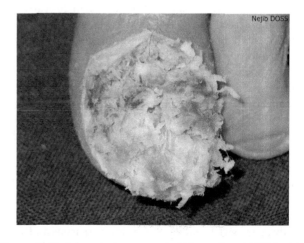

Figure 27.8 Advanced squamous cell carcinoma of the big toenail. (Courtesy of Prof Dr Nejib Doss, Tunis.)

40 years.[36] Treatment of choice of subungual SCC is microscopically controlled surgery (Figure 27.7).

Histopathologically, periungual SCC is similar to SCC in other locations.[37] Large atypical epithelial proliferations extend into the dermis. A variable degree of keratinization and superficial ulceration is present. The basal as well as spinous-appearing cells display a high degree of atypia with large and hyperchromatic nuclei. Atypical mitoses occur in the entire tumor thickness. The orderly stratification is lost. In long-standing SCC, deep invasion down to the bone may be seen, but this is rare subungually. It appears that two types of subungual SCC exist: one derived from HPV-induced Bowen disease, another developing *de novo*. Whereas the former often shows small cells, koilocytosis and clear cells, the latter is devoid of koilocytes and has larger cells thus resembling SCC of the skin.[2]

Bowen's carcinoma derives from Bowen's disease and commonly retains some similarity with in situ Bowen's lesions.[38] Clear cells are more often observed.[39] Whereas p16 is positive in in situ carcinoma it is negative in most invasive ones.[40]

Carcinoma cuniculatum

Carcinoma cuniculatum is a very slow-growing neoplasm and virtually never metastasizes. It is most frequently found in the webspace between the toes where it causes channels and sinuses often releasing a smelly material upon pressure. Some cases were observed in the nail apparatus with distal-lateral onycholysis and paronychia, nail bed inflammation, and discharge of a foul-smelling yellow-white cheese-like material from the nail bed with loss of the nail plate,[41] verrucous tumor of the distal part of the thumb, and subungual tumor with deep holes in the nail bed.[42] The big and the little toes were involved with loss of the nail. Even though metastases do not occur (except for lesions developing after radiotherapy), bone erosion is frequent probably because of the long duration before treatment.[43] The etiology of this particular type of low-grade carcinoma is not known, but one patient was an internist who had performed X-ray screening examinations over a period of more than 20 years.[42] The clinical differential diagnosis includes warts and keratoacanthoma, papillomatosis, eccrine porocarcinoma, and a variety of sinus-forming and fistulating processes.

Histopathology requires a sufficiently large and deep diagnostic or excisional biopsy. The localization and the architecture are important keys to the diagnosis. There is a proliferation of squamous cells with epithelium-lined sinuses and tracts containing keratinous debris. The deep border is pushing rather than invasive. There is a well-organized stratification of the epithelium, often with marked focal hypergranulosis. Cellular atypia is absent to mild.[44]

Differential diagnosis includes warts (even histologically) and keratoacanthoma, which exhibits rapid growth and clinically aggressive behavior. SCC is less verrucous and shows considerable dysplasia. Pseudoepitheliomatous hyperplasia is even more regular, does not form epithelium-lined channels, and has a very irregular papillomatous and jagged deep border.[2] However, sometimes several biopsies are necessary to make the correct diagnosis.[45]

Basal cell carcinoma

BCC is the most frequent malignant neoplasm of humanity. However, only about 25 cases have been described in the nail region.[46] BCC presents as a periungual eczema or chronic paronychia that may be associated with granulation tissue, erosion or ulceration, and pain.[47] Jagged borders were observed in superficial BCC.[48] One case in a white patient presented as an acquired longitudinal melanonychia.[49] Fingers are the most common location, ten of them were described in the thumb, only seven BCCs were observed in the ungual region of toes.[50,51] The diagnostic delay ranges from one to 40 years.[52] The treatment of choice is microscopically controlled surgery. The clinical differential diagnosis comprises of trauma, onychomycosis, bacterial infection, eczema, chronic paronychia, pyogenic granuloma, SCC, and amelanotic melanoma.

The pathogenesis of BCC is an inappropriate activation of the hedgehog signaling pathway, but mutations of the tumor-suppressor gene p53 may also play a role. The sonic hedgehog (SHH) protein links with the tumor-suppressing protein-patched homologue 1 (PTCH1), which arrests the smoothened (SMO) intracellular signal inhibitor regulating the GLI family of transcription factors. A mutation inactivating PTCH1 was found in Gorlin's syndrome and in 30%–40% of sporadic cases of BCC. SMO is thus constitutionally active and responsible for a permanent activation of the target genes. This is the basis for the new chemotherapy of BCC with the hedgehog pathway inhibitor vismodegib.

Histologically, BCC is an adnexal carcinoma allegedly arising from the outer root sheath of the hair follicle. Histopathologic examination shows a basophilic tumor with palisaded basal cells and small cuboid cells in the center. There is often a split formation between the epithelial carcinomatous component and its surrounding soft tissue. Mitoses are rare.[2]

Immunohistochemistry reveals an identical cytokeratin profile in the hair follicle and BCC[53] confirming the relation of BCC with embryonal hair follicle formation by the demonstration of the epithelial adhesion molecule Ep-CAM in all BCCs, the human embryonic hair follicle, the secondary hair germ, and the outer root sheath of the vellus hair follicle, but not the adult anagen hair follicles. In contrast, the embryonic nail organ completely lacks Ep-CAM reactivity.[54] This may be an explanation why BCC is so exceptional in the nail region. Ep-CAM demonstrated with the antibody Ber-EP4, allows the differentiation of BCCs from actinic keratoses and SCC, which are negative.[55]

Aggressive digital papillary adenocarcinoma

Aggressive digital papillary adenocarcinoma (ADPAC) was also called aggressive digital papillary adenoma but due to its propensity to recur and metastasize the distinction into aggressive digital papillary adenoma and adenocarcinoma[56] is no longer justified.[57] ADPAC occurs almost exclusively on the fingers, palms, toes, and soles, with preponderance of the hands of men between 40 and 70 years of age,[58] but it was also observed in adolescents.[59] It is usually an insidiously growing, firm, tan-gray to white-pink, rubbery, sometimes cystic or ulcerated, deep-seated nodule or infiltration in a finger, specifically on the volar surface or between the nail bed and the distal interphalangeal joint. One case mimicked an acquired digital fibrokeratoma.[60] Even when reaching a diameter of several centimeters joint mobility is not impeded. Nail bed involvement is rare.[61,62] The nail unit is secondarily affected in most cases. Pain may be a sign of extension to the bone, joint, or nerves. Metastasis as the presenting sign is rare. Radiographs are unremarkable as long as the bone is not invaded. Almost 50% of the carcinomas recur after initial surgical removal and 40% metastasize with the lung being the most frequent site followed by lymph nodes, brain, kidneys, bone, and retroperitoneum. Although sentinel lymph node biopsy may detect metastases earlier, the survival benefit of this procedure is not clear.[63] Radical excision or preferably amputation of the digit are the treatment of choice.[64] The clinical differential diagnoses comprise various cysts and pseudocysts, calluses, pyogenic and foreign body granulomas, SCCs, hemangiomas, giant cell tumors, osteomyelitis, soft tissue infections, or gout.[59]

Histopathology reveals multilobular aggregates of cuboid to low columnar basophilic cells with round to oval nuclei. Spaces are formed into which tumor cell proliferations protrude giving the appearance of a papillary lesion. A cribriform pattern is sometimes seen. A fibrovascular core may be seen in some areas whereas other projections lack stromal support. Although mitoses and necrotic areas are frequent there is little cytologic atypia. Cysts contain necrotic debris or eosinophilic material similar to secretory material. Tumors are well-circumscribed or show an infiltrative border. ADPAC is thought to derive from eccrine sweat glands[65] and an important differential diagnosis is papillary eccrine adenoma. Other histologic differential diagnoses are eccrine acrospiroma, hidradenoma, chondroid syringoma, and, rarely, metastatic papillary adenocarcinoma of the breast, lung, thyroid, or ovary.[66] No specific histologic features have been identified to predict recurrence or metastasis.[59]

Eccrine porocarcinoma

Eccrine porocarcinoma is a rare tumor mainly of the palms and soles of elderly persons.[67] It is rare in the tip of the digit.[68] One case was apparently induced by chronic exposure to Roentgen rays as the ulcerating tumor developed in the middle finger of a chronic radiodermatitis of both hands.[69] When occurring in the lateral nail fold it may simulate SCC.[70] One of our patients had a large eccrine porocarcinoma of the fifth metatarsal-fifth toe area completely overgrowing the nail of the little toe with a massively hyperkeratotic verrucous growth.[2] Most porocarcinomas appear to arise de novo although one fifth to one half of them may develop by malignant transformation of a benign pre-existing poroma.[71]

Histopathologically, eccrine porocarcinoma derives from the eccrine sweat ducts. It grows as intraepidermal and dermal, solid cords and nests of cuboid to polygonal cells with pale cytoplasm. The cell nuclei are pleomorphic with irregular shape, prominent nucleoli, and multiple mitoses. Intraepithelial tumor cells are sharply demarcated from the adjacent keratinocytes. They are seen as single cells in the epidermis in a pagetoid pattern or form nests.[72] Keratinization is lacking despite the occasional clinically verrucous appearance. When the tumor contains glycogen, the cytoplasm appears pale.[73] Lymphatic invasion in the deep dermis is probably the reason for the sometimes-catastrophic course.[74]

Immunohistochemistry shows positivity for pancytokeratin; intraepithelial porocarcinoma cells are usually weaker stained than the surrounding epithelium.[75] Ductal formations in the tumor stain with antibodies to carcinoembryonic antigen and epithelial membrane antigen. Whereas p53 is expressed in both eccrine poroma as well as porocarcinoma,[76,77] p16 is negative throughout eccrine porocarcinoma.[78] The main differential diagnoses are benign eccrine poroma, hidracanthoma simplex, and Paget's disease.[79] Although eccrine poroma and hidracanthoma simplex may show some focal atypicality they are symmetrical and well delimited.

Adenocystic sweat gland carcinoma

Adenocystic sweat gland carcinoma is a rare neoplasm of which one case of a mucinous variant was observed in the tip of the great toe of a 30-year-old black female. The tumor was tender and movable.[80] Its relation to adenoid cystic carcinoma and microcystic adnexal carcinoma is not entirely clear.[2]

Histopathology demonstrates an adenoid, tubular, or cribriform differentiation with abundant small epithelial islands. The adenocystic sweat gland carcinoma of the nail was composed of solid, papillary, and trabecular tumor cell aggregates focally exhibiting abundant mitoses. Microcystic adnexal carcinoma, adenoid cystic carcinoma, ADPAC, eccrine porocarcinoma are all anticipated to origin from eccrine sweat glands and may show some similarities. Immunohistochemistry is usually not helpful as these carcinomas display the same antigen profile.[2]

Spiradenocarcinoma

Spiradenocarcinoma is suggested to result from malignant degeneration of a benign spiradenoma.[81] It is an extremely rare neoplasm. Middle-aged persons are mainly affected. It develops from a long-standing lesion that abruptly enlarges to a neoplasm of 8 mm to 10 cm, ulcerates, changes its color, and becomes tender. Spiradenocarcinoma is an aggressive tumor that may metastasize to lymph nodes, lung, and bones.[82,83] A history of multiple eccrine spiradenomas may be present. A single case was described in the big toe involving the nail bed that had developed over a period of approximately 10 years from a benign spiradenoma of the dorsolateral aspect of the toe after multiple cauterizations and a local excision.[84]

Histopathology demonstrates well-circumscribed nodules of typical benign eccrine spiradenoma with its characteristic two cell types of peripheral cuboid basal cells and luminal cells. The carcinomatous change may be seen as a gradual transition to a malignant area in the tumor where the two-layered spiradenoma architecture changes to monomorphous carcinoma with ill-defined nests and cords of tumor cells. Duct-like structures may be completely missing and glandular components as well as hyaline globules are decreased. The other type usually presents as a spiradenocarcinoma adjacent to the benign tumor without transition. There may be Bowenoid, squamous, ductal carcinoma-like, tubular, histiocytoid, and carcinosarcomatous changes with rhabdomyoblastic and osteosarcomatous differentiation.[85] Necrosis and hemorrhage are found in advanced spiradenocarcinoma. The most important differential diagnosis is benign spiradenoma as the diagnosis of malignant transformation may be missed in case of an insufficient biopsy.

Hidradenocarcinoma

This rare neoplasm has been described under various terms, such as clear-cell papillary carcinoma, clear-cell hidradenocarcinoma, malignant clear-cell hidradenoma, malignant clear-cell acrospiroma, malignant eccrine acrospiroma, nodular hidradenocarcinoma, clear-cell eccrine carcinoma, mucoepidermoid hidradenocarcinoma, and malignant nodular clear-cell hidradenoma;[2] whether the term primary mucoepidermoid carcinoma of the skin is justified remains disputed. Most patients are around 50 years of age. A slight female preponderance was noted. There is no characteristic appearance allowing a clinical diagnosis to be made. It is a slow-growing, asymptomatic solitary tumor. Two cases were described in the nail apparatus. One was that of 77-year-old black man with a slowly growing mass on the right middle fingernail bed, which began as a pigmented band rapidly enlarging in size in the last months prior to consultation. Clinically, it presented as an ulcerated dome-shaped red nodule involving most of the nail bed. The nail plate was destroyed and partially lost. The remaining nail plate on both sides of the lesion was hyperpigmented.[86] Another hidradenocarcinoma of the nail apparatus appeared clinically as a recurrent onychomycosis in a 72-year-old man.

Histopathology reveals one or several tumor nodules of variable shapes and sizes, frequently with tubular and ductal structures as well as mass necrosis. Although the overlying epithelium may be eroded or ulcerated there is no connection with the epidermis. The tumor proliferations are made up of pale to clear cells with a distinct cytoplasmic

membrane, pleomorphic nuclei, and many mitoses. Nuclear atypia was described in the ungual hidradenocarcinoma. Benign clear-cell hidradenoma with focal degenerative changes has to be differentiated. Other differential diagnoses include other clear-cell tumors such as clear-cell Bowen's carcinoma, but also rhabdoid and tumors with a granular cytoplasm.[2]

Sebaceous carcinoma

Sebaceous carcinoma is a malignant neoplasm with sebocytic differentiation. There is one report of a sebaceous gland carcinoma of the lateral aspect of the right index finger in a 46-year-old man. It presented as a painless swelling without bony alterations on X-ray. The excision was carried out under the clinical diagnosis of an epidermoid cyst and showed an irregular, well-circumscribed lesion with a pseudocapsule. The lesion was treated by amputation.[87]

Histopathology showed vacuolated and multivesicular clear cells characteristic of sebaceous carcinoma. The periungual sebaceous carcinoma had many atypical mitoses and the nuclei were hyperchromatic and pleomorphic. Immunohistochemically, EMA staining makes the vacuolar cell changes stand out even more clearly although this is not seen in all sebaceous carcinomas.

MALIGNANT FIBROUS TUMORS

Malignant fibrous tumors are by definition sarcomas. They are very rare in the nail region. Their diagnosis is not possible on clinical grounds alone, and even histopathology often requires special stains, immunohistochemistry, and molecular biologic techniques.[2]

Fibrosarcoma

This is the prototype of sarcoma. It is extremely uncommon in the nail apparatus.[88] In the skin, it is a firm nodule or plaque, first slow-growing, then rapidly increasing. In the nail, its appearance is totally non-specific. It destroys almost the entire distal phalanx. Histology showed a proliferation of uniform spindle cells with few mitoses. Immunohistochemistry was only positive for vimentin. Amputation led to recurrence-free survival for the following three years. In the differential diagnosis, all spindle cell neoplasms have to be considered.

Low-grade myofibroblastic sarcoma

This is a recently defined malignant mesenchymal tumor that most commonly occurs in the head and neck region. A case of a 5-year-old female patient with a myofibroblastic sarcoma of the distal phalanx of a finger was described. R-0 amputation with a 28-month follow-up showed no recurrence. Histopathology revealed sheets of spindle cells arranged in bundles, whorls, short fascicles and storiform pattern, some atypical mitoses, and areas of necrosis with a mixed inflammatory infiltrate. In addition to vimentin, muscle markers were positive.[89]

Dermatofibrosarcoma protuberans

Dermatofibrosarcoma protuberans (DFSP), a low-to-medium-grade sarcoma, is the most common sarcoma of the skin. Most cases occur on the trunk in young to middle-aged males. Acral localization is rare but relatively more common in children.[90] The neoplasm is ill-defined and recurrences are frequent. Three cases were reported to involve the distal phalanx, all patients were women. They appeared as hard lobulated painful mass on the pulp, as a dark hyperkeratotic plaque, or as a pigmented thickened nail.[91-93] The differential diagnosis comprises hypertrophic scar, keloid, chronic fibrotic paronychia, and recurrent infantile digital fibromatosis.[2]

A t(17:22)(q22:q13), somatic mutation is found in DFSP, which fuses the collagen 1A1 gene to the platelet-derived growth factor B chain gene resulting in a chimeric COL1A1-PDGFB gene. Treatment is wide local excision with 3-cm safety margin, which means amputation for the digit in case of ungual DSFP.

Histologically, fusiform cells are seen with arrangement in cords, strands, and sometimes whorls. Mitoses and atypias are rare. The nail is a particular region rendering the histopathological diagnosis very difficult. Immunohistochemistry is positive for CD34 and negative for CD68. Synovial sarcoma shows monomorphic spindle cells that may be mistaken for DFSP or superficial acral fibromyxoma. It is positive for the fusion product of SYT-SSX from a t(X:18), which can be demonstrated by PCR.[94]

Epithelioid sarcoma

Epithelioid sarcoma is a rare, clinically non-specific lesion often diagnosed only very late. Although a slow-growing neoplasm, the 5-year survival rate is barely 50%. At the distal digit, it appears as a tender swelling or firm myxoid pseudo-cyst. Most patients are young persons and the predominant localization is near a joint. Treatment of choice is amputation, but even then, the recurrence rate is high.[95,96]

Histologically, there is a proliferation of plump, often epithelioid cells resembling a granuloma annulare in the beginning. Ulceration may occur. Immunohistochemistry is positive for vimentin and focally also for cytokeratin and epithelial membrane antigen.[2]

OTHER SARCOMAS

Other sarcomas are even more uncommon and there are only some anecdotal reports.

Angiosarcomas

There are many different types of angiosarcomas, most of which were not described in the nail apparatus. Histologically, they are difficult to differentiate and require special historical and anatomical data to be diagnosed.[2]

KAPOSI SARCOMA

Kaposi sarcoma (KS) is now divided into three subtypes: classical KS occurring mainly on the lower extremity of elderly men, epidemic KS seen in Africa, and immune deficiency-associated KS observed in patients with acquired immunodeficiency syndrome and other immunosupressions. All are associated with human herpes virus type 8. Clinically, it starts as a macular bruise-like area developing into a hemorrhagic plaque. After a variable period of evolution, ulcerating and bleeding nodules are formed, particularly on the feet. They may overgrow the nail unit or lift the nail when occurring in the nail bed. In AIDS patients, small bruises may appear in the nail area and the distal phalanx of the toe may enlarge.[97,98] Hyperplastic acroangiodermatitis and pseudo-KS in acral hyperstomy syndrome are the main clinical differential diagnoses.

Histopathology depends on the stage of the disease; however, in the nail apparatus, usually nodules or plaques are biopsied allowing a clear-cut diagnosis to be made. Slit-like capillary vessels separate the collagen bundles, and many extravasated erythrocytes dominate the histologic picture. Cellular atypia is sparse. HHV8 is positive, CD34 negative, and podoplanin-positive, hinting at a lymphatic origin of the lesion.[2]

EPITHELIOID HEMANGIOENDOTHELIOMA

Epithelioid hemangioendothelioma (EHEA) is a rare low-to-medium-grade angiosarcoma. One case in the nail apparatus appeared as a paronychia developing into a diffuse swelling of the big toe, which became bluish-red with an overcurved nail. The distal phalanx bone was lytic.[99] Two more cases presented with violaceous nodules of the finger and toe tips, one with nail destruction and one thought to be due to prolonged exposure to vinyl chloride.[100-103]

EHEA is a vascular neoplasm with solid and vascular components that stand out by their epithelioid appearance. Pathologic mitoses and pleomorphism may be marked focally. Vascular markers such as CD 31, CD34, and factor VIII are positive.

GLOMANGIOSARCOMA

Glomangiosarcoma is an extremely rare neoplasm. One case was observed in the distal phalanx of the thumb. It has a similar symptomatology as a benign glomus tumor but the diagnosis should be suspected when its diameter is larger than 20 mm.[104]

Subungual liposarcoma

A case of a subungual liposarcoma with metastases to the brain was reported.[105]

Leiomyosarcoma

Leiomyosarcoma derives from smooth muscle cells. It is mainly seen in elderly men. Subungual localization was observed once in a 63-year-old male and was associated with pain. Histologically it displayed interlacing bundles of large spindle cells with pleomorphic nuclei. The cytoplasm was eosinophilic and the cell borders ill defined. Muscle antigens stain positive.[106]

Chondrosarcoma

Chondrosarcoma is common in the hand, but localization in the distal phalanx is exceptional. The prognosis of distal lesion is better than that of proximal lesion.[107–110] Whereas benign chondromas are painless chondrosarcomas are symptomatic and present with swelling and enlargement of the distal phalanx. X-rays may show speckles thought to represent active growth. Chondrosarcomas also develop in up to 50% of Ollier's multiple enchondroma syndrome,[111] in 18% of Maffucci–Kast syndrome, and in hereditary multiple exostosis syndrome.

Histologically, chondrosarcomas are divided into grades 1–3. Grade 1 chondrosarcoma exhibits only slight atypia of the chondrocytes and an evenly hyaline ground substance. Grade 2 has more pronounced cellular atypia and a less homogeneous ground substance. Grade 3 stands out by marked cellular atypia. One case of subungual clear-cell chondrosarcoma in the distal phalanx was reported and characterized by large tumor cells with a clear cytoplasm and distinct cell membranes.[112] Chondroid differentiation was also observed in a case of subungual melanoma.[113]

MALIGNANT NEUROGENIC AND NEUROENDOCRINE TUMORS

These malignant tumors are very rare in the nail apparatus. They cannot be diagnosed on clinical grounds and require a sufficiently large biopsy for histopathological examination.[2]

Malignant schwannoma

Swelling and nail dystrophy were the leading signs of distal digital malignant schwannomas.[114] Histologically, they are mostly low-grade malignant schwannomas with few Verocay bodies and a low mitotic rate. Benign neurilemmoma and neurofibroma have to be ruled out.

Malignant granular cell tumor

Most granular cell tumors derive from modified Schwann cells. Malignant granular cell tumor is exceedingly rare. One subungual case was seen in the right index finger of a 51-year-old woman. It recurred two years after surgery, presented with 2.5 cm diameter erosion. Despite finger amputation, the patient developed metastases and died shortly thereafter.

Histopathologically, the subungual malignant granular cell tumor exhibited polygonal eosinophilic granular cells with mitoses and some multinucleated giant cells. In the metastasis, anaplastic cells were seen in addition.[115]

Merkel cell carcinoma

Merkel cell carcinoma (MCC) was first termed trabecular carcinoma of the skin, but also cutaneous neuroendocrine carcinoma, cutaneous APUDoma, and primary small cell carcinoma of the skin. It is mainly localized in chronically light-exposed skin and hence most patients are Caucasians. A specific virus associated with MCC, the Merkel cell polyomavirus (MCPyV), was recently identified.[116] It can be found in approximately 80% of patients. Localization on fingers is very rare. The neoplasm is solitary, round to dome-shaped, red to violaceous, and painless. They grow fast to about 2 cm in diameter or larger, but ulceration is uncommon.[117] A case was described on the left great toe of a teenage girl associated with an ingrown nail. We have seen a large ulcerated nodule on the distal dorsal aspect of the distal middle finger phalanx in a 73-year-old woman. The treatment of choice is radical surgery, often with postoperative radiotherapy. The recurrence rate is very high; metastases occur in the regional lymph nodes and finally hematogenously.

Histopathology of MCC is characteristic with densely packed cells with light round to oval nuclei, small nucleoli, little cytoplasm, often many mitoses, and apoptoses. They may form solid tumor strands or trabeculae. Immunohistochemistry is positive for Merkel cell markers such as cytokeratin 20, epithelial membrane antigen, and a variety of other neural markers. CK20 is positive as paranuclear small granules, which are also seen in electron microscopy.[118,119]

Ewing sarcoma

Ewing sarcoma is a rare tumor almost exclusively seen in persons under 20 years of age. Only about 1% occur in the small bones of the hands and feet. Pain and swelling with low-grade fever are the leading symptoms. Two forms are distinguished: skeletal and extraskeletal Ewing sarcoma. The extraskeletal Ewings sarcoma is cytogenetically and molecular genetically identical to peripheral primitive neuroectodermal tumor (PNET), but is less well differentiated histologically. Its clinical presentation is a neoplasm with a diameter of 5–10 cm. One case of probable skeletal Ewing sarcoma was observed in the tip of a toe radiographically causing lytic lesions.[120] The pulp was swollen and ulcerated. A subungual Ewing sarcoma was observed by F. Facchetti (unpublished 2012). Treatment was successful by amputation.[121] Another recent case showed complete destruction of the nail unit.[122] The clinical differential diagnosis includes osteomyelitis, tuberculosis, enchondroma, and a variety of benign tumors. Treatment is by generous local excision and chemotherapy.

Histopathology is the method of diagnosis. It reveals a neoplasm made up of tumor cells that are arranged in lobules, nests, trabeculae, or sheets. Their nuclei are uniformly small, round to oval, vesicular, or hyperchromatic and the cytoplasm is scant, pale eosinophilic, or vacuolated without a clearly visible cell membrane. Nucleoli are small or not visible. Mitoses vary in number. Apoptotic cells are abundant and many are dark. Intracytoplasmic glycogen stains with PAS. Reticulin stain demonstrates fibers around cell groups. Immunohistochemistry is positive for membranous CD99 (MIC2) and some neural markers such as neuron-specific enolase, neurofilament proteins, Leu-7, PGP9.5, and synaptophysin. Roughly 85% of skeletal and extraskeletal Ewing sarcomas as well as PNETs show a characteristic chromosomal translocation t(11;22)(q24;q12).

LANGERHANS CELL HISTIOCYTOSIS

This malignant systemic disease is also known as histiocytosis X or malignant histiocytosis. It is rare with an estimated incidence of 1 case per 200,000 children and 1–2 cases per million adults. The skin is the second most frequent site of involvement with 39% of the cases showing skin involvement. Three clinical variants are known: the acute generalized Letterer–Siwe disease mainly seen in children, the chronic multifocal form of Hand–Schüller–Christian,[123] and the localized form called eosinophilic granuloma. Although nail involvement is rare it is seen as a marker of systemic or generalized cutaneous disease.[124–126] Nail lesions may show small periungual nodules, onycholysis, subungual hyperkeratosis, thick nails, pits, nail splitting, subungual bleedings, nail loss, paronychia, and nail fold destruction.[127–132]

Histopathology of nail Langerhans histiocytosis reveals a dense infiltrate of relatively large cells with a reniform nucleus and abundant cytoplasm that invade the dermis and may form large intraepithelial sheets. Invasion of the matrix causes nail dystrophy and that of the nail bed often subungual splinter hemorrhages. The cells display all characteristics of Langerhans cells both immunohistochemically as well as electron microscopically, such as protein S100, langerin (CD207), CD1a, peanut agglutinin as well as Birbeck granules.[2,133] Recent research showed evidence of mutations involving the Ras/Raf/MEK/ERK pathway with almost half of the patients having a BRAF V600E mutation. This may indicate that B-Raf-MEK inhibition might be a treatment for cases not responding to standard cytostatic therapy.[134]

HEMATOGENOUS NEOPLASMS INVOLVING THE NAIL

Hematogenous tumors of the nail are rare and mostly malignant lymphomas or leukemias. Benign pseudolymphomas are extremely rare.

T-cell lymphomas

Mycosis fungoides (MF) and Sézary's syndrome (SS) are the classical cutaneous T-cell lymphomas. They may involve the nail primarily or nail lesions may occur as part of widespread skin disease. However, compared with folliculotropic MF, ungueotropic MF and SS are rare. Nail changes occur late, are non-specific and unpredictable, mostly affect several digits. Particularly in erythrodermic MF/SS, nail changes may also be non-specific histopathologically. The nails are brittle, thickened, yellow, opaque, rough, ridged, with subungual hyperkeratosis. This feature is also seen in pityriasis rubra pilaris and erythrodermas of different etiologies.[135,136] Pterygium and acquired anonychia as well as massive lymphomatous involvement are rare.[137] Periungual blistering occurred in cases of MF bullosa.[138] Other rare events are single-digit tumor stage MF of a nail and childhood nail MF.[2] Clinically, nail involvement may look bland like a mild inflammation, psoriasis, pityriasis rubra pilaris, or eczema. An HTLV-1 infection looked like MF of the nail.[139]

The histopathology of specific nail alterations is similar to that of the cutaneous lesions, but may be very discrete. Epitheliotropism of lymphocytes with slightly larger and hyperchromatic nuclei is characteristic, and occasionally, Pautrier's microabscesses are seen. Nail plate changes are the result of matrix involvement.[140] Immunohistochemistry shows mainly T-cell markers with variable percentages of CD4 and CD8 cells. Small-cell anaplastic carcinoma and melanoma has to be differentiated.

Treatment is according to the stage of MF or SS.

B-cell lymphoma of the distal digit

Cutaneous B-cell lymphomas are rare. Chronic lymphocytic leukemia (CLL) is the prototype, occurs in elderly persons, and runs a protracted, relatively benign appearing course. Soft nodular acral infiltrates over the finger joints, rarely the distal phalanx are characteristic. Involvement of the nail unit mimics chronic paronychia, causes nail plate elevation, overcurvature, or clubbing.[141–144] Onychomycosis-like nail alterations plus small sub- and periungual tumors were reported once.[145] Non-specific nail dystrophy is seen in roughly one quarter of CLL patients.[146] The infiltrates respond rapidly to X-irradiation.

Histopathology shows monomorphic infiltrates of mature B lymphocytes. The differential diagnoses include lupus erythematosus profundus, small-cell carcinomas, and melanomas including metastases.[2]

Plasmocytoma

Plasmocytoma is a type of B-cell lymphoma with differentiation toward plasma cells. It is rare in the skin and even less common in the nail unit. Skin infiltrates are seen as red plaques or nodes. Ungual involvement may cause nail elevation, onychoschizia and onycholysis.[147,148] A patient with POEMS (Crow-Fukase) syndrome plus plasmocytoma developed clubbing.[149] Lichen planus-like nail dystrophy as the sole sign of multiple myeloma was also described.[150] Acquired cutis laxa was observed in a patient with multiple myeloma and primary systemic amyloidosis; she developed marked loss of elasticity of the thumb pulps without further visible nail changes.[151]

Histologically, a dense infiltrate of immature to mature plasma cells, is seen. They produce one class of immunoglobulin.[2]

Hodgkin's disease

Although Hodgkin's disease is probably the most frequent type of malignant lymphoma, nail involvement is rare and it is not clear whether the reported cases were due to specific infiltrates, treatment-induced, or non-specific.[152–154] Several publications describe transverse leukonychia and Beau's lines as therapy-induced.

Leukemia

Most nail changes in patients suffering from leukemia are non-specific. The nail bed may appear pale, nails tend to split and break, hemorrhages are a sign of clotting abnormalities.[155] Pernio-like lesions in the acral parts including the digits of hands and feet occurred in the preleukemic phase of myelomonocytic leukemia.[156–158] An infiltrate of the distal thumb phalanx with bone involvement and pachydermoperiostosis developed in acute myelomonocytic leukemia.[159,160] A brownish infiltrated spot occurred on the proximal nail fold of the left middle finger in chronic myeloid leukemia.[2]

Histopathology of early acute myelogenic leukemia reveals an angiocentric and interstitial infiltrate of relatively monotonous myeloperoxidase positive cells. Their nuclei are round to oval with inconspicuous nucleoli. Epidermotropism is lacking. The cells of myelogenous leukemia are bone marrow derived and positive for myeloperoxidase, chloroacetate esterase, Leder stain, and Sudan black B as well as for the myeloid markers CD13, CD15, CD33, and CD117.[2] Myeloperoxidase is a very reliable stain to exclude T- and B-cell lymphomas. All monotonous round-cell infiltrates may be considered. Sweet syndrome, in particular neutrophilic dermatosis of the dorsal hands,[161] may mimic skin lesions of acute myelogenous leukemia and vice versa.[162] Bilateral ingrown toenails demonstrating sheets and solid nodules of neoplastic cells with scanty cytoplasm and hyperchromatic round nuclei that were positive for myeloperoxidase and CD43, revealed the diagnosis of a granulocytic sarcoma.[163]

MELANOMA OF THE NAIL APPARATUS (NAIL UNIT MELANOMA)

Ungual melanoma is undoubtedly the most serious nail condition. It has attracted much attention in the last 25 years as evidenced by the many publications on all aspects of nail unit melanoma (NUM). The first subungual melanoma was reported in 1834 of a patient with a decades-long history of a pigmented nail that eventually turned into a "bleeding fungus."[164] Melanomas in general still remain an enigmatic skin tumor in dermatology, dermatopathology, and clinical medicine. Misconceptions as to its diagnosis, natural course, and treatment abound, and this is particularly the case for nail melanomas.[165]

Localization

NUMs belong to the subgroup of acral lentiginous melanomas, which display a somewhat different behavior compared to melanomas of other skin sites. They are localized under and around the nail (matrix, nail bed, nail folds, hyponychium, pulp); in fact, they comprise virtually all melanomas of the distal phalanx. Thumbs and big toes are the most frequent site of NUM, followed by middle, index, ring and little fingers, and the lesser toes.[2]

Localization-dependent frequency

It is commonly claimed that NUMs are rare; however, this is not true: Approximately 1.5% to 2.5% of all melanomas in light-skinned Caucasians are nail melanomas[166,167] but the entire surface of all nails taken together is far below 1%—thus, the nail is clearly overrepresented as a localization for melanoma.[2,164,168] Further, by far most nail melanomas arise in the matrix, which then appears to be a hot spot of melanoma development. The percentage, not the absolute number, of melanomas localized in the nail apparatus is even much higher in individuals with dark complexion where it is roughly 20% of their melanomas.[169,170] In East Asians, 50% to 77% of all melanomas were acral melanomas[171–174] as compared to only 4% to 7% of Germans.[175,176]

In contrast to cutaneous melanoma where the incidence has continuously increased, this has remained stable for acral lentiginous and nail melanomas.[177]

Patient age

The age of most nail melanoma patients is between 50 and 70 years, but the age range is very wide, from childhood to very old age.[178,179]

Gender

There is no clear cut gender dominance in light skinned individuals as some studies have reported higher prevalanec in women while others in men.[180]

Localization, trauma, and ultraviolet irradiation

Approximately 70% of all nail melanomas arise in the thumb and the great toenail, which have the biggest nail fields; but again this means an enormous concentration of melanomas for two particular localizations. It has long been anticipated that trauma plays a major role in the initiation of nail melanoma.[181–183] Most reports, however, do not support this assumption as the time between the perceived trauma and the nail melanoma was often too short.[184] Conversely, trauma is an important factor negatively influencing the prognosis.[185] Nail melanomas detected after a trauma were thicker. Artificial nails may hide a subungual melanoma or even promote its growth.[186] NUMs are not associated with ultraviolet exposure. The nail plate allows just a fraction of UV to penetrate,[3,187,188] the big toenail is usually protected from UV irradiation by shoes, and the matrix—except for the small lunula area of some digits—as the most frequent origin of nail melanomas is covered by the proximal nail fold.[2]

Clinical diagnosis of NUM

The clinical diagnosis of most NUMs is not difficult for a physician trained in nail disorders as two thirds to three quarters of them are pigmented. Nevertheless, many are overlooked or diagnosed very late. It is the **lack of suspicion** that is the most important factor for delaying or missing the correct diagnosis. In light-skinned adults, it is important to recognize that any acquired melanin pigmentation in the nail must evoke the suspicion of nail melanoma, independent of the patient's age and digit involved.[2] However, this is much more difficult to decide in dark-complexioned persons. A careful comparison of the nail pigmentation of all digits—both fingers as well as toes—is indispensable. A rule of thumb is that an acquired melanotic longitudinal streak in the nail of a light-skinned adult or of a melanotic streak standing out by its color, width, and irregular internal structure from the rest of the light brown bands in dark-skinned individuals is rather malignant than benign (Figures 27.9 and 27.10).[2,189] This is particularly true if the streak is

- Wider than 5 mm
- Located on the thumb, index, middle finger, or big toe
- Involves a single digit
- Widening proximally indicating growth of the lesion in the matrix
- Associated with nail dystrophy even if this is minute
- Accompanied by periungual pigmentation, the Hutchinson sign
- Develops a tumefaction

However, ungual melanomas were also observed in children[190–192] and even concurrently in two thumbs.[193]

Analogous to the ABC rule of cutaneous melanomas, an ABCDEF rule was proposed for NUMs:[194]

A **A**ge and race – most nail melanomas occur between the age of 40 to 70 and most patients are **A**sians, **A**fricans, **A**frican-Americans, and native **A**mericans[a]

B **B**rown to **b**lack band, **b**roader than 3–5 mm, **b**order irregular or blurred

C **C**hange: rapid increase in width and growth rate, nail dystrophy does not improve despite "adequate treatment"

D **D**igit: Thumb > big toe > index finger; usually single-digit involvement, more fingers rarely affected

E **E**xtension of pigmentation: periungual pigmentation = Hutchinson sign

F **F**amily or personal history of melanoma or so-called dysplastic nevi

---

[a] As the absolute number of NUMs is the same in Caucasians and dark-skinned individuals this assumption has to be taken with care!

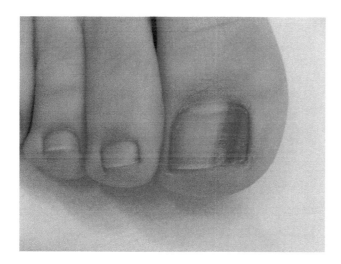

Figure 27.9 In situ melanoma of the big toenail.

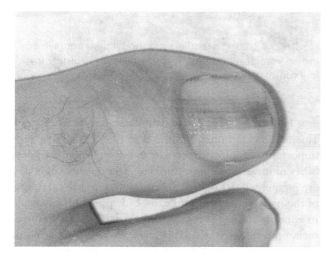

Figure 27.10 Subungual melanoma in situ: The melano-nychia is wider proximally than distally giving evidence of rapid horizontal growth.

These criteria are valid for most lesions originating in the nail matrix. However, as the absolute number of NUM is more or less equal among Caucasians and dark-skinned races, the statement that most patients are from dark-skinned races is not true, i.e., race is **not** a particular risk factor.[2] No melanocytic lesion deriving from the nail bed can give a longitudinal streak as this is due to incorporation of the melanin into the growing nail plate and the nail bed does not add to it.[2] Furthermore, most nail bed melanomas are amelanotic (Figure 27.11). The diagnosis of amelanotic NUMs is a real challenge and requires a very high degree of clinical suspicion. It is self-evident and good clinical practice to always submit every piece of a surgical specimen from the nail region for histopathologic examination, even—particularly in adults—when the clinical diagnosis was just granulation tissue or an ingrown nail.[2] Strict adherence to the ABCDEF rule might even delay the diagnosis, as many patients are younger than 30 years.[195] This rule is also not adequate to diagnose childhood nail melanoma.[2]

Laboratory examinations are, until now, not helpful to make the diagnosis of NUM.

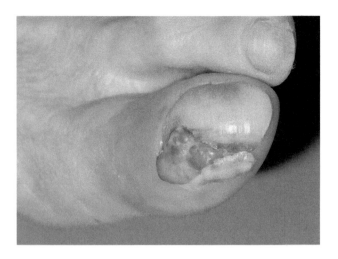

Figure 27.11 Nodular amelanotic melanoma of the nail bed breaking through the nail.

Differential diagnoses

The list of clinical differential diagnoses is enormous with warts, hematoma, pyogenic granuloma, ingrown toenail, onychomycosis,[196] keratoacanthoma, SCC, foreign body granuloma, or mole to mention just a few.[197–200] This list is even longer for amelanotic NUM.[182,201] However, onychomycosis and other conditions may co-exist with melanoma.[202]

Prognosis

NUMs have often been claimed to have a particularly poor prognosis. Large series of 100 or more cases showed a mean Breslow thickness of 4 mm and more[203,204] hinting at an enormous neglect both from the patients as well as their physicians (Figures 27.12 and 27.13). The five-year survival for invasive subungual melanoma was only 51%.[166] Several publications of pigmented NUMs misdiagnosed and mistreated as onychomycosis give evidence that even obviously pigmented nail melanomas are not correctly diagnosed.[197–200] Sixty percent of the initially unrecognized acral lentiginous melanomas were nail melanomas, and 30% of them were amelanotic.[180] The assumption that amelanotic NUMs have a poorer prognosis only reflects the fact that they are diagnosed and treated even later than non-nail acral lentiginous melanomas.[205,206] On the other side, long-term survival of stage IV subungual melanoma with spontaneous regression of metastases[207] and even complete regression of an advanced subungual melanoma with a tumor thickness of 4 mm were observed.[208]

The assumption that subungual melanomas grow faster than those in other locations is also not true. Many publications report on decade-long histories of ungual melanomas[164,209] and many of our cases were still in situ even after ten years or more that a brown streak had been noticed.[210]

Diagnosis of NUM

The diagnosis of nail melanomas ought to be straightforward if there is a recently acquired pigmented nail streak

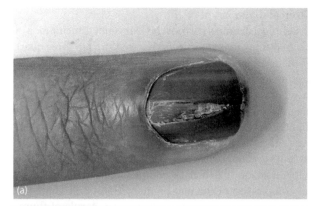

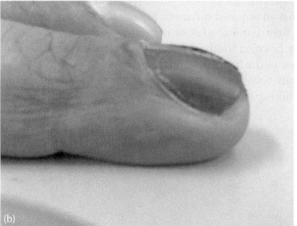

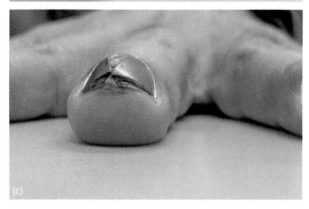

Figure 27.12 Long-standing subungual melanoma in an Indian immigrant patient. (a) Dorsal view; (b) Side view; (c) Frontal view.

or a Hutchinson sign in an individual over 30 to 35 years. This is, however, often not the case (see above). The most important "diagnostic measure" is **not to forget the possibility of melanoma**. Two-thirds to three quarters of NUMs are pigmented. Human melanin reaches into the free edge of the nail, is granular, and can be identified histologically in Fontana-stained sections (see below). In contrast, fungal melanin is diffuse and usually forms a narrow wedge pointing proximally. Blood does not reach the free nail margin, is deposited in large clumps of erythrocytes, and can easily be demonstrated using the benzidine test: A tiny piece of the nail with the pigment in question is cut or the pigment

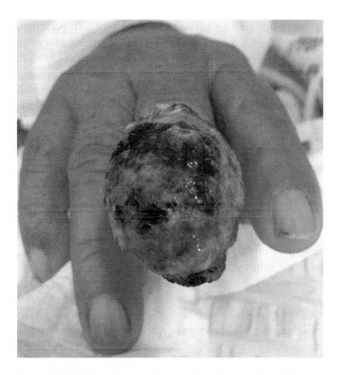

Figure 27.13 Far advanced ungual melanoma in a 67-year-old woman from Guatemala. (Courtesy of Dra Patricia Chang, Guatemala.)

is scraped into a small test tube, a drop of water is added, and after a few minutes a Hemostix® such as used for the demonstration of blood in urine or feces is dipped into the test tube: Even very few erythrocytes give a positive test.[211] Another possibility is to wipe the pigmented nail with 3% hydrogen peroxide, which removes the blood while producing white foam due to the production of atomic oxygen. Be aware that the demonstration of blood does not rule out a bleeding melanoma or another bleeding tumor![2]

Dermatoscopy

Dermatoscopy can help to make the clinical diagnosis. It should be started "dry," i.e., without an immersion medium, then "wet." Dry dermatoscopy allows surface irregularities to be seen, wet technique permits a better look into and through the nail plate. As the nail surface is curved a transparent gel staying on the curvature is recommended. The fine melanin granules are not visible whereas blood agglomerates are seen with a magnifier lens and the dermatoscope. Transungual elimination of nevus cell nests looks like brown dots. The brown band is built by lines of pigment, which are irregular in width, spacing, and color in NUM. Tiny pigmentations of the surrounding skin, the micro-Hutchinson sign, are very rare in benign nevi. A recent study found that Hutchinson's sign is associated with invasive melanoma whereas in situ NUM only shows a longitudinal melanonychia.[212] Dermatoscopy, like clinical inspection, of a melanonychia does not allow the responsible melanocyte focus to be seen as it is under the nail and the proximal nail

fold. This means that the two-dimensional dermatoscopy of a cutaneous melanocytic lesion is reduced to one-dimension only and that it is not the lesion itself, but its product melanin incorporated in the nail plate, which has to be evaluated.[2] The melanonychia is due to overproduction of melanin that cannot completely be degraded by the matrix keratinocytes and remains in the upper matrix keratinocytes. The melanin is finally incorporated in the nail plate cells. A melanocyte lesion growing in width will lead to a wider band whereas a longitudinal increase may lead to a more intense pigmentation of the streak. Growth in the transverse diameter of the melanocyte lesion within a certain time period is visible as a streak wider proximally than distally. This is usually seen as a sign of malignancy in adults, but common in nevi in children. Very even pigmentation of a melanonychia is the rule for benign lesions, but in general, dermatoscopy only gives a hint at the benignity of the lesion.[2] Most nail bed melanomas are amelanotic, but even if they produce melanin this remains under the nail making the diagnosis even more difficult. Independent of the validity of dermatoscopy, histopathology is always a must.[213]

Intraoperative matrix dermatoscopy is an invasive method but it permits direct bi-dimensional observation of the pigmented lesion in the matrix and nail bed with a multicomponent pattern of brown-black pigmentation, globules, dots, structureless areas, and thick streaks being suspicious for melanoma.[214–216] One study was able to reliably distinguish 7 of 8 matrix melanomas from a benign lentigo by immediate postoperative confocal laser scanning microscopy (CLSM) thus speeding up the diagnostic delay between extirpation and histopathology, and the one lesion not safely diagnosable by CLSM also required immunohistochemistry to make the diagnosis.[217]

X-ray fiber diffraction was claimed to be able to differentiate eight different malignancies from a single nail clipping.[218] This technique still awaits confirmation by an independent group.

The gold standard of diagnosis is histopathology,[219] which requires a biopsy. If the biopsy is insufficient, it delays the diagnosis. The responsible lesion for a longitudinal streak in the nail is in the matrix. Thus, an optimal biopsy of the matrix must be obtained. This can be a longitudinal biopsy including the proximal nail fold, the matrix, nail bed, hyponychium, and nail plate. It is the method of choice for laterally located melanonychias. A streak in the center of the nail may be biopsied with a punch with a maximal diameter of 3 mm in order not to leave a nail dystrophy in case the lesion is benign, or with a fusiform or crescentic biopsy of the matrix, which is oriented transversely in order to prevent a post-biopsy split nail. Nail bed biopsies are fusiform and performed longitudinally because of the unique longitudinal arrangement of the nail bed rete ridges. We have developed a tangential matrix and nail bed biopsy that prevents post-biopsy nail dystrophy and allows large superficial excisions.[220,221] Briefly, the proximal nail fold is detached from the nail, incised at its both sides and reflected, the proximal third of the nail is detached from the matrix and lifted up to permit the melanocytic lesion to be seen, and a shallow incision is carried around it with an adequate safety margin. Using a #15 scalpel blade, the lesion is then tangentially removed with sawing motions. The nail plate is laid back and the proximal nail fold reclined and stitched. The surgical specimen is about 0.7 to 1 mm thick.[222] It is transferred onto a piece of filter paper to stretch it out and both are immersed in formalin.

Treatment of NUM

The treatment of ungual melanomas is still somewhat controversial. Whereas amputation was and still is the rule for most surgeons[223] this is only necessary for frankly invasive nail melanomas. Since 1978, we have adopted a strategy of functional surgery: in situ and early invasive melanomas are widely excised locally and the defect repaired with a free full-thickness graft or other methods;[224,225] this has proven to be very safe[226-230] and is now more and more accepted also by other dermatosurgeons[229-232] and plastic surgeons.[233] However, a Korean study measuring the distance from the matrix to the underlying bone doubted the safety of this treatment approach whereas another Korean group stated that dermal invasion of the matrix is a late event in matrix melanoma.[234,235] A recent study from Japan on 151 nail melanomas found that local recurrences were not observed independent on the type of surgery; the prognosis was determined by the tumor thickness, not the type of surgery.[236] Amputation is held to be the treatment of choice for invasive melanomas. The role of sentinel lymph node biopsy in nail melanomas is still disputed.

Histopathology

This is not the place to give a detailed account on all aspects of NUM histopathology.[2] The histopathologic diagnosis of clinically typical nail melanomas does not usually pose any difficulties. Doubtful cases often require serial and step sections, best from a total excision. This is well achieved with the tangential biopsy technique as it is always the in situ melanoma and intraepithelial component challenging the dermatopathologist. Normal matrix melanocytes are present in the suprabasal layer of the lower matrix epithelium, they are normally dormant not producing melanin, are positive for HMB45, and their number is about 6.5 per mm stretch of basal layer.[237,238] Higher melanocyte counts were yielded when counting matrix segments.[239] Melanocyte density was counted 59/mm (39–136) for melanoma as compared to 15 (5–31) in benign melanocytic hyperplasia.[237]Another method found approximately 200 melanocytes/mm^2 in the matrix that are usually dormant, particularly in the proximal matrix whereas about half of the melanocytes in the distal matrix are active. In the nail bed, there are only up to 50/mm^2 and they are quiescent. In contrast, about 1150 melanocytes are present per mm^2 in the epidermis.[240]

NUMs vary in histologic appearance depending on their exact location within the nail unit, even when a melanoma involves different areas of the same nail unit. In periungual skin, they are similar to acral lentiginous melanoma of the palm and sole. In the periphery of lesions extending from the proximal nail fold to the dorsum of the digit, they may mimic lentigo maligna melanoma except for the epidermis usually remaining of normal thickness or being slightly acanthotic.

In the beginning, most nail melanomas show a lentiginous proliferation at the dermo-epidermal junction and just above it, particularly at the advancing margin of the NUM. Some melanoma cells may be found in clear-cut suprabasal position and sometimes migrate upwards and be included into the nail plate;[241] intraungual melanoma cells always come from the matrix and not from the nail bed as was wrongly stated.[242] Although this underlines the potential importance of attached nail plate for the diagnosis of subungual melanoma[243] we recline the detached plate and fix it as this facilitates healing of the superficial matrix wound. Usually the diagnosis is more obvious in the center of the lesion and over invasive portions. Here, cellular atypia is seen, rarely a mitosis. Most subungual melanomas we have seen did not have a marked inflammatory infiltrate although this may be present focally or at the entire lesion and occasionally be so dense or lichenoid as to mask the true nature of the lesion. The melanoma cells are rounded and spindle shaped, often demonstrating long very plump dendrites. Most NUMs deriving from the matrix are pigmented and melanophages may be abundant. The degree of pigmentation is well seen in Fontana-stained sections. The localization of the melanin in the nail plate allows its origin to be suggested: Pigment in the uppermost layer derives from melanocytes of the apical matrix, that in the middle of the nail plate from the middle of the matrix, melanin in the lowermost layers from the distal matrix and pigment in all layers reflects melanocytes in the entire length of the matrix. Melanomas originating from the nail bed often, but not always, remain amelanotic. Even if melanotic they cannot give pigment into the growing nail.

Nail dystrophy is common in long-standing lesions, which is due to the gradual substitution of nail producing matrix epithelium by melanoma cells.[244-245] Any longitudinal melanonychia be it very light or dark, narrow, or wide associated with a slight nail dystrophy is suspicious for melanoma.[246-248]

The basal and suprabasal layers of the nail bed epithelium are invaded by an excessive number of melanocytes often displaying cellular atypia. Areas of invasion show subepithelial atypical melanocytes, sometimes with mitoses. Even a pigmented nail bed melanoma cannot produce a longitudinal streak as the nail keratinocytes do not produce nail plate despite one contradictory assumption.[249] Three cases of in situ amelanotic melanoma clinically mimicking lichen planus were observed. They all had a marked increase of melanocyte density in the matrix and nail bed, which was located in the basal layer and arranged in a lentiginous fashion with only a few nests. No inflammatory infiltrate was present.[250]

NUMs of the hyponychium are similar to palmar and plantar acral lentiginous melanomas. The basal and suprabasal epidermal layers are populated with more or less atypical melanocytes that are often densely pigmented. Pagetoid spread and transepidermal elimination of single and sometimes small groups of melanoma cells is frequent. Mitoses are usually rare. In invasive areas, spindle-shaped cells often predominate.

Desmoplastic areas and completely desmoplastic ALMs do occur. They are more often amelanotic and spindle-shaped.[169] The entire dermis may show an alteration of its architecture.[251] Together with focal infiltrates of lymphocytes and occasional plasma cells in or at the periphery may be a clue to the diagnosis at scanning magnification. Higher magnification exhibits spindle cells in a markedly fibrotic stroma. In subungual localization, they are often negative for S-100 and only the superficial cells are positive for Melan-A; HMB-45 is often negative. Sox10 was found to be a reliable marker for desmoplastic melanoma. Neurotropism may be seen and neurotropic melanoma may be a variant of desmoplastic melanoma.[252] Spindle cells invade the perineurial and intraneural structures; this is very difficult to see, often only giving the aspect of hypercellularity of the nerves.[253] The neurotropism is often associated with a higher risk of metastasis.

Hutchinson's sign is the periungual extension of an in situ component of subungual melanoma.[254] It often only shows a bland proliferation of melanocytes in a lentiginous pattern. Equidistant melanocyte distribution is rather the rule than an exception making the diagnosis of clear-cut melanoma in situ very difficult although rarely it may be histologically more obvious than the matrix or nail bed melanoma.[255] Immunohistochemistry may be helpful to outline the long and plump dendrites.[19] For cases where the diagnosis is not unequivocal, crowding and nesting are lacking and melanocytic atypia is not convincing like in most cases of the advancing edge of an in situ subungual melanoma or Hutchinson sign, the term atypical melanocytic hyperplasia was coined.[256] However, Hutchinson sign is not specific for melanoma and has been described (called pseudo-Hutchinson sign) in many non-melanoma conditions as summarized in Box 27.1. Hence, blindly relying on Hutchinson sign alone for the diagnosis of NUM is not advocated.

Even long-standing subungual melanomas with a decade-long history are often still in situ. There is frequently an extension on the entire matrix, all along the adjacent ventral surface of the proximal nail fold, the nail bed and the hyponychium. In these instances, the nail bed often appears to be relatively devoid of melanoma cells as compared to the matrix and the hyponychium. As in melanomas of the palms and soles, the intraepidermal component may be more extensive than clinically anticipated. In the marginal area, it may be very difficult to see single melanocytes between the keratinocytes. This is where immunohistochemical demonstration of melanocytes is indicated.[195]

BOX 27.1: Hutchinson sign in non-melanoma conditions[254]

Racial	In dark-skinned persons
Nail unit nevi	Congenital melanocytic nevus, acquired nevus, Spitz nevus, regressing nevoid melanosis in childhood
Benign tumors of the nail unit	Onychomatricoma, superficial acral fibromyxoma
Non-melanoma nail unit cancer	Bowen's disease, basal cell carcinoma
Mycologic and bacterial pigmentation	Black molds, black dermatophytes
Trauma-induced pigmentation	Friction, nail biting and picking, subungual hematoma, post-traumatic melanonychia
Dermatological conditions	Laugier–Hunziker–Baran syndrome, epidermodysplasia verruciformis
Systemic conditions	Peutz–Jegher syndrome, pregnancy, malnutrition, pituitary tumor, and Addison's disease
Infections	Acquired immune deficiency syndrome
Drugs	Minocycline, zidovudine, amlodipine, hydroxycarbamide
Miscellaneous	Radiation therapy, silver nitrate staining

Immunohistochemistry is a diagnostic adjunct for nail melanomas.[257–261] The most commonly used antibodies are MART-1, MelanA, HMB45, and S-100p. MART-1 and MelanA are two slightly different clones of melanosomal proteins recognized by T cells and are cytoplasmic markers for melanocytes with very similar staining profiles; however, they may also stain melanosomes in keratinocytes and melanophages. S-100 has a sensitivity of 90% and specificity of 70% whereas HMB45 has a specificity of 97% and sensitivity of 75% in cutaneous melanoma. Junctional cells are more intensely marked than dermal cells.[262] HMB-45 or Melan-A do not stain 83% of spindle cell and desmoplastic melanoma. S-100p is less specific as it stains many other cells derived from the neural crest, but in nail melanomas, this antigen is often lost.[263] Furthermore, they are not really specific and also stain other neural crest derived tumors, adenocarcinomas and even lymphomas.[264] Microphthalmia transcription factor 1 (MITF-1) is less frequently used[265,266] although the staining with MITF-1 is more specific as it does not stain melanin or melanosomes, but the nuclei. Sox10 is a transcription factor necessary for the development of the neural crest and of melanocytes. It is expressed in the nuclei of melanocytes, melanoma cells, peripheral nerve sheath cells, and secretory sweat gland portions, but also some other tissues, particularly breast.[267] It is useful for the diagnosis of desmoplastic melanoma since fibroblasts and histiocytes remain unstained.[268,269] Using MelanA together with Sox10 staining, benign reactive dermal melanocytes were identified in approximately 10% of melanoma in situ cases and nearly one third of squamous and BCCs.[270] Sox10 is upregulated with melanoma progression.[271] Both Sox10 and MITF-1 allow easy distinction of pigmented keratinocytes from melanocytes and melanoma cells, but none distinguishes benign from malignant melanocytic lesions.[272]

Recently, new monoclonal antibodies against melanocytic differentiation antigens (MAGE, NKI/C3, NKI/beteb, KBA 62, BNL2) and melanocyte antibody cocktails were developed that virtually stain all melanoma cells; however, they are not melanoma-specific.[273,274] It appears that Ki67 (MiB1) is the most useful adjunct in differentiating benign from malignant melanocytic tumors.[258]

Whereas most of our patients presented with in situ and early invasive melanomas large numbers of patients from other centers showed appallingly thick and advanced tumors.[203,236,237] These cases do not present the diagnostic difficulties outlined above.

Several cases of subungual melanoma with chondroid and osseous differentiation were observed.[113,274,275]

Melanomas are characterized by heterogeneous DNA mutations leading to the activation of oncogenes and inactivation of tumor suppressor genes and by gains, losses, and amplifications of whole or partial chromosomes. These genomic aberrations lead to mutational and karyotypic profiles that differ amongst different subtypes of melanoma.[276–279]

Approximately one third of acral and mucosal melanomas as well as melanomas of chronically sun-damaged skin have c-KIT, 10% of acral melanomas have NRAS and 10%–15% BRAF V600 mutations.[280,281] Fluorescence in situ hybridization (FISH) and comparative genomic hybridization (CGH) studies have shown that molecular genetically altered cells can be found in the epidermis up to 9 mm from the visible margin of pigmented acral lentiginous melanoma, but this phenomenon was restricted to the in situ melanocytes; they were called field cells.[282] This is probably the reason that acral melanomas seemingly excised *in toto* were observed to recur. Immunohistochemical demonstration of cKIT/CD117 may be useful to identify patients that could benefit from imatinib therapy.[283]

There is now much research on potential melanoma stem cells;[284,285] however, this has not yet arrived at nail unit melanomas.

The histogenetic type of melanoma—ALM, SSM or NM—is difficult to define in the nail. It is, however, not really important as the molecular genetic investigations have not shown differences among them, but among melanomas of different localizations. Clark level and Breslow thickness are also very difficult to ascertain. This is not only due to the fact that most biopsies are only partial, but that the nail anatomy itself is different from skin. The papillary and reticular dermis are not clearly separated, and there is no cutaneous fat between the distal matrix-nail bed and the periosteum.[167] Clark level I is therefore intraepidermal, II is very superficial, III is invasion into the mid- to deep dermis, IV almost reaches the periosteum, and V is invasion to or into the bone. Measuring the vertical tumor thickness according to Breslow is challenging as there is normally no granular layer in the matrix and nail bed and the epithelium may be acanthotic and grossly thickened giving large numbers that do not really reflect the prognosis. Therefore, a division into melanomas thinner or thicker than 2.5 mm has been proposed; this gave statistically significant differences in survival after 5 years: 88% *vs.* 40%.[166] Old age, ulceration, higher mitotic index, amelanotic tumor, and higher stage of disease are further negative prognostic factors.[143]

Melanomas often show characteristic gene alterations seen in fluorescent in situ hybridization (FISH) and CGH. KIT mutations are more frequent in acral lentiginous melanomas than in those of light-exposed skin. Gene amplifications were seen in all ALMs investigated, most commonly on chromosome 11q13 where cyclin D1 is a potential candidate gene. In contrast, mutations of the BRAF oncogene are less frequent.[286–289] These changes were typical for melanomas of the palms, soles, and nail independent of their histological growth pattern.[290]

Erosive oozing tumors of the nail may be adequate for cytological diagnosis of smears. This is easily performed with a glass slide that is gently scraped over the tumor and then over another slide to spread the cells. After drying and short alcohol-acetone fixation, the cytosmear can be stained for H&E and a melanocyte marker.[2]

NAIL MELANOMA IN CHILDREN

Longitudinal melanonychia is not an uncommon finding in children, particularly in Asians, Africans, native Americans, and Afro-Americans. Most cases are due to either melanocyte activation, lentigo, or junctional nevi in the matrix. In attempts to use dermatoscopy of longitudinal melanonychia, great uncertainty was found.[291] In small children, the nevus may show broad pigmentation with some variegation of the brown color similar to that seen in adult nails with melanoma. The parents usually are not only concerned because of the faint risk of being an infant nail melanoma, but also the embarrassing esthetic effect. In children, the pigmentation first exhibits a rapid increase in color intensity and width and then characteristically stabilizes. At adolescence, there is often a regression or even complete disappearance.[292,293] Thus, in general, a brown streak in the nail of a child should be taken as a benign lesion. However, when the streak suddenly widens after having been present and stable for years, becomes markedly darker and wider proximally than distally, a diagnostic excision is recommended.

There are some reports in the literature on nail melanomas in children. This is generally a rare event and most dermatopathologists hesitate to make this diagnosis in children as there may be considerable nuclear atypia in infantile matrix nevi. One of our cases sent to a panel of melanoma and nail pathology specialists was not diagnosed as melanoma but as atypical melanocytic hyperplasia.[179,191] Not all lesions described in children were unanimously accepted as nail melanoma, e.g., the first case described in a child that was probably fair skinned[294] and in some of the cases reported from Japan.[295] In fact, most cases were described from Japan,[296] but also from other countries with more intensely pigmented people such as the Philippines,[297] Argentina, Brazil,[49] Colombia,[190] and the USA.[298] Two cases had positive lymph nodes.[294,299]

RARE MELANOCYTIC TUMORS

A case of a collision tumor of subungual squamomelanocytic tumor was observed with a positive sentinel lymph node. Whereas the biopsy had only shown a melanoma in situ total nail unit resection revealed a SCC in a melanoma occupying the entire matrix and nail bed with ulceration and many mitoses.[300] In contrast, a recent publication on co-occurrence of NUM and nail bed SCC showed in fact the association of subungual onycholemmal cysts with subungual melanoma.[301]

THE MELANONYCHIA PROBLEM

The diagnosis of ungual melanoma in children is often not made. Lentigines and junctional nevi of the matrix in children may exhibit very worrying features that when present in an adult nail would be diagnosed as melanoma without hesitation.

Another problem is the acquired, histopathologically often barely noticeable melanonychia in adults. As is known from the advancing edge of subungual in situ melanomas the correct diagnosis can be extremely difficult; indeed, it is often challenging to recognize melanocytes at all.[302] In our experience, an acquired melanonychia in an adult fair-skinned Caucasian should always be considered of potential biologic malignancy despite appearing morphologically bland with the exception of functional melanonychia (Table 27.1).

Table 27.1 Melanonychia and age of onset in light-skinned individuals

Babies and children	Benign
Adolescents	Usually benign
Adults < 30 years	Probably benign
Adults > 30 years	Suspicious
Adults > 40 years	Probably malignant
Adults > 50 years	Usually malignant

Differential diagnoses

Generally accepted criteria for the diagnosis of early nail melanoma do not (yet) exist.[2] A clinico-pathologic correlation is necessary. However, in general, the clinical appearance of a pigmented streak is of little help in establishing the correct diagnosis.[303] The most important differential diagnosis of ungual melanoma is a benign melanocytic proliferation.[304] In longitudinal melanonychia, the responsible melanocytic lesion may be an activation of normal matrix melanocytes without a higher number of melanocytes, called functional melanonychia, or a numerical increase in the number of normal melanocytes, i.e., a lentigo or a nevus. The histopathologic changes seen in functional melanonychia may be very subtle and require immunohistochemistry to visualize the melanocytes and special pigment stains such as Fontana–Masson to see the melanin. A lentigo is usually visible in H&E stained sections as it contains more melanin and some single melanophages may be seen in the superficial matrix dermis. A melanocytic nevus of the matrix is defined by the presence of nests of melanocytes without cellular atypia and with slender dendrites. Whereas some authors claim that a melanonychia in a child as well as a very light-brown band in adults do not require histopathologic examination it is our policy to excision-biopsy all cases as the tangential matrix biopsy avoids post-operative nail dystrophy.

Particularly in subjects with dark skin, an ungual Bowen's disease may cause a longitudinal pigmentation.[21,305–308] This is histopathologically seen as a population of the lesion by normal melanocytes. Also, SCC may be pigmented.[219]

Fungal melanonychia presents a diffuse light yellow-brown staining of the nail. Many different species have been isolated; *Trichophyton rubrum* is the most common cause in Central Europe, but a number of non-dermatophytic molds were also found to produce brown-to-black nails.[309] One case of longitudinal melanonychia in three toenails with fumagoid cells (Medlar bodies), a peculiar pattern of chromoblastomycosis, was described.[310]

METASTASES

Metastases to the nail apparatus are very rare. They are usually a late sign and the life expectancy of most patients is short, usually between 3 and 6 months. Men are twice as often affected as women and fingers are five times more frequently involved than toes. Bronchial carcinoma is the most common malignancy metastasizing to the distal phalanx and nail region, but many other malignancies were also found.[305,306] Distal phalangeal metastases are often mistaken for an inflammation or infection. Usually, they are little symptomatic compared to their size, but painful subungual metastases have also been described. The histopathology depends on the type of primary neoplasm and often only permits a "group" diagnosis if the primary tumor is not known. Treatment is by distal amputation if it is not too late anyway.

REFERENCES

1. Haneke E. Important malignant and new nail tumors. *J Dtsch Dermatol Ges* 2017; 15: 367–386.
2. Haneke E. *Histopathology of the Nail—Onychopathology.* Boca Raton, FL: CRC Press, 2017.
3. Stern DK, Creasey AA, Quijije J, Lebwohl MG. UV-A and UV-B penetration of normal human cadaveric fingernail plate. *Arch Dermatol* 2011; 147: 439–441.
4. Potter GK. Neoplasia in the toes and toenail areas. *Clin Podiatr Med Surg* 1995; 12: 287–297.
5. Perrin C, Langbein L, Ambrossetti D, Erfan N, Schweizer J, Michiels JF. Onychocytic carcinoma: A new entity. *Am J Dermatopathol* 2013; 35: 679–684.
6. Wang L, Gao T, Wang G. Invasive onychocytic carcinoma. *J Cutan Pathol* 2015; 42: 361–367.
7. Chaser BE, Renszel KM, Crowson AN, Osmundson A, Shendrik IV et al. Onycholemmal carcinoma: A morphologic comparison of 6 reported cases. *J Am Acad Dermatol* 2013; 68: 290–295.
8. Alessi E, Zorzi F, Gianotti R, Parafioriti A. Malignant proliferating onycholemmal cyst. *J Cutan Pathol* 1994; 21: 183–188.
9. Maity JP, Nath B, Kar S, Chen CY, Banerjee S, Jean JS, Liu MY et al. Arsenic-induced health crisis in peri-urban Moyna and Ardebok villages, West Bengal, India: An exposure assessment study. *Environ Geochem Health* 2012; 34: 563–574.
10. Haneke E. Arsenverbindungen - eine Gefahr für den biologischen Präparator. *Präparator* 1978; 24: 131–135.
11. Khandpur S, Malhotra AK, Bhatia V, Gupta S, Sharma VK, Mishra R, Arora NK. Chronic arsenic toxicity from Ayurvedic medicines. *Int J Dermatol* 2008; 47: 618–621.
12. Elmariah SB, Anolik R, Walters RF, Rosenman K, Pomeranz MK, Sanchez MR. Invasive squamous-cell carcinoma and arsenical keratoses. *Dermatol Online J* 2008; 14(10): 24.
13. Hundeiker M, Petres J. Morphogenese und Formenreichtum der arseninduzierten Präkanzerosen. *Arch Klin Exp Dermatol* 1968; 231: 355–365.
14. Gunjan M, Jacobs AA, Orengo IF, McClunga A, Rosen T. Combination therapy with imiquimod, 5-fluorouracil, and tazarotene in the treatment of extensive radiation-induced Bowen's disease of the hands. *Dermatol Surg* 2009; 35: 1–7. doi:10.1111/j.1524-4725.2009.01325.x.
15. Haneke E. Morbus Bowen und Plattenepithelkarzinom der Nagelregion – klinisches Spektrum und Therapie. In: Winter H, Bellmann K-P, eds. *Fortschritte der Operativen und onkologischen Dermatologie - Operative Dermatologie - Möglichkeiten und Grenzen.* Berlin, Germany: Springer, 1995; 9: 187–190.
16. Haneke E. Epidermoid carcinoma (Bowen's disease) of the nail simulating acquired ungual fibrokeratoma. *Skin Cancer* 1991; 6: 217–221.
17. Haneke E, Bragadini LA, Mainusch O. Enfermedad de Bowen de células claras del aparato ungular. *Act Terap Dermatol* 1997; 20: 311–313.
18. Baran R, Perrin C. Longitudinal erythronychia with distal subungual keratosis. Onychopapilloma of the nail bed and Bowen's disease. *Br J Dermatol* 2000; 143: 132–135.
19. Guitart J, Bergfeld WF, Tuthull RJ, Tubbs RR, Zienowicz R, Fleegler EJ. Squamous cell carcinoma of the nail bed: A clinicopathological study of 12 cases. *Br J Dermatol* 1990; 123: 215–222.
20. Haneke E. Bowen's disease of the nails. *4th Cong Eur Acad Dermatol Venereol, Brussels,* Oct 10–15, 1995: Abstracts on CD-ROM EADV 1995:S75.
21. Baran R, Eichmann A. Longitudinal melanonychia associated with Bowen disease. *Dermatology* 1993: 18: 159–160.
22. Baran R, Gormley D. Polydactylous Bowen's disease of the nail. *J Am Acad Dermatol* 1987; 17: 201–204.
23. Perruchoud DL, Varonier C, Haneke E, Hunger RE, Beltraminelli H, Borradori L, Ehnis Pérez A. Bowen disease of the nail unit: A retrospective study of 12 cases and their association with human papillomaviruses. *J Eur Acad Dermatol Venereol* 2016; 30(9): 1503–1506.
24. Shim WH, Park HJ, Kim HS, Kim SH, Jung DS, Ko HC, Kim BS, Kim MB, Kwon KS. Bowenoid papulosis of the vulva and subsequent periungual Bowen's disease induced by the same mucosal HPVs. *Ann Dermatol* 2011; 23: 493–496.
25. Turowski CB, Ross AS, Cusack CA. Human papillomavirus-associated squamous cell carcinoma of the nail bed in African-American patients. *Int J Dermatol* 2009; 48: 117–120.
26. Shimizu A, Tamura A, Abe M, Amano H, Motegi S, Nakatani Y, Hoshino H, Ishikawa O. Human papillomavirus type 56-associated Bowen's disease. *Br J Dermatol* 2012; 167: 1161–1164.
27. Stetsenko GY, McFarlane RJ, Chien AJ, Fleckman P, Swanson P, George E, Argenyi ZB. Subungual Bowen disease in a patient with epidermodysplasia verruciformis presenting clinically as longitudinal melanonychia. *Am J Dermatopathol* 2008; 30: 582–585.
28. Ongenae K, Van De Kerckhove M, Naeyart J. Bowen's disease of the nail. *Dermatology* 2002; 204: 348–350.
29. Young LC, Tuxen AJ, Goodman G. Mohs' micrographic surgery as treatment for squamous dysplasia of the nail unit. *Australas J Dermatol* 2012; 53: 123–127.
30. Gómez Vázquez M1, Navarra Amayuelas R. Periungual Bowenoid papulosis due to human papillomavirus type 42. *Actas Dermosifiliogr* 2013; 104: 932–934.

31. Papadopoulos AJ, Schwartz RA, Lefkowitz A, Tinkle LL, Jänniger CK, Lambert WC. Extragenital Bowenoid papulosis associated with atypical human papillomavirus genotypes. *J Cut Med Surg* 2002; 6: 1117–1119.

32. Sung W, Sam H, Deleyiannis FW. Subungual squamous cell carcinoma after organ transplantation. *J Am Podiatr Med Ass* 2010; 100: 304–308.

33. Patel PP, Hoppe IC, Bell WR, Lambert WC, Fleegler EJ. Perils of diagnosis and detection of subungual squamous cell carcinoma. *Ann Dermatol* 2011; 23(Suppl 3): S285–287.

34. Mauro JA, Maslyn R, Stein AA. Squamous-cell carcinoma of nail bed in hereditary ectodermal dysplasia. *N Y State J Med* 1972; 72: 1065–1066.

35. Canovas F, Dereure O, Bonnel F. A propos d'un cas de carcinoma épidermoïde du lit unguéal avec métastase intraneurale du nerf médian. *Ann Chir Main* 1998; 17: 232–235.

36. Batalla A, Feal C, Roson E, Posada C. Subungual squamous cell carcinoma: A case series. *Ind J Dermatol* 2014: 59: 352–354.

37. Figus A, Kanitkar S, Elliot D. Squamous cell carcinoma of the lateral nail fold. *J Hand Surg [Br]* 2006; 31: 216–220.

38. Mii S, Amoh Y, Tanabe K, Kitasato H, Sato Y, Katsuoka K. Nestin expression in Bowen's disease and Bowen's carcinoma associated with human papillomavirus. *Eur J Dermatol* 2011; 21: 515–519.

39. Misago N, Toda S, Narisawa Y. Tricholemmoma and clear cell squamous cell carcinoma (associated with Bowen's disease): Immunohistochemical profile in comparison to normal hair follicles. *Am J Dermatopathol* 2012; 34: 394–399.

40. Corbalán-Vélez R, Oviedo-Ramírez I, Ruiz-Maciá JA, Conesa-Zamora P, Sánchez-Hernández M, Martínez-Barba E, Brufau-Redondo C, López-Lozano JM. Immunohistochemical staining of p16 in squamous cell carcinomas of the genital and extragenital area. *Actas Dermosifiliogr* 2011; 102: 439–447.

41. McKee R, Wilkinson JD, Black MM, Whimster IW. Carcinoma (epithelioma) cuniculatum: A clinico-pathological study of nineteen cases and review of the literature. *Histopathology* 1981; 5: 425–436.

42. Baran R, Haneke E. *Epithelioma cuniculatum. XIth Congress of the International Society of Dermatologic Surgery*, Florence, Italy, Book of Abstracts 1990.

43. Kurashige Y, Kato Y, Hobo A, Tsuboi R. Subungual verrucous carcinoma with bone invasion. *Int J Dermatol* 2013; 52: 217–219.

44. Haneke E, Baran R. Epithelioma cuniculatum, histopathology, immuno and lectin histochemistry. *XIth Congress of the International Society of Dermatologic Surgery*, Florence, Italy, Book of Abstracts 1990.

45. Badani H, Abi Ayad Y, Saleh H, Kadi A, Mahammedi M, Zaidi N, Serradj A. Carcinome verruqueux de l'orteil: La difficulté de diagnostic. *Ann Dermatol Vénéréol* 2013; 140: S120–S121.

46. Forman SB, Ferringer TC, Garrett AB. Basal cell carcinoma of the nail unit. *J Am Acad Dermatol* 2007; 56: 811–814.

47. Martinelli PT, Cohen PR, Schulze KE, Dorsey KE, Nelson BR. Periungual basal cell carcinoma: Case report and literature review. *Dermatol Surg* 2006; 32: 320–323.

48. Brasie RA, Patel AR, Nouri K. Basal cell carcinoma of the nail unit treated with Mohs micrographic surgery: Superficial multicentric BCC with jagged borders—A histopathological hallmark for nail unit BCC. *J Drugs Dermatol* 2006; 5: 660–663.

49. Rudolph RI. Subungual basal cell carcinoma presenting as longitudinal melanonychia. *J Am Acad Dermatol* 1987; 16: 229–233.

50. Waldman MH, Jacobs LA. Malignant tumors of the foot. A report of 2 cases. *J Am Podiatr Med Ass* 1986; 76: 345.

51. Matsushita K, Kawada A, Aragane Y, Tezuka T. Basal cell carcinoma on the right hallux. *J Dermatol* 2003; 30: 250–251.

52. Herzinger T, Flaig M, Diederich R, Röcken M. Basal cell carcinoma of the toenail unit. *J Am Acad Dermatol* 2003; 48: 277–278.

53. Krüger K, Blume-Peytavi U, Orfanos CE. Basal cell carcinoma possibly originates from the outer root sheath and/or the bulge region of the vellus hair follicle. *Arch Dermatol Res* 1999; 291: 253–259.

54. Sellheyer K, Krahl D. Basal cell (trichoblastic) carcinoma. Common expression pattern for epithelial cell adhesion molecule links basal cell carcinoma to early follicular embryogenesis, secondary hair germ, and outer root sheath of the vellus hair follicle: A clue to the adnexal nature of basal cell carcinoma? *J Am Acad Dermatol* 2008; 58: 158–167.

55. Ansai SI, Takayama R, Kimura T, Kawana S. Ber-EP4 is a useful marker for follicular germinative cell differentiation of cutaneous epithelial neoplasms. *J Dermatol* 2012; 39: 688–692.

56. Kao GF, Helwig EB, Graham JH. Aggressive digital papillary adenoma and adenocarcinoma. A clinicopathological study of 57 patients with histochemical, immunopathological and ultrastructural observations. *J Cutan Pathol* 1987; 14: 129–146.

57. Duke WH, Sherod TT, Lupton GP. Aggressive digital papillary carcinoma (aggressive digital papillary adenoma and adenocarcinoma revisited). *Am J Surg Pathol* 2000; 24: 775–784.

58. Ferrándiz-Pulido C, Fernández-Figueras MT, Marco V, Combalia A, Ferrándiz C. An intertriginous lesion on the foot of a 74-year-old man: Aggressive digital papillary adenocarcinoma. *Clin Exp Dermatol* 2014; 39: 102–104.

59. Frey J, Shimek C, Woodmansee C, Myers E, Greer S, Liman A, Adelman C, Rasberry R. Aggressive digital papillary adenocarcinoma: A report of two diseases and review of the literature. *J Am Acad Dermatol* 2009; 60: 331–339.

60. Chi CC, Kuo TT, Wang SH. Aggressive digital papillary adenocarcinoma: A silent malignancy masquerading as acquired digital fibrokeratoma. *Am J Clin Dermatol* 2007; 8: 243–245.

61. Inaloz HS, Patel GK, Knight AG. An aggressive treatment for aggressive digital papillary adenocarcinoma. *Cutis* 2002; 69: 179–182.

62. Gorva AD, Mohil R, Srinivasan MS. Aggressive digital papillary adenocarcinoma presenting as a paronychia of the finger. *J Hand Surg [Br]* 2005; 30: 534.

63. Bogner PN, Fullen DR, Lowe L, Paulino A, Biermann JS, Sondak VK, Su LD. Lymphatic mapping and sentinel lymph node biopsy in the detection of early metastasis from sweat gland carcinoma. *Cancer* 2003; 97: 2285–2289.

64. Singla AK, Shearin JC. Aggressive surgical treatment of digital papillary adenocarcinoma. *Plast Reconstr Surg* 1997; 99: 2058–2060.

65. Cebellos PI, Penneys NS, Acosta H. Aggressive digital papillary adenocarcinoma. *J Am Acad Dermatol* 1990; 23: 331–334.

66. Borradori L, Hertel R, Balli-Antunes M, Zala L. Metastatic eccrine sweat gland carcinoma: Case report. *Dermatologica* 1988; 177: 295–299.

67. Pinkus H, Mehregan AH. Epidermotropic eccrine carcinoma. *Arch Dermatol* 1963; 88: 597–606.

68. Van Gorp J, van der Putte SC. Periungual eccrine porocarcinoma. *Dermatology* 1993; 187: 67–70.

69. Requena L, Sanchez M, Aguilar P, Ambrojo P, Sánchez Yus E. Periungual porocarcinoma. *Dermatologica* 1990; 180: 177–180.

70. Moussallem CD, Abi Hatem NE, El-Khouri ZN. Malignant porocarcinoma of the nail fold: A tricky diagnosis. *Dermatol Online* 2008; 14: 8.

71. Zina AM, Bundino S, Pippione MG. Pigmented hidroacanthoma simplex with porocarcinoma. Light and electron microscopic study of a case. *J Cutan Pathol* 1982; 9: 104–112.

72. Landa NG, Winkelmann RK. Epidermotropic eccrine porocarcinoma. *J Am Acad Dermatol* 1991; 24: 27–31.

73. Rütten A, Requena L, Requena C. Clear-cell porocarcinoma in situ: A cytologic variant of porocarcinoma in situ. *Am J Dermatopathol* 2002; 24: 67–71.

74. Robson A, Green J, Ansari N, Kim B, Seed PT, McKee PH, Calonje E. Eccrine porocarcinoma (malignant eccrine poroma): A clinicopathologic study of 69 cases. *Am J Surg Pathol* 2001; 25: 710–720.

75. Huet P, Dandurand M, Pignodel C, Guillot B. Metastasizing eccrine porocarcinoma: Report of a case and review of the literature. *J Am Acad Dermatol* 1996; 35: 680–684.

76. Akalin T, Sen S, Yucetürk A, Kandiloglu G. P53 expression in eccrine poroma and porocarcinoma. *Am J Dermatopathol* 2001; 23: 402–406.

77. Tateyama H, Eimoto T, Toda T, Inagaki H, Nakamura T, Yamauchi R. p53 protein and proliferating cell nuclear antigen in eccrine poroma and porocarcinoma, an immunohistochemal study. *Am J Dermatol* 1995; 17: 457–464.

78. Gu LH, Ichiki Y, Kitayama Y. Aberrant expression of p16 and RB protein in eccrine porocarcinoma. *J Cutan Pathol* 2002; 29: 473–479.

79. Gschnait F, Horn F, Lindlbauer R, Sponer D. Eccrine porocarcinoma. *J Cutan Pathol* 1980; 7: 349–353.

80. Geraci TL, Janis L, Jenkinson S, Stewart R. Mucinous (adenocystic) sweat gland carcinoma of the great toe. *J Foot Surg* 1987: 26: 520–523.

81. Argenyi ZB, Nguyen AV, Balogh K, Sears JK, Whitaker DC. Malignant eccrine spiradenoma. A clinicopathologic study. *Am J Dermatopathol* 1992; 14: 381–390.

82. Ishikawa M, Nakanishi Y, Yamazaki N, Yamamoto A. Malignant eccrine spiradenoma: A case report and review of the literature. *Dermatol Surg* 2001; 27: 67–70.

83. Meyer TK, Rhee JS, Smith MM, Cruz MJ, Osipov VO, Wackym PA. External auditory canal eccrine spiadenocarcinoma: A case report and review of literature. *Head Neck* 2003; 25: 505–510.

84. Engel CJ, Meads GE, Joseph NG, Stavraky W. Eccrine spiradenoma: A report of malignant transformation. *Can J Surg* 1991; 34: 477–480.

85. McCluggage WG, Fon LJ, O'Rourke D, Ismail M, Hill CM, Parks TG, Allen DC. Malignant eccrine spiradenoma with carcinomatous and sarcomatous elements. *J Clin Pathol* 1997; 50: 871–873.

86. Nash J, Chaffins M, Krull E. Hidradenocarcinoma. *59th Ann Meet Am Acad Dermatol*, Washington, DC, March 2–7, 2001.

87. Kasdan ML, Stutts JT, Kassan MA, Clanton JN. Sebaceous gland carcinoma of the finger. *J Hand Surg* 1991; 16A: 870–872.

88. Inoue A, Hasegawa T, Ikata T, Hizawa K. Fibrosarcoma of the toe: A destructive lesion of the distal phalanx. *Clin Orthop Relat Res* 1996; 333: 239–244.

89. San Miguel P, Fernández G, Ortiz-Rey JA, Larrauri P. Low-grade myofibroblastic sarcoma of the distal phalanx. *J Hand Surg Am* 2004; 29: 1160–1163.

90. Tsai YJ, Lin PY, Chew KY, Chiang YC. Dermatofibrosarcoma protuberans in children and adolescents: Clinical presentation,

histology, treatment, and review of the literature. *J Plast Reconstr Aesthet Surg* 2014; 67: 1222–1229.

91. Coles M, Smith M, Rankin EA. An unusual case of dermatofibrosarcoma protuberans. *J Hand Surg* 1989; 14A: 135–138.

92. Hashiro M, Fujio Y, Shoda Y, Okumura M. A case of dermatofibrosarcoma protuberans on the right first toe. *Cutis* 1995; 56: 281–282.

93. Dumas V, Euvrard S, Ligeron C, Ronger S, Chouvet B, Faure M, Claudy A. Dermatofibrosarcome de Darier–Ferrand sous-unguéal. *Ann Dermatol Vénéréol* 1998; 125(Suppl 3): S93.

94. Norlelawati AT, Mohd Danial G, Nora H, Nadia O, Zatur Rawihah K, Nor Zamzila A, Naznin M. Detection of SYT-SSX mutant transcripts in formalin-fixed paraffin-embedded sarcoma tissues using one-step reverse transcriptase real-time PCR. *Malays J Pathol* 2016; 38: 11–18.

95. Carloz B, Bioulac P, Gavard J, Baudet J, Doutre MS, Beylot C. Récidives multiples d'un sarcome épithélioïde. *Ann Dermatol Vénéréol* 1991; 118: 623–628.

96. Khapake DP, Jambhekar NA, Anchan C, Madur BP, Chinoy RF, Agarwal M, Puri A. Epithelioid sarcoma of the foot with subsequent lesion in hand: Metastatic lesion or second primary? *Indian J Pathol Microbiol* 2007; 50: 563–565.

97. Zaias N. *The Nail in Health and Disease*. Norwalk, CT: Appleton, 1990.

98. Aïm F, Rosier L, Dumontier C. Isolated Kaposi sarcoma of the finger pulp in an AIDS patient. *Orthop Traumatol Surg Res* 2012; 98: 126–128.

99. Kennedy CT, Burton PA, Cook P. Swollen toe due to epithelioid haemangioma of bone. *Br J Dermatol* 1990; 123(Suppl 37): 85–89.

100. Bessis D, Sotto A, Roubert P, Chabrier PE, Mourad G, Guilhou JJ. Endothelin-secreting angiosarcoma occurring at the site of an arteriovenous fistula for haemodialysis in a renal transplant recipient. *Br J Dermatol.* 1998; 138: 361–363.

101. Kikuchi K, Watanabe M, Terui T, Ohtani N, Ohtani H, Tagami H. Nail destroying epithelioid haemangioendothelioma showing an erythematous scar-like appearance on the finger. *Br J Dermatol* 2003; 148: 834–836.

102. Davies MFP, Curtis M, Howat JMT. Cutaneous haemangioendothelioma, possible link with chronic exposure to vinyl chloride. *Br J Indust Med* 1990; 47: 65–67.

103. Laskowski J, Bamberg C, Zimmermann R, Gross G. Multifokales Hämangioendotheliom der unteren Extremität. *Hautarzt* 1999; 50(Suppl 1): S74.

104. Wetherington RW, Lyle WG, Sangüeza OP. Malignant glomus tumor of the thumb: A case report. *J Hand Surg Am* 1997; 22: 1098–1102.

105. Bailey SC, Bailey B, Smith NT, Van Tassel P, Thomas CR Jr. Brain metastasis from a primary liposarcoma of the digit: Case report. *Am J Clin Oncol* 2001; 24: 81–84.

106. Bryant J. Subungual epithelioid leiomyosarcoma. *South Med J* 1992; 85: 560–561.

107. Sivridis E, Verettas D. Chondrosarcoma in the distal phalanx of the ring finger. A case report. *Acta Orthop Scand* 1990; 61: 183–184.

108. Debruyne PR, Dumez H, Demey W, Gillis L, Sciot R, Schöffski P. Recurrent low- to intermediate-grade chondrosarcoma of the thumb with lung metastases: An objective response to trofosfamide. *Onkologie* 2007; 30: 201–204.

109. Tos P, Artiaco S, Linari A, Battiston B. Chondrosarcoma in the distal phalanx of index finger: Clinical report and literature review. *Chir Main* 2009; 28: 265–269.

110. Masuda T, Otuka T, Yonezawa M, Kamiyama F, Shibata Y, Tada T, Matsui N. Chondrosarcoma of the distal phalanx of the second toe: A case report. *J Foot Ankle Surg* 2004; 43: 110–112.

111. Nakajima H, Ushigome S, Fukuda J. Case report 482: Chondrosarcoma (grade 1) arising from the right second toe in patient with multiple enchondromas. *Skeletal Radiol* 1988; 17: 289–292.

112. Engels C, Werner M, Delling G. Clear-cell chondrosarcoma. *Pathologe* 2000; 21: 449–455.

113. Cachia AR, Kedziora AM. Subungual malignant melanoma with cartilaginous differentiation. *Am J Dermatopathol* 1999; 21: 165–169.

114. Wood MK, Erdmann MW, Davies DM. Malignant schwannoma mistakenly diagnosed as carpal tunnel syndrome. *J Hand Surg Br* 1993; 18: 187–188.

115. Urabe A, Imayama S, Yasumoto S, Nakayama J, Hori Y. Malignant granular cell tumor. *J Dermatol* 1991; 18: 161–166.

116. Kassem A, Schöpflin A, Diaz C, Weyers W, Stickeler E, Werner M, Zur Hausen A. Frequent detection of Merkel cell polyomavirus in human Merkel cell carcinomas and identification of a unique deletion in the VP1 gene. *Cancer Res* 2008; 68: 5009–5013.

117. Engelmann L, Kunze J, Haneke E. Giant neuroendocrine carcinoma of the skin (Merkel cell tumour). *Skin Cancer* 1991; 6: 211–216.

118. Haneke E, Schulze HJ, Mahrle G. Immunohistochemical and immunoelectron microscopic demonstration of chromogranin A in formalin-fixed tissue of Merkel cell carcinoma. *J Am Acad Dermatol* 1993; 28: 222–226.

119. Haneke E. Electron microscopy of Merkel cell carcinoma from formalin-fixed tissue. *J Am Acad Dermatol* 1985; 12: 487–492.

120. Steens SC, Kroon HM, Taminiau AH, de Schepper AM, Watt I. Nail-patella syndrome associated with Ewing sarcoma. *J Belge Radiol – Belg T Radiol* 2007; 90: 214–215.

121. San-Juan M, Dölz R, Garcia-Barrecheguren E, Noain E, Sierrasesumaga L, Canadell J, Limb salvage in bone sarcomas in patients younger than 10 years. A 20-year experience. *J Pediatr Orthop* 2003; 23: 753–762.

122. Binesh F, Sobhanardekani M, Zare S, Behniafard N. Subungual Ewing sarcoma/PNET tumor family of the great toe: A case report. *Electron Physician* 2016; 8: 2238–2242.

123. Harper JI, Staughton R. Letterer-Siwe disease with nail involvement. *Cutis* 1983; 31: 493, 498.

124. Kahn G. Nail involvement in histiocytosis-X. *Arch Dermatol* 1969; 100: 699–701.

125. Mataix J, Betlloch I, Lucas-Costa A, Pérez-Crespo M, Moscardó-Guilleme C. Nail changes in Langerhans cell histiocytosis: A possible marker of multisystem disease. *Pediatr Dermatol* 2008; 25: 247–251.

126. Kumar V, Angappan D, Scott J, Munirathnam D, Vij M, Shanmugam N. Extensive nail changes in a toddler with multisystemic Langerhans cell histiocytosis. *Pediatr Dermatol* 2017; 34: 732–734.

127. Chander R, Jaykar K, Varghese B, Garg T, Seth A, Nagia A. Pulmonary disease with striking nail involvement in a child. *Pediatr Dermatol* 2008; 25: 633–634.

128. Sabui TK, Purkait R. Nail changes in Langerhans cell histiocytosis. *Indian Pediatr* 2009; 46: 728–729.

129. Tallon B, Rademaker M. Asymptomatic papules over the proximal nail fold in a child. *Arch Dermatol* 2008; 144: 105–110.

130. Berker DL, Lever LR, Windebank K. Nail features in Langerhans cell histiocytosis. *Br J Dermatol* 1994; 1 30: 523–527.

131. Jain S, Sehgal VN, Bajaj P. Nail changes in Langerhans cell histiocytosis. *J Eur Acad Dermatol Venereol* 2000; 14: 212–215.

132. Ashena Z, Alavi S, Arzanian MT, Eshghi P. Nail involvement in Langerhans cell histiocytosis. *Pediatr Hematol Oncol* 2007; 24: 45–51.

133. Peters K-P, Vigneswaran N, Hornstein OP, Haneke E. Peanut agglutinin in the diagnosis of skin tumours. *17th World Congr Dermatol* 1987; II: 368.

134. Tran G, Huynh TN, Paller AS. Langerhans cell histiocytosis: A neoplastic disorder driven by Ras-ERK pathway mutations. *J Am Acad Dermatol* 2017. doi:10.1016/j.jaad.2017.09.022.

135. Sonnex TS, Dawber RP, Zachary CB, Millard PR, Griffiths AD. The nails in adult type 1 pityriasis rubra pilaris. A comparison with Sézary syndrome and psoriasis. *J Am Acad Dermatol* 1986; 15: 956–960.

136. Dalziel KL, Telfer NR, Dawber RP. Nail dystrophie in cutaneous T-cell lymphoma. *Br J Dermatol* 1989; 120: 571–574.

137. Tosti A, Fanti PA, Varotti C, Massive lymphomatous nail involvement in Sézary syndrome. *Dermatologica* 1990; 181: 162–164.

138. Fränken J, Haneke E. Mycosis fungoides bullosa. *Hautarzt* 1995; 46: 186–189.

139. Wolter M, Schleussner-Samuel P, Marsch WC. HTLV-I-Infektion: Unguales T-Zell-Lymphom als Primärlokalisation. *Hautarzt* 1991; 42: 50–52.

140. Parmentier L, Dürr C, Vassella E, Beltraminelli H, Borradori L, Haneke E. Specific nail alterations in cutaneous T-cell lymphoma: Successful treatment with topical mechlorethamine. *Arch Dermatol* 2010; 146: 1287–1291.

141. High DA, Luscombe HA, Kauh YC. Leukemia cutis masquerading as chronic paronychia. *Int J Dermatol* 1985; 24: 595–597.

142. Yagci M, Sucak GT, Haznedar R. Red swollen nail folds and nail deformity as presenting findings in chronic lymphocytic leukaemia. *Br J Haematol* 2001; 112: 1.

143. Stanway A, Rademaker M, Kennedy I, Newman P. Cutaneous B-cell lymphoma of the nails, pinna and nose treated with chlorambucil. *Australas J Dermatol* 2004; 45: 110–113.

144. Simon CA, Su WP, LiCY. Subungual leukemia cutis. *Int J Dermatol* 1990; 29: 636–639.

145. Pedersen LM, Nordin H, Nielsen H, Lisse I. Non-Hodgkin malignant lymphoma in the nails in the course of a chronic lymphocytic leukaemia. *Acta DermVenereol* 1992; 72: 277–278.

146. Beck CH. Skin manifestations associated with lymphatic leukemia. *Dermatologica* 1948; 96: 350–356.

147. Borrego L, Rodríguez J, Bosch JM, Castro V, Hernández B. Subungual nodule as a manifestation of multiple myeloma. *Int J Dermatol* 1996; 35: 661–662.

148. Von der Helm D, Ring J, Schmoeckel C, Braun-Falco O. Erworbene Hyalinosis cutis et mucosae bei Plasmocytom mit monoklonaler IgG-lambda-Gammopathie. *Hautarzt* 1989; 40: 153–157.

149. Dispenzieri A, Kyle RA, Lacey MQ, Rajkumar SV, Therneau TM, Larson DR, Greipp PR et al. POEMS syndrome: Definitions and long-term outcome. *Blood* 2003; 101: 2496–2506.

150. Mancuso G, Fanti PA, Berdonini, RM. Nail changes as the only skin abnormality in myeloma-associated amyloidosis. *Br J Dermatol* 1997; 137: 471–472.

151. Lee MY, Byun JY, Choi YW, Choi HY. Multiple myeloma presenting with acquired cutis laxa and primary systemic amyloidosis. *Eur J Dermatol* 2017; 27: 654–655.

152. Mullens GM, Lenhard RE Jr. Digital clubbing in Hodgkins disease. *Hopkins Med J* 1971; 128: 153–157.

153. Shahani RT, Blackburn EK. Nail anomalies in Hodgkin's disease. *Br J Dermatol* 1973; 89: 457–458.

154. Raffle EJ. Letter: Nail anomalies in Hodgkin's disease. *Br J Dermatol* 1974; 90: 585–586.

155. Hirschfeld H. Leukämie und verwandte Zustände. In Schittenhelm A, ed. *Handbuch der blutbildenden Organe*. vol 1. Berlin, Germany: Springer, 1925.

156. Marks R, Lim CC, Borrie PF. A perniotic syndrome with monocytosis and neutropenia: A possible association with a preleukaemic state. *Br J Dematol* 1969; 81: 327–332.

157. Kelly JW, Dowling JP. Pernio: A possible association with chronic myelomonocytic leukemia. *Arch Dermatol* 1985; 121: 1048–1052.

158. Cliff S, James SL, Mercieca JE, Holden CA. Perniosis: A possible association with a preleukemic state. *Br J Dermatol* 1996; 135: 330–345.

159. Chang DY, Whitaker LA, La Rossa D. Acute monomyelocytic leukemia presenting as a felon. *Plast Reconstr Surg* 1975; 56: 623–624.

160. Mackenzie CR. Pachydermoperiostosis: A paraneoplastic syndrome. *N Y State J Med* 1986; 86: 153–154.

161. Walling HW, Snipes CJ, Gerami P, Piette W. The relationship between neutrophilic dermatosis of the dorsal hands and Sweet syndrome. *Arch Dermatol* 2006; 142: 57–63.

162. Hirai I, Sakiyama T, Konohana A, Takae Y, Matsuura S. A case of neutrophilic dermatosis of the back of the hand in acute leukemia—A distributional variant of Sweet's syndrome. *J Dtsch Ges Dermatol* 2015; 13: 1033–1035.

163. Kausar S, Holloway M, Wiseman D, Cahalin P. A strange case of ingrowing toenails. *Am J Hematol* 2012; 87: 819.

164. Boyer. Fongus hématodes du petit doigt. *Gaz Méd Paris* 1834; 212.

165. Haneke E. Ungual melanoma - controversies in diagnosis and treatment. *Dermatol Ther* 2012; 25: 510–524.

166. Banfield CC, Redburn JC, Dawber RP. The incidence and prognosis of nail apparatus melanoma. A retrospective study of 105 patients in four English regions. *Br J Dermatol* 1998; 139: 276–279.

167. O'Leary JA, Berend KR, Johnson JL, Levin LS, Seigler HF. Subungual melanoma. A review of 93 cases with identification of prognostic variables. *Clin Orthop Relat Res* 2000; 378: 206–212.

168. Ragnarsson-Olding BK. Spatial density of primary malignant melanoma in sun-shielded body sites: A potential guide to melanoma genesis. *Acta Oncol* 2011; 50: 323–328.

169. Kato T, Suetake T, Sugiyama Y, Tabata N, Tagami H. Epidemiology and prognosis of subungual melanoma in 34 Japanese patients. *Br J Dermatol* 1996; 134: 383–387.

170. Thai KE, Young R, Sinclair RD. Nail apparatus melanoma. *Australas J Dermatol* 2001: 42: 71–81.

171. Seui M, Takematsu H, Hosokawa M, Obata M, Tomita Y, Kato T, Takahashi M, Mihm MC Jr. Acral melanoma in Japan. *J Invest Dermatol* 1983: 80(1 Suppl): 56s–60s.

172. Ishihara K, Saida T, Otsuka F, Yamazaki N. Prognosis and statistical investigation committee of the Japanese Skin Cancer Society. Statistical profiles of malignant melanoma and other skin cancers in Japan: 2007 update. *Int J Clin Oncol* 2008; 13: 33–41.

173. Roh MR, Kim J, Chung KY. Treatment and outcomes of melanoma in acral location in Korean patients. *Yonsei Med J* 2010; 51: 562–568.

174. Chang JW-C. Cutaneous melanoma: Taiwan experience and literature review. *Chang Gung Med J* 2010; 33: 602–612.

175. Lichte V, Breuninger H, Metzler G, Haefner HM, Moehrle M. Acral lentiginous melanoma: Conventional histology vs. three-dimensional histology. *Br J Dermatol* 2009; 160: 591–599.

176. Haenssle HA, Hofmann S, Buhl T, Emmert S, Schön MP, Bertsch HP, Rosenberger A. Assessment of melanoma histotypes and associated patient related factors: Basis for a predictive statistical model. *J Dtsch Dermatol Ges* 2015; 13: 37–45.

177. Bradford PT, Goldstein AM, McMaster ML, Tucker MA. Acral lentiginous melanoma: Incidence and survival patterns in the United States, 1986–2005. *Arch Dermatol* 2009; 145: 427–434.

178. Kiryu H. Malignant melanoma in situ arising in the nail unit of a child. *J Dermatol* 1998; 25: 41–44.

179. Tosti A, Piraccini BM, Cagalli A, Haneke E. In situ melanoma of the nail unit in children: Report of 2 cases in Caucasian fair skinned children. *Pediatr Dermatol* 2012; 29: 79–83.

180. Phan A, Touzet S, Dalle S, Ronger-Savlé S, Balme B, Thomas L. Acral lentiginous melanoma: A clinicoprognostic study of 126 cases. *Br J Dermatol* 2006; 155: 561–569.

181. Möhrle M, Häfner HM. Is subungual melanoma related to trauma? *Dermatologica* 2002; 204: 259–261.

182. Rangwala S, Hunt C, Modi G, Krishnan B, Orengo I. Amelanotic subungual melanoma after trauma: An unusual clinical presentation. *Dermatol Online J* 2011; 17(6): 8.

183. Lesage C, Journet-Tollhupp J, Bernard P, Grange F. Mélanome acral post-traumatique: une réalité sous-estimée? *Ann Dermatol Venereol* 2012; 139: 727–731.

184. Fanti PA, Dika E, Misciali C, Vaccari S, Barisani A, Piraccini BM, Cavrin G, Maibach HI, Patrizi A. Nail apparatus melanoma: Is trauma a coincidence? Is this peculiar tumor a real acral melanoma? *Cutan Ocul Toxicol* 2013; 32: 150–153.

185. Bormann G, Marsch WC, Haerting J, Helmbold P. Concomitant traumas influence prognosis in melanomas of the nail apparatus. *Br J Dermatol* 2006; 155: 76–80.

186. Keitea M, Keita AM, Traoré B, Thiam I, Soumah MM, Diané BF, Tounkara TM, Baldé H, Camara A, Camara AD, Cissé M. Mélanome du pouce et faux ongles chez une fille de 29 ans infectée par le VIH. *Ann Dermatol Vénéréol* 2013; 140: S112–S113.

187. Micu E, Baturaite Z, Juzeniene A, Bruland ØS, Moan JE. Superficial-spreading and nodular melanomas in Norway: A comparison by body site distribution and latitude gradients. *Melanoma Res* 2012; 22: 460–465.

188. Moan J, Baturaite Z, Porojnicu AC, Dahlback A, Juzeniene A. UVA, UVB and incidence of cutaneous malignant melanoma in Norway and Sweden. *Photochem Photobiol Sci* 2012; 11: 191–198.

189. Kopf AW, Waldo E. Melanonychia striata. *Australas J Dermatol* 1980; 21: 59–70.

190. Motta A, López C, Acosta A, Peñaranda C. Subungual melanoma in situ in a Hispanic girl treated with functional resection and reconstruction with onychocutaneous toe free flap. *Arch Dermatol* 2007; 143: 1600–1602.

191. Iorizzo M, Tosti A, Di Chiacchio N, Hirata SH, Misciali C, Michalany N, Dominguez J, Toussaint S. Nail melanoma in children: Differential diagnosis and management. *Dermatol Surg* 2008; 34: 974–978.

192. Bonamonte D, Arpaia N, Cimmino A, Vestita M. In situ melanoma of the nail unit presenting as a rapid growing longitudinal melanonychia in a 9-year-old white boy. *Dermatol Surg* 2014; 40: 1154–1157.

193. Rotunda AM, Graham-Hicks S, Bennett RG. Simultaneous subungual melanoma in situ of both thumbs. *J Am Acad Dermatol* 2008; 58: S42–S44.

194. Levit EK, Kagen MH, Scher RK, Grossman M, Altman E. The ABC rule for clinical detection of subungual melanoma. *J Am Acad Dermatol* 2000; 42: 269–274.

195. Rosendahl C, Cameron A, Wilkinson D, Belt P, Williamson R, Weedon D. Nail matrix melanoma: Consecutive cases in a general practice. *Dermatol Pract Concept* 2012; 2(2): 13: 63–70.

196. Elloumi-Jellouli A, Triki S, Driss M, Derbel F, Zghal M, Mrad K, Rhomdhnane KhB. A misdiagnosed nail bed melanoma. *Dermatol Online J* 2010; 16(7): 13.

197. Wallberg B, Hansson J. Delayed diagnosis of subungual melanoma. Two cases were misjudged as onychomycosis [In Swedish]. *Läkartidningen* 1997; 94: 2543–2544.

198. Braham C, Fraiture AL, Quatresooz P, Piérard-Franchimont C, Piérard GE. Des "dermatomycoses banales" qui ne pardonnent pas. "Banal onychomycosis" that cannot be overlooked [In French]. *Rev Med Liège* 2002; 57: 317–319.

199. Soon SL, Solomon AR Jr, Papadopoulos D, Murray DR, McAlpine B, Washington CV. Acral lentiginous melanoma mimicking benign disease: The Emory experience. *J Am Acad Dermatol* 2003; 48: 183–188.

200. De Giorgi V, Sestini S, Massi D, Panelos J, Papi F, Dini M, Lotti T. Subungual melanoma: A particularly invasive "onychomycosis." *J Am Geriatr Soc* 2007; 55: 2094–2096.

201. Shukla VK, Hughes LE. Differential diagnosis of subungual melanoma from a surgical point of view. *Br J Surg* 1989; 76: 1156–1160.

202. Blum A. Onychomykose mit Onychodystrophie oder akrolentiginöses Melanom mit Onychomykose und Onychodystrophie? *Hautarzt* 2012; 63: 341–343.

203. Blessing K, Kernohan NM, Park KG. Subungual malignant melanoma: Clinicopathological features of 100 cases. *Histopathology* 1991; 19: 425–429.

204. Cohen T, Busam KJ, Patel A, Brady MS. Subungual melanoma: Management considerations. *Am J Surg* 2008; 195: 244–248.

205. Chow WT, Bhat W, Magdub S, Orlando A. In situ subungual melanoma: Digit salvaging clearance. *J Plast Reconstr Aesthet Surg* 2013; 66: 274–276.

206. Graf RM, Tolazzi AR, Colpo PG, de Oliveira e Cruz GA. Sentinel lymph node detection in a patient with subungual melanoma after transaxillary breast augmentation. *Plast Reconstr Surg* 2011; 127: 65e–66e.

207. Wantz M, Antonicelli F, Derancourt C, Bernard P, Avril MF, Grange F. Long-term survival and spontaneous tumor regression in stage IV melanoma: Possible role of adrenalectomy and massive tumor antigen release. *Ann Dermatol Venereol* 2010; 137: 464–467.

208. Dominguez-Cherit J. Spontaneous regression of subungual melanoma. *XXVI Cong Soc Mex Dermatol*, Leon Gto, Aug 5–9, 2014.

209. Sundell J. Mystery of the swollen leg [Finnish]. *Duodecim* 2010; 126: 1827–1830.

210. Haneke E. Operative therapie akraler und subungualer melanome. In: Rompel R, Petres J, eds. *Operative und onkologische Dermatologie. Fortschritte der operativen und onkologischen Dermatologie*. Berlin, Germany: Springer, 1999; 15: 210–214.

211. Haneke E, Baran R. Subunguale Tumoren. *Z Hautkr* 1982: 57: 355–362.

212. Starace M, Dika E, Fanti PA, Patrizi A, Misciali C, Alessandrini A, Bruni F, Piraccini BM. Nail apparatus melanoma: Dermoscopic and histopathologic correlations on a series of 23 patients from a single centre. *J Eur Acad Dermatol Venereol* 2018; 32: 164–173.

213. Braun RP, Gutkowicz-Krusin D, Rabinovitz H, Cognetta A, Hofmann- Wellenhof R, Ahlgrimm-Siess V, Polsky D et al. Agreement of dermatopathologists in the evaluation of clinically difficult melanocytic lesions: How golden is the "gold standard"? *Dermatology* 2012; 224: 51–58.

214. Hirata SH, Yamada S, Almeida FA, Almeida FA, Tomomori-Yamashita J, Enokihara MY, Paschoal FM, Enokihara MM, Outi CM, Michalany NS. Dermoscopy of the nail bed and matrix to assess melanonychia striata. *J Am Acad Dermatol* 2005; 53: 884–886.

215. Hirata SH, Yamada S, Almeida FA, Enokihara MY, Rosa IP, Enokihara MM, Michalany NS. Dermoscopic examination of the nail bed and matrix. *Int J Dermatol* 2006; 45: 28–30.

216. Di Chiacchio N, Hirata SH, Enokihara MY, Michalany MS, Fabbrocini G, Tosti A. Dermatologists' accuracy in early diagnosis of melanoma of the nail matrix. *Arch Dermatol* 2010; 146: 382–387.

217. Debarbieux S, Hospod V, Depaepe L, Balme B, Poulalhon N, Thomas L. Perioperative confocal microscopy of the nail matrix in the management of in situ or minimally invasive subungual melanomas. *Br J Dermatol* 2012; 167: 828–836.

218. James VJ. Fiber diffraction of skin and nails provides an accurate diagnostic test for 8 malignancies. *Int J Cancer* 2009; 125: 133–138.

219. Ruben BS. Pigmented lesions of the nail unit: Clinical and histopathology features. *Semin Cutan Med Surg* 2010; 29: 148–158.

220. Haneke E, Lawry M. Nail surgery. In: Robinson JK, Hanke WC, Sengelmann RD, Siegel DM, eds. *Surgery of the Skin*. Philadelphia, PA: Elsevier, 2005: 719–742.

221. Haneke E. Cirugía ungueal. In: Torres Lozada V, Camacho Martínez FM, Mihm MC, Sober AJ, Sánchez Carpintero I, eds. *Dermatología Práctica Ibero-Latinoamericana. Atlas, enfermedades sistémicas asociadas y terapéutica*. Chapter 142. México: Nieto Editores, 2005: 1643–1652.

222. Di Chiacchio N, Refkalefsky Loureiro W, Schwery Michalany N, and Kezam Gabriel FV. Tangential biopsy thickness versus lesion depth in longitudinal melanonychia: A pilot study. *Dermatol Res Pract* 2012; 2012: 353864.

223. Glat PM, Spector JA, Roses DF, Shapiro RA, Harris MN, Beasley RW, Grossman JA. The management of pigmented lesions of the nail bed. *Ann Plast Surg* 1996; 37: 125–134.

224. Haneke E, Binder D. Subunguales Melanom mit streifiger Nagelpigmentierung. *Hautarzt* 1978; 29: 389–391.

225. Duarte AF, Correia O, Barros AM, Azevedo R, Haneke E. Nail matrix melanoma in situ: Conservative surgical management. *Dermatology* 2010; 220: 173–175.

226. Möhrle M, Metzger S, Schippert W, Garbe C, Rassner G, Breuninger H. "Functional" surgery in subungual melanoma. *Dermatol Surg* 2003; 29: 366–374.

227. Möhrle M, Lichte V, Breuninger H. Operative therapy of acral melanomas. *Hautarzt* 2011; 62: 362–367.

228. Duarte AF, Correia O, Barros M, Ventura F, Haneke E. Nail melanoma in situ: Clinical, dermoscopic, pathologic clues, and steps for minimally invasive treatment. *Dermatol Surg* 2015; 41: 59–68.

229. Ángeles LB, Lacey Niebla RM, Guevara Sanginés E. Subungual melanoma: Functional treatment with Mohs Surgery. *Dermatol Cosm Med Quir* 2007; 5: 136–143.

230. Sohl S, Simon JC, Wetzig T. Finger stall technique skin graft for reconstruction of fingers after extensive excisions of acral lentiginous melanomas. *J Dtsch Dermatol Ges* 2007; 5: 525–526.

231. Sureda N, Phan A, Paoulalhon N, Balme B, Dalle S, Thomas L. Conservative surgical management of subungual (marix derived) melanoma: Report of seven cases and literature review. *Br J Dermatol* 2011; 165: 852–858.

232. Montagner S, Belfort FA, Belda W Jr, Di Chiacchio N. Descriptive survival study of nail melanoma patients treated with functional surgery versus distal amputation. *J Am Acad Dermatol* 2018; 79: 147–149.

233. Smock ED, Barabas AG, Geh JL. Reconstruction of a thumb defect with Integra following wide local excision of a subungual melanoma. *J Plast Reconstr Aesthet Surg* 2010; 63: e36–e37.

234. Kim JY, Jung HJ, Lee WJ, Kim DW, Yoon GS, Kim DS, Park MJ, Lee SJ. Is the distance enough to eradicate in situ or early invasive subungual melanoma by wide local excision? from the point of view of matrix-to-bone distance for safe inferior surgical margin in Koreans. *Dermatology* 2011; 223: 122–123.

235. Shin HT, Jang KT, Mun GH, Lee DY, Lee JB. Histopathological analysis of the progression pattern of subungual melanoma: Late tendency of dermal invasion in the nail matrix area. *Mod Pathol* 2014; 27: 1461–1467.

236. Ogata D, Uhara H, Tsutsumida H, Yamazaki N, Mochida K, Amano M, Yoshikawa S, Kiyohara Y, Tsuchida T. Nail apparatus melanoma in a Japanese population: A comparative study of surgical procedures and prognoses in a large series of 151 cases. *Eur J Dermatol* 2017; 27: 620–626.

237. Amin B, Nehal KS, Jungbluth AA, Zaidi B, Brady MS, Coit DC, Zhou Q, Busam KJ. Histologic distinction between subungual lentigo and melanoma. *Am J Surg Pathol* 2008; 32: 835–843.

238. Tosti A, Piraccini BM, Cadore de Farias D. Dealing with melanonychia. *Semin Cutan Med Surg* 2009; 28: 49–54.

239. Perrin C. Tumors of the nail unit. A review. Part I. Acquired localized longitudinal melanonychia and erythronychia. *Am J Dermatopathol* 2013; 35: 621–636.

240. Perrin C, Michiels JF, Pisani A, Ortonne JP. Anatomic distribution of melanocytes in normal nail unit: An immunohistochemical investigation. *Am J Dermatopathol* 1997; 19: 462–467.

241. Lee D-Y. Variable sized cellular remnants in the nail plate of longitudinal melanonychia: Evidence of subungual melanoma. *Ann Dermatol* 2015; 27: 328–329.

242. Kerl H, Trau H, Ackerman AB. Differentiation of melanocytic nevi from malignant melanomas in palms, soles, and nail beds solely by signs in the cornified layer of the epidermis. *Am J Dermatopathol* 1984: 6(Suppl.): 159–160.

243. Ruben BS, McCalmont TH. The importance of attached nail plate epithelium in the diagnosis of nail apparatus melanoma. *J Cut Pathol* 2010; 37: 1028–1029.

244. Haneke E. Pathogenese der Nageldystrophie beim subungualen Melanom. *Verhandlungen der Deutschen Gesellschaft für Pathologie* 1986; 70: 484.

245. Ohata C, Nakai C, Kasugai T, Katayama I. Consumption of the epidermis in acral lentiginous melanoma. *J Cutan Pathol* 2012; 39: 577–581.

246. Baran R, Haneke E. Diagnostik und Therapie der streifenförmigen Nagelpigmentierung. *Hautarzt* 1984; 35: 359–365.

247. Haneke E, Baran R. Longitudinal melanonychia. *Dermatol Surg* 2001; 27: 580–584.

248. Gosselink CP, Sindone JL, Meadows BJ, Mohammadi A, Rosa M. Amelanotic subungual melanoma: A case report. *J Foot Ankle Surg* 2009; 48: 220–222.

249. Johnson M, Shuster S. Continuous formation of nail along the bed. *Br J Dermatol* 1993; 128: 277–280.

250. André J, Moulonguet I, Goettmann-Bonvallot S. In situ amelanotic melanoma of the nail unit mimicking lichen planus: Report of 3 cases. *Arch Dermatol* 2010; 146: 418–421.

251. Ha JM, Yoon JH, Cho EB, Park GH, Park EJ, Kim KH, Kim KJ. Subungual desmoplastic malignant melanoma. *J Eur Acad Dermatol Venereol* 2016; 30: 360–362.

252. Quinn MJ, Crotty KA, Thompson JF, Coates AS, O'Brien CJ, McCarthy WH. Desmoplastic and desmoplastic neurotropic melanoma: Experience with 280 patients. *Cancer* 1998; 83: 1128–1135.

253. Innominato PF, Libbrecht I, van den Oord JJ. Expression of neurotrophins and their receptors in pigment ell lesions of the skin. *J Pathol* 2001; 194: 95–100.

254. Baran LR, Ruben BS, Kechijian P, Thomas L. Non-melanoma Hutchinson sign: A reappraisal of this important, remarkable melanoma simulant. *J Eur Acad Dermatol Venereol* 2018; 32.

255. Miranda BH, Haughton DN, Fahmy FS. Subungual melanoma: An important tip. *J Plast Reconstr Aesthet Surg* 2012; 65: 1422–1424.

256. Cho KH, Kim BS, Chang SH, Lee YS, Kim KJ. Pigmented nail with atypical melanocytic hyperplasia. *Clin Exp Dermatol* 1991; 16: 451–454.

257. Sheffield MV, Yee H, Dorvault CC, Weilbaecher KN, Eltoum IA, Siegal GP, Fisher DE, Chhieng DC. Comparison of five antibodies as markers in the diagnosis of melanoma in cytologic preparations. *Am J Clin Pathol* 2002; 118: 930–936.

258. Mahmood MN, Lee MW, Linden MD, Nathanson SD, Hornyak TJ, Zarbo RJ. Diagnostic value of HMB-45 and anti-Melan A staining of sentinel lymph nodes with isolated positive cells. *Mod Pathol* 2002; 15: 1288–1293.

259. Ohsie SJ, Sarantopoulos GP, Cochran AJ, Binder SW. Immunohistochemical characteristics of melanoma. *J Cutan Pathol* 2008; 35: 433–444.

260. Jing X, Michael CW, Theoharis CG. The use of immunocytochemical study in the cytologic diagnosis of melanoma: Evaluation of three antibodies. *Diagn Cytopathol* 2013; 41: 126–130.

261. Orchard GE. Comparison of immunohistochemical labelling of melanocyte differentiation antibodies melan-A, tyrosinase and HMB 45 with NKIC3 and S100 protein in the evaluation of benign naevi and malignant melanoma. *Histochem J* 2000; 32: 475–481.

262. Pluot M, Joundi A, Grosshans E. Contribution of monoclonal antibody HMB45 in the histopathologic diagnosis of melanoma. *Ann Dermatol Venereol* 1990; 117: 691–699.

263. Kiuru M, McDermott G, Berger M, Halpern AC, Busam KJ. Desmoplastic melanoma with sarcomatoid dedifferentiation. *Am J Surg Pathol* 2014; 38: 864–870.

264. Friedman HD, Tatum AH. HMB-45-positive malignant lymphoma. A case report with literature review of aberrant HMB-45 reactivity. *Arch Pathol Lab Med* 1991; 115: 826–830.

265. Theunis A, Richert B, Sass U, Lateur N, Sales F, André J. Immunohistochemical study of 40 cases of longitudinal melanonychia. *Am J Dermatopathol* 2011; 33: 27–34.

266. Mohamed A, Gonzalez RS, Lawson D, Wang J, MD, Cohen C. SOX10 expression in malignant melanoma, carcinoma, and normal tissues. *Appl Immunohistochem Mol Morphol* 2013; 21: 506–510.

267. Palla B, Su A, Binder S, Dry S. SOX10 expression distinguishes desmoplastic melanoma from its histologic mimics. *Am J Dermatopathol* 2013; 35: 576–581.

268. Shin S, Vincent JG, Cuda JD, Xu H, Kang, S, Kim J, Taube JM. Sox10 is expressed in primary melanocytic neoplasms of various histologies but not in fibrohistiocytic proliferations and histiocytoses. *J Am Acad Dermatol* 2012; 67: 717.

269. Danga ME, Yaar R, Bhawan J. Melan-A positive dermal cells in malignant melanoma in situ. *J Cutan Pathol* 2015; 42(6): 388–393. doi: 10.1111/cup.12473.

270. Rönnstrand, Phung B. Enhanced SOX10 and KIT expression in cutaneous melanoma. *Med Oncol* 2013; 30: 648–649.

271. Buonaccorsi JN, Prieto VG, Torres-Cabala C, Suster S, Plaza JA. Diagnostic utility and comparative immunohistochemical analysis of MITF-1 and SOX10 to distinguish melanoma in situ and actinic keratosis: A clinicopathological and immunohistochemical study of 70 cases. *Am J Dermatopathol* 2014; 36: 124–130.

272. Kaufmann O, Koch S, Burghardt J, Audring H, Dietel M. Tyrosinase, melan-A, and KBA62 as markers for the immunohistochemical identification of metastatic amelanotic melanomas on paraffin sections. *Mod Pathol* 1998; 11: 740–746.

273. Kazakov DV, Kutzner H, Rütten A, Michal M, Requena L, Burg G, Dummer R, Kempf W. The anti-MAGE antibody B57 as a diagnostic marker in melanocytic lesions. *Am J Dermatopathol* 2004; 26: 102–107.

274. Katenkamp K, Henke R-P, Katenkamp D. Dermales chondroides Melanom. *Pathologe* 2005; 26: 149–152.

275. Sundersingh S, Majhi U, Murhekar K, Krishnamurthy R. Malignant melanoma with osteocartilaginous differentiation. *Indian J Pathol Microbiol* 2010; 53: 130–132.

276. Curtin JA, Fridlyand J, Kageshita T, Patel HN, Busam KJ, Kutzner H, Cho KH et al. Distinct sets of genetic alterations in melanoma. *N Engl J Med* 2005; 353: 2135–2147.

277. Blokx WA, van Dijk MC, Ruiter DJ. Molecular cytogenetics of cutaneous melanocytic lesions - diagnostic, prognostic and therapeutic aspects. *Histopathology* 2010; 56: 121–132.

278. Pleasance ED, Cheetham RK, Stephens PJ, McBride DJ, Humphray SJ, Greenman CD, Varela I et al. A comprehensive catalogue of somatic mutations from a human cancer genome. *Nature* 2010; 463: 191–196.

279. Glitza IC, Davies MA. Genotyping of cutaneous melanoma. *Chin Clin Oncol* 2014; 3(3): 27.

280. Curtin JA, Busam K, Pinkel D, Bastian BC. Somatic activation of KIT in distinct subtypes of melanoma. *J Clin Oncol* 2006; 24: 4340–4346.

281. Yeh I, Bastian BC. Genome-wide associations studies for melanoma and nevi. *Pigment Cell Melanoma Res* 2009; 22: 527–528.

282. North JP, Kageshita T, Pinkel D, Leboit PE, Bastian BC. Distribution and significance of occult intraepidermal tumor cells surrounding primary melanoma. *J Invest Dermatol* 2008; 128: 2024–2030.

283. Junkins-Hopkins JM. Malignant melanoma: Molecular cytogenetics and their implications in clinical medicine. *J Am Acad Dermatol* 2010; 63: 329–332.

284. Lang D, Mascarenhas JB, Shea CR. Melanocytes, melanocyte stem cells, and melanoma stem cells. *Clin Dermatol* 2013; 31: 166–178.

285. Redmer T, Welte Y, Behrens D, Fichtner I, Przybilla D, Wruck W, Yaspo M-L, Lehrach H, Schäfer R, Regenbrecht CRA. The nerve growth factor receptor CD271 is crucial to maintain tumorigenicity and stem-like properties of melanoma cells. *PLoS ONE* 2014; 9(5): e92596.

286. Bastian BC, Kashani-Sabet M, Hamm H, Godfrey T, Moore DH 2nd, Bröcker EB, LeBoit PE, Pinkel D. Gene amplifications characterize acral melanoma and permit the detection of occult tumor cells in the surrounding skin. *Cancer Res* 2000; 60: 1968–1973.

287. Bauer J, Bastian BC. Distinguishing melanocytic nevi from melanoma by DNA copy number changes: Comparative genomic hybridization as a research and diagnostic tool. *Dermatol Ther* 2006; 19: 40–49.

288. Fargnoli MC, Pike K, Pfeiffer RM, Tsang S, Rozenblum E, Munroe DJ, Golubeva Y et al. MC1R variants increase risk of melanomas harboring BRAF mutations. *J Invest Dermatol* 2008; 128: 2485–2490.

289. Gerami P, Jewell SS, Morrison LE, Blondin B, Schulz J, Ruffalo T, Matushek P IV et al. Fluorescence in situ hybridization (FISH) as an ancillary diagnostic tool in the diagnosis of melanoma. *Am J Surg Pathol* 2009; 33: 1146–1156.

290. Viros A, Fridlyand J, Bauer J, Lasithiotakis K, Garbe C, Pinkel D, Bastian BC. Improving melanoma classification by integrating genetic and morphologic features. *PLoS Med* 2008; 5(6): e120.

291. Di Chiacchio N, Farias DC de, Piraccini DM, Hirata SH, Richert B, Zaiac M, Daniel R et al. Consensus on melanonychia nail plate dermoscopy. *An Bras Dermatol* 2013; 88: 309–313.

292. Kikuchi I, Inoue S, Sakaguchi E, Ono T. Regressing nevoid nail melanosis in childhood. *Dermatology* 1993; 186: 88–93.

293. Koga H, Saida T, Uhara H. Key point in dermoscopic differentiation between early nail apparatus melanoma and benign longitudinal melanonychia. *J Dermatol* 2011; 38: 45–52.

294. Lyall D. Malignant melanoma in infancy. *J Am Med Assoc* 1967; 202: 93.

295. Kato T, Usuba Y, Takematsu H, Kumasaka N, Tanita Y, Hashimoto K, Tomita Y, Tagami H. A rapidly growing pigmented nail streak resulting in diffuse melanosis of the nail. A possible sign of subungual melanoma in situ. *Cancer* 1989; 64: 2191–2198.

296. Hori Y, Yamada A, Tanizaki T. Pigmented small tumors. *Jpn J Pediatr Dermatol* 1988; 7: 117–120.

297. Antonovich DD, Grin C, Grant-Kels JM. Childhood subungual melanoma in situ in diffuse nail melanosis beginning as expanding longitudinal melanonychia. *Ped Dermatol* 2005; 22: 210–212.

298. Jean-Gilles Jr J, Bercovitch L, Jellinek N, Robinson-Bostom L, Telang G. Subungual melanoma in-situ arising in a 9-year-old child. *J Cut Pathol* 2011; 38: 185.

299. Uchiyama M, Minemura K. Two cases of malignant melanoma in young persons. *Nippon Hifuka Gakkai Zasshi* 1979; 89: 668.

300. Haenssle HA, Buhl T, Holzkamp R, Schön MP, Kretschmer L, Bertsch HP. Squamomelanocytic tumor of the nail unit metastasizing to a sentinel lymph node: A dermoscopic and histologic investigation. *Dermatology* 2012; 225: 127–130.

301. Boespflug A, Debarbieux S, Depaepe L, Chouvet B, Maucort-Boulch D, Dalle S, Balme B, Thomas L. Association of subungual melanoma and subungual squamous cell carcinoma: A case series. *J Am Acad Dermatol* 2018; 78: 760–768.

302. Weedon D, Van Deurse M, Rosendahl C. "Occult" melanocytes in nail matrix melanoma. *Am J Dermatopathol* 2012; 34: 855.

303. Husain S, Scher RK, Silvers DN, Ackerman AB. Melanotic macule of nail unit and its clinicopathologic spectrum. *J Am Acad Dermatol* 2006; 54: 664–667.

304. Tomizawa K. Early malignant melanoma manifested as longitudinal melanonychia: Subungual melanoma may arise from suprabasal melanocytes. *Br J Dermatol* 2000; 143: 431–434.

305. Baran R, Simon C. Longitudinal melanonychia: A symptom of Bowen's disease. *J Am Acad Dermatol* 1988; 18: 1359–1360.

306. Lemont H, Haas R. Subungual pigmented Bowen's disease in a nineteen-year-old black female. *J Am Podiatr Med Assoc* 1994; 84: 39–40.

307. Sass U, André J, Stene JJ Noel JC. Longitudinal melanonychia revealing an intraepidermal carcinoma of the nail apparatus: Detection of integrated HPV-16 DNA. *J Am Acad Dermatol* 1998; 39: 490–493.

308. Lambiase MC, Gardner TL, Altman CE, Albertini JG. Bowen disease of the nail bed presenting as longitudinal melanonychia: Detection of human papillomavirus type 56 DNA. *Cutis* 2003; 72: 305–309.

309. Kim DM, Suh MK, Ha GY, Sohng SH. Fingernail onychomycosis due to Aspergillus niger. *Ann Dermatol* 2012; 24: 459–463.

310. Ko CJ, Sarantopoulos GP, Pai G, Binder SW. Longitudinal melanonychia of the toenails with presence of Medlar bodies on biopsy. *J Cutan Pathol* 2005; 32: 63–65.

PART 9

Psychocutaneous Nail Disorders

28

Nail tic disorders

ISHMEET KAUR AND ARCHANA SINGAL

INTRODUCTION

Tic disorders generally start in childhood and are characterized by multiple sudden, rapid, recurrent, and non-rhythmic movements (motor tics) or utterances (vocal tics), or both. They are mostly transient and may fade away in adolescence. However, sometimes they may be chronic and tend to persist lifelong. Tic disorders have been classified under neuropsychiatric disorders. Nail tic disorders are tics pertaining to nail unit.[1] Their occurrence is not only limited to cosmetic disfigurement of the nail but is associated with psychopathological states that can affect a patient's quality of life. Nail tic disorders are poorly understood and often pose a management challenge.

This chapter will aim to provide a comprehensive understanding on various nail tic disorders and will help broaden the concept of psycho-cutaneous medicine.

TYPES OF PSYCHO-CUTANEOUS DISORDERS

For a better understanding of nail tic disorders, basic awareness about psycho-dermatological disorders is necessary. These are classified into the following broad categories[2]:

1. **Physio-psychological Disorders:** In physio-psychological disorders, the dermatological manifestations are not caused by stress but appear to be precipitated

by stress factor. These include disorders such as psoriasis, atopic dermatitis, acne excoriee, urticaria, hyperhidrosis, and seborrheic dermatitis.[2]

2. **Primary Psychiatric Disorders:** In primary psychiatric disorders, patients develop dermatological manifestations as a result of psychiatric illness. They include broad categories: disorders of dermatological beliefs, body awareness, impulse control disorders, factitious disorders, psychogenic pruritus, cutaneous phobias, and atypical pain disorders. Among these, a few nail tic disorders such as onychotillomania fall into the group of impulse control disorders.[3]

Body-focused repetitive behaviors (BFRBs) is another entity recognized under the Diagnostic and Statistical Manual 5th edition (DSM-5) and is defined as motoric acts that become habitual and cause functional impairment.[4] These nervous habits become problematic when they interfere with the person's everyday functioning. When these BFRBs cross this line, then they are classified as impulse control disorders.[5] Nail tic disorders such as onychophagia are included in this category as "Other Unspecified Obsessive-Compulsive and Related Disorders."[4] On the other hand, according to the International Classification of Diseases and Health Related Problems – 11th Revision (ICD-11), these are classified under emotional and behavioral problems.[6,7]

3. **Secondary Psycho-cutaneous Disorders:** In secondary psycho-cutaneous disorders, patients have psychiatric symptoms as a result of the skin disease. These include alopecia areata, vitiligo, chronic eczema, ichthyosiform syndromes, severe acne, rhinophyma, neurofibroma, and albinism.[2]

The following nail common disorders will be discussed in this chapter (Box 28.1):

Onychophagia

Onychophagia is defined as chronic nail biting. It usually presents in early childhood, although adult cases are known to occur. Besides biting of the nail, it includes biting of the cuticle as well as the soft tissue around the nail.[7-9] Onychophagia is a stress-relieving habit where the patient has an urge to bite the nail when in an emotional state of anxiety. As mentioned earlier, its classification according to ICD 11 and DSM-5 remains unclear, but it is closely related to obsessive-compulsive disorders.[7]

EPIDEMIOLOGY AND PREVALENCE

Onychophagia is seen in 20%–30% of the population.[10] Prevalence of onychophagia is age dependent. It increases from early childhood to adolescence and may persist into adulthood, while the prevalence decreases thereafter. It is more commonly seen in girls than boys.[9] In an Indian study, the prevalence of onychophagia among school children was 12.7%, with a female predilection.[11]

TRIGGER FACTORS

Nail biting can be triggered by factors such as boredom, as a form of self-stimulation, anxiety/stress, anguish, or handling a difficult task. Others tend to have it as an automatic behavior while doing some other activity such as watching television, working on a computer, or learning/reading.[6,9] It is usually less seen during a social interaction. The complete nature of onychophagia is unclear and varies between an anxiety disorder or obsessive–compulsive disorder to an emotional and behavioral problem.[9,12] Some patients get a sense of relief with the act of nail biting that further develops an urge for the behavior.[9,13] Psychiatric disorders in parents also play a role as onychophagia was found to be more prevalent in children whose mothers had schizophrenia or major depressive disorder.[14]

CLINICAL FEATURES

Onychophagia causes damage to both nail and the cuticle. Nails appear shortened and irregular (Figures 28.1 and 28.2).

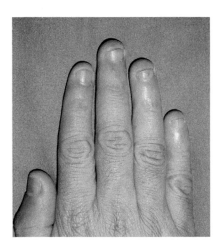

Figure 28.1 Shortening of nail plates of fingernails in a young man with onychophagia.

> **BOX 28.1: Nail tic disorders**
>
> **Well-Known Nail Tic Disorders**
>
> 1. Onychophagia
> 2. Onychotillomania
> 3. Perionychotillomania
> 4. Habit tic deformity
> 5. Onychotemnomania
> 6. Onychotieromania
> 7. Onychodaknomania
>
> **Lesser Known**
>
> 8. Bidet nails or worn-down nails
> 9. Onycholysis seminularis
> 10. Lacquer nail

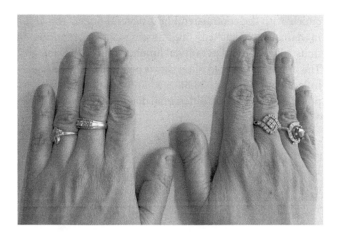

Figure 28.2 Onychophagia in a 55-year-old woman persisting since childhood.

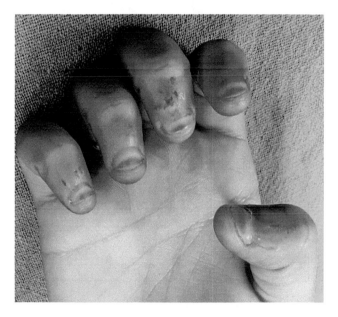

Figure 28.3 Pigmentation and hangnails secondary to onychophagia.

This may be accompanied by hangnails (Figure 28.3) and acute or chronic paronychia. Surrounding skin may show erythema, edema, or even scarring. Fingernails are affected more commonly. Severe cases may present with irreversible shortening (Figure 28.4) or complete loss of nail.[1,6,15]

COMORBIDITIES

Onychophagia is commonly associated with other psychiatric conditions such as obsessive-compulsive disorders, anxiety, major depressive disorders, and attention deficit hyperactivity disorders.[6,8]

OUTCOME

The act of onychophagia involves putting the nail into the mouth in such a manner that contact occurs between a fingernail and one or more teeth. This may damage nail, teeth, gum, and the fingers and also lead to dentofacial and dentoalveolar complications.[1,6,8]

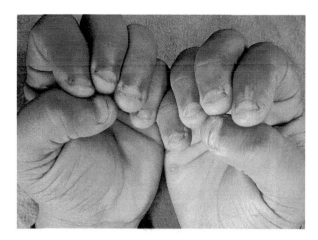

Figure 28.4 Marked, irreversible shortening of fingernails in an adult with persistent onychophagia.

Nail complications include longitudinal melanonychia that occurs due to activation of nail matrix melanocytes, nail dystrophy, and shortening of nail bed.[10]

Infections: Recurrent damage to the nail folds exposes the underlying soft tissue and predisposes the nail to various infections. Paronychia is the most common infection seen in onychophagia. Besides paronychia, herpetic whitlow and osteomyelitis can also be a complication.[9,10]

Oral and Dental: Repeated contact of the nail with the teeth and gingiva leads to gingival infections and dental malocclusion.[8–10] An increased oral carriage of Enterobacteriaceae is also found in patients of onychophagia, predominantly *Escherichia coli*.[16]

Social Outcomes: Besides the physical outcomes, onychophagia can also have a social impact on the patient as well as the family as this habit is considered as a sign of immaturity or under-confidence.[9,10,17]

Onychotillomania

Onychotillomania is a self-induced disorder characterized by a compulsive urge to pick or pull off the nails, unlike onychophagia, where the patient has tendency to bite the nails. According to International Classification of Diseases-10, onychotillomania is classified along with the other impulse control disorders. According to DSM-5, it is recognized as a BRBF as "Other Specified Obsessive-Compulsive and Related Disorders."[18]

EPIDEMIOLOGY AND PREVALENCE

Prevalence studies of onychotillomania are scarce in the literature; however, it is less common than onychophagia. In a study by Pacanet et al., out of 160 patients, 46.7% had onychophagia while only 0.9% prevalence suffered from onychotillomania. Age of onset of onychotillomania was found to be in early childhood, 6–10 years being the average age at presentation. They noted a male predominance, with male-to-female ratio of 1.5:1.[6]

TRIGGER FACTORS

Onychotillomania results from recurrent nail picking or frequent manicuring of nails. This can be triggered by anxiety or stress.

It is also associated with various self-mutilation diseases like Lesch–Nyhan Syndrome and Smith-Magenis Syndrome.[18]

CLINICAL FEATURES

Onychotillomania involves picking of the nail that may cause damage to the nail matrix. This may present with loss of cuticle, erythematous nail folds, subungual hematoma, or loss of nail plate, with or without ulcerations. A characteristic median nail dystrophy can also be seen as a result of injury to the nail matrix.

COMORBIDITIES

Onychotillomania is associated with various psychiatric disorders such as obsessive-compulsive disorders, anxiety, and major depressive disorders.[6,17]

OUTCOMES

Onychotillomania involves nail picking, which leads to trauma to the nail fold and exposure of the underlying soft tissue. This predisposes the nail unit to recurrent infections, paronychia, and herpetic infections. Frictional melanonychia is another complication seen as a result of activation of nail matrix melanocytes.[6,18]

Perionychotillomania

Also known as perionychophagia, this term includes picking or tearing of the periungual skin. Presence of hangnails acts as both a trigger factor and a consequence of perionychotillomania, thereby creating a vicious cycle.[1] Onychotillomania may be considered as an exaggerated form of perionychotillomania.[19]

Habit tic deformity

Habit tic deformity is a condition where there is repeated external trauma to the nail matrix that causes multiple transverse ridges in the nail. The patient tends to manipulate the proximal nail fold with the adjacent finger. This condition most commonly affects the thumbnails (Figure 28.5) but fingernails may also be involved. Simultaneous involvement of finger- and toenails has also been described (Figure 28.6).[20] As expected, patient is generally unaware of the act of pushing

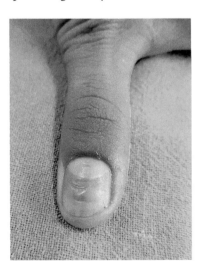

Figure 28.5 Characteristic habit tic deformity of the fingernail.

cuticle with the contralateral or ipsilateral finger. This results in damaged, detached, and missing cuticle exposing the unusually large and pyramidal lunula (Figures 28.6 and 28.7). The proximal nail fold often shows pigmentation and signs of inflammation (Figure 28.8). Median canaliform nail dystrophy (MCND) is a close differential diagnosis and presents with

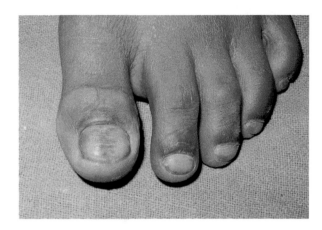

Figure 28.6 Habit tic deformity of the toenail.

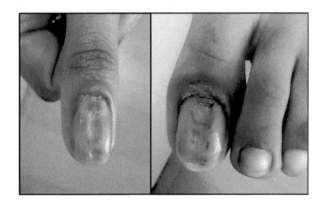

Figure 28.7 Habit tic deformity of both thumb and big toenails in a young girl (note the absent cuticle and enlarged pyramidal lunula due to pushing back of the cuticle).

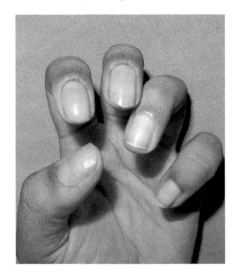

Figure 28.8 Detached, damaged, and missing cuticle on thumb, index, and middle finger in a young boy.

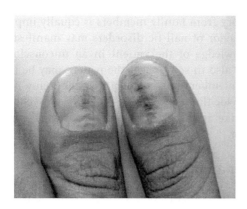

Figure 28.9 Classical "Washboard" nail of habit tic deformity with parallel transverse ridging and damaged cuticle.

a series of transverse ridges with a central depression mimicking a fir tree pattern. It is considered closely related to habit tic deformity but may have a normal cuticle (Figure 28.9). Both are considered different variants of nail disorder secondary to trauma.[21,22]

OTHER NAIL TIC DISORDERS

Onychotemnomania

Onychotemnomania means cutting the nails too short leading to damage to nail fold and nail bed. It is considered as a severe variant of nail factitious disorder, which may involve the use of scissors, razor blade, or cutter.[23] It is found to be associated with body dysmorphic disorders, self-mutilation disorders, and other psychiatric diseases like hypochondriasis and depression.[19]

Onychotieromania

In onychoteiromania, patient feels the urge to rub or file the nails leading to thin and cracked nails. In severe cases, excessive rubbing may lead to vanishing of the nails.[19] However, this should not be confused with shiny nails in atopic patients where the patients rub the itchy lesions with the help of distal aspect of the phalanges instead of the terminal part of the nails.[23]

Onychodaknomania

It is defined as psychopathological condition where patient tends to bite the nails to attain lustful pain. It is a rare condition and may result in depression and cracks in the nail, punctate or striate leukonychia. It is usually associated with underlying psychiatric disorders. Severe cases may cause resorption of the terminal phalynx.[19,23]

Bidet nails

Also known as **worn-down nail syndrome**, presents with a classic triangular defect in the nail with its base at the free edge of the nail. It is usually seen in females who are obsessed with genital hygiene and tend to scratch or rub the nails against the porcelain of the bidet while cleaning their genital area. It was first reported by Baran and Moulin in three homemakers who were overly concerned with vaginal hygiene, which led to repeated trauma to their middle three fingers of dominant hand.[24,25]

Onycholysis semilunaris

It is a common but often missed nail tic disorder that usually presents with a sharply delimited distal onycholysis in a semilunar shape (Figure 28.10). It is more commonly seen in women and in fingernails and results from overzealous manicuring with hard brushes and application of chemicals to clean the space under the free margin of the nail. The damage caused to the hyponychium creates an empty recess, for accumulation of dirt, bacterial colonization like Pseudomonas aeruginosa, and sometimes even leading to biofilm formation that further worsens the onycholysis. Onycholysis semilunaris must be differentiated from nail psoriasis by the absence of inflammation and red-brown discoloration that is commonly seen in psoriasis (Figure 28.11). To break the cycle of onycholysis, regular trimming of the nails and cleaning of the hyponychium is necessary.[1,23]

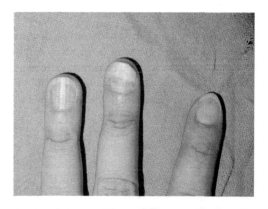

Figure 28.10 Onycholysis seminularis with white onycholytic nail plate and regular margin in a young woman.

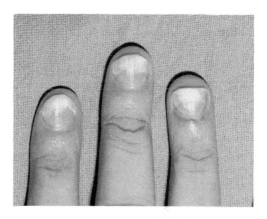

Figure 28.11 Red-brown discoloration at the proximal onycholytic margin of nail psoriasis.

Lacquer nails

This is considered as a variant of worn-down nail syndrome. As the name suggests, lacquer nails is a tic disorder that occurs due to frequent rubbing of the nail plate with nail filers or the applicators provided with the topical antifungal nail lacquers.[1]

APPROACH TO A PATIENT WITH NAIL TIC DISORDERS

The approach involves detailed history taking, examination of nails, and muco-cutaneous examination and psychiatric evaluation in some as outlined in Box 28.2.

History

A detailed history is of extreme importance in arriving at a diagnosis of nail tic disorders. Onset, duration, and symptoms of the condition must be noted.[1,10] Nail tic disorders usually start in early childhood and tend to decrease as the age advances. There may be trigger factors that may be associated with the habit such as boredom, anxiety, stress, or difficult task. A chronological order and evolution of the nail tic behavior and any trigger factor like depression or mental trauma should be noted. The habit may tend to subside with social interaction.[6,9]

History of evolution of the act should be discussed with the patient. Usually patients with neurotic excoriations and onychotillomania give history of a feeling of tension followed by picking of the nail that may or may not be accompanied by itching. This eventually provides a sense of relief to the patient.[26]

History suggestive of other psychiatric disorders such as anxiety, depression, obsessive-compulsive disorder, and attention deficit hyperactivity disorder should also be included.[1,7,8] History of medication for the same or for any other indication should also be asked to rule out drug-induced nail changes. Nail changes associated with other cutaneous dermatosis such as psoriasis, lichen planus, atopy, paronychia, and dermatophytosis, which may mimic nail tic disorders, should also be excluded. A possibility of systemic diseases like liver, kidney diseases, and malignancy known to cause nail manifestations should also be considered.

BOX 28.2: Approach to a patient with nail tic disorders

- History
- Examination – Nails, skin, mucous membranes, oral cavity
- Histopathology
- Psychiatric Evaluation
- Treatment:
  a. Non-pharmacological
  b. Pharmacological

History from family members is equally important as the behavior of nail tic disorders may manifest without the knowledge of the patient in an unconscious manner and also in some cases the patient may be in denial. Family members must be inquired about any indication of behavior that may suggest underlying psychiatric disorders like anxiety, depression, or obsessive-compulsive behavior.

Examination

Examination of nail along with rest of the body, skin, and mucosa should be done for all the patients.

- All 20 finger- and toenails should be examined in proper light.
- Secondary complications such as paronychia, splinter hemorrhages, melanonychia, and damage to cuticle and periungual region should be looked for.[10]
- Certain nail tic disorders such as onychophagia and onychotillomania may closely mimic other nail dermatosis like onychomycosis, nail psoriasis, nail lichen planus, paronychia, and twenty-nail dystrophy and pose a diagnostic challenge.[6,18]
- Body and scalp hair should be examined to rule out related disorders like trichotillomania.
- Oral cavity should be checked in case of onychophagia to rule out oral dental carriers, gingival infection, and malocclusion.[8,16]
- Vaginal examination in case of bidet nails is important to look for suspected obsession with genital hygiene.[24,25]
- Systemic examination should be done for all the patients to rule out secondary systemic causes of the nail changes as well as to look for systemic associations of the psychiatric disorders.

Histopathology

Nail biopsy is not routinely done in nail tic disorders as the diagnosis is usually made on clinical grounds. However, in diagnostic dilemma, where the history is not supportive or unreliable, biopsy may be required. Histopathology usually shows non-specific features such as focal hyperkeratosis, hypergranulosis, and papillomatosis seen in onychophagia.[10] In addition to these findings, onychotillomania may show acanthosis and elongation of rete ridges. However, absence of features of other differentials like nail psoriasis, onychomycosis, and lichen planus would aid in ruling out these dermatoses.[18]

Psychiatric evaluation

Psychodermatology involves interaction between skin and mind. On one hand, skin reflects the visible part of the disease, while on the other hand the psychiatric state of the patient reflects the invisible part and needs a detailed evaluation.

- A proper psychiatric analysis of the patient should be done including the underlying psychiatric disorder such as anxiety, depression, obsessive-compulsive disorder, or psychosis.
- History suggestive of other associated co-morbidities commonly seen with nail tic disorders should be asked like trichotillomania, dermatitis artefacta, acne excoriee that may be seen in patients with impulse control disorders.
- A patient of anxiety disorder may give history of frequent washing of hands.
- Patients affected with psychosis may give history suggestive of delusions like body dysmorphism or delusion of parasitosis.
- Those with depression will have symptoms such as easy fatigability, anhedonia, erratic sleep, and feeling of excessive guilt.[26]

It should also be kept in mind that nail tic disorders like onychophagia are more common in children whose parents are affected with psychiatric disorders like schizophrenia; therefore, psychiatric assessment of the family and its management should not be neglected.[13]

Treatment

Treatment of nail tic disorders should be a two-pronged approach:

- **Non-pharmacological:** Non-pharmacological methods such as hypnosis, biofeedback, and cognitive behavioral therapy should be combined with pharmacological treatment.
- **Pharmacological**

NON-PHARMACOLOGICAL

1. Counseling
   - The first step towards management is to build a rapport with the patient. The patient has to be educated about the mechanism of the damage to the nail and they have to be encouraged to quit this behavior.
   - The next and most important step is counseling, to stop the tic habit. The latter can be achieved by educating the patient about the consequences and building up self-esteem and confidence. Mild cases may be treated with proper counseling alone.
   - Children should be encouraged and given positive reinforcement from their loved ones and efforts should be made to remove the triggering stress factor.
   - Counseling of the patient must be accompanied with counseling of the family members.
2. Cognitive behavioral therapy accounts for a major part in the treatment. Patients can be encouraged to start some tension-relieving activities such as arts and crafts or outdoor activities that may distract the child from the tic. Habit reversal can be achieved with the

help of awareness of warning signs and development of competing responses, object manipulation, and certain non-removable reminders like wrist bands that may help in avoidance of the habit.[10,18,26]
3. Physical measures
   - Severe cases may require measures like frequent application of emollient (olive oil) to make the nails soft and trimming the nails short.
   - Application of a bitter-tasting material over the nails has been found to be very useful in onychophagia.[1,9,10]
   - Application of band-aids, glue, micropore dressing, and Unna boots has been found effective in onychotillomania as well.[6,18]
   - Habit tic deformity too requires cessation of the repeated trauma, with the help of proper counseling as well as measures like application of instant cyanoacrylate glue or tape to the nail folds. However, care must be taken about the risk of developing contact allergic dermatitis to the cyanoacrylate glue.[21]

PHARMACOLOGICAL

The choice of the pharmacological agent depends on the type of co-existent psychiatric disorder, which includes four broad categories: anxiety, depression, psychosis, and obsessive-compulsive disorder. Accordingly, patient may require sedatives, antidepressants, or antipsychotic treatment.[3]

- Disorders like onychophagia and onychotillomania are treated in line with obsessive-compulsive disorders.
- **Selective serotonin re-uptake inhibitors** (SSRIs) such as sertraline, which are used in the treatment of OCD, can be added in severe cases of onychophagia and onychotillomania.[10,18]
- **N-acetyl Cysteine** has also been found to be effective in some cases by regulation of reward/reinforcement system through glutamine.[27]
- Nail tic disorders associated with bipolar disorders can be treated with drugs like **lithium**, while those associated with depression may require **anti-depressants** like norepinephrine-dopamine reuptake inhibitor such as bupropion and tricyclic antidepressants like amitriptyline.
- Severe or refractory cases of habit tic deformity can also be treated in terms of obsessive-compulsive disorders with drugs like SSRIs.
- Treatment with multivitamin supplements including biotin has also shown to be effective in some cases.[21,22]

CONCLUSION

Nail tic disorder is a commonly missed and underdiagnosed condition. There is very little literature on clinical features and treatment guidelines of nail tic disorders. However, due to its impact on both cosmetic and social aspect of the patient, more awareness is required among dermatologists about the subtle signs that point towards its diagnosis as well as how to form a refined approach to such patients.

KEY POINTS

- Nail tic disorders are tics pertaining to nail unit that can have variable presentation.
- Nail tic disorders are not uncommon but are probably under-diagnosed and under-reported as patients seldom seek active intervention.
- Their management requires a systematic and holistic approach: detailed history and psychological evaluation followed by proper counseling.
- In addition, various physical measures like application of occlusive dressing to avoid access to the nail may be required.
- In severe cases, SSRIs, tricyclic antidepressants, N-acetyl cysteine, and multivitamins have shown a promising role.
- A thorough understanding of the pathogenesis, clinical presentation, and management is of paramount importance to address timely intervention.

REFERENCES

1. Singal A, Daulatabad D. Nail tic disorders: Manifestations, pathogenesis and management. *Indian J Dermatol Venereol Leprol* 2017;83(1):19–26.
2. Jafferany M. Psychodermatology: A guide to understanding common psychocutaneous disorders. *Prim Care Companion J Clin Psychiatry* 2007;9(3):203–213.
3. Yadav S, Narang T, Kumaran MS. Psychodermatology: A comprehensive review. *Indian J Dermatol Venereol Leprol* 2013;79:176–192; Chamberlain SR, Odlaug BL. Body focused repetitive behaviors (BFRBs) and personality features. *Curr Behav Neurosci Rep* 1(1):27–32.
4. Siddiqui EU, Naeem SS, Naqvi H, Ahmed B. Prevalence of body-focused repetitive behaviors in three large medical colleges of Karachi: A cross-sectional study. *BMC Res Notes* 2012;5(1):614.
5. Pacan P, Grzesiak M, Reich A, Kantorska-Janiec M, Szepietowski JC. Onychophagia and onychotillomania: Prevalence, clinical picture and comorbidities. *Acta Derm Venereol* 2014;94(1):67–71.
6. Pacan P, Grzesiak M, Reich A, Szepietowski JC. Onychophagia as a spectrum of obsessive-compulsive disorder. *Acta Derm Venereol* 2009;89(3):278–280.
7. Sachan A, Chaturvedi TP. Onychophagia (nail biting), anxiety, and malocclusion. *Indian J Dent Res* 2012;23(5):680–682.
8. Ghanizadeh A. Nail biting: Etiology, consequences and management. *Iran J Med Sci* 2011;36(2):73–79.
9. Halteh P, Scher RK, Lipner SR. Onychophagia: A nail-biting conundrum for physicians. *J Dermatolog Treat* 2017;28(2):166–172.
10. Shetty SR, Munshi AK. Oral habits in children: A prevalence study. *J Indian Soc Pedod Prev Dent* 1998;16(2):61–66.
11. Wells JH, Haines J, Williams CL. Severe morbid onychophagia: The classification as self-mutilation and a proposed model of maintenance. *Aust N Z J Psychiatry* 1998;32(4):534–545.
12. Ghanizadeh A. Association of nail biting and psychiatric disorders in children and their parents in a psychiatrically referred sample of children. *Child Adolesc Psychiatry Ment Health* 2008;2(1):13.
13. Vafaei B, Seidy A. A comparative study on the prevalence of emotional and behavioral symptoms in children and adolescents born to mothers with schizophrenia and other psychotic disorders. *Acta Medica Iranica* 2003;41(4):254–259.
14. Lee DY. Chronic nail biting and irreversible shortening of the fingernails. *J Eur Acad Dermatol Venereol* 2009;23(2):185.
15. Kamal FG, Bernard RA. Influence of nail biting and finger sucking habits on the oral carriage of Enterobacteriaceae. *Contemp Clin Dent* 2015;6(2):211–214.
16. Bhardwaj A, Agarwal S, Koolwal A, Bhardwaj C, Sharma R. Onychotillomania as manifestation for underlying depressive disorder. *Indian J Psychiatry* 2016;58(1):98–99.
17. Halteh P, Scher RK, Lipner SR. Onychotillomania: Diagnosis and management. *Am J Clin Dermatol* 2017;18(6):763–770.
18. Haneke E. Management of the aging nail. *J Women's Health Care* 2014;3:204.
19. Singal A. Habit tic deformity of bilateral thumb and toenails in a young boy: An unusual occurrence. *Skin Appendage Disord* 2017;3(4):186–187.
20. Perrin AJ, Lam JM. Habit-tic deformity. *CMAJ* 2014;186(5):371.
21. Gloster H Jr, Kindred C. Habit-tic-like and median nail-like dystrophies treated with multivitamins. *J Am Acad Dermatol* 2005;53(3):543–544.
22. Haneke E. Trastornos de autoagresión hacia la suñas. *Dermatol Rev Mex* 2013;57(4):225–234.

23. Baran R, Moulin G. The bidet nail: A French variant of the worn-down nail syndrome. *Br J Dermatol* 1999;140(2):377.

24. Dogra S, Yadav S. What's new in nail disorders? *Indian J Dermatol Venereol Leprol* 2011;77(6):631–639.

25. Ghosh S, Behere RV, Sharma PSVN, Sreejayan K. Psychiatric evaluation in dermatology: An overview. *Indian J Dermatol* 2013;58(1):39–43.

26. Ghanizadeh A, Derakhshan N, Berk M. N-acetylcysteine versus placebo for treating nail biting, a double blind randomized placebo controlled clinical trial. *Antiinflamm Antiallergy Agents Med Chem* 2013;12(3):223–228.

27. Berk M, Jeavons S, Dean OM, Dodd S, Moss K, Gama CS, Malhi GS. Nail-biting stuff? The effect of N-acetyl cysteine on nail-biting. *CNS Spectr* 2009;14(7):357–360.

Surgical Management of Nail Diseases

29

Basics of nail surgery

SHILPA KAPANIGOWDA AND BIJU VASUDEVAN

INTRODUCTION

Nail surgeries are commonly done in day-to-day practice by dermatologists. Various indications for nail surgeries include ingrown toenail, periungual or subungual abscess, nail tumors, nail deformities, and nail biopsies for diagnostic purposes. Nail surgeries should be done with precise techniques to avoid untoward complications. Apart from the surgical skills, basic requirements that are essential for optimum outcome in nail surgeries have been covered in this chapter.

CLEANING OF NAIL BEFORE PROCEDURE

A common problem associated with toenail removal surgery is the accompanying bacterial infection that often ensues. The foot has a particularly difficult anatomy to prepare antiseptically for surgery, which contributes to this widespread problem.[1] Adequate removal of bacteria from the nail folds and web spaces of the foot presents a challenge, as it is seen that an aerobic bacterial culture rate higher than 70% exists for foot specimens after treatment with standardized methods involving povidone-iodine.[2]

Studies using phenol for ingrown toenail surgery have reported infection rates up to approximately 15%.[3] This suggests that while the addition of phenol to the nail avulsion procedure dramatically decreases symptomatic recurrence, it is at the cost of increased post-operative infection.[4]

In a study conducted by Becerro de Bengoa Vallejo et al., four methods of skin and nail preparation were evaluated for their efficiency in eliminating bacteria from the hallux nail fold and first web space of the foot. It was shown that an alcohol pre-wash (prewash with 70% isopropyl alcohol for 3 minutes followed by 7.5% povidone-iodine scrub for 5 minutes and 10% povidone iodine paint) (Figure 29.1) plays an important role in decreasing the bacterial load when undergoing nail avulsion surgery. The foot-preparation solutions that may be used are 4% chlorhexidine gluconate, 70% isopropyl alcohol, and 7.5% or 10% povidone-iodine.

Additionally, it was determined that immersion of the foot in a solution of water and 4% chlorhexidine gluconate before the skin and nail preparation protocol further increased the treatment efficacy. It was established that the addition of alcohol to povidone-iodine increased the efficacy of the nail preparation method prior to nail avulsion surgery. Consistently incorporating this pre-operative step may aid in the prevention of increased bacterial load often associated with this type of nail surgery.[5]

In another study by Becerro de Bengoa Vallejo, incorporation of intraoperative irrigation of sterile saline solution (Figure 29.2) after nail avulsion surgery reduces potential bacterial load. Every effort should be made to lower the risk of contamination after nail plate avulsion.[2] The important steps to be followed for cleaning before nail surgery have been given in Box 29.1.

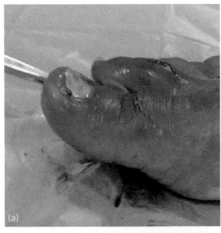

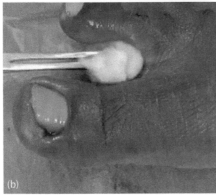

Figure 29.1 Surgical preparation of nail unit **(a)** Povidone iodine paint followed by **(b)** alcohol paint.

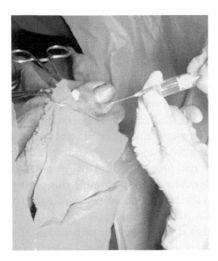

Figure 29.2 Intraoperative irrigation with saline to reduce bacterial load.

DRESSINGS

An ideal dressing after nail surgery should allow functional mobility of the digit, protect the surgical site, absorb any discharge, and at the same time should not be too heavy and should not slip off easily.[6]

According to Henderson HP, the best dressing for a nail bed is the nail itself. The replacement of a surgically avulsed nail

(Figure 29.3) as a splint and dressing with "Superglue" provides a painless cover for the sterile matrix and facilitates the dressing of fingertip injuries. A few drops of "Superglue" around the margin of the nail is sufficient to keep it in place for long enough to provide time for adequate healing of the underlying tissues.[7]

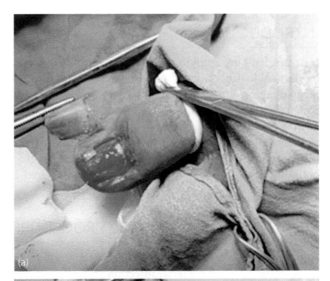

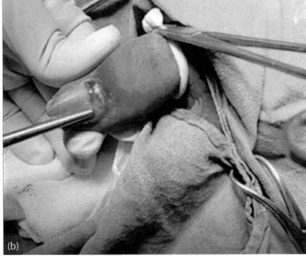

Figure 29.3 **(a and b)** Nail plate being replaced as natural dressing.

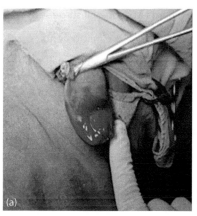 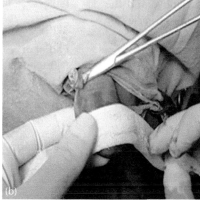 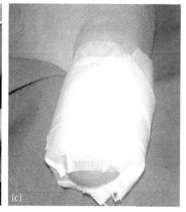

Figure 29.4 Dressing with **(a)** first layer of topical antibiotic like povidone iodine ointment, **(b)** followed by non-adherent sterile gauze, **(c)** which is secured later with micropore.

The most common dressing applied is with first layer of topical antibiotic like povidone iodine ointment followed by non-adherent sterile gauze, which is secured later with micropore or adhesive plaster (Figures 29.4 and 29.5). A bulky dressing provides a cushion against local trauma. However, bulky dressing is prone to slip away sometimes.

To overcome this and standardize nail dressing, a unique Y technique has been designed by Dr Ashique KT. The first step is winding the base layer of this paraffin gauze (i.e., the stem of the Y), which provides adequate grip for the dressing and prevents dislodgement (Figure 29.6). The second layer is the adsorbent gauze, which is also cut in the same "Y" shape and wound over the first layer in the same fashion. This layer further promotes the grip.

The authors have found this dressing to be extra-stable and limit the use of multiple layers of bandages. In addition, this dressing does not require much expertise, is small-sized, and hence increases the post-operative functionality of the operated digit.[8]

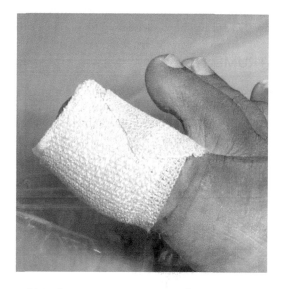

Figure 29.5 Same as Figure 29.4. Adhesive plaster being used.

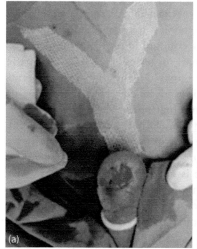 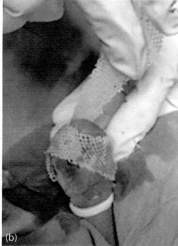 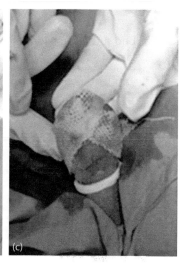

Figure 29.6 Y Technique – **(a)** Paraffin gauze cut in the shape of a Y and vertical stem of Y is placed below the great toe; **(b** and **c)** The oblique limbs are then made to cover the nail bed.

After 24 hours, the dressing is safe to remove and the toe should be soaked in warm water following surgeries for ingrown toenail. If persistent oozing is there, dressing may be continued for 48–72 hours.

SUTURES

Sutures are rarely required in day-to-day nail surgeries. Sutures are used when:

- Repairing lacerated nail unit injuries
- Removal of tumor
- Lateral nail fold excision for advanced stages of ingrown toenail (rarely done nowadays)
- Flap surgeries for correction of pincer nail
- Following elliptical matrix biopsy

Absorbable Vicryl sutures 4–0 and 5–0 are used for matrix and nail bed surgeries. Non-absorbable sutures like Prolene (Figure 29.7) or Ethilon 5–0 are used for nail fold suturing.

INSTRUMENTS

Nail surgery requires very meticulously designed instruments that suit the nail architecture. Depending on the type of surgery, the required instruments (Figure 29.8) are tabulated in Table 29.1.

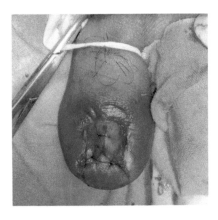

Figure 29.7 Nail bed sutured with Prolene.

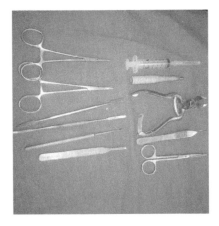

Figure 29.8 Instruments commonly used in nail surgeries.

Table 29.1 Instruments used in nail surgeries

Surgery	Instruments
Partial or total nail avulsion	Freer's nail elevators, nail splitter, clippers, straight scissors, straight artery forceps, Phenol or sodium hydroxide, Radiofrequency/electrocautery/curette (for matricectomy)
Nail tumors	Single- or double-pronged skin hooks, pointed scissors (Gradle scissors), curved iris scissors, small-nosed hemostats, mosquito forceps
Nail biopsy	Disposable biopsy punches, scalpel blades, BP handles, mosquito forceps
Common for all procedures	Luer-Lok syringe, 30-gauge needles, tourniquet

TOURNIQUET

A tourniquet is a mechanical device used for the temporary control of the blood circulation, especially used in surgeries of extremities. The nail derives its blood supply from the lateral digital arteries, which give rise to numerous branches and proximal and distal arcades, which anastomose extensively.[9] All nail surgical procedures require the use of a tourniquet. The nail bed, being a very vascular structure, needs to be exsanguinated at the start and then a tourniquet needs to be tied at the base. A number of tourniquets have been described, including a Foley's catheter, a Penrose drain, a rubber strip, or a rubber band.[10] An ideal material for use as tourniquet should not be thin, twisted, and constrictive like a rubber band. It should be sterile as it comes in close contact with the operative field.

For brief intraoperative hemostasis (e.g., nail avulsion, punch biopsy of the nail bed), squeezing the sides of the digits is effective but it is not practical for long surgeries.

The most commonly used tourniquet is the surgical gloves. For nail surgeries of the hand, the patient is made to wear the glove. On the digit to be operated glove is cut at the tip and rolled over till the base of the digit, slowly exsanguinating the digit (Figure 29.9). This technique, apart from providing a bloodless field, also provides sterile environment in the adjacent digits. However, in toenail surgeries, instead of full gloves a part of the finger glove is cut like a tube, encircled over digit, and slowly exsanguinated till the base and then further tightened with hemostat (Figure 29.10). The use of hemostat to secure the tourniquet at the base may also interfere with the operative field or may loosen out during the procedure. The movement and manipulation of the digit during surgery are also restricted by attaching a hemostat at its base.

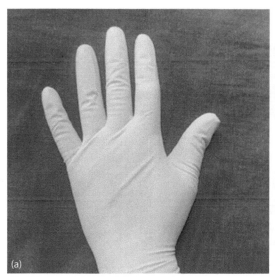
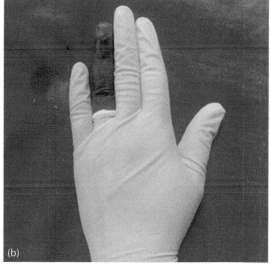

Figure 29.9 Surgical glove being used as tourniquet in fingernail surgeries. **(a)** Wearing of glove on the hand **(b)** Cutting glove of digit of nail to be operated on at distal end and rolling it proximally.

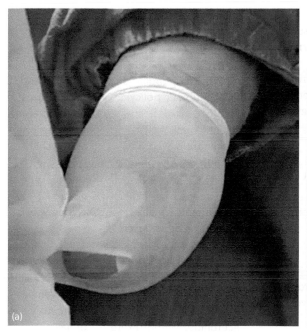
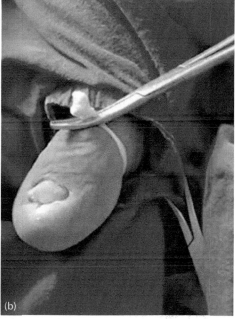

Figure 29.10 Surgical glove being used as tourniquet in toenail surgeries. **(a)** Cutting out a tube like part of one glove finger and putting it on to the great toe **(b)** Rolling up from distal to proximal and application of hemostat.

To overcome these difficulties, a refined and standard-ized method was devised by Chander Grover et al., in which a sterile gauze was used for exsanguination in addition to a tourniquet during nail surgery. A 25-inch long piece of autoclaved gauze is folded on itself to form a flat strip (half-an-inch wide). The strip is then used to exsanguinate the digit, if deemed necessary. It is wrapped tightly around the digit from the distal to the proximal end, achieving extrava-sation. For this, each loop should partially overlap the pre-vious loop. When the base of the finger is reached, two extra loops are wound to secure the strip at the base. Thereafter,

one should start unwrapping from the distal end until you reach the lower 1/3rd of the digit. At this stage, both the free ends are tied in a secure knot to form a tourniquet at the base of the finger (Figure 29.11). The use of gauze strip tourniquet offers several advantages over the other tourni-quets described. The requisite gauze strips are cost effective and easily available to every surgeon and do not require any special procurement of material or sterilization. Being a flat strip, it does not cause uneven or undue pressure on the underlying digital nerves or arteries. Above all, a knot and not a hemostat holds the tourniquet at the base, helping in

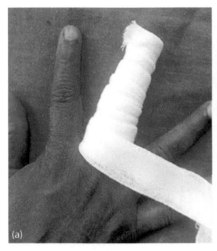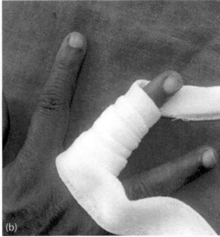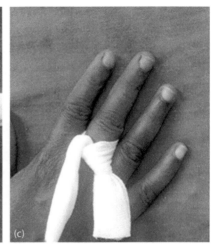

Figure 29.11 Sterile gauze strip being used as tourniquet. (a) Gauze strip being wrapped from distal to proximal end with partial overlap, (b) unwrapping from distal to proximal end, (c) knot being tied at the base.

maintaining easy maneuverability of the digit during surgery. It also avoids chances of accidental slippage of tourniquet during surgery.[10]

Tourniquet use has been recommended for about 20 minutes at a stretch without any complications. For longer procedures, the tourniquet can be intermittently loosened and then tied tightly at the base.

Potential risks associated with tourniquets include:

- Local skin damage under a poorly applied tourniquet
- Compromised circulation caused by extended use
- Peripheral nerve and vessel damage

CONTROL OF BLEEDING

Nail bed, being a highly vascular structure, can pose a problem of intra- and post-operative bleeding. This can be overcome by using anesthetic agent combined with epinephrine as vasoconstrictive agents. Apart from the pharmacological agents, bleeding in nail surgeries is controlled using a tourniquet as described above.

Sometimes bleeding may be seen after the tourniquet is removed, but it can be stopped by compressing the lateral edges of the distal interphalangeal joint. In cases of persistent bleeding, 35% aluminum chloride solution or a cellulose application should be applied.

DRUGS BEST SUITED FOR NAIL

The commonly used drugs and their indication have been tabulated in Table 29.2. However, details of the drugs, dose, and duration have been covered in respective chapters.

Table 29.2 List of common drugs used in nail disorders

Drugs	Indications
Antibiotics (depending on local antibiotic policy)	Periungual and subungual abscess, post-operative period, paronychia
Oral antifungals – Itraconazole, Terbinafine, Fluconazole	Onychomycosis, chronic paronychia
Analgesics	Periungual and subungual abscess, paronychia
Topical agents – nail lacquers like Ciclopirox olamine, Amorolfine	Onychomycosis
Potent topical steroids	Inflammatory conditions of nail
Chemical peels like glycolic acid	Dystrophic nails for cosmetic improvement
Injectables – Triamcinolone acetonide, Methotrexate	Inflammatory conditions of nail
Bleomycin	Periungual and subungual wart

REFERENCES

1. Becerro De Bengoa Vallejo R, LIM, Alou Cervera L, Sevillano Fernández D, Prieto Prieto J. Efficacy of preoperative and intraoperative skin and nail surgical preparation of the foot in reducing bacterial load. *Dermatol Surg* 2010;36(8):1258–1265.
2. de Bengoa Vallejoa RB, Iglesiasb MEL, Cerverac LA, Sevillano DF, Prieto JP. Importance of pre-operative skin and nail preparation of the foot and intra-operative surgical irrigation in reducing infection after

surgical nail avulsion. In *Science Against Microbial Pathogens: Communicating Current Research and Technological Advances.* Méndez-Vilas A (Ed.) FORMATEX 2011-448-51.

3. Felton PM, Weaver TD. Phenol and alcohol chemical matrixectomy in diabetic versus nondiabetic patients. A retrospective study. *J Am Podiatr Med Assoc* 1999;89(8):410–412.

4. Rounding C, Bloomfield S. Surgical treatments for ingrowing toenails. *Cochrane Database Syst Rev* 2005;2:CD001541.

5. Becerro de Bengoa Vallejo R, Iglesias LM, Cervera L, Fernández LS, o Prieto JP. Preoperative skin and nail preparation of the foot: Comparison of the efficacy of 4 different methods in reducing bacterial load. *J Am Acad Dermatol* 2009;61(6):986–992.

6. Khunger N, Kandhari R. Ingrown toenails. *Indian J Dermatol Venereol Leprol* 2012;78:279–989.

7. Henderson HP. The best dressing for a nail bed is the nail itself. *J Hand Surg Br Eur Vol* 1984;9(2):197–198.

8. Ashique KT, Grover C. The 'Y' technique: An attempt to standardize nail dressing. *J Am Acad Dermatol* 2018;78(5):e103-e104.

9. Hale AR, Burch GE. The arteriovenous anastomoses and blood vessels of the human finger. Morphological and functional aspects. *Medicine* 1960;39:191–240.

10. Grover C, Nanda S, Nagi Reddy BS. Gauze strip tourniquet for nail surgery. *J Cutan Aesthet Surg* 2014;7:164–166.

30

Anesthesia of the nail unit

SHEKHAR NEEMA AND DIPALI RATHOD

INTRODUCTION

Anesthesia is an important therapeutic tool and without a good anesthesia many of the dermatologic surgeries considered routine today become difficult to perform. It is of paramount importance for the physician to spend adequate time in learning the science and art of anesthesia, so as to make the process of performing surgery as painless as possible. To achieve adequate anesthesia, it is imperative to understand the anatomy of the digit, pathophysiology of pain and pathology of the nail unit. In this chapter, we will discuss different types and techniques of local anesthesia used in nail surgery.

NERVE SUPPLY TO DIGITS

Each digit is supplied by two pairs of digital nerves. The paired palmar digital nerve supplies palmar aspect of digit and nail bed and the paired dorsal digital nerve supplies dorsal aspect of digit (Figure 30.1). In hands, these nerves arise from the median, ulnar, and radial nerves while in feet they arise from the tibial and peroneal nerves.[1]

Infiltrative anesthesia results in blockage of initial transmission of nociception in small nerve fibers, whereas nerve blocks affect larger and more proximal nerve fibers that require longer time to diffuse into the nerves and block depolarization.

CHEMICAL STRUCTURE OF ANESTHETIC AGENTS

Most of the synthetic anesthetic agents comprise a benzene ring and a short aliphatic chain with a secondary or tertiary amine. They are bound together with either an ester or an amide bond. Both these groups are different in their chemical stability, allergenicity, and metabolism. Esters are metabolized by pseudocholinesterases in plasma and the amides are metabolized in the liver. Esters are unstable in solution and more likely to cause allergic reaction. Commonly used amide local anesthetic agents are lignocaine, bupivacaine, and prilocaine. Tetracaine, chloroprocaine, and cocaine are examples of ester local anesthetic agents. For all practical purposes, local anesthetic agents most commonly used are those of the amide type.

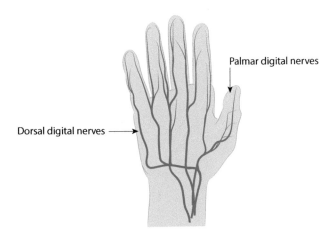
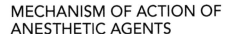

Figure 30.1 Schematic diagram showing nerve supply of hand.

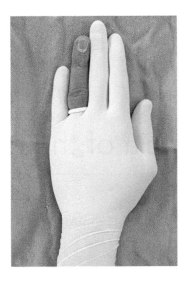

Figure 30.2 Use of sterile glove to exsanguinate the digit and prepare the sterile surgical field.

MECHANISM OF ACTION OF ANESTHETIC AGENTS

Local anesthetics work by diffusing into the nerve cells through hydrophobic cell membranes and block the voltage-gated sodium channels of the free nerve endings. Blocking of sodium channels prevents nerve depolarization, blocking propagation of nerve impulse and thus retarding the transmission of pain. They act on all types of nerve cells as well as the peripheral nervous tissue, on efferent motor and afferent sensory and autonomic nerves.

FACTORS INFLUENCING THE POTENCY OF LOCAL ANESTHESIA (LA)

Following anesthesia, the pain and discomfort experienced by the patients may be affected by several factors, which include specific characteristics of the anesthetic agent (molecular composition, temperature, pH, addition of epinephrine), choice of syringe and needle size, technique of injection, and the distracting stimuli used.

Addition of epinephrine

Epinephrine prolongs the anesthetic effect and causes vasoconstriction, which decreases bleeding and provides a better and longer duration of pain control during digital surgeries.[2] It further reduces the need for the use of tourniquet and larger volume of anesthetic agent.

There have been contradictory opinions regarding the use of epinephrine in the extremities due to the risk of ischemia. However, numerous studies support the use of lidocaine with epinephrine, as the combination is safe in digits.[3,4] In the absence of contraindications, combination is safe and is not associated with increased risk of digital infarction or permanent ischemia.[5,6]A concentration of 1:2,00,000 is deemed safe. Proper injection technique and

adequate selection of the patients are recommended to minimize complications. However, epinephrine is not recommended in patients with peripheral vascular disease. In case of prolonged ischemia, nitroglycerine ointment or phentolamine injection may be used to reverse it.[7]

In case epinephrine is contraindicated or not available, tourniquet may be applied to minimize bleeding. An easy and efficient way of applying a tourniquet is by cutting a tiny hole into the corresponding finger after donning a sterile glove and then rolling it back. This technique not only exsanguinates the finger but also gives a sterile field[8] (Figure 30.2). Another advantage of this technique is that in case the surgery takes longer than 20 to 30 minutes, the tourniquet may be released or changed every 15 minutes for a few minutes to prevent gangrene.[3] It is important to keep a track of the tourniquet time during surgery, and to minimize the tourniquet time, it should be applied once adequate anesthesia has been achieved. It is also prudent to avoid use of LA with epinephrine and tourniquet in same patient.

Choice of syringe and needle size

Due to the compact structure of the nail unit apparatus, the use of a Luer-Lock syringe is advisable, because anesthetic injections used during nail surgeries provide high resistance due to little expansion of the tissues. The rationale for the use of very thin needles (27-gauge for toes, 30-gauge for fingers and for children in all locations) is that it reduces pain due to the needle puncture and the flow of the anesthetic agent is controlled better with a gradual development of the soft tissue swelling.

COMMONLY USED ANESTHETIC AGENTS

The two main anesthetic agents commonly used in digital anesthesia are lidocaine and bupivacaine (Table 30.1).

Table 30.1 Common anesthetics used during nail unit surgery

Sr. No.	Anesthetic agent	Action onset (mins)	Duration of action (mins) without/with adrenaline	Tolerability/ toxicity	Pregnancy category	Recommended dose without/with adrenaline per Kg body weight
1.	Lidocaine	<1	30–120/60–400	Good/Low	B	4.5mg/7mg/Kg
2.	Bupivacaine	2–5	120–240/240–480	Good/Medium	C	2mg/2.5mg/Kg

Lidocaine

Lidocaine (1% or 2%) is the most widely used local anesthetic. It is also known as lignocaine or xylocaine. It is characterized by quick absorption and near instantaneous anesthesia, i.e., the onset is faster (<1–3 min) than that of the other agents. Its duration of action is 60 minutes. It is available in 1% or 2% strength, as plain or in combination with adrenaline.

Maximum safe dose of lignocaine is 4.5 mg/Kg (7 mg/Kg if used with epinephrine). For a 60 Kg individual, the maximum dose of lignocaine is 270 mg (420 mg with adrenaline). 2% lignocaine contains 21.3 mg lignocaine/mL. Hence, the maximum of 12 mL 2% lignocaine without adrenaline can be administered (270/21.3). With adrenaline, 20 mL can be given. If we use 1% lignocaine instead of 2%, the amount of LA that can be safely used is doubled. Since anesthetic action of lignocaine can be achieved at even 0.5% dilution, it is better to use it at 1% strength especially if use of larger amount is contemplated.

Bupivacaine

Bupivacaine (0.5%) has a slower onset of action and a longer duration of action (480 min).[7] It may be added to provide post-operative analgesia. It is available in 0.25% or 0.5% strength. The recommended maximum safe dose for bupivacaine without adrenaline is 2 mg/Kg and with adrenaline is 2.5 mg/Kg. For a 60 Kg individual, the maximum bupivacaine that can be administered is 120 mg (150 mg—with adrenaline). 0.5% bupivacaine contains 5mg/mL of bupivacaine, so a maximum of 24 mL of 0.5% bupivacaine (30 mL with adrenaline) can be administered safely in a 60 Kg adult without other comorbidities.[8]

TECHNIQUES OF ADMINISTRATION OF LA

During the administration of anesthesia, it is best to have the patient in a reclined position in the event of a vasovagal episode. In addition, to avoid a dangerous reflex jerk, it is best to inform the patient when the needle stick is expected. The nerve blocks have the advantage of achieving larger areas of anesthesia with fewer injections as compared to infiltration anaesthesia.[1,9,10]

Distal nail block

Distal nail block is easier to perform and plain 2% lidocaine is usually preferred. Distal nail anesthesia offers immediate anesthesia of the total nail unit and is appropriate for biopsies, but the anesthesia is short lived. The injection is given very slowly to minimize the pain. The injection may be performed as a wing block or approached either through the proximal nail fold (PNF) or the hyponychium.

DISTAL WING BLOCK

Local infiltrative anesthesia, termed the distal wing block, is the technique of choice in nail surgery; is well-tolerated, rapid, and an efficient form of anesthesia provided if it is performed properly and rate of injection is slow. The junction of the PNF and the lateral nail fold is identified, and the anesthetic injection is given approximately 5 to 8 mm proximal and lateral to this point. The needle is introduced at a 45° angle and directed distally down towards the bone, and approximately 0.3 to 0.5 mL of the anesthetic agent is slowly injected, which distends and blanches both the nail folds and anaesthetizes the dorsal nerves (especially the terminal, transverse, and descending branches) (Figure 30.3). Since the folds distend distally and medially from the point of injection, a "wing-like" appearance is noted. To ensure complete anesthesia, the PNF and the lateral nail fold need to be infiltrated along their entire width right up to the hyponychium, and the procedure should be repeated on the opposite side as this injection provides anesthesia for only half of the nail apparatus.

If more advanced surgery (i.e., flaps) is planned, anesthesia of the ventral roots is necessary. In order to anaesthetize the ventral nerve roots, the needle is inserted at the initial puncture site and pushed downwards gliding along the lateral aspect of the phalanx and approximately 0.5 mL solution is injected into the pulp. In case the needle tip penetrates the periosteum, resistance to the injection may occur and careful withdrawal of the needle results in a free flow.

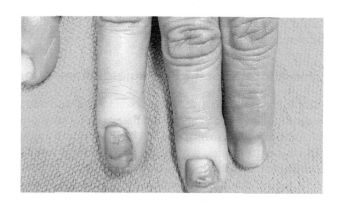

Figure 30.3 Distal wing block resulting in blanching of proximal nail fold and lateral nail folds.

It is faster and provides volumetric compression, thus achieving better hemostasis as compared to proximal block. Distal block is more painful as compared to proximal block.

DISTAL ANESTHESIA THROUGH THE PROXIMAL NAIL FOLD

It is also known as matricial block. It provides anesthesia to the nail matrix, PNF, and proximal half of the nail bed. The needle is inserted at mid-point of PNF, at an angle of 60°, 5–7 mm proximal to cuticle. It is pushed until it touches the bone, then withdrawn slightly and 0.5–1 mL of anesthetic agent is slowly injected. The lunula and the nail bed blanches, which roughly indicates the territory of anesthesia.

DISTAL ANESTHESIA THROUGH THE HYPONYCHIUM

This technique is useful for anesthesia of the hyponychium, the bed, and most of the matrix. However, it is rarely performed because it is more painful. The needle is inserted in the lateral hyponychial area and directed horizontally in the nail bed to avoid trauma to the prominent distal phalangeal ungual process. Then, the anesthetic agent is injected, which roughly blanches the territory of anesthesia.

Proximal field block/ring block

Regional anesthesia of a single digit is commonly achieved by the proximal block. It was traditionally known as ring block as it involved injection all around the digit. This technique has a potential hazard of compression and trauma to the neurovascular bundles with subsequent postoperative edema that may cause long-lasting pain compared to the other techniques and it may require up to 20 minutes for the anesthetic effect to develop.[17] That is why a modified form of proximal block is now used. Injection is given in midline on lateral aspect of digit, 1 cm distal to interdigital web. The needle is inserted at an angle of 45° until it touches the bone and approximately 1.5–2 mL of anesthetic solution is deposited. The same process is repeated on the medial aspect. Anesthesia is achieved in approximately 10 min (Figure 30.4).

It has slower onset of action, requires mechanical tourniquet for hemostasis, and has potential for neurovascular damage. However, proximal block is less painful as compared to distal block and complete anesthesia of the digit is achieved with this block.

Transthecal anesthesia/single-digit injection

This technique is effective for the second, third, and fourth fingers (index, middle, and ring fingers). It is a very good alternative to the proximal field block and provides complete anesthesia. Its greatest advantage is that the neurovascular bundles of the digits are exempted from injury.

A total of 3 mL 2% lignocaine with 27 G needle is used. Hand is kept in supine position and needle is inserted at palmar metacarpal crease through flexor tendon sheath to reach bone (Figure 30.5). Needle is then slowly withdrawn

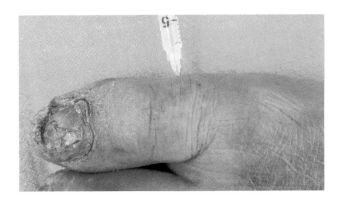

Figure 30.4 Proximal nail fold block: Injection is given in midline on lateral aspect of digit, 1 cm distal to interdigital web.

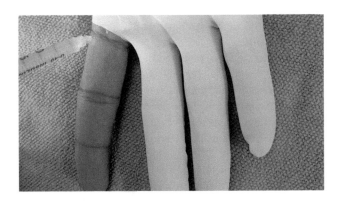

Figure 30.5 Transthecal block: Hand is kept in supine position and needle is inserted at palmar digital crease through flexor tendon sheath to reach bone. Needle is then slowly withdrawn and anesthetic solution is pushed in space of flexor tendon sheath.

and anesthetic solution is pushed in space of flexor tendon sheath. Anesthetic solution diffuses centrifugally and blocks the digital nerves. During the injection, nondominant hand is used to apply pressure just proximal to the injection site, to direct the flow of anesthetic agent distally.

It is an excellent technique as it requires single injection, and complete anesthesia is achieved. However, it can be used only for index, middle, and ring fingers.

PREFERENCE OF THE ANESTHETIC TECHNIQUE

The technique of digital anesthesia usually depends upon the type of surgery and the personal preference of the surgeon. Each technique has its own benefit and surgeons involved in routine nail surgery should include more than one technique in their armamentarium. Proximal digital block gives excellent anesthesia for virtually all types of nail surgery and is the preferred technique in presence of infection of nail unit. Distal anesthesia works faster and results in blanching of the tip of the digit, requires less volume of anesthetic agent, and provides better hemostasis. Transthecal anesthesia requires only single injection and is especially useful for intramatricial injections.

METHODS TO ALLEVIATE THE PAIN ASSOCIATED WITH LA INJECTION

It is important that the process of anesthesia is minimally painful, as patient remembers this process rather than surgery. All efforts should be made to make patient comfortable. The following methods have been suggested to reduce the pain while injecting a local anesthetic agent.[11]

Decrease pain due to infiltration

1. Injection of an acidic solution is more painful.
   - Lignocaine plain has a pH of 6.09. Lignocaine mixed with adrenaline has a pH of 4.24 and is an acidic solution.
   - Buffering 10 mL of lidocaine premixed with adrenaline by adding 1 to 1.8 mL of 8.4% sodium bicarbonate produces a mixture with a near physiologic pH. This neutral pH solution is not only less painful while injecting, but also yields more efficient anesthesia. However, mixture should be prepared just before injection.[12]
2. The anesthetic agent should be warmed to 37°C or should be left outside fridge to come to room temperature.[13]
3. The needle with a smaller size (30 gauge for fingers, 27 G for toes) decreases pain due to puncture and limits the flow of anesthetic agent, further reducing discomfort and pain from rapid tissue distention.
4. Use a small-volume syringe and inject slowly in deeper dermis.
5. Use of strong, distinct, physical stimulus proximal to the site of injection by repetitive, rapid pinching or tapping the skin or using a massager may decrease pain by creating sensory noise.

Decrease pain from needle stick

1. Topical anesthesia—Especially in children EMLA should be applied 60 minutes prior to surgery and needle should be introduced through anesthetized area.
2. Ice application—Ice should be applied to make area numb and removed just before needle insertion.
3. Use of small-gauge needle (27 or 30 G).
4. Distraction—While injecting, talk to patient.
5. Keeping needle out of sight is important, especially in children.

Sedation

1. For anxious patients, benzodiazepines like diazepam or alprazolam can be given orally. It reduces fear of injection. It also produces retrograde amnesia, which is helpful in reducing any perceived trauma from the experience.[14]

LA DURING PREGNANCY

Lignocaine is a pregnancy category B drug, while bupivacaine is a pregnancy category C drug. During pregnancy, the blood volume increases as a result of increase in the plasma volume, thus decreasing the plasma protein concentration. Therefore, the biologically active drug concentration rises. Various studies have suggested that risk to mother and fetus on exposure to lignocaine for dermatologic surgery is minimal.[15]

Epinephrine belongs to pregnancy category C. High doses have been shown to cause uterine artery spasm and decreased placental perfusion and, therefore, has been associated with slightly higher risk of developing congenital malformations.

CONTRAINDICATIONS OF LA

Absolute and relative contraindications for nail unit anesthesia are outlined as follows:

Absolute contraindication

- History of allergy to the LA or other constituents of the local anesthetic solution

Relative contraindications

- Diabetes mellitus
- Disorders of hemostasis
- Peripheral vascular disease

Acute infection or inflammation of the nail unit

COMPLICATIONS DURING LOCAL ANESTHESIA

Digital anesthesia for nail surgery is remarkably well tolerated. Complications are rare. However, complications may be avoided by adequate preventive measures, such as judicious patient selection, aseptic technique, and gentle handling of the nail matrix. Proper patient examination prior to nail surgery and correct technique usually avoid the most common complications and rule out high-risk patients. Complications to LA have been discussed in Table 30.2.

Adverse reaction to local anesthetic agents: Local anesthetic agents are generally considered safe and life-threatening reactions resulting from LA are fortunately rare. LA belong to two groups: amide and esters. Most commonly used anesthetic agents like lignocaine and bupivacaine belong to amide groups. Allergic reactions can be classified as IgE-mediated or non-IgE-mediated reactions.[16]

Immediate hypersensitivity (Type I) reaction is an IgE-mediated reaction and is mediated by mast cells and basophils. These reactions are idiosyncratic reactions and are usually caused by ester anesthetic because of formation of para amino benzoic acid (PABA) through hydrolysis. It occurs within minutes up to 1 hour after exposure and is characterized by pruritus, urticarial

Table 30.2 Complications during LA and the measures to tackle them

Sr. No.	Complication	Cause	Treatment
1.	Vasovagal reaction—nausea, hyperventilation, diaphoresis, bradycardia, and hypotension	Anxiety	• Most crucial step is prevention • Preoperative anxiolytic • All procedures to be performed in recumbent position • If signs of vasovagal reaction evident—place the patient in the Trendelenberg position immediately and place a cool cloth over the head. • If loss of consciousness present—supplemental oxygen and spirits of ammonia may help in reviving the patient.
2.	Bleeding	• Occurs after releasing the tourniquet • Patient on anticoagulants	• Ice application • Direct pressure without release for at least 20 mins • Coagulation of the vessel • Suturing
3.	Pain during operation	• Poor anesthesia	• Dressing—absorbs blood and avoids further pain from inadvertent injury • Elevation of extremity for 24 to 48 hours • Analgesics
4.	Edema	• Fluid redistribution	• The limb is elevated to 30° and the patient kept recumbent for 48 hours • Cool compresses
5.	Infections	• Septic technique	• Adhere to strict asepsis and atraumatic surgery • Outer surface of the anesthetic bottle to be cleansed by alcohol prior to each puncture of the needle • Avoid infiltration in a contaminated or purulent wound, instead a nerve or field block should be preferred. • Antibiotic prophylaxis
6.	Nerve laceration	• Compartment syndrome due to infiltration within the epineurium, causing axonolysis	• Regular use of 30-gauge needle as permanent nerve damage is unlikely with this size • Anesthetic agent not to be injected into a nerve or foramen • In case the patient complains of electric sensation, needle should be withdrawn slightly until the *paraesthesia* resolves, taking care to avoid any lateral motion.
7.	Necrosis	• Sutures are too tight and not removed in time	• More superficial injection • Avoid too-tight sutures. Release them at appropriate time.
8.	Permanent residual defects	• Type of surgery undertaken or may result from one of the complications mentioned	• Proper history and examination of the patient prior to surgery rules out high-risk individuals. • One should carry out appropriate LA technique and possess adequate knowledge of digital anatomy.

rash, angioedema, bronchospasm, wheezing, dyspnea, cyanosis, laryngeal edema, nausea, vomiting, abdominal cramping, and shock. Patient should be treated with 0.3–0.5 mg Epinephrine (1: 1000) intramuscular and basic life support should be started.

Differential diagnosis: Vasovagal response, reaction to epinephrine, and overdose of LA can mimic anaphylaxis.[17]

a. Vasovagal reaction presents with diaphoresis, palpitation, nausea, bradycardia, and hypotension. Patient should be placed in the Trendelenburg position and in case of no response atropine 0.4 mg subcutaneously can be administered.

b. Epinephrine reaction presents with palpitation, flushing, and tachycardia. Patients on propranolol can have severe reaction to epinephrine due to unopposed alpha-adrenergic activation. Epinephrine reaction resolves spontaneously and does not require any treatment. Epinephrine should be avoided in patients with uncontrolled hyperthyroidism, severe hypertension, and pheochromocytoma.

c. Systemic toxicity resulting from overdose of LA is central nervous system (CNS) and cardiovascular (CVS) toxicity. Early features of CNS toxicity include light headedness, dizziness, tinnitus, and drowsiness. It is followed by shivering, twitching, tremors, and generalized tonic-clonic seizure. CVS toxicity is due to negative inotropic action on cardiac muscle. Bupivacaine is a more potent cardiac depressant than lignocaine. Ventricular arrhythmia can also occur resulting from intravenous administration. It is mandatory to prevent toxicity as it is very difficult to treat CVS collapse resulting from overdose of LA.

Type IV (i.e., delayed-type hypersensitivity) reactions account for most of the allergic reactions to local anesthetics and are characterized by erythema, plaques, and pruritus. They are seen with the both amide and ester subtypes of anesthetics. However, it is more common with the ester subtype of anesthetics. Although an anesthetic agent itself can rarely cause allergic reaction, more commonly preservatives like paraben or sulfite are the cause of allergy.

Approach to a case of patient with or history of suspected LA allergy

Though allergic reactions to LA are quite rare, any history of allergic reaction to LA or allergic reaction during a procedure puts the dermatologic surgeon in a tough situation.

1. The first step is to confirm the diagnosis of LA allergy. The test depends on whether allergy is Type I or Type IV mediated reaction. If patient develops Type I reaction, skin prick testing (SPT) can be done to confirm the diagnosis. If patient tolerates SPT, intradermal test can be done in increasing concentration until it is determined that patient can tolerate LA. Patient should be observed for reaction like wheal and flare. Systemic reaction to SPT is rare, but there is a potential risk of anaphylaxis and a resuscitation tray should be kept ready. Approximately 98% of patients who pass intradermal test tolerate LA in clinic setting.[18–20] Patients with Type IV hypersensitivity reaction should undergo patch testing to determine the exact nature of the allergen.[21]

2. In patients with allergy to one class of LA, another class of LA can be used. In case a patient is allergic to both ester and amide-type local anesthetics, alternative agents include isotonic sodium chloride solution and antihistamines. An intradermal injection of 0.9% sodium chloride solution can provide temporary anesthesia resulting from physical pressure on the nerve endings due to the volume injected. A bacteriostatic solution that contains benzyl alcohol may be used for limited procedures such as punch biopsy.[22]

- Injectable 1% diphenhydramine can be used as an alternative anesthesia in patients with allergy to LA. The mechanism of anesthetic action of injectable antihistamines, such as diphenhydramine, is unknown. Injectable diphenhydramine is effective, but it is painful, has a short duration of activity, and causes sedation. It should be diluted to 1% by mixing one vial of 50 mg diphenhydramine with 4 mL of bacteriostatic sodium chloride solution.[23]

Preoperative evaluation of patients

- A thorough patient history and clinical examination may help to avoid unnecessary complications and identify potential contraindications.
- History of drug allergy should be taken. History of previous procedures under local anesthesia and outcome should be specifically mentioned.
- Various surgical and non-surgical treatment options need to be discussed with the patient, including the pain and inconvenience expected postoperatively.
- Any treatable condition, e.g., acute infections, should be tackled prior to the surgery.
- Patients on antidiabetic and antihypertensive medications should continue their medications. Patients on antiplatelet or anticoagulant drugs do not need to stop these medications for routine nail surgery. In case of advanced nail surgery like flap surgery, these medications need to be stopped in consultation with physician.
- Smoking should be stopped before and after surgery, as it increases the risk of ischemic complications and delays wound healing.
- Investigations are generally not necessary in routine nail surgery, but it is prudent to perform baseline hematological and biochemical investigations.

Pre-operative checklist

1. Informed consent
2. Ask about systemic medication and whether patient has taken his daily medication
3. History of allergy to any drug
4. Pre-operative photograph
5. Antibiotic prophylaxis in high-risk cases
6. Confirm the identity of the patient and the site of surgery
7. Disinfection of surgical field

Post-operative checklist

1. Non-adherent dressing
2. Antibiotics
3. Analgesic
4. Instruction to change dressing after three days and restrict activity for a week
5. Time for suture removal

CONCLUSION

Complete anesthesia is a prerequisite for a successful digital and nail surgery. The usefulness of anesthesia during nail unit surgery is indisputable. The successful application of techniques of local anesthesia is pre-requisite to good outcome in nail surgery.

KEY POINTS

- Knowledge of the pain pathways, understanding of the anatomy, and described injection techniques provide the surgeon with comfort to tailor local anesthesia for each patient, digit, and procedure.
- Several techniques exist for obtaining good nail unit anesthesia.

REFERENCES

1. Richert B. Anesthesia of the nail apparatus. In: Richert B, Di Chiacchio N, Haneke E, editors. *Nail Surgery*. New York: Informa Healthcare; 2010. pp. 24–30.
2. Schnabi SM, Unglaub F, Leitz Z et al. Skin perfusion and pain evaluation with different local anaesthetics in a double blind randomized study following digital nerve block anaesthesia. *Clin Hemorheol Microcirc* 2013; 55(2): 241–253.
3. Krunic AL, Wang LC, Soltani K, Weitzul S, Taylor RS. Digital anesthesia with epinephrine: An old myth revisited. *J Am Acad Dermatol* 2004; 51: 755–759.
4. Wilhelmi BJ, Blackwell SJ, Miller JH et al. Do not use epinephrine in digital blocks: Myth or truth? *Plast Reconstr Surg* 2001; 107: 393–397.
5. Harness NG. Digital block anesthesia. *J Hand Surg Am* 2009; 34(1): 142–145.
6. Andrade A, Here HG. Traumatic hand injuries: The emergency clinician's evidence-based approach. *Emerg Med Pract* 2011; 13(6): 1–24.
7. Denkler K. A comprehensive review of epinephrine in the finger: To do or not to do. *Plast Reconstr Surg* 2001; 108: 114–124.
8. Alhelail M, Al-Salamah M, Al-Mulhim M et al. Comparison of bupivacaine and lidocaine with epinephrine for digital nerve blocks. *Emerg Med J* 2009; 26: 347–350.
9. Flarity-Reed K. Methods of digital block. *J Emerg Nurs* 2002; 28: 351–354.
10. Richert B. Basic nail surgery. *Dermatol Clin* 2006; 24(3): 313–322.
11. Strazar AR. Leynes PG, Lalonde DH. Minimizing the pain of local anesthesia injection. *Plast Reconstr Surg* 2013; 132(3): 675–684.
12. Frank SG. Lalonde DH. How acidic is the lidocaine we are injecting, and how much bicarbonate should we add? *Can J Plast Surg* 2012; 20(2): 71–73.
13. Davidson JA, Boom SJ. Warming lidocaine to reduce pain associated with injection. *BMJ* 1992; 305: 617–618.
14. Ravitskiy L, Phillips PK, Roenigk RK et al. The use of oral midazolam for perioperative anxiolysis of healthy patients undergoing Mohs surgery: Conclusions from randomized controlled and prospective studies. *J Am Acad Dermatol* 2011; 64(2): 310–322.
15. Gormley DE. Cutaneous surgery and the pregnant patient. *J Am Acad Dermatol* 1990; 23: 269–279.
16. Batinac T, Sotosek Tokmadzic V, Peharda V, Brajac I. Adverse reactions and alleged allergy to local anesthetics: Analysis of 331 patients. *J Dermatol* 2013; 40: 522–527.
17. Fathi R, Serota M, Brown M. Identifying and managing local anesthetic allergy in dermatologic surgery. *Dermatol Surg* 2016; 42(2): 147–156.
18. Jacobsen RB, Borch JE, Bindslev-Jensen C. Hypersensitivity to local anaesthetics. *Allergy* 2005; 60: 262–264.
19. McClimon B, Rank M, Li J. The predictive value of skin testing in the diagnosis of local anesthetic allergy. *Allergy Asthma Proc* 2011; 32: 95–98.
20. Troise C, Voltolini S, Minale P, Modena P et al. Management of patients at risk for adverse reactions to local anesthetics: Analysis of 386 cases. *J Investig Allergol Clin Immunol* 1998; 8: 172–175.
21. Mackley CL, Marks JG Jr, Anderson BE. Delayed-type hypersensitivity to lidocaine. *Arch Dermatol* 2003; 139: 343–346.
22. Campbell-Jones V. A comparison of lidocaine versus normal saline for local anesthesia before intravenous cannula insertion. *J Natl Black Nurses Assoc* 2010; 21(2): 27–33.
23. Pavlidakey PG, Brodell EE, Helms SE. Diphenhydramine as an alternative local anesthetic agent. *J Clin Aesthet Dermatol* 2009; 2(10): 37–40.

31

Biopsy of the nail unit

SUSHIL TAHILIANI AND HARSH TAHILIANI

INTRODUCTION

Nail unit biopsy is a useful and simple procedure that helps in the treatment and diagnosis of various nail diseases. Newer imaging techniques like high-resolution Magnetic resonance imaging (MRI), ultrasound, confocal laser microscopy, and onychoscopy are available but they cannot substitute the information that can be obtained by histopathology.[1,2] Therefore, nail unit biopsy must be a part of every dermatologist's armamentarium. Many dermatologists appear reluctant to perform nail biopsy because of risk of scarring, but if standard procedures are followed, risk of scarring is minimal and not prohibitive. Sometimes, when isolated nail involvement without any skin/mucosal lesions is the presentation, nail biopsy is the only diagnostic tool available.

INDICATIONS

A nail unit biopsy may be required when medical history, clinical examination, and other diagnostic tests fail to establish a diagnosis. The common indications are listed in Box 31.1.[3]

BOX 31.1: Indications of nail biopsy

- Isolated nail disease without any mucocutaneous clues
- To differentiate between infective and inflammatory disorders of the nail apparatus
- To establish the cause of nail dystrophy and plan further course of management
- To diagnose the nail tumors
- To excise small benign tumors

PRE-REQUISITES

Knowledge of surgical anatomy of the nail

The detailed discussions on nail anatomy can be found in the chapters "Nail anatomy and physiology (chapter 2)" and "Basics of onychopathology (chapter 8)". In short, mostly nail matrix and, to some extent, nail bed contribute to the formation of nail plate. Proximal and two lateral nail folds help keep the growing nail plate in position and proximal nail fold, in addition, protects the germinative nail matrix.

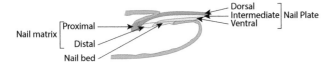

Figure 31.1 Diagram showing relationship between nail matrix and nail plate. (Courtesy of Dr. Mamta Yadav and Dr. Piyush Kumar.)

The changes in nail plate reflect the pathology of nail matrix and help us in deciding the site for biopsy. The changes due to proximal nail matrix pathology are both visible and palpable; changes due to distal nail matrix result in changes in intermediate part of the nail plate that are visible, but not palpable (Figure 31.1). Nail plate is tightly attached to nail bed; the attachment may be lost in various infective and inflammatory conditions and due to growth of various space-occupying lesions.[4]

The nail unit is supplied by two lateral digital arteries, running along the sides of digits. The pressure on each side of finger ensures adequate hemostasis. If a tourniquet is used, one should not leave it in place for more than 20 minutes.

The insertion of extensor tendon lies around 12 mm proximal to the cuticle; adequate care should be taken during the procedure not to damage it.[4,5]

Table 31.1 Selection of site for nail biopsy

Nail changes	Site for nail biopsy
Pitting, onychorrhexis,	Proximal nail matrix
True leukonychia	Distal nail matrix
Onycholysis, subungual hyperkeratosis	Nail bed
Longitudinal melanonychia	Nail matrix
Pseudoleukonychia (onychomycosis)	Nail plate
Nail fold lesions, paronychia, cuticle damage	Nail fold
Space occupying lesion	Lesion (after partial/total nail plate avulsion)

Source: Braun, R.P. et al., J. Am. Acad. Dermatol., 56, 835–847, 2007.

Patient selection

Proper patient selection is a key step in ensuring minimal peri- and post-operative complications. A complete history with a focus on potential vascular compromise, altered hemostasis, diabetes, cardiovascular diseases, and the use of drugs that could interfere with anesthesia or coagulation is mandatory. In addition, history of allergy to antibiotics, and topical anesthetics such as lidocaine, bupivacaine, ropivacaine, or parabens should be sought. Relative contraindications have been summarized in Box 31.2.[1,2]

Clinical examination should include palpation of peripheral pulses and mucocutaneous signs of vascular compromise. A thorough evaluation of fingernails and toenails is needed to select the site as well as type of nail biopsy. A rough guide to site selection is mentioned in Table 31.1.

The patient should be explained the details of technique and need for nail biopsy, alternative options and risks, expected course after the biopsy, potential risks of nail dystrophy, and other complications like bleeding, pain, and infection. Informed consent should be obtained before performing the nail biopsy. The pre-operative evaluation of the patient has been summarized in Box 31.3.

Nail anesthesia

Nail unit biopsies should be performed under local anesthesia. Lignocaine 2% is the preferred anesthetic agent. Injection bupivacaine 0.5% can be used for large longitudinal wedge excisional biopsies to prevent post-procedure pain.

Proximal digital nerve block works well for most cases. A distal digital nerve block or transthecal digital block may also be used.[1] The detailed discussion on various techniques of nail anesthesia and their merits and demerits can be found in the chapter on anesthesia of the nail unit (chapter 30).

BOX 31.3: Pre-nail biopsy evaluation[1,4,5]

- History
  - Drugs: anticoagulants
  - Cardiovascular diseases, peripheral arterial diseases, connective tissue diseases with vasculitis, or Raynaud's disease
  - Diabetes or other causes of immunosuppression
  - History of allergy to drugs and local anesthetics or their constituents
- Clinical examination
  - All 20 nails
  - Mucous membranes
  - Skin and hair
- Onychoscopy
- Laboratory
  - X-ray if required
  - Microbiology including mycological assessment
- Patient counseling and education
  - Possible permanent dystrophy – degree of risk with the type of procedure
  - Possibility of inconclusive findings and no diagnosis
  - Length of time for nail to regrow
  - Bleeding, pain, and risk of infection
- Clinical photographs of the nails

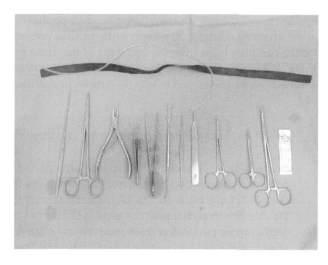

Figure 31.2 Instruments trolley for nail plate avulsion and longitudinal nail unit biopsy. (Courtesy of Dr. Sushil S. Savant.)

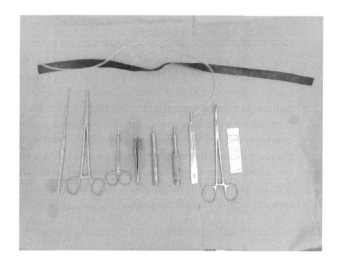

Figure 31.3 Instruments trolley for punch biopsy. (Courtesy of Dr. Sushil S. Savant.)

Instruments

Nail biopsy requires few specific instruments as mentioned in Box 31.4 (Figures 31.2 and 31.3).[3,5]

BOX 31.4: Instruments required for nail biopsy

- Magnifying loupe
- Adson's forceps, Castroviejo's forceps
- Biopsy punch, surgical blade, and handle
- Skin hook
- Stevens scissors, Gradle scissors
- Mosquito forceps
- Curette
- Tourniquet
- Nail elevator, Freer septum elevator, dental spatula
- Nail splitter
- Nail nipper
- Sutures

TYPES OF NAIL BIOPSY

Nail bed biopsy

Nail bed biopsies are useful for diagnosing various infective (onychomycosis), inflammatory (psoriasis, lichen planus), and neoplastic disorders (benign nail bed tumors such as glomus tumor, fibroma; premalignant and malignant conditions like Bowen's disease, squamous cell carcinoma, melanoma, etc.). Part of nail plate should be sent to the laboratory especially if mycotic diseases are being considered in clinical differentials. An experienced onychopathologist could pick up a few other diagnoses through histopathologic examination of nail plate alone.

For nail bed biopsy, the specimen should be punched/excised up to the periosteum of distal phalanx. Nail bed specimens are delicate and should be handled carefully to avoid crushing. Using a 30-gauge needle or firm pressure on the nail plate helps in upward popping of the tissue cylinder. A fine-tip scissors like Gradle scissors or fine, curved Castroviejo's scissors is used to snip the base of the specimen at the level of periosteum. A 3 mm or even 4 mm defect in the nail bed usually heals well with secondary intention and without nail deformities. Larger defects should be sutured with absorbable sutures. Various techniques of nail bed biopsy have been summarized in Box 31.5.[1,4,5]

BOX 31.5: Techniques of nail bed biopsy (Figure 31.4)[1,4-6]

a. **Punch biopsy**: The nail bed is exposed after partial (or rarely, complete) nail plate avulsion. After removal of the nail plate, the nail bed is inspected to select a site for biopsy and a sample is collected with a 3 mm punch. Soaking the nail in tepid water for 10–15 minutes just prior to punching softens the nail plate.

b. **Double punch technique**: This technique obviates the need of nail plate removal. A hole in the nail plate is created with a bigger punch, 5 or 6 mm, and the nail plate disc is removed with the help of a scalpel. Next, a 3 mm punch is used to get a nail bed sample through this hole. The punched-out nail plate is placed in its original position as dressing after the specimen has been obtained (Figure 31.5a–d).[5]

c. **Elliptical excision**: This technique is used when larger sample is desirable. The nail bed is exposed by partial or complete nail plate avulsion and the sample is collected by longitudinal elliptical excision. The defect is closed by 6–0 absorbable suture after undermining the edges. Relaxing incisions on the lateral margins of the nail bed may assist in achieving proper approximation of the edges. Transverse excision is not done to avoid scarring and subsequent onycholysis. For diagnosis of nail bed tumors this method is preferred over punch biopsies.

d. **Trap door/"pop the bonnet" technique**: The nail plate is separated from the underlying nail bed, but not from the proximal nail fold, and then lifted like a car bonnet/hood. The sample is collected from the exposed nail bed by punch biopsy or elliptical excision, and then the nail plate is placed back on the nail bed and secured with suture.

e. **Submarine hatch technique**[6]: This technique is used for distal nail matrix or proximal nail bed lesions and can be considered a modification of the double punch technique. A 4 or 5 mm punch is applied obliquely to the nail plate overlying the lesion at an approximately 70° angle, and is withdrawn when the nail matrix/nail bed is reached. Gentle pressure allows the nail plate to hinge open, like a submarine hatch. The sample is collected with a 3 mm punch (distal nail matrix) or 4 mm punch (proximal nail bed). The hinged nail plate is pushed back into its original position and is glued with ethyl cyanoacrylate. This technique provides an excellent cosmesis and requires no additional wound care other than regular hygiene.

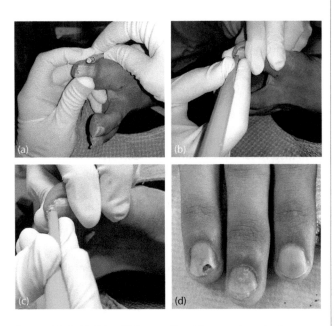

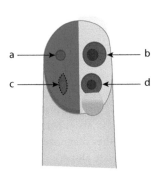

Figure 31.4 Different techniques of nail bed biopsy. (a) punch biopsy (b) double punch technique (c) elliptical excision (d) Trap door technique. (Courtesy of Dr. Mamta Yadav and Dr. Piyush Kumar.)

Figure 31.5 Nail bed biopsy- Double punch technique. (a) Punch used to remove the nail plate; (b) 3 mm punch through the circular defect to obtain nail bed specimen; (c) Punch inserted up to the periosteum; (d) 2 weeks post-biopsy; circular defect grows out without nail deformity.

Nail matrix biopsy

The nail matrix biopsy carries the highest risk of scarring as compared to biopsy of other locations within the nail unit. Whenever possible, distal matrix biopsies should be preferred over proximal matrix biopsy. To expose the nail matrix, releasing incisions are made at the junction of the proximal and lateral nail folds and the proximal nail fold and cuticle are carefully reflected proximally with the help of skin hooks. The proximal-most part of the nail plate is cut to allow complete visualization of the nail matrix (Figure 31.6). In general, a transverse nail matrix biopsy should be performed to obtain adequate specimen from the matrix compared to a longitudinal matrix biopsy. Longitudinal nail matrix biopsy may result in split nails later on, and hence is not preferred. The distal curved configuration of the lunula should not be disturbed while performing the biopsy. A transversely oriented wedge excision of the matrix up till the periosteum followed by undermining and primary closure with absorbable 5–0 or 6–0 sutures should be done. There is a thinning of the nail plate and no fissures after a wedge biopsy of the matrix as long as the proximal part of the matrix is not disturbed.[1,5,7]

Even a 3 mm punch biopsy of the matrix may not produce an easily noticeable deformity but it is not a preferred method.[1,7] Various types of nail matrix biopsy are summarized in Box 31.6.

Lateral longitudinal biopsy

This technique is best suited for the biopsy of suspected malignant lesions located in the lateral one-third of the nail. It is also useful for the diagnosis of inflammatory conditions

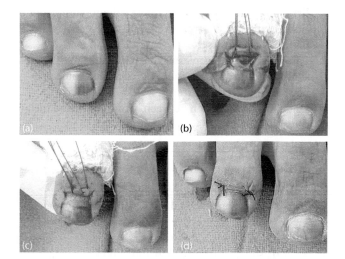

Figure 31.6 **(a)** Longitudinal melanonychia of right third toe; **(b)** Nail matrix is exposed by retracting proximal nail fold with stay sutures and by removing the proximal most part of the nail plate; **(c)** After collecting sample from nail matrix, the proximal nail fold is repositioned; **(d)** and sutured. (Courtesy of Dr. Archana Singal.)

BOX 31.6: Nail matrix biopsy types (Figure 31.7)[1,7]

a. **Punch biopsy**: A punch biopsy of the nail matrix is usually indicated for melanonychia with <3 mm width. The specimen is collected at the origin of the pigmented band.
b. **Longitudinal elliptical excision**: This technique is an alternative to punch biopsy when one intends to excise the lesions of <3 mm in width.
c. **Transverse matrix excision**: This technique is used to excise matrix lesions that are >3 mm in width. One should ensure that the distal margin of the excision matches the shape of the lunula. The defect is then closed by 6-0 absorbable suture.
d. **Tangential (shave) excision**: This technique is preferred when one needs a sample from the proximal nail matrix or the lesion of more than 3 mm size is located in the middle of the nail matrix.

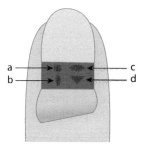

Figure 31.7 Various types of nail matrix biopsy (a) punch biopsy (b) longitudinal elliptical excision (c) transverse elliptical excision (d) tangential excision. (Courtesy of Dr. Mamta Yadav and Dr. Piyush Kumar.)

---

in which the nail bed, nail matrix, nail plate, and nail folds are affected simultaneously.

A lateral longitudinal biopsy helps to obtain an adequate specimen without the risk of split nail deformity, which occurs after a median longitudinal biopsy. A wedge excision with one incision starting from the hyponychium of the lateral nail groove extending proximally to the midway between the cuticle and the distal-most crease of the distal interphalangeal joint along the groove between the nail plate and the lateral nail fold and the other incision 3 mm medial to the former incision through the nail plate is made (Figure 31.8). The cutting through the nail plate is facilitated by pre-operative soak in warm water mixed with antiseptics for 10 minutes. The specimen is excised up to the bone to include the hyponychium, a full thickness fragment of nail bed, matrix along with the lateral horn, and proximal nail fold. Before closure, debridement of the lateral matrix pocket is done with a small curette to ensure

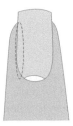

Figure 31.8 Incisions for lateral nail unit biopsy. The lateral incision should be made through the lateral nail groove so that anatomy of lateral nail fold is not disturbed. (Courtesy of Dr. Mamta Yadav and Dr. Piyush Kumar.)

complete removal of matrix remnants. Complete removal of matrix remnants is needed to avoid postoperative cysts, spicules, and/or pain. 4–0 sutures are placed on the proximal nail fold and hyponychium and left in place for 10–14 days. Back stitches are placed along the lateral nail fold and nail plate to achieve reconstruction of the lateral nail fold.[8,9]

Nail fold biopsy

Biopsy of the proximal nail fold is indicated for diagnosis of tumors of the nail fold, for systemic diseases with periungual lesions like multicentric reticulo-histiocytosis, and for collagen vascular diseases. A 3 mm punch biopsy can be performed by advancing the punch down to the nail plate. The distal margin of the proximal nail fold should be preserved during this procedure.[1,2]

Alternatively, a shave biopsy can be performed by the razor blade technique. A razor blade is broken into two longitudinal halves. One half is held between the thumb and index finger to slice out the proximal nail fold.[1]

A crescent excision 4 mm wide at its greatest width can be performed for collagen diseases and treatment of some tumors.[4,5] Hemostasis can be achieved by sliding gauze pressure or application of topical hemostatic agents.

Small wedge excisions in the median or lateral part of proximal nail fold may sometimes be indicated to acquire a larger specimen or for treatment of certain tumors.

For any procedure on the proximal nail fold, it is preferable to insert a nail spatula underneath the proximal nail fold, to avoid any inadvertent damage to the underlying nail matrix.

Lateral nail fold biopsy may be required in cases with focal lesions or tumors and may be performed using punch, elliptical excision, or shave excision techniques, similar to those used for cutaneous surfaces.[1]

Nail plate biopsy

This may be done in cases with onycholysis where there is strong clinical suspicion of onychomycosis. The altered nail is just clipped or the specimen of nail plate proximal to onycholysis is collected by punch after distal block, and the sample is sent for histopathological examination including Periodic Acid–Schiff (PAS) stain. The nail plate sample can be sent directly without fixation as keratin material does not decompose easily. The care should be taken to ensure that subungual hyperkeratotic tissue too is collected and sent along with biopsy specimen. The nail plate may also show intraungual melanocytes in subungual melanoma, blood inclusions in subungual hematoma, bacterial biofilms, and nail cosmetics. Onychomatricoma, a nail matrix tumor, can be diagnosed by nail plate biopsy alone.[1,4]

POST-BIOPSY CARE

A simple dressing with topical antibiotic or antibiotic tulle gauze should be done. The initial dressing should be bulky and padded to prevent pain from minor inadvertent trauma. Prophylactic oral antibiotics may be added in certain circumstances. Wound infection is the most common complication, but it is rare if proper aseptic precautions have been followed. The initial dressing should be changed and the wound should be examined after 48 hours. Analgesics may be needed for 1–2 days.[4,5]

LIMITATIONS OF NAIL BIOPSY

Awareness of these limitations helps in better utilization of nail biopsy as a tool.[1,4,5]

- Dystrophic nails due to multiple causes often share a similar clinical and histological picture.
- The histopathologic picture from a particular disease with nail involvement may differ from its corresponding cutaneous counterpart. For example, spongiosis and hypergranulosis are not the common features of psoriasis lesions affecting skin. On the contrary, spongiosis and hypergranulosis are frequent in nail psoriasis.[10] Hence, the interpretation of nail biopsy findings requires a separate, dedicated training.
- Organisms particularly fungi are often secondary colonizers and may not be the primary cause of dystrophic nails.
- Primary trauma may mimic/mask inflammatory conditions, and recurrent trauma may obscure neoplastic nature of the disease.
- Late diagnosis of neoplasms due to insufficient tissue sample or difficult discrimination between some neoplasms and reactive patterns.
- Difficult differentiation between hemosiderin and melanin and inability to assess the source of pigment.

KEY POINTS

- Nail unit biopsy is vital in correct and early diagnosis of many infective and inflammatory nail disorders, and nail unit tumors.
- A reasonable surgical skill and good knowledge of anatomy is mandatory.
- Hemostasis can be achieved with the use of tourniquet and hemostatic gels/solutions.
- Most routine biopsies can be performed in the dermatologist's office.

REFERENCES

1. Braun RP, Baran R, Le Gal FA, Dalle S, Ronger S, Pandolfi R et al. Diagnosis and management of nail pigmentations. *J Am Acad Dermatol* 2007;56(5):835–847.
2. Hirata SH, Yamada S, Almeida FA, Enokihara MY, Rosa IP, Enokihara MM, Michalany NS. Dermoscopic examination of the nail bed and matrix. *Int J Dermatol* 2006;45(1):28–30.
3. Grover C, Bansal S. Nail biopsy: A user's manual. *Indian Dermatol Online J* 2018;9:3–15.
4. Haneke E. Anatomy of the nail unit and the nail biopsy. *Semin Cutan Med Surg* 2015;34(2):95–100.
5. Rich P. Nail biopsy: Indications and methods. *Dermatol Surg* 2001;27(3):229–234.
6. Zaiac MN, Norton ES, Tosti A. The "submarine hatch" nail bed biopsy. *J Am Acad Dermatol* 2014;70(6):e127–e128.
7. André J, Sass U, Richert B, Theunis A. Nail pathology. *Clin Dermatol* 2013;31(5):526–539.
8. Zaias N. The longitudinal nail biopsy. *J Invest Dermatol* 1967;49(4):406–408.
9. de Berker D. Lateral longitudinal nail biopsy. *Australas J Dermatol* 2001;42:142–144.
10. Fernandez-Flores A, Saeb-Lima M, Martínez-Nova A. Histopathology of the nail unit. *Rom J Morphol Embryol* 2014;55(2):235–256.

32

Injection therapy for nail disorders

B.B. MAHAJAN, JYOTISTERNA MITTAL, KHAYATI SINGLA, AND PARUL CHOJER

INTRODUCTION

Nail disorders have always remained a therapeutic challenge for the dermatologist. Deformed and unhealthy nails cause a psychological setback and may have significant impact on a patient's daily life, social functioning, and mental health—hence, the quality of life. So, nails form a vital part of the individual's personality.[1-3]

A wide range of topical and systemic modalities have been used for treating various nail disorders, but response is often unsatisfactory. One of the aims in treating nail disorders is to make the drug available to the site of pathology (nail matrix or nail bed or both) in an effective concentration. Systemic drugs have to be given in high doses, which may result in toxicity, and they still may not effectively reach the nail matrix in the requisite concentration. Topical therapies for nail disorders have their own drawbacks like the potential for local adverse effects on the skin, need for prolonged occlusion, repeated applications, and limited efficacy due to low permeability into the nail plate. Various hurdles encountered in the treatment of nail diseases by drugs—topical or systemic—have been summarized in

Box 32.1. Delivering the drug directly into the nail matrix by intramatricial injection therefore seems to be the best option for treating various nail disorders. Intramatricial injections have been used in Psoriasis, Lichen Planus, Trachyonychia, and other inflammatory nail disorders with good outcomes.[4]

APPLIED ANATOMY OF THE NAIL UNIT

Complete knowledge of the detailed anatomy of the nail unit is important for learning the injectable therapies in various nail disorders.

According to Zaias, the nail consists of four distinct epidermal parts: nail matrix, nail bed, proximal and lateral nail folds, and hyponychium (Figure 32.1). One needs to identify the major site of pathology by carefully analyzing the various nail signs (described in chapters on nail anatomy and physiology, and nail biopsy techniques) and then choose the type of nail injection. Intramatricial injections and nail bed injections are the most commonly used techniques and have been described in this chapter.

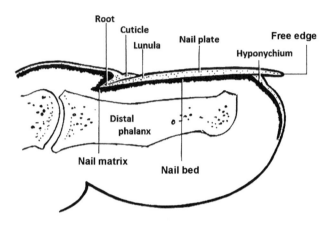

Figure 32.1 Diagrammatic representation of nail unit.

NAIL DISORDERS THERAPY

Therapeutic options may be topical, systemic and injection therapy. This chapter focuses on the various aspects of injection therapy.

Topical

Topical therapies are indicated when only nails are affected.

Topical treatment includes high-potency corticosteroid (cream, ointment, or lotion), retinoids like tazarotene 0.1% gel, Vitamin D analogues like calcipotriol, topical 1%, 5% 5-FU cream or solution, topical methotrexate, topical cyclosporine, etc.

Systemic therapy

Systemic therapy is usually indicated when there is nail as well as cutaneous involvement and includes PUVA therapy, methotrexate, cyclosporine, and retinoids. But these modalities are not usually advocated for cases with nail involvement only.

INJECTION THERAPY

Drugs that can be used systemically whether subcutaneous (S/C), intramuscular (I/M), intravenous (I/V), or intra-articular (I/A), can be given as intramatricial or nail bed injections. This therapy can be given in any inflammatory disorder affecting nails.

Indications

- Nail psoriasis
- Nail lichen planus
- Trachyonychia
- Nail dystrophy due to eczemas, atopic dermatitis, etc.
- Traumatic onychodystrophy
- Other causes of onychodystrophy include antineoplastic drugs, and contact dermatitis due to cyanoacrylate used as adhesive on artificial plastic fingernails.
- Traumatic onychodystrophy
- Viral wart- intra lesional injection therapy bleomycin has been discussed in chapter 18.

Contraindications

There are no absolute contraindications for this procedure except if there is known hypersensitivity to the drugs used.

Relative contraindications

- Peripheral vascular disease
- Collagen vascular disease
- Bleeding disorders
- Uncontrolled diabetes mellitus
- Previous history of allergy to anesthetic agent
- Active infection at the injection site

Drugs

Drugs used for nail disorders are enumerated in Box 32.2 (Figure 32.2).

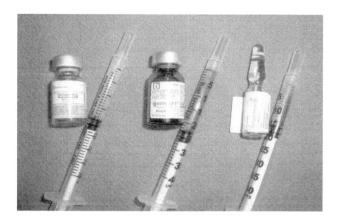

Figure 32.2 Common drugs used for injection.

Intramatricial corticosteroid injections have been used for many years in nail psoriasis with good results, the steroid molecule of choice being Triamcinolone acetonide.

Methotrexate, in the form of intra articlular (I/A) injections, has been widely used in psoriatic arthritis in doses of 10–20 mg/mL. The drug has also been tried for intramatricial injections and injections in the nail bed.

Intramatricial cyclosporine has not been widely used in nail psoriasis and various nail disorders. However, in a study by Burns et al. (1992), intralesional cyclosporine (17 mg/mL) yielded significant improvements in chronic plaque psoriasis, suggesting that cyclosporine is capable of exerting beneficial effects by local mechanism.[5]

Similarly, there are various studies regarding the use of etanercept in the form of intralesional injections in the treatment of keloids and I/A injections in the treatment of rheumatoid arthritis and various small joint arthritis. In a study by Bliddal et al. (2006), 25 out of 26 patients of small joint arthritis were successfully treated with I/A injections of Etanercept without any adverse effects. Though experience with etanercept in nail diseases is limited, it can emerge as a promising treatment modality in the near future.[6]

The authors have experience with injecting Triamcinolone acetonide in all three concentrations—2.5, 5, and 10 mg/mL—in psoriasis and lichen planus nails with excellent results. Also, injections of methotrexate and cyclosporine give equally good results in psoriatic nails. Injection etanercept is being evaluated as a new therapeutic modality in nail psoriasis.

PROCEDURE

Preoperative

- Detailed history, examination, and clinical diagnosis.
- Detailed history of any systemic disorders like bleeding disorders, diabetes mellitus, and collagen vascular disorders.
- History of any drug intake—NSAIDs, acetylsalicylic acid, and blood thinners—need to be stopped 5–6 days prior to the procedure.
- History of any vaso-vagal syncope and hypersensitivity reaction/anaphylaxis to local anesthesia or methotrexate or cyclosporine.
- Discontinuation of smoking a few weeks prior to the procedure.
- Diagnosis needs to be established by onychoscopy, imaging and/or histopathology prior to the procedure.
- Appropriate premedication and antibiotic prophylaxis if needed.
- Proper explanation about the procedure to the patient, time needed and expected therapeutic response.
- Detailed informed consent for the procedure and photographic evaluation for assessing the response of the treatment.

Operative

- Under aseptic precautions, the digit is cleaned and draped in a sterilized sheet.
- Digital nerve block with lignocaine (2%) is administered in the web spaces on either side of the digit.
- An insulin syringe is used for the intramatricial injection.
- The needle is inserted from the lateral angle of the proximal nail fold into the proximal nail matrix (Figure 32.3).
- On entering the proximal nail matrix, loss of resistance is felt, which is a sign of having reached the nail matrix.
- A volume of 0.05 mL is injected from each lateral angle, forming a "V" (Figure 32.3).
- Immediate blanching of the lunula (Figure 32.4a) indicates that the injection is being given correctly into the proximal nail matrix.

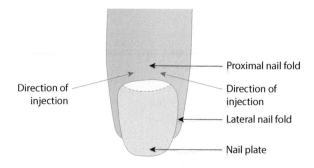

Figure 32.3 Intramatricial injection: positioning of injections.

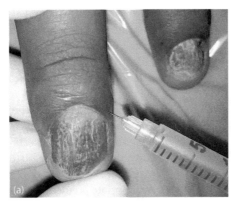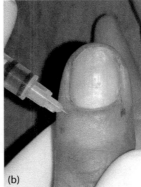

Figure 32.4 (a) Blanching of the lunula seen immediately after giving an intramatricial triamcinolone acetonide injection (Courtesy of Sushil S. Savant) (b) Yellowish discoloration of the lunula seen immediately after an intramatricial injection of methotrexate.

- In case of injection Methotrexate, yellowish discoloration of the lunula is seen because of the yellow color of the injection (Figure 32.4b).
- A needle-free jet injector, such as derm-o-jet or port-o-jet, can also be used. There is less injection pain, but it is not recommended owing to the difficulty in sterilizing the apparatus. Also, there is theoretical possibility of transferring infection from one patient to the next with the gun due to splash-back of blood on to the instrument and the physician.[7]
- **Technique for nail bed injection** – Nail matrix injections are easier than nail bed injections. However, the nail bed diseases (e.g., onycholysis, subungual hyperkeratosis, oil drop sign in nail psoriasis) are less responsive to intramatricial injections. Such cases require injection of the drug into the nail bed. So, careful examination of nail diseases is required to determine whether the patient requires nail matrix injection or nail bed injection or both.
- Approaches for nail bed injections are enumerated in Box 32.3.[7,8]
- More recent publications prefer a higher concentration of triamcinolone acetonide (10 mg/mL), 0.1 mL administered in each of the four periungual sites, ensuring symmetrical delivery of the steroid to the nail matrix and nail bed, and administered less frequently, such as every 2 months.[7,9]

BOX 32.3: Different approaches for nail bed injections

1. Direct penetration of the nail plate
2. Injection via hyponychium
3. Injection via the lateral nail fold, directing the needle medially towards the nail bed
4. More recently, a new approach via proximal nail fold, with needle directed medially and distally to enter the nail bed via nail matrix[8]

Postoperative instructions

- Patient is advised to clean the treated digits twice daily with povidone-iodine lotion.
- Analgesics with serratio peptidase may be given for 3–5 days if required.
- Regular moisturization of the nail unit.

Complications

Injection therapies in nails, whether nail bed or intramatricial injection, are relatively safe procedures, especially when done in expert hands, and complications are rare. However, sometimes a few side effects can occur, which are as follows:

- Post-injection numbness in fingers
- Pain, severe and persistent, with injection cyclosporine
- Subungual hematoma (Figure 32.5)

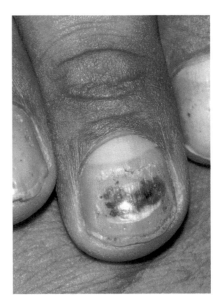

Figure 32.5 Subungual hematoma after intramatricial triamcinolone acetonide. (Courtesy of Piyush Kumar.)

- Paronychia
- Onychomadesis
- Nail splitting
- Distortion of nail plate, rarely
- Atrophy, depigmentation, secondary infection, inclusion cysts, subungual hemorrhage, and tendon rupture[7]
- Nicolau syndrome – sudden onset of severe painful local necrosis at the site of injection[10]

Results

These injection therapies have been found to be most effective in reversing nail abnormalities due to matrix disease, namely, pitting, ridging, and leukonychia. Nail bed disease including subungual hyperkeratosis, distal onycholysis, and oil drop changes have been found to respond less favorably.[11,12,14] A further report by Abell and Samman revealed that dystrophies involving nail matrix improved markedly, but onycholysis was frequently unaffected.[13,14] This can be overcome by simultaneous injection of drug into nail bed as described earlier.

CLINICAL USAGE

Nail psoriasis

NAPSI score is used at baseline and during treatment period to assess the treatment response in nail psoriasis. Details of NAPSI scores are given in chapter on nail psoriasis (Chapter 13).

Different treatment modalities (topical, systemic and injection therapy) for nail psoriasis have been summarized in Table 32.1. The evidence for safety and efficacy of different injectable treatments for nail psoriasis has been summarized in Table 32.2.

Based on our experience, injection triamcinolone acetonide (Figure 32.6) showed 100% improvement in 8 nails out of 30 at 24 weeks. On the other hand, intramatricial injection of methotrexate (Figure 32.7) and cyclosporine showed 100% improvement in 9 out of 30 and 4 nails out of 30, respectively, at 24 weeks. A total of two injections were given 6 weeks apart in all 3 groups. Thus, based on our experience, injection therapy with methotrexate is the most accepted drug by the patient, showing a minimum number of side effects and maximum number of nails having improvement.[25]

Table 32.1 Treatment modalities for nail psoriasis

Therapies for nail psoriasis						
Author	Year	N	Intervention	Comparison	Protocol	Results	LoE
Rigopoulos et al.[15]	2007	46	0.1% tazarotene cream	0.05% clobetasol propionate	Once daily under occlusion for 3 months	Similar efficacy in both the groups	A2
Tzung et al.[16]	2008	40	0.005% calcipotriol + 0.05% betamethasone dipropionate	0.005% calcipotriol	Calcipotriol twice daily and calcipotriol + betamethasone once daily for 3 months	Similar efficacy in both groups, significant reduction in NAPSI scores	B
Nakamura et al.[17]	2012	15	Clobetasol propionate at concentrations 0.05%, 1%, and 8%	Placebo	Twice weekly for 3 months	5% improvement in treatment group	N/A
Tosti et al.[18]	2009	36	Acitretin	—	0.2–0.3 mg/kg/day, for 6 months	41% reduction in NAPSI scores	N/A
Sanchez-Regana et al.[19]	2011	84	Classical treatment	Biological treatment	Classical: MTX, CsA, PUVA, NUVB, REPUVA Biological: Infliximab, etanercept, adalimumab. Up to 8 months	Significant reduction in NAPSI scores with all except NBUVB	N/A
Van den Bosch et al.[20]	2010	259	Adalimumab	—	40 mg, sc, at every other week through week 12	Mean NAPSI scores are reduced by 44% at week 12.	N/A

(Continued)

Table 32.1 (*Continued*) Treatment modalities for nail psoriasis

Therapies for nail psoriasis							
Author	Year	N	Intervention	Comparison	Protocol	Results	LoE
Fabroni et al.[21]	2011	48	Infliximab	—	5 mg/kg infusion at weeks 0, 2, 6, and every 8 weeks through week 38	NAPSI-50 is achieved in 85% of patients at week 14, 96% at week 22, 98% at week 38; NAPSI-75 is achieved in 23% of patients at week 14, 65% at week 22, 81% at week 38; NAPSI-90 is achieved in 29% of patients at week 38.	N/A
Ortonne et al.[22]	2012	69	Etanercept	Etanercept	First group 50 mg weekly for 24 weeks and second group 50 mg twice weekly for the first 12 weeks, 50 mg weekly for the other 12 weeks, sc	Both dose regimens are effective for nail psoriasis and significant improvement in NAPSI scores in both groups at week 24.	N/A
Berker et al.[7]	1997	19	Triamcinolone acetonide	—	0.4 mL, 10 mg/mL, with 0.1 mL injected into four periungual sites	20% of digits were cured of pitting, thickening cleared in 67% of cases, and subungual hyperkeratosis resolved partially in 75% of digits.	—
Saricaoglu et al.[23]	2011	1	Methotrexate	—	2.5 mg injected into proximal nail fold on each side of nail, repeated once a week for 6 weeks	Subungual hyperkeratosis and pitting improved.	Case report-based
Daulatabad et al.[9]	2017	Four (30 psoriatic nails)	Methotrexate	—	0.1 mL of 25 mg/mL into nail bed	Mean NAPSI of nails with nail bed changes declined from 4.19 to 2.56 and nails with both nail bed and nail matrix changes declined from 5.0 to 3.14.	Case series-based

MTX: Methotrexate, CsA: Cyclosporine, PUVA: Psoralen with UVA, NBUVB: Narrow-band UVB, REPUVA: Etretinate with PUVA, TA: Triamcinolone acetonide.

Table 32.2 Injection therapy for nail psoriasis

Parameter studied	Gerstein[24] (1962)	Abell[14] (1972)	Bleeker[11] (1972)	Peachey[12] (1976)	De Berker and Lawrence[7] (1998)	Author's experience[25]
Technique used	Needle	Port-o-jet	Port-o-jet	Port-o-jet	Needle	Needle
Drug used	TA	TA	TA	TA	TA	TA: 10 mg/mL
Strength	10 mg/mL	5 mg/mL	5 mg/mL	5 mg/mL	10 mg/mL	MTX: 25 mg/mL
						CsA: 50 mg/mL
Site of injection	Matrix	PNF	PNF	PNF	Matrix and bed	Matrix
No. of patients	4	58	400	28	19	18
No. of nails	17	N/A	569	28	46	90
Follow up period (months)	14	Up to 24	5–20	1	9	6

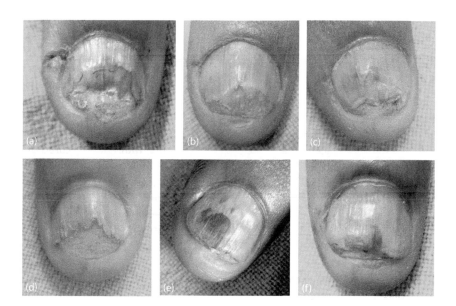

Figure 32.6 (a) Intramatrix Triamcinolone acetonide 10 mg/mL (0 weeks) and (b) response on follow up at weeks 6, (c) 12, (d) 16, (e) 20 (f) and 24.

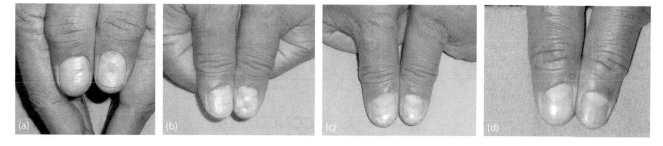

Figure 32.7 (a) Nails treated with intramatricial methotrexate (0 weeks) (b) and follow-up at weeks 12, (c) 16, and (d) 20.

Table 32.3 Injection therapy for the treatment of various nail dystrophies

Author	Year	N	Intervention	Comparison	Protocol	Results	Comment
Abell et al.[14]	1973	100 (693 nails)	Triamcinolone acetonide	—	5 mg/mL TA Port-o-jet injection on three occasions at 2–4 weekly interval	19 out of 24 patients of psoriasis with matrix involvement improved greatly. 3 out of 14 patients with onycholysis improved markedly. 7 out of 11 patients of lichen planus improved greatly. 3 of 4 patients of alopecia fully resolved. 3 out of 15 patients of idiopathic onycholysis improved.	—
Berker et al.[7]	1997	19	Triamcinolone acetonide	—	0.4 mL, 10 mg/mL, with 0.1 mL injected into four periungual sites	20% of digits were cured of pitting, thickening cleared in 67% cases and subungual hyperkeratosis resolved partially in 75% digits.	—
Khoo BP, Giam YC[26]	2000	Four patients of lichen planus	Triamcinolone acetonide	—	2.5–10 mg/mL	Pitting decreased to mean of 15% in second month and 42% in fourth month.	Case series
Brauns B et al.[27]	2011	One patient of lichen planus	Triamcinolone acetonide	—	10 mg/mL	Complete recovery 4 months after injection	Case report
Grover C[28]	2015	2	Triamcinolone acetonide	—	5 mg/mL into proximal nail fold at 4-weekly interval	Nails improved after 16 weeks of intramatricial therapy.	Case report

Nail dystrophy

Dystrophic nails caused by various diseases can be treated by injection therapy. The evidence for the same has been summarized in Table 32.3.

CONCLUSION

The nail plate is a big hurdle to the absorption of topical medicines, thereby limiting the utility of topical medications. With injection therapy, one can deposit the drug where it is needed, thereby obviating the need for systemic therapy. Hence, injection therapy is particularly valuable in cases with isolated nail diseases. It has been proven to be a safe and effective treatment modality in the management of various nail disorders. Considering its low cost, fewer treatment visits, minimal adverse effects in skilled hands, and possibility of avoiding systemic drugs, injection therapy is a great option for the treatment of nail disorders.

KEY POINTS

- Injection therapy provides the opportunity of depositing drugs at the site of pathology.
- Understanding of the nail anatomy and correct assessment of the site of pathology are essential for successful treatment outcome.
- Various complications of injection therapy are avoided by proper patient selection and correct injection techniques.
- Nail psoriasis, nail lichen planus and nail dystrophies due to different inflammatory conditions are the most important indications for injection therapy.
- Triamcinolone acetonide and methotrexate are most commonly used drugs for injection therapy of inflammatory nail diseases. Cyclosporine and biologicals like etanercept are being evaluated.

REFERENCES

1. Dogra S, Yadav S. Psoriasis in India: Prevalence and pattern. *Indian J Dermatol Venereol Leprol* 2010;76:595–601.
2. Ghosal A, Gangopadhyay DN, Chanda M, Das NK. Study of nail changes in psoriasis. *Indian J Dermatol* 2004;49:18–21.
3. de Jong EM, Seegers BA, Gulinck MK, Boezeman JB, van de Kerkhof PC. Psoriasis of the nails associated with disability in a large number of patients: Results of a recent interview with 1,728 patients. *Dermatology* 1996;193:300–303.
4. Richert B, Lorizzi M, Tosti A, Andre J. Nail bed lichen planus associated with Onychopapilloma. *Br J Dermatol* 2007;156:1071–1072.
5. Burns MK, Ellis CN, Eisen D, Duell E, Griffiths CE, Annesley TM et al. Intralesional cyclosporine for psoriasis. Relationship of dose, tissue levels, and efficacy. *Arch Dermatol* 1992;128:786–790.
6. Bliddal H, Terslev L, Qvistgaard E, vd Recke P, Holm CC, Danneskiold-Samsoe B, Savnik A, Torp-Pedersen S. Safety of intra-articular injection of etanercept in small joint arthritis: An uncontrolled, pilot study with independent imaging assessment. *Joint Bone Spine* 2006;73:714–717.
7. de Berker DA, Lawrence CM. A simplified protocol of steroid injection for psoriatic nail dystrophy. *Br J Dermatol* 1998;138(1):90–95.
8. Daulatabad D, Grover C, Singal A. Role of nail bed methotrexate injections in isolated nail psoriasis: Conventional drug via an unconventional route. *Clin Exp Dermatol* 2017. doi:10.1111/ced.13087.
9. Saleem K, Azim W. Treatment of nail psoriasis with a modified regimen of steroid injections. *J Coll Physicians Surg Pak* 2008;18(2):78–81.
10. Grover C, Kharghoria G, Daulatabad D, Bhattacharya SN. Nicolau syndrome following intramatricial triamcinolone injection for nail lichen planus. *Indian Dermatol Online J* 2017;8:350–351.
11. Bleeker JJ. Intradermal triamcinolone acetonide treatment of psoriatic nail dystrophy with port-o-jet. *Br J Dermatol* 1975;92:479–489.
12. Peachey RDG, Pye RJ, Harman RRM. The treatment of psoriatic nail dystrophy with intradermal steroid injections. *Br J Dermatol* 1976;95:75–78.
13. Bedi TR. Intradermal triamcinolone treatment of psoriatic onychodystrophy. *Dermatologica* 1977;155:24–27.
14. Abell E, Samman PD. Intradermal triamcinolone acetonide treatment of nail dystrophies. *Br J Dermatol* 1973;89:191–197.
15. Rigopoulos D, Gregoriou S, Katsambas A. Treatment of psoriatic nails with tazarotene cream 0.1% vs. clobetasol propionate 0.05% cream: A double-blind study. *Acta Derm Venereol* 2007;87(2):167–168.
16. Tzung TY, Chen CY, Yang CY, Lo PY, Chen YH. Calcipotriol used as monotherapy or combination therapy with betamethasone dipropionate in the treatment of nail psoriasis. *Acta Derm Venereol* 2008;88(3):279–280.
17. Nakamura RC, Abreu LD, Duque-Estrada B, Tamler C, Leverone AP. Comparison of nail lacquer clobetasol efficacy at 0.05%, 1% and 8% in nail psoriasis treatment: Prospective, controlled and randomized pilot study. *An Bras Dermatol* 2012;87(2):203–211.
18. Tosti A, Ricotti C, Romanelli P, Cameli N, Piraccini BM. Evaluation of the efficacy of acitretin therapy for nail psoriasis. *Arch Dermatol* 2009;145(3):269–271.
19. Sánchez-Regaña M, Sola-Ortigosa J, Alsina-Gibert M, Vidal-Fernández M, Umbert-Millet P. Nail psoriasis: A retrospective study on the effectiveness of systemic treatments (classical and biological therapy). *J Eur Acad Dermatol Venereol* 2011;25(5):579–586.

20. Van den Bosch F, Manger B, Goupille P, McHugh N, Rødevand E, Holck P et al. Effectiveness of adalimumab in treating patients with active psoriatic arthritis and predictors of good clinical responses for arthritis, skin and nail lesions. *Ann Rheum Dis* 2010;69(2):394–399.

21. Fabroni C, Gori A, Troiano M, Prignano F, Lotti T. Infliximab efficacy in nail psoriasis. A retrospective study in 48 patients. *J Eur Acad Dermatol Venereol* 2011;25(5):549–553.

22. Ortonne JP, Paul C, Berardesca E, Marino V, Gallo G, Brault Y, Germain JM. A 24-week randomized clinical trial investigating the efficacy and safety of two doses of etanercept in nail psoriasis. *Br J Dermatol* 2013;168(5):1080–1087.

23. Saricaoglu H, Oz A, Turan H. Nail psoriasis successfully treated with intralesional methotrexate: Case report. *Dermatology* 2011;222:5–7.

24. Gerstein W. Psoriasis and lichen planus of the nails. *Arch Dermatol* 1962;86:419–421.

25. Mittal J, Mahajan BB. Intramatricial injections for nail psoriasis: An open-label comparative study of triamcinolone, methotrexate, and cyclosporine. *Indian J Dermatol Venereol Leprol* 2018;84:419–423.

26. Khoo BP, Giam YC. A pilot study on the role of intralesional triamcinolone acetonide in treatment of pitted nails in children. *Singapore Med J* 2000;41:66–68.

27. Brauns B, Stahl M, Schon MP, Zutt M. Intralesional steroid injection alleviates nail lichen planus. *Int J Dermatol* 2011;50(5):626–627.

28. Grover C, Vohra S. Onychomadesis with lichen planus: An under-recognised Manifestation. *Indian J Dermatol* 2015;60(4):420.

Surgery of benign nail tumors

ECKART HANEKE

There is a great number of benign tumors of the nail unit (see chapter on benign nail tumors) that require surgery for their treatment.[1] They will not be dealt with here individually as the principle of surgery of many tumors is fundamentally similar: try to completely remove the lesion without interfering with the anatomy, function, and cosmesis of the nail apparatus as much as possible. It is also beyond the scope of this chapter to mention all approaches ever described to treat a particular benign nail tumor.

Different surgical methods are available and should be adapted to the type of nail tumor, its size, signs, and symptoms as well as its functional and esthetic consequences.[2-4] Further, the preoperative diagnostic certainty is important as surgery of a malignant neoplasm should be different from the beginning. Whether or not a prior diagnostic biopsy is necessary has to be evaluated in each case. The most common surgical excision techniques for benign nail tumors are curettage, punch excisions for very small lesions, scalpel excision for all sizes, and horizontal excision ("shave") for superficial ones with special excision techniques for some tumors and Mohs surgery being reserved mainly for malignant neoplasms. Sometimes, a tumor reduction technique or serial excision may be considered if the lesion is very big, but slowly growing and it has no tendency to degenerate to a malignant neoplasm.

CURETTAGE

Curettage is not a favorite surgical technique for nail tumors, whether benign or malignant. Two types of curettes are available: the sharp spoon and the ring scalpel. The former is sometimes used to reduce the wart load in peri- and subungual *verrucae*, rarely as a treatment of its own. It has to be considered that DNA of human papillomavirus may be found 15 mm around the visible wart and that surgical removal of viral warts would require a "safety margin" of more than 15 mm all around the warts, leaving a defect larger than for a nail apparatus melanoma. Further, warts are said to have a natural life span of 2 years and a maximum life span of 5 years and are benign infectious lesions. After curettage, a conservative treatment with necrotizing agents or topical immunotherapy, such as imiquimod or sensitization with diphencyprone, has to follow. In case of patients older than 30 years, the differential diagnosis is Bowen disease and therefore a histopathological examination of the curettage material is essential!

Pyogenic granuloma may be seen around the nail or even penetrating the nail plate. They may be curetted and, in case of a pulsating feeder artery, this is gently cauterized with ferrichloride, aluminum chloride or by cautious electrocautery. The exuberant lesion is sent for histopathology.

LASER THERAPY

Laser treatment of benign tumors can be done in different ways; however, it has to be kept in mind that they are blind methods not permitting the diagnosis to be made and margins of laser treatment to be determined.

The *carbon dioxide* laser (Figure 33.1a–e) is probably the most widely used laser for tumor treatment. It allows all tissues including the overlying nail plate to be vaporized or carbonized and to be cut out more or less bloodlessly. As it has a heat damage of 40 μ after several passes or shots, the wound margin is black, not allowing it to be evaluated. Further, the laser plume contains hazardous material including intact virus particles. The carbon dioxide laser allows warts to be vaporized.[5] The erbium-YAG laser is also ablating[6] but with a very thin layer of tissue removed with each pass and with no blood coagulation.

The tunable pulsed dye laser was used to more or less selectively coagulate the blood capillaries of viral warts.[7]

The recommended fluence is 9–9.5 J/cm^2. The success rate varies from zero to 80%.[8]

The neodymium-YAG laser can be used to achieve hyperthermia (10W, 8 mm spot size, continuous wave up to 20 seconds)[9] or destroy the warts (spot size 5 mm, fluence 150–185 J/cm^2, pulse duration 15 msec).[10]

Ingrown nails have been treated with the CO$_2$ laser (this author deems chemocautery of the matrix horn easier, less expensive, and more effective with a higher cure rate). The lateral nail strip is avulsed and the matrix horn vaporized with the laser.[11] Staining of the matrix with methylene blue avoids leaving matrix rests behind and reduces the risk of recurrence.[12] Some authors use lasers of different kinds to reduce or ablate the granulation tissue.

ELECTROSURGERY

Electrosurgery is a method that generates heat. It can be used to "boil" and carbonize as well as cut out tissue. The collateral damage due to heat convection is considerable

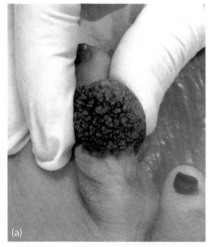
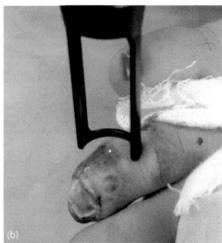
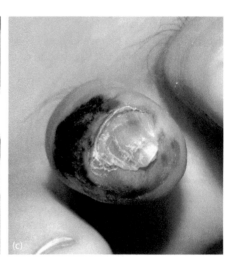
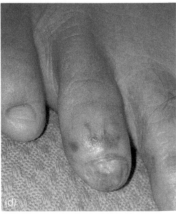
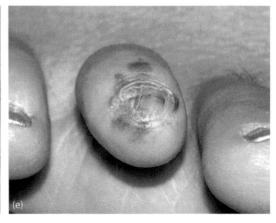

Figure 33.1 **(a)** Congenital melanocytic nevus affecting the distal part of right fourth toe in a circumferential manner; **(b)** Carbon dioxide laser followed by manual dermabrasion was done; **(c)** Follow up photograph after 1 month; **(d)** Follow up clinical photograph after two sessions of carbon dioxide laser and manual dermabrasion, followed by two sessions of q-switched Nd:YAG laser; **(e)** Final follow up photograph. (Courtesy of Dr Sushil S. Savant.)

and it is therefore not recommended for nail surgery. Matrix electrocoagulation may cause thermal (peri) ostitis. Keloids have been observed after its use.

RADIOSURGERY

Radiosurgery is similar to electrosurgery in principle, but due to its higher frequency heat development is much less. Its indications are very similar if not identical to those of a CO_2 laser.

CRYOSURGERY

Cold is another blind method used for a variety of lesions. However, it is difficult to confine it to a specific small region, and peritherapeutic damage may be deleterious to nail growth.[13]

Cryosurgery is still used for wart treatment in many clinics, but post-cryo nail dystrophy is not rare, particularly when warts on the proximal nail fold are frozen so deep that the matrix was also reached. Cryosurgery has also been used for myxoid pseudocysts. In expert hands, it has shown good results.[14,15]

Some authors use cryosurgery for the treatment of ingrown nails, either to reduce the granulation tissue or to freeze the matrix. The results are variable and range from failure to over 75% cure. Pain is considerable.[16,17]

A mallet finger, which is due to the disruption of the extensor tendon insertion, was seen twice after cryotherapy of warts on the dorsal aspect of the distal phalanx.[18]

PUNCH EXCISION

Punches for the nail apparatus should not be too large. The maximum acceptable size of the punch is 4 mm and 3 mm for nail bed and nail matrix respectively. In our experience, punches are not the ideal tools for tumor removal as even small ones are rarely perfectly round. Their main indications are diagnostic biopsies. The round defect of a punch excision is usually not sutured in the nail bed as this is so firmly attached to the bone that only sharp dissection from the phalanx allows the defect diameter to be reduced by a maximum of 50%. In the matrix, a punch defect of 3 mm is said to leave no postoperative nail dystrophy although a reddish streak and slightly thinner nail plate may result. If a suture is tried the matrix connective tissue is dissected from the underlying bone with sharp pointed curved iris scissors and sutured with 6–0 absorbable stitches in a transverse manner. A so-called double stitch distributes the tension on the matrix and prevents cutting of the suture through the fragile matrix. Even if a complete wound closure cannot be achieved it must not be forced as wound margin necrosis is worse than a narrow surgical defect.

TANGENTIAL EXCISION

This technique, colloquially called shave excision, was developed in order to prevent post-biopsy nail dystrophies in case of diagnostic interventions for matrix melanocytic foci. It proved to be applicable for all superficial lesions of both the matrix and nail bed. It is ideal for the removal of melanocyte foci of *functional melanonychia*, *matrix lentigines* and *nevi*, *onychocytic matricomas*, *onychopapillomas*, *subungual filamentous tumors*, and other superficial matrix and nail bed lesions. A more saucer-like excision is often adequate in case of *onychomatricoma*.

Depending on the exact localization of the subungual lesion, the overlying nail plate is partially separated and lifted from the matrix and nail bed to expose them; in case of a matrix lesion, the proximal nail fold has also to be reclined. It is important to permit sufficient perilesional matrix and nail bed to be seen in order to allow the horizontal excision without difficulty. A shallow perilesional incision is made around the lesion and the scalpel is laid on the neighboring matrix or nail bed and pressed flat on it. Then, the lesion is tangentially removed with sawing back-and-forth movements. While doing this, the scalpel blade is seen shining through the thin tissue slice. When fully excised the tissue is laid on filter paper, gently flattened and transferred to the jar with 4% neutral buffered formalin. The shallow defect is covered with the nail plate again as this is the best physiologic dressing and facilitates wound healing, which takes place within a few days. Whether or not the plate is fixed with stitches or sutures strips is a matter of personal preference. The nail plate cannot reattach, which has to be explained to the patient. After removal of the stitches, it can be left on and fixed with instant glue or tape and may be cut some more weeks later. Healing is usually without postoperative nail dystrophy.[19–21]

Concerning tangential excisions in curved and deep matrix areas, horizontal excisions can be difficult with common scalpels as the matrix is soft and may give in when the scalpel tries to cut; an ophthalmic or microblade may be beneficial in such an instance.

SCALPEL EXCISION OF GLOMUS TUMORS

Scalpel excisions are possible for virtually all nail neoplasms. In the surgery of benign tumors, they should follow certain rules: Nail bed lesions are excised with a longitudinal axis, matrix tumors with a transverse axis. Laterally located lesions may be excised as a lateral longitudinal nail biopsy in which the proximal nail fold may be spared in case the apical matrix is not involved.

Glomus tumors are very characteristic for the nail unit. They present as small violaceous spots under the nail plate in the matrix or, less frequently, nail bed from which a reddish band may extend to the hyponychium. The symptomatology of intense pain upon slightest trauma and cold, often radiating to the shoulder, disappearance of the pain when an arm tourniquet is inflated to about 300 mm Hg, and maximum pain over the center of the area of origin upon probing allow the diagnosis to be made. Ultrasonography, arteriography, and particularly magnetic resonance imaging are useful adjuncts, but their relatively low resolution requires at least a 2 mm diameter of the glomus tumor to be seen. A very small glomus tumor visible before surgery and localizable by probing may virtually disappear after anesthesia and placing a tourniquet. In such a case, temporary opening of the tourniquet helps to re-localize the glomus tumor. The method of extirpation depends on its exact localization: centrally located glomus tumors require separation of the overlying nail plate with an incision of the nail bed or matrix whereas those in the lateral third may be approached from the lateral aspect of the distal phalanx.

Glomus tumor in central localization of the nail bed and matrix

The nail plate is gently separated from the nail bed and/or matrix exposing at least 5–8 mm more of the underlying structure. In most cases, the glomus tumor is now visible as a violaceous spot of 3–8 mm diameter. When it is localized in the matrix, a gently curved superficial incision parallel to the lunula border is made that often already allows the glassy greyish tumor to be seen. Using very fine iris scissors it is freed from the surrounding, relatively soft matrix connective tissue leaving it otherwise intact. When it is completely dissected it presents as a round grey lesion of the size of a peppercorn to a pea or rarely larger.[22] The matrix is then sutured with 6–0 or 7–0 absorbable stitches (Figure 33.2a–f). In case of a nail bed glomus tumor, the incision over it is made in a longitudinal fashion. As the nail bed dermis is much firmer than that of the matrix the incision is begun very superficially, spread with fine scissors, and deepened until the glomus tumor becomes visible. Most nail bed glomus tumors are smaller than matrix ones and may not so easily be seen as a round lesion; also, they may appear violaceous red or grey. They are usually discernable as the nail bed dermis is whiter than that of the matrix. Again, the lesion is dissected from the dermis and the incision sutured with 6–0 absorbable material. None of our glomus tumors required excision of the overlying matrix or nail bed epithelium. Finally, the elevated portion of the nail plate is laid back and sutured to the nail apparatus. Healing is fast and uneventful. The pain disappears within a few days. A normal nail regrows without postoperative dystrophy.

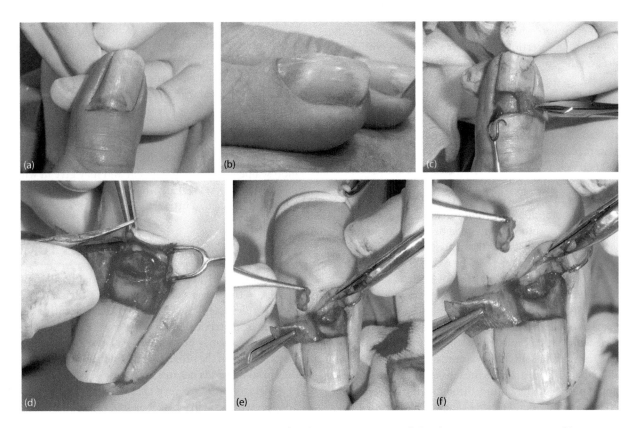

Figure 33.2 (a and b) Clinical image of glomus tumor of nail matrix area; (c and d) Glomus tumor is exposed by retracting proximal nail folds, and lateral nail plate curl. Glomus tumor is visible as bluish lesion; (e and f) Glomus tumor is gently dissected out from the surrounding tissue.

Glomus tumor in lateral position

The lateral approach is adequate for laterally localized lesions. An incision is made about 4 mm below the level of the nail plate in the lateral aspect of the distal phalanx to get under the matrix and nail bed to the level between the dermis and the periosteum (the term "subperiosteal approach"[23] is wrong as the glomus tumor is never under the periosteum!). By gently lifting the upper wound margin, the glomus tumor will become visible as a greyish glassy nodule against the more whitish nail bed-matrix dermis and can be dissected. Skin sutures terminate this operation. This surgery was called "nail-preserving" as comparing it with the excision of the overlying matrix and nail bed epithelium, which is virtually never necessary but leaves defects with subsequent nail dystrophy, gave better esthetic results; its recurrence rate was, however, 15%. We have never encountered a glomus tumor requiring Mohs surgery.[24,25]

Subungual lipoma

Subungual lipoma is a rare event. It grows slowly and insidiously usually causing an atypical nail overcurvature. As they are mainly located in the distal matrix and nail bed a longitudinal nail bed incision is made. Normally, the nail bed has no adipose tissue and the lipoma therefore stands out, but may resemble a subungual cyst in the beginning of the dissection. It then leaves a relatively large "empty space," which, however, does not require any particular closing technique. The nail plate is unbent, trimmed to the size of the nail field, and sutured to the now flat nail bed. Healing is uneventful with a normal nail again.

Oncholemmal horn

Oncholemmal horn, proliferating oncholemmal tumor, and *proliferating oncholemmal cyst* are only diagnosed by histopathology after their excision as their clinical aspect is non-specific. The surgical technique depends on the size and suspected diagnosis, whether benign or malignant, and defect closure has to be adapted to each particular case.

Cysts

Cysts are heterogeneous. Multiple small *oncholemmal cysts* are usually a chance observation in larger surgical specimens or may clinically mimic onychopapilloma and are then removed with a horizontal excision from the nail bed. The bigger cysts are either post-surgical or post-traumatic *epidermal* or *hybrid epidermal-matrix cysts*, rarely pure *matrix* cysts.[26] When the diagnosis is made before the surgery, the overlying tissue is cautiously incised until the cyst wall is visible and then bluntly dissected. However, most post-surgical cysts are the result of insufficient ingrown nail surgery and are deeply buried in the lateral region of the base of the distal phalanx, often in chronic granulomatous and scar tissue. They may require opening of the overlying skin and sharp dissection, sometimes followed by curettage of remaining cyst and keratin granuloma tissue. Wound closure depends on the size of the wound and whether there is an infection or not. Antibiotic prophylaxis may be necessary.

Myxoid pseudocysts

Myxoid pseudocysts are the most common pseudotumors of the nail apparatus. Histopathology shows a circumscribed mucinosis that turns into a lake of mucin when the lesion matures.[1] Most occur in the proximal nail fold and cause a longitudinal canaliform depression in the nail due to pressure on the matrix (type A myxoid pseudocyst). When the cystic lesion ruptures into the nail pocket and the pressure is released an irregular depression results (type B). Subungual localization causes a hemi-overcurvature of the nail and a violaceous color of the matrix, which is positive for transillumination (type C). Up to 80% of the lesions develop a connection with the distal interphalangeal joint, which can be made visible by intraarticular injection of 0.05–0.1 mL of sterile 1% methylene blue into the distal joint. In case this was successful and there is a connecting stalk, the lesions stain bluish. Simple excision and suture has a very high recurrence rate. We therefore prefer to dissect the entire myxoid tissue. The skin over the cyst is raised like a U-shaped flap or the entire lesion is excised with the overlying skin and a U-shaped transposition flap is raised from the adjacent skin. If present the stalk opening is seen as a dark blue spot and ligated like a bleeding artery. The flap is laid back or transposed into the primary defect and stitched with 6–0 suture material.[27] In case of a subungual myxoid pseudocyst, the proximal nail fold is incised at the junction to the lateral fold and separated from the nail, the overlying nail plate is cut transversely from one side in the middle of the nail, and the proximal half is gently separated to expose the pseudocyst. An arched incision is made to dissect the pseudocyst. As there is no real fibrous capsule, the lesion often ruptures during dissection and the remaining myxoid tissue has to be removed. The matrix is stitched with 6–0 absorbable sutures, the nail laid back and fixed with a stitch, and finally the nail fold is sutured again. A thick padded dressing terminates the surgery. No finger splinting is necessary. The dressing is changed after 48 hours. Healing is uneventful and a normal nail without depression regrows. Postoperative finger stiffness is very rare.

It has to be noted that there are many other ways to treat these lesions: injection of corticosteroid crystal suspension or sclerosant agent, cryosurgery, infrared and laser coagulation, vaporization, etc. They may be useful for multiple myxoid pseudocysts.

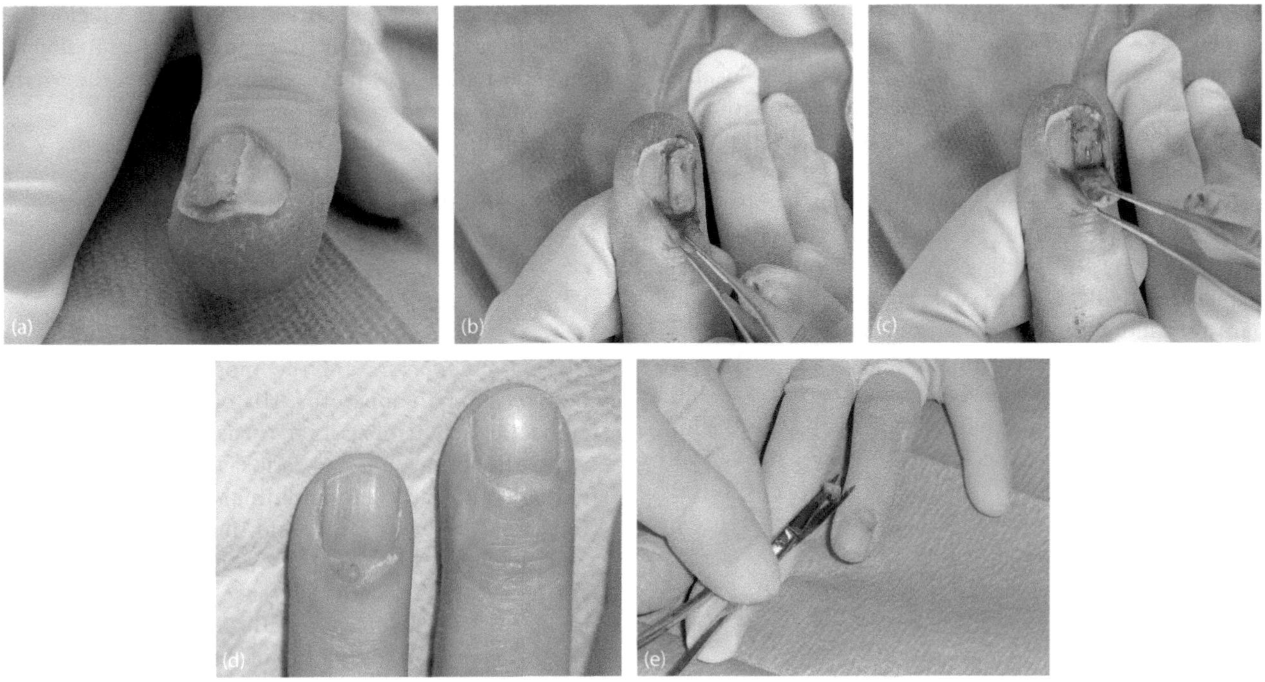

Figure 33.3 Ungual fibrokeratoma (a) is not firmly attached to underlying nail plate and can be easily removed (b and c). Acquired fibrokeratoma too behaves in similar manner (d and e).

Ungual fibrokeratomas

Ungual fibrokeratomas occur in association with the tuberous sclerosis complex as multiple lesions or sporadically. The latter are usually longer and slenderer, whereas the former occur as multiple Koenen tumors in many to all digits. Depending on their specific localization within the nail organ, their clinical appearance is different. On the nail fold, they look like a garlic clove. Those arising in the depth of the nail pocket under the nail fold are long and slender, have a hyperkeratotic, often dark tip and cause a narrow deep longitudinal canal. Fibrokeratomas originating from the mid-matrix grow in the nail plate until the overlying lamella breaks off and the tip of the lesion is visible. Nail bed fibrokeratomas cause a rim. None of these fibrokeratomas are firmly attached to the nail plate, and they can be lifted up from it. The treatment is similar for the matrix-derived tumors: a pointed scalpel blade is held parallel to the tumor and nail and gently advanced to the bone while cutting around its base. Using pointed curved iris scissors, the base is dissected from the bone (Figure 33.3a–e). No suture is necessary. Nail bed lesions require prior elevation of the nail plate.

In patients with tuberous sclerosis, the fibrokeratomas should be removed before the nail is severely damaged by the multitude of lesions. If the patient has already many Koenen tumors, they are cut at their base informing the patient that they will regrow.

MOHS MICROGRAPHIC SURGERY

Mohs surgery is not generally used for the treatment of benign tumors, and in the cases described in the literature it remains debatable whether Mohs surgery was really necessary in these particular cases.

Two publications deal with Mohs surgery for recurrent glomus tumors resulting from insufficient primary excision.[24,25] One group treated an onychomatricoma with Mohs surgery.[28]

Probably the only benign tumor indication for Mohs surgery is recurrent ungual *keratoacanthoma* (KA), although KA is held to be a particular type of squamous cell carcinoma in the USA. Nail KAs mainly occur in the lateral nail groove and hyponychium and on the proximal nail fold. They are characteristically painful and fast growing. Their hallmark is the central keratotic plug. In contrast to KAs on hairy skin, distal digital KAs do not show a tendency to spontaneous involution. Surgery is by wide excision with adaptive sutures. In case of recurrence, Mohs surgery is indicated.[29] The tumor is excised with clear clinical margins and a three-dimensional histopathological margin control is performed. This is the method with the highest cure and lowest recurrence rate while saving most of the surrounding normal skin.

REFERENCES

1. Haneke E. *Histopathology of the Nail–Onychopathology.* CRC Press, Boca Raton, FL; 2017.
2. Haneke E, Baran R. Nail surgery. *Clin Dermatol* 1992;10:327–333.
3. Haneke E. Nail surgery. *Eur J Dermatol* 2000;10:237–241.
4. Haneke E. Nail surgery: Indications and outcome. *Expert Rev Dermatol* 2006;1:93–104.
5. Lim JT, Goh CL. Carbon dioxide laser treatment of periungual and subungual viral warts. *Australas J Dermatol* 1992;33:87–91.
6. Wollina U, Konrad H, Karamfilov T. Treatment of common warts and actinic keratoses by Er:YAG laser. *J Cutan Laser Ther* 2001;3:63–66.
7. Park HS, Choi WS. Pulsed dye laser treatment for viral warts: A study of 120 patients. *J Dermatol* 2008;35:491–498.
8. Huilgol SC, Barlow RJ, Markey AC. Failure of pulsed dye laser therapy for resistant verrucae. *Clin Exp Dermatol* 1996;21:93–95.
9. Pfau A, Abd-el-Raheem TA, Bäumler W, Hohenleutner U, Landthaler M. Nd:YAG laser hyperthermia in the treatment of recalcitrant verrucae vulgares (Regensburg's technique). *Acta Derm Venereol* 1994;74:212–214.
10. Kimura U, Takeuchi K, Kinoshita A, Takamori K, Suga Y. Long-pulsed 1064-nm neodymium: Yttrium-aluminum-garnet laser treatment for refractory warts on hands and feet. *J Dermatol* 2014;41:252–257.
11. André P. Ingrowing nails and carbon dioxide laser surgery. *J Eur Acad Dermatol Venereol* 2003;17:288–290.
12. Ozawa T, Nose K, Harada T, Muraoka M, Ishii M. Partial matricectomy with a CO_2 laser for ingrown toenail after nail matrix staining. *Dermatol Surg* 2005;31:302–305.
13. Caravati CM Jr, Wood BT, Richardson DR. Onychodystrophies secondary to liquid nitrogen cryotherapy. *Arch Dermatol* 1969;100:441–442.
14. Kuflik EG. Cryosurgical treatment of periungual warts. *J Dermatol Surg Oncol* 1984;10:673–676.
15. Kuflik EG. Specific indications for cryosurgery of the nail unit: Myxoid cyst and periungual verrucae. *J Dermatol Surg Oncol* 1992;18:702–706.
16. Masters N. Cryotherapy ineffective for ingrowing toenails. *Br J Gen Pract* 1991;41(351):433–434.
17. Küçüktaş M, Kutlubay Z, Yardimci G, Khatib R, Tüzün Y. Comparison of effectiveness of electrocautery and cryotherapy in partial matrixectomy after partial nail extraction in the treatment of ingrown nails. *Dermatol Surg* 2013;39:274–280.
18. Al-Qattan MM, Al-Arfaj N. Mallet finger as a complication of liquid nitrogen cryosurgery for verruca vulgaris. *J Hand Surg Eur Vol* 2009;34:546–548.
19. Haneke E. Diagnostische Biopsien am Nagelorgan. *Z Hautkr* 1999;74:493–494.
20. Haneke E. Advanced nail surgery. *J Cutan Aesthet Surg* 2011;4:167–175.
21. Haneke E. Anatomy of the nail unit and the nail biopsy. *Semin Cut Med Surg* 2015;34:95–100.
22. Duarte AF, Correia O, Barreiros H, Haneke E. Giant subungual glomus tumor: Clinical, dermoscopy, imagiologic and surgery details. *Dermatol Online J* 2016;22(10).
23. Garg B, Machhindra MV, Tiwari V, Shankar V, Kotwal P. Nail-preserving modified lateral subperiosteal approach for subungual glomus tumour: A novel surgical approach. *Musculoskelet Surg* 2016;100:43–48.
24. Tehrani H, Shah D, Sidhu S, May K, Morris A. Treatment of recurrent glomus tumor using Mohs surgery. *Dermatol Surg* 2012;38:502–503.
25. Chuang GS, Branch KD, Cook J. Intraosseous subungual glomus tumor: A cautionary tale. *J Am Acad Dermatol* 2012;67:e58–e60.
26. Chavaillaz O, Borradori L, Haneke E. Subungual epidermoid cyst: Report of a case with rapid growth and nail loss mimicking a malignant tumor. *J Clin Dermatol* 2010;1(2):73–75.
27. Haneke E. Operative Therapie der myxoiden Pseudozyste. In: Haneke E, Ed. *Gegenwärtiger Stand der operativen Dermatologie. Fortschritte der operativen Dermatologie* 4, Springer, Heidelberg, Germany; 1988: pp. 221–227.
28. Graves MS, Anderson JK, LeBlanc KG Jr, Sheehan DJ. Utilization of Mohs micrographic surgery in a patient with onychomatricoma. *Dermatol Surg* 2015;41:753–735.
29. Cecchi R, Troiano M, Buralli L, Innocenti S. Recurrent distal digital keratoacanthoma of the periungual region treated with Mohs micrographic surgery. *Australas J Dermatol* 2012;53:e5–e7.

Nail Cosmetics

34

Nail care and nail cosmetics

SONI NANDA AND SONAL BANSAL

INTRODUCTION

Nail has historically been an important tool in protecting terminal phalanx against injury, improving touch discrimination, and the ability to pick up small objects. Nail adornment by painting it in various colors has been practiced by ancient civilizations like Egypt and China. Lately, nail beautification has started including hardening the nails for increased firmness and longevity, thereby also providing a palette for different forms of nail arts. This kind of nail embellishment has always been an indicator of social status, even more so these days. The plethora of nail care products and cosmetics available in the market these days stand testimony to their increasing demand. With an increase in awareness and spending power of today's consumer, the desire for healthy skin and hair has now extended to the nails as well. With the advent of increasingly chemical-laden products and the complications associated with them,

the need for understanding the basics of the nail unit and its upkeep becomes important for a dermatologist to provide clear and accurate counsel to the patient.

CHARACTERISTICS OF AN ATTRACTIVE NAIL[1]

Attractive nails are considered to be good indicators of internal health as well as attention to personal hygiene and fashion trends. In general, healthy fingernails are longer than wide, whereas most toenails are wider than long. Essential features of a healthy and attractive nail have been described in Box 34.1.

Various cosmetic procedures are employed to enhance these characteristics, and they shall be discussed in detail in the chapter along with potential complications that can arise with their use.

NAIL CARE AND GROOMING

Dermatologists often come across discolored and damaged nails because of improper grooming techniques and exposure to irritants. An important component of treatment then constitutes educating the patients regarding personal hygiene and nail care. Pertinent points are as follows[2]:

1. Chemicals, soaps, and detergents exposure should be kept to a minimum.
2. Excessive wetting is counterproductive.
3. Avoid nail biting and skin picking.
4. Wear gloves as much as possible while doing gardening, household chores, and such.
5. Avoid cutting nails too short or pointed; they should always be cut parallel to the free edge of the nail plate.
6. Soaking before cutting nails decreases the mechanical stress.
7. Be wary of over-aggressive nail technicians; too much cuticle manipulation or over buffing can lead to irreversible nail plate changes.
8. Avoid sharing nail care instruments in a salon.
9. Be cautious with extra-long nails; they may easily result in substantial injury to the nail unit and its components.
10. Filing should be optimally performed in a single direction.

MANICURE AND PEDICURE

They are most popular grooming procedures for hands and feet.

Definition – Manicuring is a process by which fingernails are cleaned, shaped, and sometimes augmented by the application of a nail lacquer or other nail enhancement. The pedicure is analogous to the manicure, but involves toenails and the smoothening of the sole or filing of any calluses on the plantar surface of the foot.[3]

Steps of a manicure/pedicure and their implications[4]

1. Hands or feet are soaked in warm, soapy water to remove any debris from under the nails and to soften the nails and cuticles, which helps in easier clipping or filing. Filing with a disposable nail file is the preferred method as it reduces the chances of onychoschizia (Figure 34.1).
2. Existing nail paint, if any, is removed and the nails are then trimmed and filed to the ideal shape. The ideal nail possesses a central, delicate arc without any sharp corners, so as to create the illusion of a long, slender finger.[3] However, this can be a predisposing cause of hangnails, nail plate fractures, and ingrown nails.[5] So, preferably, nails should be shaped with a very slight curve with corners left untouched. The nail shape in vogue changes frequently and often square nails are the trend, which do not commonly cause ingrown nails.
3. A foot scraper or a pumice stone is used to buff the rough skin of palms and soles and any thick calluses are softened.
4. Cuticles are softened by either applying a chemical cuticle remover (alkaline substance like 0.4% sodium or potassium hydroxide) or soaking in warm water. Once soft and malleable, the cuticles are pushed proximally and/or clipped away with a metal or wood implement. This is the most damaging step in the whole procedure as it predisposes the nail folds to environmental insult and secondary infections. Use of unsterilized instruments can help transmit fungal and viral infections from one nail to another, and from one person to another. Pedicure tubs in which hands and feet are

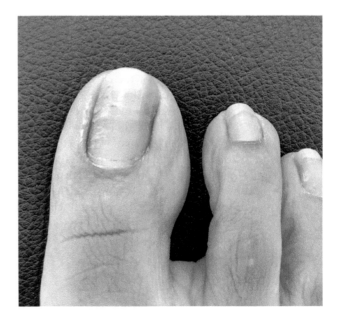

Figure 34.1 Onychoschizia due to incorrect and frequent pedicure techniques.

BOX 34.2: Recommended manicure/pedicure practices

Do's and don'ts of manicure/pedicure[7]:

1. Distal nail plate filing is preferred over clipping, because the latter can sometimes cause cracking and layering.
2. When clipping is necessary, the nails should first be softened by soaking, and the cutting implement should be held perpendicular to the nail plate to prevent onychoschizia.[8]
3. Many manicurists prefer to remove the cuticles as this step allows even application of nail lacquer and prevents nail lacquers, gels, and shellacs from chipping. As discussed above, cuticular manipulation should be strictly avoided. If client insists, it is recommended that just the distal end be removed and then gently rubbed with a washcloth daily.
4. Corner of nails should be left untouched to avoid ingrown nails and paronychia.
5. Over-aggressive buffing of the nail plate should be avoided.

BOX 34.3: Patient information on safe use of nail products and salons[5,9]

1. Use a licensed nail technician and licensed salon.
2. Wash hands before any nail salon services.
3. Look for cleanliness in the salon.
4. Ask about sanitization and sterilization in the salon.
5. Bring your own instruments, particularly files that cannot be sterilized.
6. Inform the staff immediately if you experience any itching or burning after a service; it could signal a reaction.
7. Allergy to nail polish can show up on the face, eyelids, and neck.
8. Keep nail extensions short.
9. Do not allow the technician to file the surface of the nail plate in preparation for extensions.
10. Do not over-buff the nails, which can weaken them.
11. Wear gloves for all wet work chores to protect the manicure and help prevent infections associated with artificial enhancements.
12. If you experience a nick or cut during a salon procedure, seek medical attention to avoid infections.

soaked have been reported to cause *Mycobacterium fortuitum* infections from a nail salon in California.[6]

5. Surface of the nail plate is then buffed to smooth any ridges and to improve adhesion of nail lacquer or other nail enhancement. Over-aggressive buffing can lead to thinning of the nail plate, which in turn can lead to frequent breakage and risk of infections.

Thus, an apparently simple and routine enhancement procedure has the potential to irreversibly destroy the cosmesis of the nail unit, or give rise to chronic infections with a long recovery period. Good manicure/pedicure practices have been summarized in Boxes 34.2 and 34.3.

NAIL POLISH AND NAIL POLISH REMOVERS

The science of nail polish and nail polish remover has been discussed in Chapter 35.

ARTIFICIAL NAILS

Artificial nails are very commonly used for both medical and cosmetic purposes. These are more durable than nail polish. Preformed nails are useful for breaking the habit of nail biting and also for lengthening/reinforcing soft, brittle, or damaged nails. These can be partially attached as nail tips or used to reinforce the entire length as sculpted nails (acrylic or gel based) (Figure 34.2).

Nail shellacs[4,5]

Shellac is the brand name for a new, patent-pending nail product created by Creative Nail Design (CND). It is a hybrid, meaning half nail polish, half gel. It can be a transparent or pigmented polymer of any color desired.

The product can be applied similarly to nail polish on natural nails (no sculpting or filing). It is applied in three layers with exposure to UV light to cause polymerization to occur. Advantages:

- Thin and strong product that gives it both flexibility and durability
- Natural look combined with the shine associated with gel nails
- Lasts up to 14 days

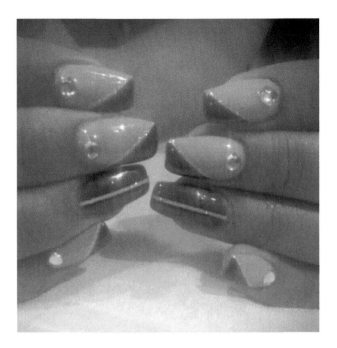

Figure 34.2 Nail adornments.

Disadvantages:

- Unlike other artificial nails, this cannot be used to lengthen nails.
- It is only sold to licensed professionals and requires a special removal process. So, no home corrections are possible.
- It requires a healthy nail bed for application.
- Removal technique uses acetone wraps, which may potentially dry and weaken the nail plate.
- It is possible that patients on photosensitizing oral medications, such as tetracycline or doxycycline, may experience photo-onycholysis when exposed to the UV radiation required to cure the polymer.

Nail tips/nail extensions[4,9]

Usually used to elongate nails, these are available at nail salons as ready-to-use plastic plates. They are available in a variety of styles: colored or uncolored, precut or uncut, press-on, pre-glued forms, and in forms requiring glue application. The nails also come in a variety of sizes and shapes to match the patient's natural nail plate. These are glued to the free edge of the nails after a rough filing with adhesives containing methacrylate or ethyl 2-cyanoacrylate. The glued-on tips may then be painted or decorated with nail art and finally coated with acrylic or gel. They can be removed with acetone.

Despite of wide variety of options available, people sometimes do not find a suitable preformed nail, accounting for the increasing popularity of custom-made nail prostheses.

Custom nail prostheses

Custom nail prostheses, also known as sculptured nails, are an increasingly popular method of obtaining long, hard nails. Sculptured nails can be *acrylic, gel, or nail wraps* (silk, linen, and fiberglass).

ACRYLIC NAILS[10]

Acrylic nails are a combination of a liquid monomer (ethyl methacrylate) and a powder polymer (poly-methacrylate). Hence, in common parlance, they are referred to as "liquid and powder" nails. The powder contains benzoyl peroxide, which acts as a catalyst, while hydroquinone acts as an inhibitor of polymerization. Individual brands may add titanium dioxide and permitted colors. A uniform thin layer is applied quickly as it hardens on air exposure. Acrylic is transparent after setting and provides a robust canvas for further nail adornment. They last long and can be removed easily. Small breaks or fractures can almost always be corrected at home. But they require more care than natural fingernails. They need filing every 2–3 weeks where the loose acrylic is clipped from the nail edges and new acrylic applied proximally. Otherwise, a lever arm gets created that predisposes the natural nail plate to traumatic onycholysis. They are losing popularity because they look less natural, especially if applied incorrectly. The application involves strong chemicals and fumes, which inhibit its use in pregnancy. They also have a real potential to damage the nail bed after 2–4 months of continued use. The natural nail plate may become yellowed, dry, and thin. It is highly recommended that the patient's natural nail be allowed to grow and act as a support by **resting them every 3 months**.

NAIL WRAPS[11]

Developed in the early 1980s, these wraps are thin products made from paper, silk, linen, fiberglass, mesh, or other fabrics applied to the nail for extra reinforcement. They can be embedded within acrylics and gels or used as a natural nail coating or extension and sealed with resin.

They cannot be used to lengthen the nails, so an ideal candidate would be someone who is looking to keep their short nails strong. These are also a possible alternative for those who are allergic to chemicals used in the acrylic or gel process. Another common use of these in the Western world is for "transitioners" or clients who are giving up acrylics and want to grow out their nails. These people have weaker nails and are subjected to a higher chance of breakage along the road to recovery, so nail wraps are a good way to keep these nails stronger.

GEL NAILS[4,5,9]

Introduced in the nail industry sometime in 1980s, they are currently the most popular type of sculptured nails (Figure 34.3).

There are two types of gel: hard gel and soft gel. Hard gel gets its name because, once cured, it is tough enough to be made into a nail extension. Soft gel refers to the gel products that are too soft to create a nail extension. This includes gel polishes and thicker gels meant for gel-overlay services.

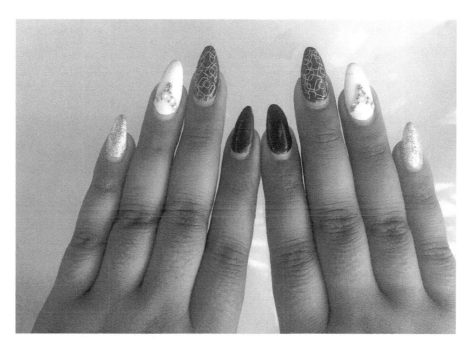

Figure 34.3 Gel nails.

Table 34.1 Acrylic and gel nail

	Acrylic nail	Gel nail
Look and feel	Less natural	Very natural
Initial and upkeep cost	Less	More; especially in-fills
Flexibility	Less; strong but not flexible	More; not thick but strong and flexible
Time required for application	More	Less
Longevity	More	Less, about 14 days
Reparability	Easy at home	Not possible
Discomfort to the patient	Strong fumes	None
Safe in pregnancy	No	Yes
Curing	Air curing	UV curing, not feasible at home
Removal process	Usually soaked in acetone	Usually filed off
Nail damage	High potential	Less potential

Gel polishes are used for the increasingly popular gel polish manicures.

All forms of gel require curing, or hardening, under an ultraviolet (UV) light, which can be either a conventional bulb or LED lamp.

The advantages of gel nails are that they look more natural and glossier, they are safer and eco-friendlier, and the procedure causes no fumes. But they are not durable, self-fixing is difficult, and they are more expensive. Acrylic and gel nails have been compared in Table 34.1.

Gel nails, though a very common cosmetic procedure, have not been evaluated adequately by dermatologists. As a matter of fact, they have been mostly shunned by us because of the reported side effects, including dryness of nails, contact allergic dermatitis of surrounding skin,

paronychia, brittleness, masking of underlying nail disorders, and reported cases of non-melanoma skin cancer possibly associated with their use.[10,12,13] On analysis, however, it can be seen that most of these side effects are technique dependent.

In the author's experience, with a correct technique, these can be used to improve the appearance of cosmetically disfigured nails where other treatment options are not warranted, either because the condition is self-limiting or irreversible or to avoid possible drug side effects.[14]

The authors have used them in various indications like trachyonychia or sand-papered nails, superficial nail pitting, onychorrhexis, onychoschizia, idiopathic Beau's lines, and longitudinal ridging with rewarding results (Figures 34.4 through 34.6).[14]

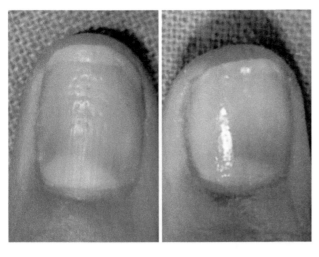

Figure 34.4 Superficial nail pitting. Pre and post procedure photograph showing improvement in nail pitting with gel nails.

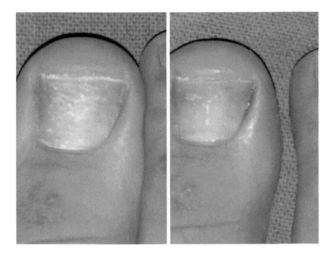

Figure 34.5 Crumbling of nail plate. Improvement in crumbling of nail plate after gel nail application.

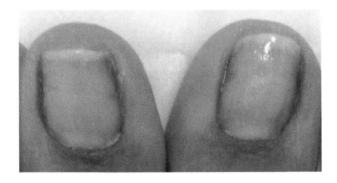

Figure 34.6 Idiopathic Beau's lines. Improvement in Beau's line on application of gel nail.

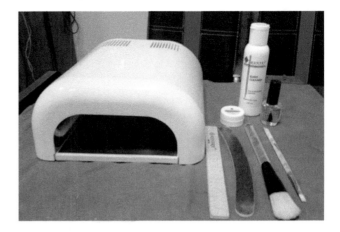

Figure 34.7 Apparatus required for gel nail application.

BOX 34.4: Steps of gel nail procedure[15]

1. Clean with antiseptic
2. Apply thin gel coat
3. Cure under UV lamp
4. Clean any remains

Steps for removal of gel nails:

1. Apply nail polish-soaked cotton
2. Cover with foil for 5–7 minutes
3. Apply moisturizer

The apparatus required for gel nails is depicted in Figure 34.7. The steps of gel nail application and removal has been summarized in Box 34.4.

There are various precautionary measures (summarized in Box 34.5) that can be taken to avoid any complications with gel nails.

Contraindications to gel nails are onychomycosis, melanonychia, paronychia, and allergy to the gel.

Sculptured nails can lead to paresthesias, eczematous reactions, onycholysis, temporary and permanent nail loss, contact dermatitis, onychomycosis (apply antifungal solution such as Thymolize™ under free edge) and paronychia, thin and brittle nail, and increased risk of transmitting bacteria.

NAIL COSMETICS: COMPLICATIONS AND THEIR MANAGEMENT

Nail cosmetics, if used judiciously, could be an effective adjunct to medical treatment in certain nail conditions like trichotillomania, twenty-nail dystrophy, pitting, brittle nails, etc. The common adverse reactions and their management have been summarized in Table 34.2.

BOX 34.5: Rational use of gel nails[10,12,15]

1. Choose your patient wisely; use of gel nails on cosmetically disfigured nails could be more rewarding as compared to their use over apparently normal nails. As the rate of growth of dermatologically compromised nails is relatively slower, gel nail lasts longer (i.e., around 4 weeks as opposed to 2 weeks in normal nails).
2. Avoid manipulation of the cuticle to reduce risk of paronychia.
3. Do nail buffing only where required, to avoid nail plate thinning.
4. Avoid doing in-fills (to avoid missing underlying nail disease).
5. The time of exposure in the UV lamp should be 2 minutes maximum (roughly equivalent to an extra sun exposure of 26 seconds per day for 5 days/week).
6. Avoid using acetone as it causes acquired brittleness of nails and contact dermatitis of surrounding skin. Preferably use normal nail polish.
7. Advise the patient to apply sunscreen regularly on hands.
8. While putting the hand in the UV lamp, cover the rest of the hand with a white cloth.
9. Avoid multiple cycles of curing. Single sitting of curing suffices (Figures 34.8 and 34.9).
10. If the lamp does not cure in 2 minutes, it needs cleaning or the bulbs need to be changed. Normally, the lamp should be cleaned once a week and bulbs need to be replaced after 6 months.

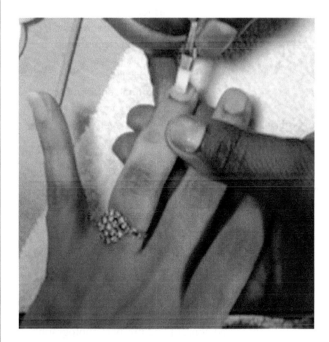

Figure 34.8 Gel application.

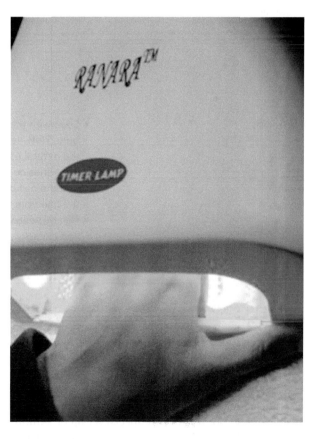

Figure 34.9 UV curing.

Table 34.2 Adverse reactions and complications due to nail cosmetics

Adverse reaction	Cause and procedure	Precaution and management
Acute bacterial paronychia	Trauma to the nail folds during pedicure or manicure	Avoid cutting of cuticles and sterilize the equipment properly.
Chronic paronychia	Cuticle damage during manicure/ pedicure, irritant contact dermatitis, water exposure	Protect cuticle. If proven yeast infection-antifungal, swollen nail folds – topical corticosteroid
Brittle nails	Dehydration due to solvent exposure, used in removing nail polish, gel nails	Avoid harsh chemicals. Do not use nail polish remover frequently.
Allergic contact dermatitis	Acrylates, formaldehyde, TSFR in nail polish	Use hypoallergenic formaldehyde-free nail polish.
Fracture of nail plate	Long and rigid extensions	Keep nail enhancements short and thin enough to be flexible.
Infections – Bacterial: Mycobacterium Fungal: Yeast (candida), dermatophyte Viral: Herpetic, verruca, other systemic viral diseases	Infections caused by improper sterilization of instruments used on multiple clients in nail salons	• Ensure antisepsis and sterilize instruments. • Use disposable files only. • Pedicure baths should be washed and all suction screens cleaned between nail clients. • Nail technicians should be screened for various infections periodically. • Antifungal, antibiotic, or antiviral as per the nature of infection.
Onycholysis	• Seen with the use of artificial nails as bond between the artificial nail and the natural nail plate is stronger than the adhesion between the natural nail and the nail bed. Minor trauma rips the nail from the nail bed. • Can be seen with overzealous manicure and excessive use of nail cosmetics.	• Rest nails every 3 months.

Source: Mattos Simoes Mendonca, M. et al., *Skin Appendage Disord.*, 1, 91–94, 2015; Dahdah, M.J., and Scher, R.K., *Dermatol. Clin.*, 24, 233–239, 2006; Iorizzo, M. et al., *J. Cosmet. Dermatol.*, 6, 53–58, 2007; Chang, R.M. et al., *Dermatol. Ther.*, 20, 54–59, 2007.

NAIL PEELS[18,19]

Chemical peels have been an important tool at dermatologists' disposal for a long time. Facial and body peels are widely used and most dermatologists have extensive experience; applying that to nails can be very beneficial if the choice of candidate and the peel is correct. They are easily available and do not require any special set up or skill. As chemical peels are cheap and painless, patient acceptance is high.

In the authors' experience, almost any patient who has a nail surface abnormality and is consenting can be taken up for peels. Only patients who are pregnant/ breastfeeding, do extensive manual work, have a known allergy to phenol, or have unrealistic expectations should not be advised peels. Any nail unit disease like paronychia or onychomycosis is an absolute contraindication. An extensive history, including any history of previous nail treatments or cosmetic procedures, should be asked before the peels are started.

Steps of the peel:
- Take informed consent and pre-peel photographs.
- Apply Vaseline on the cuticles and on nail folds.
- Clean the affected nail with alcohol/pre-peel cleanser.
- Apply single coat of the peel with nylon brush/ear bud.
- Ask the patient to wash hands after 10 minutes.
- Liberally moisturize the nails in between sessions.
- Repeat sessions at 2–4 week intervals.
- The peels most commonly used are medium-depth peels such as 70% glycolic acid, and a combination of 8% phenol with 15% trichloroacetic acid.

Good to excellent results were seen in most patients in the authors' experience. Conditions treated were nail pitting, onychogryphosis, onychorrhexis, and onychoschizia (Figure 34.10). Utmost care should be taken to avoid any side effects, which are usually limited to irritation of the cuticle and splitting of nail (with phenol).[19]

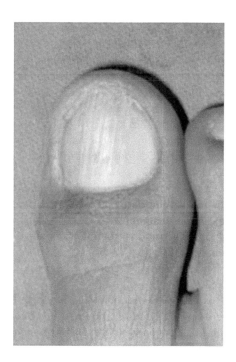

Figure 34.10 Excellent result in onychorrhexis after 70% glycolic acid peels.

ONYCHOCOSMECEUTICALS[17,20,21]

There are many preparations in the market made up of a variety of vitamins, sulfur-containing amino acids or proteins, hormones, calcium, iron, zinc, selenium, and other "essential" elements and minerals, medicinal yeast, crushed egg shells, and even organic food. Scientific evidence in support of use of these agents is limited and, hence, their supplementation cannot be recommended. In addition, the beneficial effects appear to be mainly psychological as some patients report miraculous improvement within a few days or weeks, whereas most others do not observe any benefits. Though overt deficiency of nutrients causes brittle, fragile, or soft nails, routine supplementation of these nutrients to improve the nails of an otherwise healthy person is not recommended. For example, zinc deficiency is known to cause soft, fragile nails, longitudinal ridging, striations, and gray discoloration in addition to periungual blistering and chronic paronychia. Acute-onset zinc deficiency as observed in acquired zinc deficiency syndromes also causes transverse leukonychia and/or Reil–Beau lines. But zinc supplementation in healthy adults does not necessarily improve the growth or quality of nail plates. Some of the nutrients used as supplementation in various nail diseases have been summarized in Table 34.3.

Table 34.3 Common onycho-cosmeceuticals

Agent	Indications	Dose	Comment
Biotin	Brittle nails	2.5–10 mg	
Vitamin A	Egg shell nails		Overdoses have a considerable onycho-destructive effect comparable to that of synthetic retinoids.
Vitamin E	Yellow nail syndrome	usually 600 and 1200 EU	Better results are obtained if combined with weekly 300 mg Fluconazole.
Sulfur-containing amino acids and proteins	Improve nail quality	Not established	No evidence
Calcium			No evidence
Iron	Brittle nails Koilonychia		
Zinc	Brittle nails		
Selenium	Soft nails		Selenium intoxication-caused transverse lines, nail loss, swelling of the fingertip, and purulent discharge
Silica	Brittle nails and psoriatic onychopathy		Improvement was noted in 5 of 10 evaluable patients.
Pyridoxine and ascorbic acid	Brittle nails	Pyridoxine 25–30 mg and Vitamin C 2–3 gm	It was used in combination of evening primrose oil (two capsules three times daily).
Thiamine	Improve nail quality	Thiamine mononitrate 60 mg, calcium D-pantothenate 60 mg, medicinal yeast 100 mg, L-cystine 20 mg, keratin 20 mg, and p-amino benzoic acid 20 mg	

NAIL CARE OILS[20]

Many nail oils containing jojoba oil, bisabolol, panthenol, vitamins, and amino acids have been promoted for various nail abnormalities and are considered to act by holding humidity. In general, oils as well as creams and ointments make the nail more elastic by preventing water loss, and thus prevent nail splitting.

CONCLUSION

Beautiful nails have been the privilege of rich and noble people for more than 3000 years. Nowadays, beautiful nails are affordable for almost everybody. Nail care clinics and salons are now seen everywhere and they have professional manicurists. The upward trend of this industry is here to stay and its expansion requires the dermatologist to be aware of the procedures and techniques applied. A mindful customer may want to consult a dermatologist to know more about the pros and cons of the nail products and adornment techniques. Complications and side effects associated would invariably be treated by a dermatologist and hence a thorough knowledge of the probable ingredients and processes involved is imperative. Nail cosmetics offer a way to protect weak, brittle, or soft nails from trauma. These techniques, if done correctly, can help in camouflaging any underlying nail disorder whose treatment is otherwise either futile or does not justify the associated side effects. Nail enhancements also help conceal the nail disfigurement until the treatment takes effect, which we know can be weeks to months. The authors have tried gel polish-based smoothening of nail plate with extremely gratifying results in most patients.

Pleasing appearance of otherwise brittle and lusterless nails helps boost the confidence of the patient. It can be the treatment of choice in conditions like onychotillomania, onychophagia, or even in-grown nails.

The nail cosmetics are generally safe, but substandard practices can promote disease, deformity, and allergic and irritant contact dermatitis. Therefore, it is a dermatologist's duty to provide clear recommendations regarding safe nail care practices and to recognize cosmetic causes of nail disease.

REFERENCES

1. Madnani NA, Khan KJ. Nail cosmetics. *Indian J Dermatol Venereol Leprol* 2012;78:309–317.
2. Scher RK. Nail cosmetics. *Cutis* 2012;89(4):154–155.
3. Lawry M, Rich P. The nail apparatus: A guide for basic and clinical science. *Curr Probl Dermatol* 1999;11:202–204.
4. Jefferson J, Rich P. Update on nail cosmetics. *Dermatol Ther* 2012;25(6):481–490.
5. Draelos ZD. Nail cosmetics. Medscape reference. Available at http://emedicine.medscape.com/article/1067468-overview#showall, 2011. Accessed on May 4, 2018.
6. Vugia DJ, Jang Y, Zizek C, Ely J, Winthrop KL, Desmond E. Mycobacteria in nail salon whirlpool footbaths, California. *Emerg Infect Dis* 2005;11(4):616–618.
7. Rieder EA, Tosti A. Cosmetically induced disorders of the nail with update on contemporary nail manicures. *J Clin Aesthet Dermatol* 2016;9(4):39–44.
8. Draelos ZD. Cosmetic treatment of nails. *Clin Dermatol* 2013;31(5):573–577.
9. Rich P. Nail cosmetics. *Dermatol Clin* 2006;24:393–399.
10. Mattos Simoes Mendonca M, LaSenna C, Tosti A. Severe onychodystrophy due to allergic contact dermatitis from acrylic nails. *Skin Appendage Disord* 2015;1(2):91–94.
11. Beauty Resource. Nail extensions & nail overlays. Available at https://www.beautyresource.org.uk/articles/nail-extensions-overlays.html. Accessed on May 4, 2018.
12. Dahdah MJ, Scher RK. Nail diseases related to nail cosmetics. *Dermatol Clin* 2006;24:233–239.
13. Hwang S, Kim M, Cho BK, Park HJ. Case of various nail changes induced by gel polish. *J Dermatol* 2016;43(11):1381–1382.
14. Nanda S, Grover C. Utility of gel nails in improving the appearance of cosmetically disfigured nails: Experience with 25 cases. *J Cutan Aesthet Surg* 2014;7(1):26–31.
15. Wang JV, Korta DZ, Zachary CB. Gel manicures and ultraviolet a light: A call for patient education. *Dermatol Online J* 2018;24(3).
16. Iorizzo M, Piraccini BM, Tosti A. Nail cosmetics in nail disorders. *J Cosmet Dermatol* 2007;6(1):53–58.
17. Chang RM, Hare AQ, Rich P. Treating cosmetically induced nail problems. *Dermatol Ther* 2007;20(1):54–59.
18. Banga G, Patel K. Glycolic Acid peels for nail rejuvenation. *J Cutan Aesthet Surg* 2014;7(4):198–201.
19. Daulatabad D, Nanda S, Grover C. Intra-individual right-left comparative study of medium depth peels in superficial nail abnormalities. *J Cutan Aesthet Surg* 2017;10(1):28–32.
20. Haneke E. Onychocosmeceuticals. *J Cosmet Dermatol* 2006;5(1):95–100.
21. Scheinfeld N, Dahdah MJ, Scher R. Vitamins and minerals: Their role in nail health and disease. *J Drugs Dermatol* 2007;6(8):782–787.

35

The science of nail polish, nail polish remover, and nail moisturizers

SOMODYUTI CHANDRA AND ANUPAM DAS

With the advent of modern technologies and recent advances in the field of medical sciences, there is no question of what is left unanswered when it comes to clinical or aesthetic point of view, nail care being no exception. In this chapter, we have briefly discussed the scientific rationale behind the use of nail moisturizers, nail polishes, and nail polish removers, with a comprehensive overview of the agents available in the market.

NAIL POLISH

Nail polish, also called nail enamel or nail varnish, is a viscous lacquer that is applied on the surface of nail plate of fingernails and toenails to form a water-resistant coating, primarily for cosmetic enhancement. It is one of the most widely used cosmetics throughout the world and it was estimated that in 2011, US consumers spent around 6.6 billion dollars only for nail enhancement.[1] The use of nail polishes can be traced back to 3000 B.C. when Chinese and Egyptian women used an "herbal-concoction" made of egg-white, gelatin, beeswax, gum Arabic, and vegetable dyes (like henna or mashed rose) to embellish their nails. Bright colors like red, black, and gold were symbolic of power, superiority, and prosperity and were generally reserved for the elite class, while the commoners were allowed only pale shades.[2]

Michelle Menard, partnering with Charles Revson, is generally credited as the first person to conceptualize nail polish based on automobile paint. In 1932 Revson went on to found the cosmetic company that we now know as Revlon. Since then, nail polish formulations have evolved to provide a platform for the variety of nail colors and effects desired by the consumers.[3]

Although the main purpose of using nail enamel is undoubtedly beautification and grooming, it is also used for camouflaging nail surface textural abnormalities (like pitting, lines, ridges) and discolorations (yellow or white). It is also used to temporarily strengthen thin and brittle nails.[4]

The basic components include film forming agents, resins, plasticizers, solvents, and coloring agents as summarized in Table 35.1. Nitrocellulose is the main film-forming agent in nail lacquer, which, along with resins like toluene sulphonamide formaldehyde, ensures adhesion of the nail paint to the surface of the nail plate.[5] This film is oxygen-permeable, which helps maintain nail health while providing strength and gloss. Plasticizers like camphor, dibutyl phthalate, or dioctyl phthalate provide flexibility and adhesiveness to the lacquer by linking to polymer chains and increasing the distance between them. Colorants (D&C Red no. 6/7/19) and pearlizers (guanine, bismuth oxychloride, titanium dioxide, ground mica) give the desired color and shimmer. All these ingredients are dissolved or suspended in a solvent, such as butyl acetate or ethyl acetate, which evaporate to leave behind the colorful finish.[6]

Some polishes contain additional constituents like thickening agents to make the polish easier to apply and ultraviolet filters (benozophenone-1), which help prevent discoloration when the polish is exposed to sunlight or other forms of ultraviolet light. Some brands have added natural oils like argan oil that acts as a nail-moisturizer and makes damage less noticeable and perfumes to counteract the unpleasant odor of the solvents.[7]

Nail polish application is described in Box 35.1.

Nail polish is a relatively safe cosmetic with only 3% of the users experiencing one or more untoward effects to it.[10] The most common side-effects include allergic contact dermatitis (ACD) and nail-plate staining. The most commonly identified allergen is tosylamide formaldehyde resin (TSFR), which is implicated in around 6.6% of the patch test-positive users.

Table 35.1 Constituents of a nail polish

Class of constituent	Purpose	Agents
Film-forming agent	When the nail polish is applied the solvent evaporates, leaving the polymer to form a film on the nail	Nitrocellulose, dissolved in a solvent, usually ethyl acetate or butyl acetate
Plasticizers	To make sure that nail polish stays flexible when it dries, making the nail polish last longer and be less prone to chipping	Dibutyl phthalate and camphor, trimethyl pentanyl diisobutyrate, triphenyl phosphate, ethyl tosylamide, glyceryl tribenzoate
Adhesive polymer resins	To ensure that the nitrocellulose adheres to the nail plate's surface	Tosylamide-formaldehyde resin [a] polyester resin or cellulose acetate butyrate
Dyes and pigments	To impart color	Chromium oxide greens, chromium hydroxide, ferric ferrocyanide, stannic oxide, titanium dioxide, iron oxide, carmine, ultramarine, and manganese violet
Opalescent pigments	To add glittery/shimmer look	Mica, bismuth oxychloride, natural pearls, and aluminum powder
Thickening agents	To maintain the sparkling particles in suspension while in the bottle	Stearalkonium hectorite
Ultraviolet stabilizers	Resist color changes when the dry film is exposed to sunlight	Benzophenone-1

[a] In nail polishes with label "hypoallergenic", polyester resin or cellulose acetate butyrate is used as adhesive polymer resin.

BOX 35.1: Nail polish application technique

The ideal nail polish application technique includes the following steps[8]:

1. Base coat[9]: This is the first layer, meant to strengthen the nail plate. It is transparent with high resin content, leading to stronger adherence of nail polish to the nail. It also restores moisture to the nail and helps in filling ridges.
2. Nail polish: Pigmented nail polish applied as 2–3 coats.
3. Top coat: Again, a transparent coat that contains more of nitrocellulose than resin. This prevents nail polish chipping and fading and may contain sunscreen. It adds shine to the polish.
4. Nail polish drier: Liquid that speeds up drying of the nail polish by encouraging evaporation of the solvent. Usually consists of vegetable oils, alcohols, and silicone derivatives.

Other allergens identified include formaldehyde, polyester resin, dichloroethylene, amyl acetate, phthalates, guanine, acrylate, sulfonamide, nitrocellulose, and shellac. Of late, "hypoallergic nail polishes" have become popular and have replaced TSFR with cellulose, acetate, butyrate, and polyester resin. Patch-testing is done to confirm ACD to nail polish components, using the standard patch-test tray or by using the patient's own bottle of polish. Contact dermatitis can occur locally, around the nail unit or at a distant site, such as face, eyelids, lips, and neck.[11,12] Rarely, contact dermatitis in and around genitals and perianal region,[10] and desquamative gingivitis,[13] have been reported. The common adverse effects and their management have been summarized in Table 35.2.

In addition, certain pigments in the polish, particularly when they are in a dissolved state rather than in suspension, stain the nail plate yellow. This mostly occurs with the deep red polishes containing D&C Reds No. 6, 7, 34, or FD and C yellow no. 5 Lake. The staining usually develops after 7 days of wearing the polish, is more pronounced distally than proximally, and fades spontaneously by about 14 days; however, it can be removed by scraping the nail plate with a scalpel.[4]

In instances when the nail polish is kept undisturbed for several months, when a base coat is applied prior to the varnish, or when the polish is reapplied without removing the previous layers, it results in extreme dryness and crumbling of the nail plate with whitish discoloration, mimicking white superficial onychomycosis. This change was described by Baran et al. as "keratin granulations" (Figure 35.1), and a KOH mount can differentiate it.[14]

Other reported adverse effects include onychodystrophy, onycholysis, and paronychia. Sometimes nail varnish, used as a barrier against nickel allergy, can itself lead to its sensitization.[11] An uncommon but potentially serious adverse effect has been reported with dibutyl phthalate (used as a plasticizer) including decreased sperm mobility and viability[15] and endocrine disruption leading to altered development of fetal testes.[16]

Table 35.2 Common adverse effects and management

Adverse reaction	Explanation/mechanism	Precaution and management
Brittle nails	Dehydration due to solvent exposure, used in removing nail polish, gel nails	Avoid harsh chemicals. Do not use nail polish remover frequently
Allergic contact dermatitis	Acrylates, formaldehyde, TSFR in nail polish	Use hypoallergenic formaldehyde-free nail polish
Onycholysis	Excessive use of nail cosmetics	Rest nails every 3 months
Yellow staining		Scraping with scalpel
Keratin granulations	Dehydration of nail plate, leading to clumping of keratin proteins	Take several week-long breaks from nail polish, nail polish remover, and chemicals in conjunction with using moisturizers and/or hand creams to replenish the moisture balance of the nail

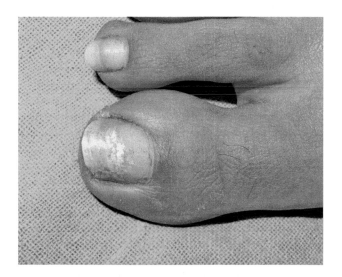

Figure 35.1 Keratin granulations. (Courtesy of Prof. Archana Singal.)

Nail hardeners[17]

These are modified nail polishes applied as a base coat for the purpose of strengthening the nail plate. This base coat moves through porous structure of nail plate, decreasing loss of water through nail plate significantly and hence providing strength and flexibility to the nail plate. These nail hardeners are used in cases where nails are soft, brittle, or prone to splitting.

They may contain titanium-silicone-zirconium polymers, polytef, nylon, calcium, and biotin. Addition of keratin, vitamins, calcium fluoride, natural oils, nylon fibers, Teflon, and silk can be done. Prolonged usage can lead to brittle nails (cross-link density rises and flexibility is reduced). The patient should be advised to periodically remove nail hardeners with nail polish remover. Other adverse effects include contact allergic dermatitis, onycholysis, and subungual hyperkeratosis.

NAIL POLISH REMOVER

Nothing in the world is constant, including the nail paints that change with a person's clothes and moods. Nail polish removers are organic solvents that break down and dissolve the polish, thus removing it from the nail plate.

An ideal lacquer remover should not be volatile enough to evaporate during application, should neither have strong degreasing effect nor leave the nails sticky, and should be non-irritating to surrounding skin.

The solvents used in nail enamel removers include acetone; gamma butyrolactone; and amyl, butyl, or ethyl acetate, which are mixed with fatty materials such as cetyl alcohol, lanolin, castor oil, or other synthetic oils.

The acetone in the remover is harsh on the nails and periungual skin and is the most common cause of irritant contact dermatitis. Excessive use of these products can also lead to dry, brittle nails. A less harsh remover contains ethyl acetate along with isopropyl alcohol. Acetonitrile, a component of the remover, has been banned in the European countries since 2000, because of its toxic and carcinogenic potential.

"Acetone-free nail polish removers" are now widely available and are generally considered safe. JJ Brown and CS Nanayakkara, however, highlighted the dangers of these "safe" acetone-free removers that contain gamma butyrolactone, which is rapidly metabolized to gamma hydroxybutyrate on ingestion, resulting in systemic toxicity. They reported a case where accidental suction of polish removing pads led to bilateral pneumothoraces, pneumomediastinum, upper respiratory obstruction, and finally cardiorespiratory collapse and coma.[18] This gamma butyrolactone has also been reported to cause fatal and non-fatal intoxication,[19] acute toxicity in 9-to-15-month olds,[20] withdrawal delirium with acute renal failure,[21] and rapid onset of coma, respiratory depression, and bradycardia.[22]

Another potentially serious adverse effect caused by accidental ingestion of nail polish removers is methemoglobinemia. Acetone, N, N-dimethyl-p-toluidine, and nitroethane are the responsible causal agents.[23]

Open-patch testing, at a concentration of 10% in olive oil, is recommended for detection of adverse effects to nail polish removers due to their high volatile solvent concentrations.[7]

NAIL MOISTURIZERS

The nail is a richly keratinized tissue with a high content of cysteine, a sulfur-containing amino acid. 10% of the dry weight of nail is constituted by sulfur, and these hard keratins attribute to the toughness of the nail and the superlative barrier function. The content of lipids and water in the nails is low, as compared to stratum corneum. But it is to be noted that nail is highly permeable to water. When the water content of nail increases, it becomes soft and opaque. However, when the water content decreases, it becomes dry and brittle. So, proper and adequate moisturization of nails is essential to prevent them from becoming brittle.[24]

Moisturizing helps maintain healthy and glistening nails. Patients must be advised to refrain from frequent use of hand sanitizers, harsh soaps and cleansers, formaldehyde-containing products, and acetone to prevent dehydration of the nail plate. Frequent soaking in water must be avoided, as this may result in brittle nails.

Urea (5%–20%) and lactic acid (5%–10%) are found to be highly efficacious in hydrating the nails. They increase the water-holding capacity of the nails by digesting the nail keratins and opening the water-binding sites. The disadvantage is that the effects are short-lived and this mandates frequent re-application for sustained effects.[25]

Other moisturizing agents found to be useful include glycerin, petrolatum, beeswax, mineral oils, natural oils (almond, avocado, jojoba, and sunflower), waxes (cetyl alcohol, stearyl alcohol, and beeswax), and humectants (aloe vera, ceramides, and glycerin).

Thus, moisturizers constitute an important part of nail care, and we should be well-acquainted with the options available in order to provide effective management to the patients.

REFERENCES

1. Jefferson J, Rich P. Update in nail cosmetics. *Dermatol Ther* 2012;25:481–490.
2. Nail polish. Available from: http://en.wikipedia.org/wiki/Nail_polish [accessed on October 30, 2017].
3. Draelos ZD. Nail cosmetic issues. *Dermatol Clin* 2000;18:675–683.
4. Rich P. Nail cosmetics. *Dermatol Clin* 2006;24:393–399.
5. Schlossman ML. Nail-enamel resins. *Cosmetic Technol* 1979;1:53.
6. Draelos ZD. Cosmetic treatment of nails. *Clin Dermatol* 2013;31:573–577.
7. Madani NA, Khan KJ. Nail cosmetics. *Indian J Dermatol Venereol Leprol* 2012;78:309–317.
8. Rich P, Kwak H. Nail physiology and grooming. In: Draelos ZD, Ed. *Cosmetic Dermatology Products and Procedures*, 1st ed. Hoboken, NJ: Wiley-Blackwell, 2010: pp. 197–205.
9. Baran R. Nail cosmetics: Allergies and irritations. *Am J Clin Dermatol* 2002;3(8):547–555.
10. Dahdah MJ, Scher RK. Nail diseases related to nail cosmetics. *Dermatol Clin* 2006;24:233–239.
11. Lazzarini R, Hafner M de FS, Lopes AS de A, Oliari CB. Allergy to hypoallergenic nail polish: Does this exist? *Anais Brasileiros de Dermatologia* 2017;92:421–422.
12. Lazzarini R, Duarte I, de Farias DC, Santos CA, Tsai AI. Frequency and main sites of allergic contact dermatitis caused by nail varnish. *Dermatitis* 2008;19:319–322.
13. Staines KS, Felix DH, Forsyth A. Desquamative gingivitis, sole manifestation of tosylamide/formaldehyde resin allergy. *Contact Dermatitis* 1998;39:90.
14. Brauer E, Baran R. Cosmetics: The care and adornment of nail. In: Baran R, Dawber RPR, de Berker D et al., Eds. *Diseases of the Nail and their Management*, 3rd ed. Oxford, UK: Blackwell; 2001: pp. 358–369.
15. Pant N, Pant A, Shukla M, Mathur N, Gupta Y, Saxena D. Environmental and experimental exposure of phthalate esters: The toxicological consequence on human sperm. *Hum Exp Toxicol* 2011;30:507–514.
16. Lorizzo M, Piraccini BM, Tosti A. Nail cosmetics in nail disorders. *J Cosmet Dermatol* 2007;6(1):53–58.
17. Habert R, Muczynski V, Lehraiki A, Lambrot R, Lécureuil C, Levacher C et al. Adverse effects of endocrine disruptors on the foetal testis development: Focus on the phthalates. *Folia Histochem Cytobiol* 2009;47:S67–S74.
18. Brown JJ, Nanayakkara CS. Acetone-free nail polish removers: Are they safe? *Clin Toxicol (Phila)* 2005;43:297–299.
19. Lenz D, Rothschild MA, Kröner L. Intoxications due to ingestion of gamma-butyrolactone: Organ distribution of gamma-hydroxybutyric acid and gamma-butyrolactone. *Ther Drug Monit* 2008;30:755–761.
20. Savage T, Khan A, Loftus BG. Acetone-free nail polish remover pads: Toxicity in a 9-month old. *Arch Dis Child* 2007;92:371.

21. Bhattacharya IS, Watson F, Bruce M. A case of γ-butyrolactone associated with severe withdrawal delirium and acute renal failure. *Eur Addict Res* 2011;17:169–171.

22. Rambourg-Schepens MO, Buffet M, Durak C, Mathieu-Nolf M. Gamma butyrolactone poisoning and its similarities to gamma hydroxybutyric acid: Two case report. *Vet Hum Toxicol* 1997;39:234–235.

23. Patra S, Sikka G, Khaowas AK, Kumar V. Successful intervention in a child with toxic methemoglobinemia due to nail polish remover poisoning. *Indian J Occup Environ Med* 2011;15:137–138.

24. Andre J, Scheers C, Baran R. Normal nail and use of nail cosmetics and treatments. In: Barel AO, Paye M, Maibach HI, Eds. *Handbook of Cosmetic Science and Technology*, 4th ed. Boca Raton, FL: CRC Press; 2014: pp. 597–608.

25. Draelos ZD, Ed. Understanding and treating brittle nails. In: *Cosmetics and Dermatologic Problems and Solutions*, 3rd ed. Boca Raton, FL: Informa Health Care; 2011: p. 262.

Miscellaneous Conditions

36

Nail degloving syndrome

ROBERT BARAN

INTRODUCTION

Nail degloving refers to partial or total avulsion of the nail and surrounding tissue (perionychium). Typically it appears as a thimble-shaped nail shedding or a partial or total loss of nail organ with soft tissue. "Fragility of dermo-epidermal junction", exploited by immune-mediated assault as in lichen planus and in toxic epidermal necrolysis and "inherent weakness due to the presence of different types of keratotic zones in nail unit" are considered responsible for this unique phenomenon. The proximal nail fold (keratinizing as cuticle) and nascent nail plate possess a different degree of strength and elasticity and hence, are vulnerable to separation from one another.

The etiology of nail degloving encompasses 4 main types: 1. Traumatic injuries; 2. Iatrogenic diseases; 3. Gangrenous conditions (streptococcal, non bacterial, and acute digital gangrene in the newborn); 4. Dermatological conditions.

TRAUMATIC INJURIES

The traumatic causes may be found in the home or in industry and in the recreation field.[1] Sometimes, the avulsion may be caused by a loop of steel wire, or by a wet cord while sailing, or a ring may be caught when the owner jumps off a trailer or a ladder.

Surgically, crushing injuries of the fingertip may be classified under tip-amputation, volar, dorsal, and circumferential injury.[2] The fingertip that has been crushed in closing a door or between two heavy objects may produce nail degloving.[3]

IATROGENIC DISEASES

Iatrogenic disease is a significant cause of nail degloving. Toxic epidermal necrolytic disease (Lyell's syndrome) provides the most typical cases and, usually, regrowth of a normal nail is obtained.[4]

GANGRENOUS CONDITIONS

Gangrene refers to a severe necrotizing and sloughing process. Dry gangrene of the digits should be allowed to demarcate by itself.

1. *Nonbacterial gangrenous conditions in adults*: Digital ischemia has been associated with many malignant neoplasms. It is frequently manifested by evidence of frank gangrene. Disseminated intravascular coagulation[5] (DIC) can result from acute leukemia. Gangrene of an extremity was reported in polycythemia.[6]
2. *Streptococcal gangrenous conditions*: Appear mainly in patients with some immune defect. Bullous manifestations surrounding the distal toes in a diabetic patient may produce progressive necrosis around the nail, leading to partially sloughed-off tissue.
3. As a secondary event, gangrene may result from trauma, secondary infection, or acropustulosis (see farther).
4. *Acute digital gangrene in the newborn*: The occurrence of acute peripheral gangrene in newborns is a rare emergency event.[7] A few hours after delivery, the newborn develops blisters on the digits. Gangrene appears the following day. Etiology includes infection,

metabolic, genetic (congenital erosive vesicular dermatosis with reticulated supple scarring[8]), drug-induced conditions, a vasculitis syndrome, or diseases related to vascular malformations. In Wollina and Verma's case,[9] the newborn had acute finger gangrene due to maternal antiphospholid syndrome.

5. *Gangrenous acral psoriasis*: In a personal case of Alan Menter, MD (USA), a 40-year-old woman presented with severe recalcitrant acropustulosis with associated bony erosions and contractures. The distal fingers were gangrenous and the patient was totally incapacitated and unable to perform day-to-day functions. Effectiveness of infliximab was dramatic.

6. *Kawasaki disease*: Ischemic necrosis of the extremities is a rare complication.[10] In a 5-month-old boy, a progressive extrusion of the entire nail apparatus was limited to the fingers. It occurred after 7 weeks and lasted 15 days.[11] The onset of psoriatic lesions during Kawasaki disease has been reported in several cases and may be considered as a Koebner phenomenon.[12]

DERMATOLOGICAL CONDITIONS

Lichen planus

A 50-year-old man from Senegal presented 10 dystrophic fingernails, some with remnants of nail keratin and others showing an onychomadesis with a normal nail plate. However, two signs were common to all the nails: a whitish material at the base of all the nail plates and a swollen proximal nail fold (PNF) (Figure 36.1a). The latter was painless but sensitive on pressure. With further progressive pressure on the PNF, the whitish material became more prominent (Figure 36.1b and c), and as pressure was kept on, it appeared totally flat. Simultaneously, this situation was accompanied by the advancing outward extrusion of the whole nail apparatus (Figure 36.2a), rigid enough to mimic a balloon fish completely opened at the rear (Figure 36.2b).

The patient refused further examination. He was otherwise in good health with normal classical blood tests. The past history was unremarkable.

The histologic examination of the lesion suggested the diagnosis of hyperkeratotic and pseudo-bullous nail lichen planus with the dramatic picture of epithelial structures

(ventral portion of the PNF, matrix, nail bed, and hyponychium) unsealed, and free from their dermal base.[13]

Epidermolysis bullosa

Autosomal dominant epidermolysis bullosa affecting finger- and toenails has been observed in a baby and his mother. All the digits were simultaneously affected by the partial or total avulsion of the nails and surrounding soft tissue[14] (Figure 36.3).

CLINICAL COURSE AND PROGNOSIS

Clinically nonsurgical nail degloving encompasses three main varieties with some possible overlapping:

1. A typical thimble-shaped nail shedding. The walls of the thimble are composed of the skin of the distal digit including the nail plate (circumferential skin shedding)
2. A partially sloughed-off nail with its surrounding tissue
3. A shedding restricted to the whole nail apparatus, sparing the surrounding epidermis of the distal digit

The initial clinical cavitary appearance depends on two factors:

1. The extension of the zone of dermal-epidermal cleavage on the PNF and the region of the pulp
2. The intensity of the reactional epithelial hyperplasia of the detached zone

As we have shown elsewhere,[13] the process of degloving followed by regeneration of the whole nail apparatus may be explained by two main mechanisms producing different aspects of nail degloving and pure gangrene, depending on the disease that may affect only the epidermis or extend to the dermal-epidermal junction.

The regeneration of the nail apparatus is explained by the sparing of its most proximal portion containing proximal matrix and retaining its attachments to the neighboring dermis. Of note, the gangrenous acral psoriasis did not clinically evolve into a cleavage of the epithelial block of the nail apparatus. The regeneration occurred progressively without dramatic shedding of the epithelial layer.

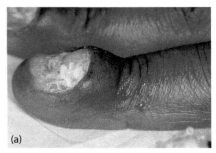 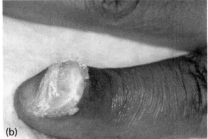 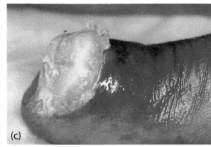

(a)   (b)   (c)

Figure 36.1 **(a)** Lichen planus involving the whole nail apparatus; **(b and c)** Partial extrusion of the nail apparatus, following a progressive pressure on the proximal nail fold. (From Baran, R., and Perrin, C., *J Am Acad Dermatol*, 58, 232–237, 2008.)

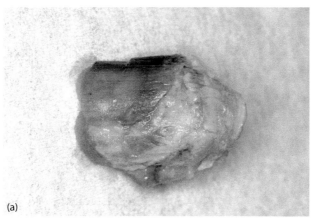
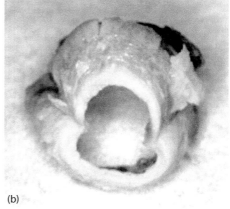

(a)   (b)

Figure 36.2 **(a)** Complete extrusion of an entire nail unit; **(b)** Appearance of balloon fish completely opened at the rear. (From Baran, R., and Perrin, C., *J Am Acad Dermatol*, 58, 232–237, 2008.)

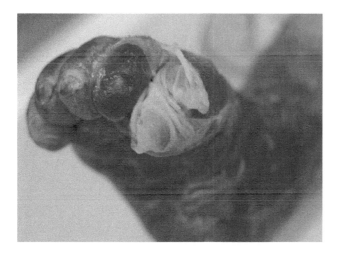

Figure 36.3 Autosomal dominant epidermolysis bullosa. (Courtesy of F. Cambazard, France.)

Finally, despite the impressive appearance of nail degloving, this condition is usually compatible with a fairly good recovery.

REFERENCES

1. Frederiks E. Treatment of degloved fingers. *Hand* 1973; 5: 140–144.
2. Tajima T. Treatment of open crushing type of industrial injuries of the hand and forearm: Degloving, open circumferential, heat-press, and nail-bed injuries. *J Trauma* 1974; 14: 995–1011.
3. Zook EG. Reconstruction of a functional and aesthetic nail. *Hand Clin* 2002; 18: 577–594.
4. Baran R, Roujeau J. New millennium, new nail problems. *Dermatol Ther* 2002; 15: 64–70.
5. Manios SG, Kanokoundi F, Miliaras-Ulachakis M. Gangrene of lower extremities in a newborn infant associated with intravascular coagulation (recession of gangrene after heparin therapy). *Helv Paediatr Acta* 1972; 27: 187–192.
6. Papageorgiou A, Stern L. Polycythemia and gangrene of an extremity in a newborn infant. *J Pediatr* 1972; 81: 985–987.
7. Askue WE, Wong R, Brooklyn NY. Gangrene of the extremities in a newborn infant. *J Pediatr* 1952; 40: 588–598.
8. Cohen BA, Esterly NB, Nelson PF. Congenital erosive and vesicular dermatosis healing with reticulated supple scarring. *Arch Dermatol* 1985; 121: 361–367.
9. Wollina U, Verma SB. Acute digital gangrene in a newborn. *Arch Dermatol* 2007; 143: 121–122.
10. Ames EI, Jones JS, Van Dommelen B *et al*. Bilateral hand necrosis in Kawasaki syndrome. *J Hand Surg* 1985; 10A: 391–395.
11. Passeron T, Olivier V, Sirvent N, Khalfi A, Boutté P, Lacour JP. Kawasaki disease with exceptional cutaneous manifestations. *Eur J Pediatr* 2002; 161: 228–230.
12. Han MH, Jang KA, Sung KJ *et al*. A case of guttate psoriasis following Kawasaki disease. *Br J Dermatol* 2000; 142: 548–550.
13. Baran R, Perrin C. Nail degloving, a polyetiologic condition with 3 main patterns: A new syndrome. *J Am Acad Dermatol* 2008; 58: 232–237.
14. Baran R, Hadj-Rabia S, Silverman R. *Pediatric Nail Disorders*, pp. 69–71. Boca Raton, FL: CRC Press; 2017.

37

Miscellaneous nail conditions

SUNIL K. KOTHIWALA AND PIYUSH KUMAR

This chapter focuses on some recently described or under-recognized conditions of clinical importance. These conditions need to be considered in clinical differentials of many common conditions (as discussed later) and awareness of these conditions helps the physicians diagnose and manage nail diseases efficiently.

ASYMMETRIC GAIT NAIL UNIT SYNDROME

Asymmetric gait nail unit syndrome (AGNUS) was first described by Zais et al. as structural changes of nail resulting from pressure on the toes and foot caused by asymmetric gait due to uneven flat foot.[1] The uneven pressure usually produces unilateral changes; when they are bilateral, one side always shows more severe changes than the other. These pressure-induced clinical signs in nail unit mimic all types of onychomycosis (OM). However, there are some additional signs that make it easy to identify AGNUS. These signs are similar to those seen in OM[2]:

- Nail plate incurved on one side due to pressure of shoe on nail matrix while walking. Associated lateral onycholysis may be present.
- Onycholysis and subungual hyperkeratosis, more pronounced at the friction point of the toe (Figure 37.1).

Surface changes of nail plate are similar to white superficial onychomycosis (WSO) (Figure 37.2).
- Abnormalities of the stratum corneum of the hyponychium (Figure 37.3).
- One important clinical clue is its waxing and waning course over time (though complete clinical resolution without intervention is not seen).
- Evidence of body asymmetry- differences between left and right shoulder height, uneven flat feet, scoliosis

AGNUS may co-exist with OM and many other diseases affecting the nail unit and results in greater clinical severity than each condition individually.[1,2] Its coexistence with fungal diseases has complicated the management of OM, as coexisting AGNUS and OM might result in erroneous clinical typing of OM, false clinical signs of drug resistance, and difficulty in assessing severity and defining complete cure.[3,4] In these patients, some clinical changes may persist even after negative KOH mount, necessitating revision of definition of cure in OM.[5]

Early recognition of signs of AGNUS may contribute to improved quality of life by early correction of skeleton abnormalities and avoiding unnecessary antifungal treatments. The cornerstone of treatment of AGNUS includes avoiding tight shoes as well as using open-toed shoes and personalized insole until complete clinical resolution is achieved.

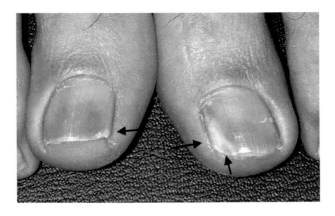

Figure 37.1 Asymmetric gait nail unit syndrome affecting toes bilaterally in an asymmetric manner. (Courtesy of Dr. Nardo Zais, Skin and Cancer Unit, Mt Sinai Medical Center, Miami Beach, FL.)

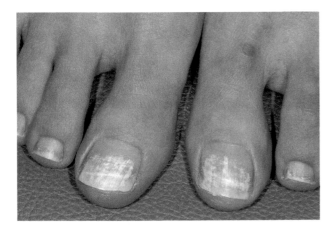

Figure 37.2 White superficial onychomycosis-like asymmetric gait nail unit syndrome. (Courtesy of Dr. Nardo Zais, Skin and Cancer Unit, Mt Sinai Medical Center, Miami Beach, FL.)

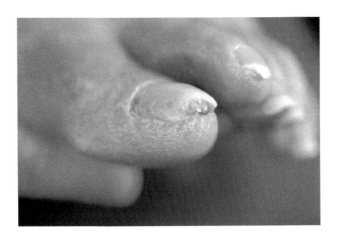

Figure 37.3 Nail plate thickening and subungual hyperkeratosis in asymmetric gait nail unit syndrome. (Courtesy of Dr. Nardo Zais, Skin and Cancer Unit, Mt Sinai Medical Center, Miami Beach, FL.)

HANGNAIL

Hangnail is a triangular-shaped overextension of the cuticle, which may separate from lateral or proximal nail folds, particularly during winter months or after prolonged exposure to water (Figures 37.4 and 37.5). Hangnails more frequently appear on the fingers than the toes. Superimposed infections in hangnail may cause swelling and redness of

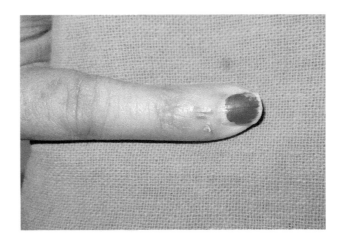

Figure 37.4 Hangnail affecting proximal nail fold in a homemaker. (Courtesy of Prof. Archana Singal.)

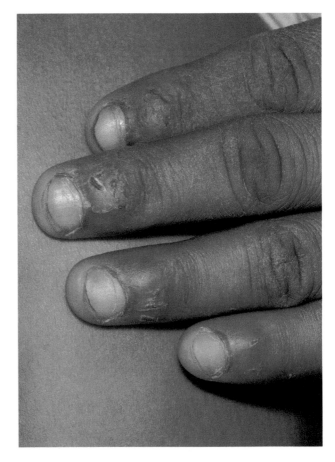

Figure 37.5 Hangnail affecting multiple digits.

nail fold. It may be associated with a habit of cuticle biting. A mild to moderate hangnail can be treated conservatively by hot fomentation, trimming hangnail straight, and constant lubrication of fingertips with skin creams. Avoidance of repeated hand immersion in water is beneficial and preventive. Attempts at removal may cause pain and extension of tear into the dermis. Infected hangnails may require a short course of topical or oral antibiotic therapy.[6]

BRITTLE NAIL SYNDROME

Brittle nail syndrome (BNS) is a heterogenous abnormality, characterized by increased fragility of the nail plate. It affects about 20% of the population and women are affected twice as frequently as men. Most patients with BNS report it as a significant cosmetic problem impairing daily activities and negative impact on the occupational abilities.[7] The brittle nails associated with dermatological conditions like lichen planus have been discussed elsewhere. This chapter focuses on brittle nails in otherwise healthy individuals, without any underlying nail diseases.

Major pathogenic factors that lead to BNS are those that impair intercellular adhesion of the corneocytes of the nail plate or abnormal nail formation by involving the matrix. The formation of the nail plate requires epidermal proliferation of both the matrix and the nail bed. Terminal differentiation with formation of layers of corneocytes involves recruitment of cycling epidermal cells. External factors like repetitive immersion or desiccation, exposure to chemicals, and interactive trauma of the nail may impair coherence of the nail plate by interfering with the intercellular adhesive factors. These factors are more harmful for nails with poor growth rate, as the cumulative exposure time to external damage is increased. Brittle nails have been found with decreased sulfur content, which implies fewer disulfide bridges among proteins forming keratin fibrils, decreased cholesterol sulfate, and decreased water binding capacity. The concentration of trace elements in brittle nails is not significantly different than normal nail. Abnormal nail formation may be caused by factors that affect epithelial growth and keratinization in the nail matrix and nail bed. Abnormal keratinization and nail growth may be impaired by systemic factors including decreased oxygenation, endocrine, metabolic factors, serious infectious diseases, decreased vascularization, irradiation, arsenic intoxication, and disorders of the keratinization.[8,9]

Clinical features of BNS are onychoschizia and onychorrhexis (Figure 37.6). The impairment of intercellular adhesive factors of nail plate is expressed clinically as onychoschizia, which is characterized by lamellar splitting of the free edge and distal portion of the nail plate. The severity of lamellar splitting may range from mild furrows of superficial layers at distal free edge to severe lamellar splitting of the complete free edge and at least one third of the distal part of the nail plate. It may also include damage of the lateral edges causing transverse splitting, which may vary from single, superficial split to multiple horizontal splits.

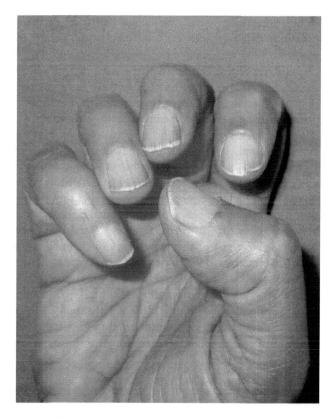

Figure 37.6 Brittle nail syndrome in a homemaker. (Courtesy of Prof. Archana Singal.)

The involvement of the nail matrix is expressed clinically as onychorrhexis, which is characterized by longitudinal thickening and thinning or ridging of the nail plate. It may vary from a few plane ridges or superficial splitting to multiple superficial or deep ones involving at least 70% of the nail surface. Another feature of onychorrhexis is triangular fragments at the free edge that can be torn off easily. Onychorrhexis may also be associated with disordered keratinization and clinical signs may be diagnostic of some particular dermatoses.[8,9]

Management of BNS should be aimed to improve quality of life and occupational abilities. First, external causative factors need to be identified and eliminated. Patients with BNS should be checked for underlying systemic disease and primary dermatologic conditions. Conservative therapeutic interventions include increasing water content by soaking nails for 15 minutes every evening followed by emollient application, as well as application of enamel to protect the nail mechanically. Also, cautious use of nail hardening agents containing formaldehyde may help to strengthen the nail plate temporarily. Among medical therapy, biotin (2.5–5 mg/d) has been shown to be a beneficial therapy but there is need of larger studies with control to support this as a treatment modality.[10]

RETRONYCHIA

Retronychia was first described by de Berker et al. and later established as an entity by the collective work of the European Nail Society in 2008.[11] Retronychia is a combination of proximal nail plate ingrowing into the proximal nail fold with old nail plates underneath the uppermost nail. It usually affects young adults with female preponderance. Many anatomical (abnormally curved nails) and behavioral factors (tight fitting footwear with increased heel height) that predispose the nail to repetitive microtrauma are thought to contribute to retronychia.[12]

Almost all cases occur in big toes as it is more prone to be traumatized. Involvement of multiple nails is unusual. Duration of having retronychia can be extended due to ignorance of patients. Early retronychia is characterized by yellow discoloration and thickening of the proximal part of the nail plate as well as inflammation of the proximal nail fold due to pressure of elevated proximal nail (Figures 37.7 and 37.8). At late stage these changes are followed by aseptic discharge; granulation tissue emerging at the junction of the proximal and lateral nail fold as well as interruption of nail growth are observed.[13]

The diagnosis of retronychia is clinical. Ultrasound imaging allows non-invasive, clear visualization of tissue changes. Recently, ultrasonographic findings were proposed as diagnostic criteria to diagnose retronychia. The findings include the following[14]:

1. Hypoechoic halo surrounding the origin of the nail plate
2. Distance between the origin of the nail plate and the base of the distal phalanx of 5.1 mm or less in big

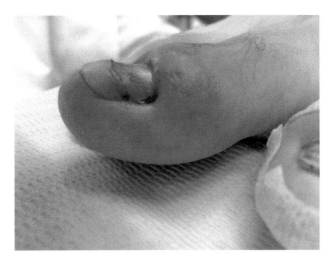

Figure 37.8 Retronychia causing inflammation of proximal nail fold in a 15-year-old girl. (Courtesy of Prof. Eckart Haneke.)

   toes and thumbs and/or a difference of 0.5 mm of this distance or greater between the affected nail and the contralateral healthy nail
3. Proximal nail fold thickness of 2.2 mm or greater for male patients or 1.9 mm or greater for female patients and/or a proximal nail fold 0.3 mm thicker or greater in comparison with the contralateral healthy nail

Histopathology is not required for diagnosis but may be helpful to rule out other proximal nail fold pathologies.

The conservative treatment of taping might be enough in early stages. It prevents retrograde movement against the proximal nail fold and allows the nail to grow distally. Nail avulsion is both diagnostic and therapeutic in most cases. It is the treatment of choice that generally resolves retronychia with no complication or recurrences.[11]

DISAPPEARING NAIL BED

Distal onycholysis refers to the separation of nail plate from the underlying nail bed; a variety of conditions (discussed elsewhere) may cause onycholysis. It has been observed that it is very difficult to achieve reattachment of nail plate to underlying nail bed in cases with long-standing onycholysis, even after adequate treatment. Daniel et al. proposed a concept of "disappearing nail bed" (DNB) to explain this observation of persisting onycholysis becoming an irreversible condition. They found that nail bed becomes keratinized with formation of a granular layer and develops dermatoglyphics, just like skin on fingertips. As a result, actual nail bed gets shortened and/or narrower (Figure 37.9). Long-standing cases of DNB may develop dorsal osteophytes due to lack of counter-pressure by the nail plate (Figure 37.10).[15,16] DNB has been considered as stage V of onycholysis, in the onycholysis grading system.[17]

In their study, Daniel et al. found DNB to be common in toenails and in older populations. When fingernails were

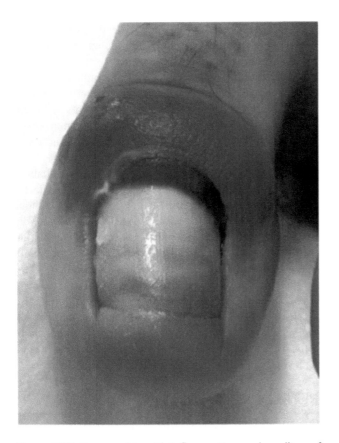

Figure 37.7 Retronychia with inflammation and swelling of proximal nail fold. (Courtesy of Dr. Michela Starace.)

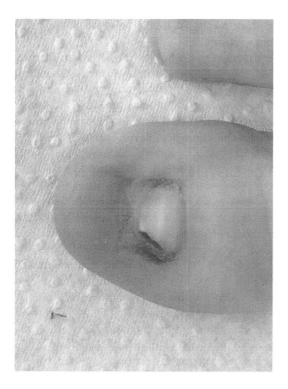

Figure 37.9 A 22-year-old woman with disappearing nail bed showing shortened nail bed (and nail plate) with presence of dermatoglyphics in distal part, similar to those of pulp of the digit. (Courtesy of Prof. Eckart Haneke.)

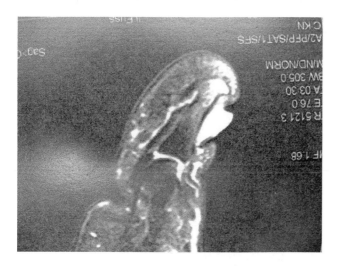

Figure 37.10 X-ray film shows the distal phalanx with the distal-dorsal osteophyte as a result of the lack of counterpressure by the hallux nail. (Courtesy of Prof. Eckart Haneke.)

involved, an association with nail biting (onychophagia) was observed. Among toes, the great toe was most frequently affected and DNB of toenails was found to be associated with OM, onychogryphosis, and same-digit surgery.[16]

Duration of onycholysis before the nail bed epithelializes is not clear. Determining this latency period is very important as once DNB develops, the nail cannot reattach to the underlying nail bed. Also, DNB has some role

in pathogenesis of ingrown nails (onychocryptosis). It has been postulated that distal non-attachment of nail plate and nail bed leads to distortion of the shape of distal digits and thus, predisposes to development of ingrown nails.[15,16]

As treatment of DNB is not established, it is prudent to prevent DNB by early identification and prompt treatment of causative factors for onycholysis.

PARAKERATOSIS PUSTULOSA

Parakeratosis pustulosa is an under-recognized non-infectious inflammatory condition affecting the distal part of the finger of a child. The condition most commonly affects a single digit of a girl child, especially the thumb, second, or third finger, and occurs more commonly on the right hand than the left one. Among toes, great toe is most frequently affected.[18]

Clinically, it starts as vesicles or pustules on the fingertip. Soon, it progresses to subacute eczema of the distal digit, characterized by erythema, scales, and fissures (Figure 37.11). The skin lesions rarely extend proximal to the distal interphalangeal joint. The nail folds may be swollen and cuticle may be absent. The lesions usually are not itchy, but some patients complain of mild pain. Nail changes follow skin lesions and include subungual hyperkeratosis; onycholysis; nail plate pitting, thickening, and discoloration; and Beau's lines (Figure 37.12).[18,19] The condition runs a chronic course; in a long-term follow up study on 20 patients, Tosti et al. reported mean duration of disease as 4 years. In the long term, clinical resolution is common; however, mild pitting or psoriasiform changes may persist indefinitely.[20]

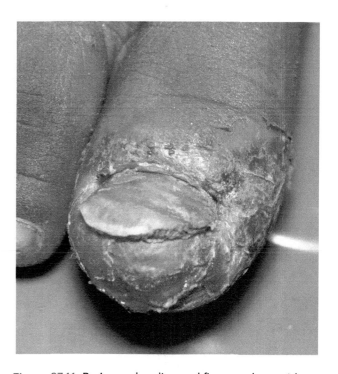

Figure 37.11 Periungual scaling and fissures along with subungual hyperkeratosis in a case of parakeratosis pustulosa.

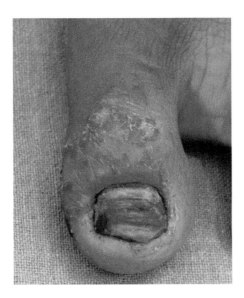

Figure 37.12 Paronychia and multiple Beau's lines in parakeratosis pustulosa.

The diagnosis is made clinically after excluding psoriasis, eczema, dermatophyte infection, and thumb sucking. Histopathological findings are similar to those of psoriasis and eczema and do not offer any diagnostic advantage. The common findings are hyperkeratosis, parakeratosis, acanthosis, mild exocytosis, papillomatosis, and polymorpho-lymphocytic infiltrate around vessels in the dermis. Some authors have reported an additional finding of dyskeratotic cells in the stratum spinosum.[19,20]

Treatment of this condition is frustrating. The frequency of recurrence or the overall duration of disease appears to be unaffected by treatment, though topical steroids and emollients provide some symptomatic relief. The disease runs a chronic non-mutilating course, interrupted by spontaneous remissions and unpredictable recurrences.[18]

WORN-DOWN NAILS/BIDET NAIL

Worn-down nails or Bidet nails result from repetitive trauma to the nail unit and are clinically characterized by a triangular area of thinning of the distal nail plate (with its base at the free edge of the nail) and erythema (Figures 37.13 and 37.14).[21] The characteristic nail changes mostly develop in the nails of the dominant hand, consistent with the role of trauma in its development. Initially, such nail changes were observed in women who had the history of frequent rubbing of nails against porcelain of the bidet while cleaning their genital area.[22] Later on, similar nail changes were noted in tailors (rubbing their nails against clothes), after nail filing for acrylic nail removal, chronic itchy conditions, and in nail tic disorders.[23–25] Considering varied etiologies, authors prefer the term worn-down nails over Bidet nails.

The diagnosis is made clinically. Histopathology findings are non-specific and biopsy is required only when one wants

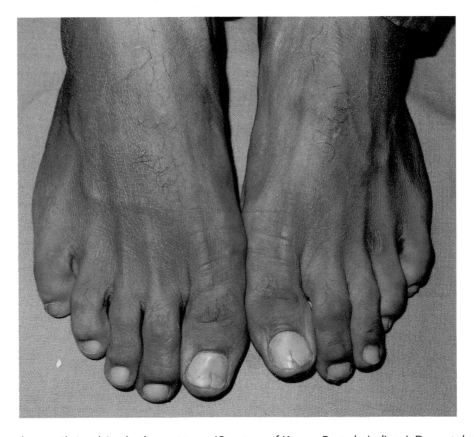

Figure 37.13 Worn-down nails involving both great toes. (Courtesy of Kumar, P. et al., *Indian J. Dermatol.*, 61, 341–342, 2016. IADVL [WB branch], Medknow Publications [Wolters Kluwer Health].)

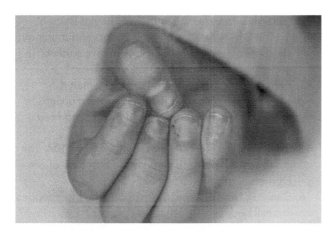

Figure 37.14 Worn-down nails affecting fingernails. (Courtesy of Dr. Michela Starace.)

to exclude clinical differentials. Onychoscopy is often helpful and shows dilated capillaries and pinpoint hemorrhages.[23] Clinical differentials include lichen planus, lichen striatus, Darier's disease, and space-occupying lesions.

A very similar presentation is "lacquer nails" described by Rigopoulos et al. and is clinically characterized by thinning of the nail plate, triangular onycholysis (with the base at the free edge of the nail, where the thinning is maximal), median longitudinal onychorrhexis, and subungual erythema. This condition has been described in women with OM, filing nails aggressively for the application of antifungal nail lacquer.[26]

The cornerstones of successful treatment are keeping the nails short (to avoid damage to the nail plate) and to avoid further trauma to the nail plate. Oral biotin may help in some cases.[21]

ECTOPIC NAIL

The ectopic nail (EN) or onychoheterotopia is a rare condition where an additional nail unit is present at an unusual location. The normal nail unit is present at the usual location, i.e., the dorsal surface of the distal part of digits. The condition may be congenital or acquired after trauma when there is implantation of part of the nail matrix in the ungula or periungual region (called post-traumatic EN). Most common presentation is small spikes of nail tissue; however, occasionally completely developed nail is noted. The continued growth is a usual feature and growth pattern may be horizontal, vertical, or circumferential, depending on the direction of the EN matrix. When in contact with underlying bone, it may block the intramembranous ossification, resulting in hypoplasia and thinning of the underlying bone.[27,28]

Many authors consider congenital EN a teratoma, developing from ectopic stray germ cells. Another school of thought believes it to be a rudimentary polydactyly. More than three-fourths of the documented cases have been reported from Japan, probably due to low awareness of the condition elsewhere. Congenital EN affects hands more than feet. The fifth finger is the most commonly affected digit,

followed by affection of the fourth digit, then of the first and third digits, and finally by the second digit. Other than digits, affection of heel, thorax, and multiple other sites is known. The condition may be familial and may be associated with other digit anomaly (e.g., syndactyly and camptodactyly), bone deformities (regressing polydactyly), ectodermal dysplasia (i.e., alopecia, anodontia), and syndromes (congenital palmar nail syndrome and Pierre Robin syndrome). The condition is usually asymptomatic and the nail is cut to avoid irritation.[27,28]

Acquired post-traumatic EN may develop after a single overwhelming traumatic event or after multiple repeated microtrauma. It usually affects the dorsal part of the finger and toe (Figures 37.15 and 37.16). In contrast to congenital EN, post-traumatic EN is more likely to be symptomatic and the patient complains of irritation, itching, pain, etc.[29]

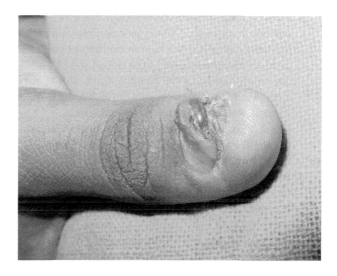

Figure 37.15 Post-traumatic ectopic nail. (Courtesy of Prof. Archana Singal.)

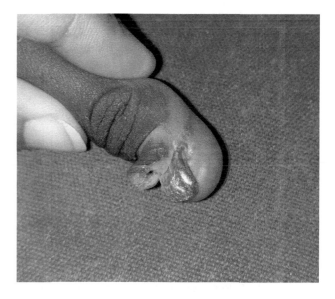

Figure 37.16 Post-traumatic ectopic nail. Note the traumatic scar of a lacerated injury. (Courtesy of Prof. Archana Singal.)

The condition needs to be differentiated from cutaneous horn, split nails (ENs have their own nail folds), and rudimentary polydactyly (differentiated by presence of Meissner body and nerve bundles that are absent in ENs). Hence, the condition requires histopathological demonstration of nail matrix tissue for the confirmation of diagnosis. However, presence of nail bed is not absolutely necessary for the diagnosis. ENs may lack nail bed, and in that case ENs grow in a vertical manner.[27]

Complete surgical excision with ablation of nail matrix is the treatment of choice. Small asymptomatic lesions may be left as such and need to be cut at regular intervals to avoid pain and irritation.[27,28]

REFERENCES

1. Zaias N, Rebell G, Casal G, Appel J. The asymmetric gait toenail unit sign. *Skinmed* 2012;10(4):213–217.
2. Zaias N, Escovar SX, Rebell G. Opportunistic toenail onychomycosis. The fungal colonization of an available nail unit space by non-dermatophytes is produced by the trauma of the closed shoe by an asymmetric gait or other trauma. A plausible theory. *J Eur Acad Dermatol Venereol* 2014;28(8):1002–1006.
3. Zaias N, Rebell G, Escovar S. Asymmetric gait nail unit syndrome: The most common worldwide toenail abnormality and onychomycosis. *Skinmed* 2014;12(4):217–223.
4. Baran R, DeDoncker P. Lateral edge nail involvement indicates poor prognosis for treating onychomycosis with systemic drugs. *Acta Derm Venerol* 1995;76:82–83.
5. Scher R, Tavakkol A, Sigurgeirsson B et al. Onychomycosis diagnosis and definition of cure. *J Am Acad Dermatol* 2007;56:939–944.
6. Lee HJ, Cho SH, Ha SJ, Ahn WK, Park YM, Byun DG, Kim JW. Minor cutaneous features of atopic dermatitis in South Korea. *Int J Dermatol* 2000;39(5):337–342.
7. Van de Kerkhof PC, Pasch MC, Scher RK, Kerscher M, Gieler U, Haneke E, Fleckman P. Brittle nail syndrome: A pathogenesis-based approach with a proposed grading system. *J Am Acad Dermatol* 2005;53(4):644–651.
8. Kechijian P. Brittle fingernails. *Dermatol Clin* 1985;3:421–429.
9. Scher RK, Bodian AB. Brittle nails. *Semin Dermatol* 1991;10:21–25.
10. Hochman LG, Scher RK, Meyerson MS. Brittle nails: Response to daily biotin supplementation. *Cutis* 1993;51:303–305.
11. deBerker DA, Rendall JR. Retronychia: Proximal ingrowing nail. *J Eur Acad Dermatol Venereol* 1999;12:S126.
12. Ventura F, Correia O, Duarte AF, Barros AM, Haneke E. Retronychia—Clinical and pathophysiological aspects. *J Eur Acad Dermatol Venereol* 2016;30(1):16–19.
13. Gerard E, Prevezas C, Doutre MS, Beylot-Barry M, Cogrel O. Risk factors, clinical variants and therapeutic outcome of retronychia: A retrospective study of 18 patients. *Eur J Dermatol* 2016;26(4):377–381.
14. Fernández J, Reyes-Baraona F, Wortsman X. Ultrasonographic criteria for diagnosing unilateral and bilateral retronychia. *J Ultrasound Med* 2018;37(5):1201–1209.
15. Daniel CR 3rd, Tosti A, Iorizzo M, Piraccini BM. The disappearing nail bed: A possible outcome of onycholysis. *Cutis* 2005;76(5):325–327.
16. Daniel R, Meir B, Avner S. An update on the disappearing nail bed. *Skin Appendage Disord* 2017;3(1):15–17.
17. Daniel CR 3rd, Iorizzo M, Piraccini BM, Tosti A. Grading simple chronic paronychia and onycholysis. *Int J Dermatol* 2006;45(12):1447–1448.
18. Pandhi D, Chowdhry S, Grover C, Reddy BS. Parakeratosis pustulosa—A distinct but less familiar disease. *Indian J Dermatol Venereol Leprol* 2003;69:48–50.
19. Mahajan VK, Ranjan N. Parakeratosis pustulosa: A diagnostic conundrum. *Indian J Paediatr Dermatol* 2014;15:12–15.
20. Tosti A, Peluso AM, Zucchelli V. Clinical features and long-term follow-up of 20 cases of parakeratosis pustulosa. *Pediatr Dermatol* 1998;15(4):259–263.
21. Kumar P, Savant SS, Hassan S, Das A, Barman PD. Worn-down nails affecting toenails. *Indian J Dermatol* 2016;61:341–342.
22. Baran R, Moulin G. The bidet nail: A French variant of the worn-down nail syndrome. *Br J Dermatol* 1999;140(2):377.
23. Patrizi A, Tabanelli M, Neri I, Pazzaglia M, Piraccini BM. Worn-down nail syndrome in a child. *J Am Acad Dermatol* 2008;59(2)(Suppl 1):S45–S46.
24. Wu TP, Morrison BW, Tosti A. Worn down nails after acrylic nail removal. *Dermatol Online J* 2015;21.
25. Tosti A, Baran R, Dawber RP, Haneke E. Nail configuration abnormalities. In: Baran R, Dawber RR, Haneke E, Tosti A, Bristow I, Eds. *A Text Atlas of Nail Disorders Techniques in Investigation and Diagnosis*, 3rd ed. London, UK: Martin Dunitz; 2003. pp. 44–46.
26. Rigopoulos D, Charissi C, Belyayeva-Karatza Y, Gregoriou S. Lacquer nail. *J Eur Acad Dermatol Venereol* 2006;20:1153–1154.
27. Riaz F, Rashid RM, Khachemoune A. Onychoheterotopia: Pathogenesis, presentation, and management of ectopic nail. *J Am Acad Dermatol* 2011;64(1):161–166.
28. Ena P, Ena L, Ferrari M, Mazzarello V. Ectopic foot nails: Clinical and dermoscopic features, treatment and outcome in 20 cases. *Dermatology* 2015;231(4):298–303.
29. Meher S, Mishra TS, Sasmal PK, Rout B, Sharma R. Post-traumatic ectopic nail: A case report and review of literature. *J Clin Diagn Res* 2016;10(11):PD01–PD02.

38

Photography of the nail unit

SANJEEV GUPTA AND KARTIKAY AGGARWAL

INTRODUCTION

Dermatology relies heavily on visual observations; thus, the old saying that "a picture is worth a thousand words" holds true for this specialty of medicine.

In dermatology, as the clinical diagnosis depends on the morphological characteristics of the lesions, visual inspection is very important in diagnosis of skin diseases. Photography offers a unique advantage of recording findings of visual inspection for various purposes.

Importance of photography in dermatology

- For disease documentation
- To know the exact evolution of the lesions as they tend to get modified over a period of time with or without treatment
- To study the atypical presentation of some diseases and their course
- To document disease relapse

- To get expert advice from peers/senior colleagues
- For monitoring treatment outcome
- Teaching and academic purposes
- For research and publication
- As an evidence for medico-legal purposes
- In teledermatology—Telemedicine is an upcoming field of medicine that is being used widely for diagnosis and treatment of many diseases in remote areas where specialist services are not available.[1]

FACTORS AFFECTING QUALITY OF CLINICAL PHOTOGRAPHS

The quality of the clinical photographs depends upon the following[2]

- Camera
- Basic photography technique and pre-requisites
- Practical skills

Camera

A camera is a basic optical instrument for recording or capturing images that may be stored locally, transmitted to another location, or both. Various parts of the camera are lens, sensor, body, viewfinder, flash, aperture, shutter release, memory card, user controls, and LCD screen. These parts are present in both compact and digital Single-lens reflex (DSLR) cameras.

- Lens—Light enters through the lens and the process of image capturing begins here. In DSLRs, the lens can be changed.
- Sensor—Sensor captures the light and converts the light in to an electronic signal.
- Body—The body houses all the components of the camera.
- Viewfinder—It lets the photographer see the shot in real time.
- Flash—To provide adequate illumination of the lesion.
- Aperture—It controls the amount of light reaching the sensor by changing the diameter of the lens opening. Aperture size can be increased for low lighting conditions and vice versa.
- Shutter release—It is the switch that releases the shutter and allows the image to be captured. Duration for which shutter remains open is decided by shutter speed and can be changed depending on photographic requirement. For example, a moving object will require fast shutter closure and hence greater shutter speed.
- Memory card—To store the data.
- User controls—To control the amount of light exposure by adjusting aperture, shutter speed, etc.
- LCD screen—Cameras now have LCD screens, which lets the photographer see the shot in real time and thus, helps plan the shot.

The quality of the image broadly depends upon the sensor quality, lens quality, flash quality, and megapixels. These factors are critical in choosing a camera for dermatology photography.[1,2]

- Sensor quality—The sensor is like the retina of the eye. It captures the light that enters through the lens. There are two types of sensors: charge-coupled device (CCD) and complementary metal oxide semiconductor (CMOS). CCD sensors produce better resolution image, are more expensive, and consume more battery while CMOS sensors are less expensive and have better battery life but quality of image is not as good as CCD sensors.
- Lens quality—A close up frame is required for nail photography that can be achieved using Macro lenses. Macro lenses vary in focal length; most common being 50mm (most economical), 80 mm and 100mm. These lenses have different magnification ratios. Lenses with short focal lengths have magnification of (1:2) which means the image produced is half the real-life size.

- Flash quality—Ring flash with adjustable intensity gives the best results.
- Megapixels—It is the unit of image-sensing capacity in a digital camera. Higher megapixel results in better resolution as number of pixels is more and image can be enlarged and printed without getting blurred. It is recommended to take clinical photographs with 8–12 megapixel cameras. The image quality also depends on other factors like spatial resolution. 8-megapixel (3264 × 2448) photos are good enough for printing a 10.88" x 8.16" image at 300 dpi. One can always enhance the brightness or change the contrast with Google apps like Snapseed. Images captured with 3-megapixel cameras and above are good for publication. Another factor that contributes to image quality is sensor size. Smartphone cameras with similar megapixel do not give the same picture quality as compact digital cameras because of the sensor size.

There are three types of cameras that can be used in clinical practice:[1,2,3]

a. Compact digital camera
b. DSLR camera
c. Smartphone camera

COMPACT CAMERAS

These are also called point-and-shoot cameras as there are no complex buttons or features in this camera and one can easily click pictures with basic knowledge. In compact cameras, focus-free lenses are used, i.e., these cameras rely on auto-focus technology. They have automatic systems for setting the exposure options and have an built-in flash unit. They do not need to be manually set before clicking a photograph. Most of the compact cameras have built-in macro modes.

Advantages: These are cost effective, compact in size, and give good image quality. These qualities make them the most practical cameras to be used in clinical practice.

Disadvantages: The image quality cannot match the ones taken by a DSLR camera and there is no option of manual settings beyond a certain limit.

DSLR CAMERAS

A digital single-lens reflex camera is a digital camera in which the optics and the mechanisms of a single-lens reflex camera are combined with a digital imaging sensor. In the reflex design, light travels through the lens and then to a mirror that alternates to send the image to either the viewfinder or the image sensor. In these cameras, one can change filters and objectives, and can add different types of flash or various lenses for photography as well as dermoscopy. Adapters for ultraviolet photographs are also available; therefore, the desired quality of dermatological photographs can be achieved and finer details of lesions can be appreciated.

White balance is very important while clicking pictures with a DSLR camera as inappropriate white balance can make the picture either look more bluish or yellowish. We recommend using the auto mode of white balance as it works best most of the time. However, if the photographer feels the auto mode is not working fine, he should calibrate the white balance with surrounding objects, so that photos of nails are not altered. For example, if we are clicking photos with dark background the auto mode will increase the warmth of the photos and thus it needs to be corrected by selecting adequate white balance from the settings.

Advantages: This is the gold standard in photography when coupled with appropriate lens, (**macro lens** in case of nail photography) and appropriate flash (**Ring flash** in case of nail photography).

Disadvantages: They are bulky and expensive.

THE SMARTPHONE CAMERAS

In the present era, there is a camera in every smartphone. The image quality of the phone's camera can even be compared to that of the digital camera in terms of megapixel count, but the sensor size is physically small so images are not comparable to DSLR camera with the same megapixel lens. However, images from good-quality smartphones are publishable provided adequate care of lighting the object has been taken.

In addition to the image quality, there is the issue of limitation of space in the body of smartphones to accommodate other components such as lenses, filters, and flash.

COMPARISON AMONG THE DIFFERENT TYPES OF CAMERAS

Benefits of a compact camera over DSLR is its compressed size, optical zoom, and built-in macro mode, and wide spectrum of focusing abilities. These features are suitable for all practical purposes. Besides, the exorbitant cost of digital SLRs and their accessories along with space constraints, especially in an outpatient clinic, are other prohibitive factors.

However, the quality of photos in the digital SLRs definitely outscores the common point-and-shoot (compact) varieties.

Technological innovations result in a periodic launching of innumerable new camera models by their manufacturers, leading to the rapid obsolescence of digital equipment.

When smartphone cameras are compared to other cameras, one of their major drawbacks is the absence or inadequacy of optical zoom. For dedicated digital cameras, lesions can be zoomed upon using the optical zoom, thus avoiding lens distortion during closeup photography. Taking the camera too close to the lesions tends to produce a spherical distortion, which might look odd, especially in facial and nail photography.

The major advantage of clinical photography using smartphones is the ease of capturing and transfer of images. The smartphone camera is now well equipped to shoot in any kind of lighting conditions. Because the smartphone is an indispensable gadget in our daily lives, it is like living with a camera 24 × 7. Different cameras have been compared in Table 38.1.

Basic photography technique and principles

One must be conversant with some basic terminology to understand basic principles of photography and to get the best image in a given set of lighting conditions. These have been described below.[2,4]

EXPOSURE

It is probably the most important factor determining the quality of image. Simply speaking, exposure means the brightness or darkness of a photo. Getting a proper exposure for a particular shot is critical and tricky, and it requires some knowledge and practice. All cameras have AUTO mode that determines the exposure automatically depending on the ambient light. However, often exposure in AUTO mode is not good enough and we need to control exposure manually to get appropriately exposed photographs. Exposure

Table 38.1 Comparison of different types of Cameras

	DSLR	Compact camera	Smartphone camera
Quality	++++	+++	+++/++
Compactness	Heavy and large	Compact	Compact
Price	Expensive	Cost effective	Variable
Accessories like macro lens	Need to be purchased separately	Not required	Not required
Photo-sharing apps	No	Present in few latest models	Present in almost all models
Macro mode	Special lens required	No special lens required	Macro capabilities in most smartphone cameras
Choice for	Professional level photos of highest grade	Practically all clinic photos	Similar to compact camera
Learning curve	Long and requires practice	Short	Short
Price range	25000 ₹ onwards	5000 ₹ onwards	4000 ₹ onwards

is manually controlled by adjusting three interdependent parameters: aperture, shutter speed, and ISO.

APERTURE

Aperture refers to the hole within the lens, through which light travels into the camera body. Understandably, wide aperture means more light entering the camera and vice versa. Aperture is represented by f-stops and the range of available f-stops depends on quality of the lens. Most lenses have f-stops ranging from f3.5 to f22, f22 being the smallest aperture and f3.5 being the widest.

In addition to exposure, aperture controls "depth of field." Wider apertures like f3.5 will give small depth of field, meaning the main subject is well-focused and everything else, including background, is blurred. Smaller apertures like f22 will result in large depth of field, meaning everything, the main subject and background, are focused. For clinical photography, where we need to have all of the face, trunk, and extremity lesions in a single frame, we must target an aperture with a large depth of field. For a single lesion on nail, small depth of field is acceptable.

SHUTTER SPEED (EXPOSURE TIME)

Shutter speed determines the length of time for which a camera shutter is open when the photographer presses the shutter button, allowing light into the camera sensor, and is usually measured in fractions of a second, such as 1/1000th or 1/60th of a second. Longer shutter speeds are required for low-light photography, but holding the camera still during long shutter speeds becomes a challenge, necessitating the use of a tripod.

ISO

Referring to light sensitivity of the image sensor ISO is usually expressed as 100, 200, 400, 800, and so on. By increasing ISO, one can increase the light sensitivity of the sensor and get better-exposed images in low-light conditions. However, increasing ISO makes the image look grainy (called noise) and is used as a last resort when everything else fails.

Other important parameters to understand and adjust are white balance, metering, composition, etc. The detailed discussion of these parameters is beyond the scope of this chapter. For clinical photography, the lesion should be placed in the center of the frame, and a non-distracting, non-reflective, uniform background is preferred.

PHOTOGRAPH EDITING SKILLS

One must learn some basic photograph editing skills as editing can improve the photograph in many ways and can correct some of the flaws. There are many desktop/laptop-based and mobile-based photograph editing apps. One must be well conversant with them to get a better outcome. Some basic editing involves cropping (to remove unwanted areas and to improve focus on the lesion), rotating the image, correcting color and saturation, and improving sharpness. These changes are acceptable in medical writing and help to bring

the best out of a given photograph. However, gross changes that deceive the viewer are unethical and unacceptable, more so in pre-intervention and post-intervention images.[5]

Practical skills

One must spend time with a camera practicing different settings to get a good exposure in a given lighting condition. Once the desired exposure is achieved, the settings should be saved for the future. To capture good images, standardization is important, i.e., the lighting should be appropriate, positioning of the subject, perspective, depth of field, and background. Photographs should be stored and presented appropriately for their use in clinical and research work.

NAIL PHOTOGRAPHY

Though the essential principles of nail photography are similar to those of dermatologic photography or photography in general, nail photography poses certain unique challenges.[6]

- Fingers are of different lengths. Thus, it is very difficult to capture all 10 fingers in a single frame.
- Thumbs are positioned in a different anatomical plane than rest of the fingers.
- Nails are a small structure, and nail pathology may be even smaller. It is very difficult to focus on such a small structure.
- Nails are convex in curvature, both longitudinally and transversally. This can mask the lesion due to the difficulty in focusing on structures with different depths.
- Nail is lustrous and hence flash may alter the lesion.

The basic principles unique to nail photography can be discussed under three broad categories:

- Preparation of the patient
- Preparation of camera and lighting
- Background

Preparation of the patient

Preparation of the patient is very important before clicking the photos. Informed consent from the patient should be taken, and the consent form should mention the purpose of the photographs.

The nails should be cleaned with spirit swab or alcohol swab to remove surface abnormalities/dust/oil or any substances that may reflect light.

If the patient has applied nail polish on nails, it should be removed with a nail polish remover.

POSES FOR NAIL PHOTOGRAPHY

As the thumb is in a different anatomical plane as compared to fingers, it is difficult to include all nails in one frame. This becomes an issue especially when the pathology involves all nails of the hand.

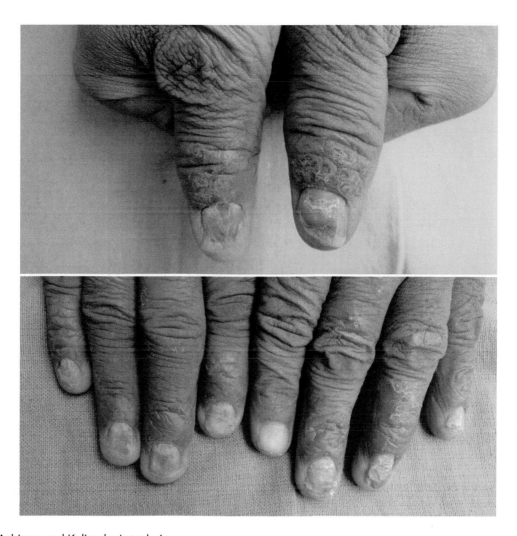

Figure 38.1 Ashique and Kaliyadan's technique.

Additionally, patients having joint problems, elderly persons, and children are unable to achieve these complex positions required for nail photography.

To address this problem, various techniques have been employed to include all nails in a single frame (or in minimum frames). Ashique and Kaliyadan described a technique in which two sets of images were obtained: one including all fingernails except the thumb and a second image including only the thumb. The images are then combined into a collage. This provides an image in which the nails are in the same plane, symmetrical, and also look aesthetically pleasing. Standardization is also easier with this technique.[7] The technique is shown in Figure 38.1. The main disadvantages of this technique are that two sets of images are required, one for the fingernails and the other for the thumb; moreover, making the collage is time consuming.

Gupta et al.[8] suggested a modification of this method where the frame could be made less broad by placing one hand over the other, in such a way that fingernails are not covered (Figure 38.2). This view provides better clarity. The overall length and width of the photograph are similar, so the chances of peripheral areas getting out of focus are less. Its drawback is that the thumbs cannot be covered in the same frame.

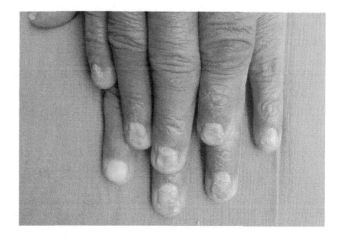

Figure 38.2 Technique described by Gupta et al.

Inamadar and Palit[9] suggested another technique (Figure 38.3) of imaging the nails in a position where the palmar aspects of both hands are kept side by side. Four fingers are flexed at proximal interphalangeal joints towards the palms. The thumbs are flexed across the palm and brought closer to the tips of other fingers in a way that the thumbnails

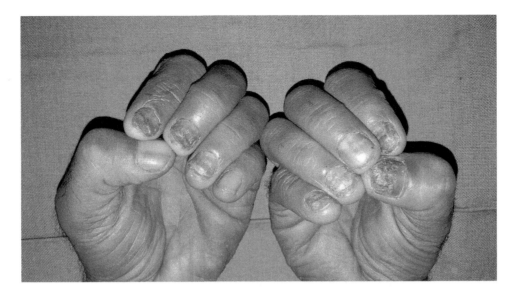

Figure 38.3 Technique described by Inamdar and Palit.

face upwards. The advantage of this technique is that all the nails can be included in a single frame. It is, however, difficult to standardize this technique and it may also pose difficulties in patients having joint problems, making flexion of the small joints difficult. To overcome this problem in elderly and for nail photography in children, use of supporting material such as clay, soft ball and empty tissue roll has been suggested.[10]

When the nail pathology is limited to one or few nails, only involved nails should be included in the frame (Figure 38.4). Nonetheless, it is recommended to click photographs of all the nails of the patient for the purpose of future records.

Some other techniques are as illustrated in Figures 38.5 and 38.6. Another technique that is being practiced by the authors is placing the patient's hand over his eye (Figure 38.7). This has the following benefits:

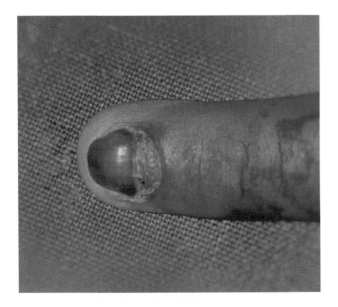

Figure 38.4 Single-nail photography.

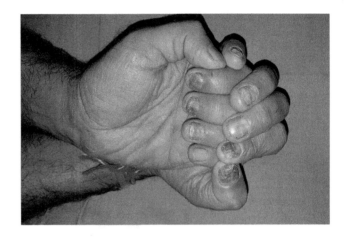

Figure 38.5 Photography of all 10 digits.

- Nails of four fingers come in one plane.
- Identity of the patient is hidden.
- The background becomes skin-colored, which is nondistracting and pleasing to the viewer.
- This is best for patients having skin pathology over the face, as both skin and nail pathology can be shown in one frame.

However, the problem of not being able to visualize the thumb remains.

Preparation of camera and lighting

Good lighting condition is the most important requirement for photography especially if you are shooting a close subject, which is the nail in our case. If the lighting conditions are not adequate, i.e., in dim light, the exposure of the camera lens will increase, which means that the aperture will be open for a longer time. This could lead to production of blur since the hand cannot remain still for a long

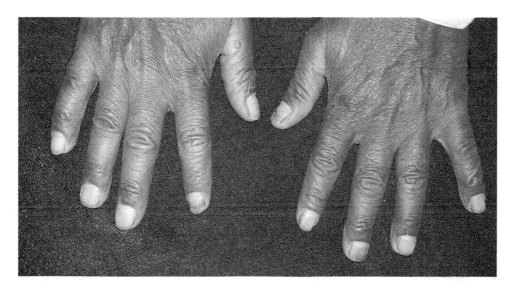

Figure 38.6 Photography of all 10 digits.

However, adequate natural sunlight is often a limiting factor in many indoor clinic setups. This problem can be overcome by using flash. Most compact camera models have a low-intensity built-in flash. With these built-in flashes, the camera lens tends to cast a shadow in close-range photographs. Furthermore, the light emitted by a built-in flash strikes the subject head-on; the resulting glare can only be avoided by changing the angle of the shot, not by rotating or moving the flash. To avoid these shadows, an external ring flash can be used.

A ring flash (Figure 38.8) is a circular photographic flash that fits around a camera lens. Its salient feature is that it provides even illumination with very few shadows visible in the resulting photographs. This is due to the origin of light being near to the optical axis of the lens. The much higher-quality results obtained with a ring (O-ring-type) flash are yet another reason for dermatologists to choose an DSLR camera over a compact or mirrorless model.

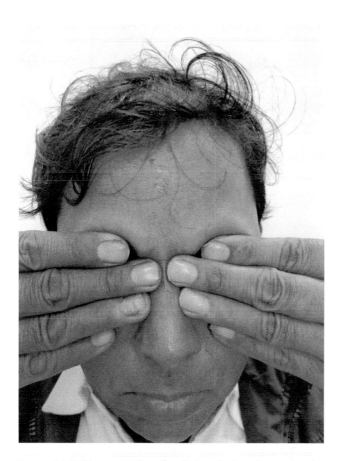

Figure 38.7 Photography of nails by placing the patient's hand over his/her eyes.

time. Using a tripod can eliminate the possibility of blurring of image due to shaking hands.

The best lighting is natural light. The benefits of natural light are that there are no distracting shadows as associated with use of flash. Additionally, nails, being lustrous, have shine and the use of flash further increases it. With natural lighting, the cost of lighting equipment is also reduced.

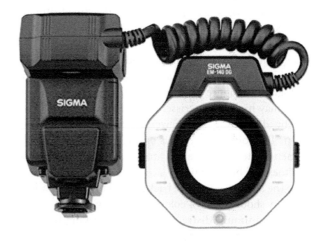

Figure 38.8 Ring flash. (Image taken from https://www.amazon.in/Sigma-EM-140-Macro-Flash-Camera/dp/B0006 4XR64?tag=googinhydr18418-21.)

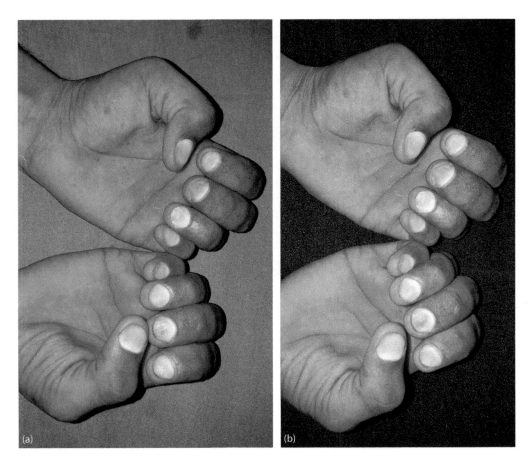

Figure 38.9 (a and b) Comparison of light and dark backgrounds in nail photography.

Background

Background of picture is an important factor in masking and illuminating nail lesions. The available data support that the background should be dark and non-distracting. While clicking skin lesions there is sufficient background of normal skin, a non-distracting background is adequate for most purposes. However, the nail is a small unit with no background of the normal skin; hence, the consideration of background becomes critical in nail photography. Dark background helps in producing good contrast to our photos. Dark blue or green sheets are commonly used in medical photography (Figure 38.9). However, the lens in autofocus mode may highlight a crisscross pattern of woven threads, thereby distracting the viewer from the nail pathology/lesion. To avoid camera focus on the background, it is recommended to keep a gap of around 2 meters between fingers/toes and background.

In the authors' view, the background in case of nail photography should be light colored matching with skin so that there is minimum distraction while observing the lesion. However, it may vary and can be customized accordingly.

Some recommendations for clinical photography and photography by smartphone camera have been summarized in Boxes 38.1 and 38.2.

BOX 38.1: Tips for clinical photography

- Take an informed consent from the patient (parents in case of minor).
- Adequate lighting is must. Natural sunlight is preferred.
- Avoid shadows. One needs to work on angles of shot and flash to avoid shadows.
- Proper support and positioning of the finger should be ensured.
- Clean the hand and nails before taking photographs.
- Use a tripod whenever possible.
- Take photos from equal distance.
- Use proper equipment (i.e., macro lens and ring flash).
- Non-distracting background with contrasting color should be used.
- Take multiple shots.
- Do not rely blindly on the LCD screen of cameras. Many a time, what appears great on these small LCD screens is not actually sharp/well focused when viewed on computer screens.

- Take an informed consent from the patient and make him understand its purpose.
- Use a non-distracting background. It is recommended to have a gap between nails and background.
- Make sure the room is well lit. Lighting is one of the most important factors in photography. Poor lighting can make even photos from the sturdiest hand look blurred.
- Make sure your camera is parallel to the nails.
- Take multiple shots.

COPYRIGHT ISSUES

Copyrights are the rights given by the law to the creators of literary, dramatic, musical, and artistic works and the producers of cinematograph films and sound recordings. The rights provided under copyright law include the rights of reproduction of the work, communication of the work to public, adaptation of the work, and translation of the work. The scope and duration of protection provided under copyright law varies with the nature of the protected work.

In India, one can use the intellectual property of someone without the fear of copyright laws for personal or private use including education and research, criticism or review, and reporting of current events and current affairs. This may include the reporting of a lecture delivered to the public.[10]

Images published in e-media or print media are considered as intellectual property of the publisher or author or both. According to the copyright law, clinical photographs cannot be used unless prior permission from the concerned author/publisher has been obtained.[11] One should not violate these rights to avoid legal implications.

STORING THE IMAGES

Image archiving

There are many image formats; JPEG, PNG, TIFF, and Raw formats are used most commonly. JPEG images are usually stored in Jpeg format with the extension .jpg or .jpeg. Almost all digital cameras save photos in this format. Image in JPEG format is of relatively lesser size as compared to TIFF or RAW format. However, many details of an image tend to get lost permanently in JPEG format.

Images in RAW format preserve most details of the shot and hence, RAW format is preferred by many. They serve the same purpose as negatives used to do in the era of film cameras. They need to be converted into a viewable format.

Storing images

It is important to save the photographs in some storage device such as personal computers. Backing up the photos just on the hard drive is not a safe option, as hard drives eventually fail. It is advisable to back up the photos to a cloud service. Google photos provide unlimited free storage for photos. Various applications (e.g., "Photos app" by Google) are also available to archive these photos.

It is advisable to save these photos on cloud services like Dropbox or Box. These provide the benefit of viewing them anywhere in addition to securing the photos in case of hard disk failure.

How to name photos

Make sure the photos are saved in a designated folder for clinical photography. It is strongly recommended that you rename your photos in such a way that they can be extracted later easily, for example by disease or with patient's name. Rename the image according to a set format such as DIAGNOSIS NAME DATE (DDMMMYYYY), e.g., "acropustulosis jagdish batra 22 oct 2017."

SUMMARY

With ever-evolving technology and new ideas for photography, it is now possible to standardize the perfect technique for nail photography. In this chapter we have tried to make it easier to identify the nail unit pathology and photograph the concerned nail area, name, and store the images.

Even with some limitations, in the present world the most practical and user-friendly camera is the point-and-shoot camera. However, the gold standard still remains the DSLR camera along with its accessories like macro lens, ring flash, and tripod.

REFERENCES

1. Kaliyadan F, Manoj J, Venkitakrishnan S, Dharmaratnam A D. Basic digital photography in dermatology. *Indian J Dermatol Venereol Leprol* 2008;74:532–536.
2. Miot HA, Paixão MP, Paschoal FM. Basics of digital photography in dermatology. *An Bras Dermatol* 2006;81:174–180.
3. Ashique KT, Kaliyadan F, Aurangabadkar SJ. Clinical photography in dermatology using smartphones: An overview. *Indian Dermatol Online J* 2015;6:158–163.
4. McClinton P. The basics of photography—introduction to photography (tutorials). Available from http://artofvisuals.com/the-basics-of-photography-introduction-to-photography-tutorials/. Accessed on April 29, 2018.

5. Kaliyadan F. Image manipulation and image plagiarism—What's fine and what's not? *Indian J Dermatol Venereol Leprol* 2017;83:519–521.

6. Thomas L, Vaudaine M, Wortsman X, Jemec GB, Drape J. Imaging the nail unit. In: Baran R, de Berker DA, Holzberg M, Thomas L, editors. *Baran and Dawber's Diseases of the Nails and Their Management.* 4th ed. Oxford, UK: Wiley-Blackwell; 2012. pp. 101–102.

7. Ashique KT, Kaliyadan F. Clinical photography of nail diseases: A simple method to include all fingernails in a frame. *J Am Acad Dermatol* 2015;72:e25.

8. Gupta S, Gupta S. A simple, novel method for nail photography. *J Am Acad Dermatol* 2015;72:e131.

9. Inamadar AC, Palit A. Nail photography: All 10 fingernails in 1 frame. *J Am Acad Dermatol* 2015;73:e143.

10. Gupta S, Singal A, Aggarwal K, Shankar Jangra R. Nail photography tricks for pediatric and geriatric patients. *J Am Acad Dermatol* 2018.

11. A hand book of copyright law. Available from http://copyright.gov.in/documents/handbook.html. Accessed on April 29, 2018.

Index

Note: Page numbers in italic and bold refer to figures and tables respectively.